GW00870702

QUICK LOOK
DRUG BOOK

TABLE OF CONTENTS

ABOUT THE AUTHORS

Leonard L. Lance, RPh

Leonard L. (Bud) Lance has been directly involved in the pharmaceutical industry since receiving his bachelor's degree in pharmacy from Ohio Northern University 23 years ago. Upon graduation from ONU, Mr Lance spent four years as a navy pharmacist in various military assignments and was instrumental in the development and operation of the first whole hospital I.V. admixture program in a military (Portsmouth Naval Hospital) facility.

After completing his military service, he entered the retail pharmacy field and has managed both an independent and a home I.V. franchise pharmacy operation. Since the late 1970s Mr Lance has focused much of his interest on using computers to improve pharmacy service and to advance the dissemination of drug information to practitioners and other health care professionals.

As a result of his strong publishing interest, he serves in the capacity of pharmacy editor and technical advisor as well as pharmacy (information) database coordinator for Lexi-Comp. Along with the *Quick Look Drug Book*, he provides technical support to Lexi-Comp's *Drug Information Handbook*, *Pediatric Dosage Handbook*, *Laboratory Test Handbook*, *Diagnostic Procedure Handbook*, and *Geriatric Dosage Handbook* publications. Mr Lance has also assisted approximately 100 major hospitals in producing their own formulary (pharmacy) publications through Lexi-Comp's custom publishing service.

L.L. Lance is a member and past president (1984) of the Summit County Pharmaceutical Association (SCPA). He is also a member of the Ohio Pharmacists Association (OPA), the American Pharmaceutical Association (APhA), and the American Society of Hospital Pharmacists (ASHP).

Charles F. Lacy, PharmD

Dr Lacy received his doctorate from the University of Southern California School of Pharmacy. With over 11 years of clinical experience at one of the nation's largest teaching hospitals, he has developed a reputation as an acknowledged expert in drug information and critical care drug therapy.

In his current capacity as Drug Information specialist at Cedar-Sinai Medical Center in Los Angeles, Dr Lacy plays an active role in the education and training of the medical, pharmacy, and nursing staff. He coordinates the Drug Information Center, the Medical Center's Intern Pharmacist Clinical Training Program, the Department's Continuing Education Program for pharmacists; maintains the Medical Center formulary program; and is editor of the Medical Center's *Drug Formulary Handbook* and the drug information newsletter — *Prescription*.

Presently, Dr Lacy holds teaching affiliations with the University of Southern California School of Pharmacy, the University of California at San Francisco School of Pharmacy, the University of the Pacific School of Pharmacy and the University of Alberta at Edmonton, School of Pharmacy and Health Sciences.

Dr Lacy is an active member of numerous professional associations including the American Society of Hospital Pharmacists (ASHP), the California Society of Hospital Pharmacists (CSHP), and the American College of Clinical Pharmacy (ACCP).

Morton P. Goldman, PharmD

Dr Goldman received his bachelor's degree in pharmacy from the University of Pittsburgh in 1983 and his doctorate from the University of Cincinnati. He completed his residency at the V.A. Medical Center in Cincinnati and subsequently began pharmacy practice at several prominent Cleveland medical centers concentrating in the area of infectious diseases.

In his capacity as infectious disease pharmacist at the Cleveland Clinic Foundation, Dr Goldman is actively involved in the continuing education of the medical and pharmacy staff. He is an editor of the foundation's *Guideline for Antibiotic Use* and has coordinated their Renal Dose Monitoring Program. Dr Goldman has authored numerous journal articles and lectures locally and nationally on the topic of infectious diseases and current drug therapies. He is currently a coauthor of an infectious diseases handbook being produced by Lexi-Comp Inc.

Dr Goldman is an active member of the Society of Infectious Disease Pharmacists, American College of Clinical Pharmacy and the American Society of Hospital Pharmacists.

EDITORIAL ADVISORY PANEL

PREFACE

Working with clinical pharmacists, hospital pharmacy and therapeutics committees, and hospital drug information centers, our editors have assisted in developing hospital-specific formulary manuals for major medical institutions in the United States and Canada. These manuals provide pertinent details on medications used within the hospital, office and other clinical settings. The most current information on drugs and medications has been reviewed, coalesced, and cross-referenced to form the *Quick Look Drug Book*.

The Indication/Therapeutic Category Index is an expedient mechanism for locating the medication of choice along with its classification. This index helps the user to, with knowledge of the disease state, identify medications which are most commonly used in treatment. All disease states are cross-referenced to a varying number of medications with the most likely or best medications noted.

All generic and brand names or synonyms appear as individual entries in the alphabetical listing of drugs. Thus, there is no alphabetical index of drugs.

This handbook gives the user quick access to data on 1283 medications. A standard, concise format was developed to ensure consistent presentation of information. Selection of medications included in this handbook was based on an analysis of medications offered in a wide range of hospital formularies.

— L.L. Lance

ACKNOWLEDGMENTS

The *Quick Look Drug Book* exists in its present form as the result of the concerted efforts of many individuals. The publisher and president of Lexi-Comp Inc, Robert D. Kerscher, deserves much credit for bringing the concept of such a book to fruition. His dedication to the project, and his support and development of the many unique and innovative features included in the book, eg, format, internal cross-references and Indication/Therapeutic Category Index, contribute substantially to the content and usefulness of the book.

Other members of the Lexi-Comp staff whose contributions were invaluable and whose patience with the editors' enumerable drafts, revisions, deletions, additions, and enhancements was inexhaustible include: Diane Harbart, MT (ASCP), medical editor; Lynn Coppinger, director of product development; Barbara F. Kerscher, production manager; Alexandra Hart, composition specialist; Jeanne Eads, Beth Daulbaugh, Julie Weekes, and Lisa Leukart, project managers; Jil R. Neuman, Julie Kelley, and Jacqueline L. Mizer, production assistants; Jeff J. Zaccagnini, Brian B. Vossler, and Jerry Reeves, sales managers; Edmund A. Harbart, vice-president, custom publishing division; and Jack L. Stones, vice-president, reference publishing division. The complex computer programming required for the typesetting of the book was provided by Dennis P. Smithers, Jay L. Katzen, David C. Marcus, Dale Jablonski, and Kenneth J. Hughes, system analysts, under the direction of Thury L. O'Connor, vice-president, and Alan R. Frasz, vice-president, editorial systems.

In addition, sincere appreciation to Vaughn W. Floutz, PhD who served as editorial consultant.

USE OF THE HANDBOOK

The *Quick Look Drug Book* is organized into a drug information section, an appendix, and indication/therapeutic category index.

The drug information section of the handbook, wherein all drugs are listed alphabetically, details information pertinent to each drug. Extensive cross referencing is provided by brand name and synonyms.

Drug information is presented in a consistent format and for quick reference will provide the following:

Generic Name	U.S. adopted name
Pronunciation Guide	
Brand Names	Common trade names
Synonyms	
Therapeutic Category	
Use	Information pertaining to appropriate use of the drug
Usual Dosage	The amount of the drug to be typically given or taken during therapy
Dosage Forms	Information with regard to form, strength and availability of the drug

Appendix

The appendix offers a compilation of tables, guidelines and conversion information which can often be helpful when considering patient care.

Indication/Therapeutic Category Index

This index provides a listing of accepted drugs for various disease states thus focusing attention on selection of medications most frequently prescribed in relation to a clinical diagnosis. Diseases may have other nonofficial drugs for their treatment and this indication/therapeutic category index should not be used by itself to determine the appropriateness of a particular therapy. The listed indications may encompass varying degrees of severity and, since certain medications may not be appropriate for a given degree of severity, it should not be assumed that the agents listed for specific indications are interchangeable. Also included as a valuable reference is each medication's therapeutic category.

SAFE WRITING

Health professionals and their support personnel frequently produce handwritten copies of information they see in print; therefore, such information is subjected to even greater possibilities for error or misinterpretation on the part of others. Thus, particular care must be given to how drug names and strengths are expressed when creating written health care documents.

The following are a few examples of safe writing rules suggested by the Institute for Safe Medication Practices, Inc.*

1. There should be a space between a number and its units as it is easier to read. There should be no periods after the abbreviations mg or mL.

Correct	Incorrect
10 mg	10mg
100 mg	100mg

2. Never place a decimal and a zero after a whole number (2 mg is correct and 2.0 mg is incorrect). If the decimal point is not seen because it falls on a line or because individuals are working from copies where the decimal point is not seen, this causes a tenfold overdose.

3. Just the opposite is true for numbers less than one. Always place a zero before a naked decimal (0.5 mL is correct, .5 mL is **in**correct).

4. Never abbreviate the word "unit." The handwritten U or u, looks like a 0 (zero), and may cause a tenfold overdose error to be made.

5. Q.D. is not a safe abbreviation for once daily, as when the Q is followed by a sloppy dot, it looks like QID which means four times daily.

6. O.D. is not a safe abbreviation for once daily, as it is properly interpreted as meaning "right eye" and has caused liquid medications such as saturated solution of potassium iodide and lugol's solution to be administered incorrectly. There is no safe abbreviation for once daily. It must be written out in full.

7. Do not use chemical names such as 6-mercaptopurine or 6-thioguanine, as 6 fold overdoses have been given when these were not recognized as chemical names. The proper names of these drugs are mercaptopurine or thioguanine.

8. Do not abbreviate drug names (5FC, 6MP, 5-ASA, MTX, HCTZ CPZ, PBZ, etc) as they are misinterpreted and cause error.

9. Do not use the apothecary system or symbols.

10. When writing an outpatient prescription, write a complete prescription. A complete prescription can prevent the prescriber, the pharmacist, and/or the patient from making a mistake and can eliminate the need for further clarification.

---

*From "Safe Writing" by Davis NM, PharmD and Cohen MR, MS, Lecturers and Consultants for Safe Medication Practices, 1143 Wright Drive, Huntingdon Valley, PA 19006. Phone: (215) 947-7566.

The legible prescriptions should contain:

    a.   patient's full name

    b.   for pediatric or geriatric patients: their age (or weight where applicable)

    c.   drug name, dosage form and strength; if a drug is new or rarely prescribed, print this information

    d.   number or amount to be dispensed

    e.   complete instructions for the patient, including the purpose of the medication

    f.   when there are recognized contraindications for a prescribed drug, indicate to the pharmacist that you are aware of this fact (ie, when prescribing a potassium salt for a patient receiving an ACE inhibitor, write "K serum leveling being monitored")

SELECTED REFERENCES

AMA Drug Evaluations Subscription, American Medical Association, Department of Drugs, Division of Drugs and Toxicology, Spring, 1990.

Drug Interaction Facts, St Louis, MO: J.B. Lippincott Co (Facts and Comparisons Division), 1993.

Facts and Comparisons, St Louis, MO: J.B. Lippincott Co (Facts and Comparisons Division), 1993.

Handbook of Nonprescription Drugs, 9th ed, Washington, DC: American Pharmaceutical Association, 1990.

Jacobs DS, DeMott WR, Finley PR, et al, *Laboratory Test Handbook with Key Word Index*, 3rd ed, Hudson, OH: Lexi-Comp Inc, 1994.

Lacy CF, Armstrong LL, Lipsy RJ, and Lance LL, *Drug Information Handbook*, Hudson, OH: Lexi-Comp Inc, 1993.

Levin D, *Essentials of Pediatric Intensive Care*, 1st ed, St Louis, MO: Quality Medical Publishing, Inc, 1990.

McEvoy GK and Litvak K, *AHFS Drug Information*, Bethesda, MD: American Society of Hospital Pharmacists, 1993.

Nelson JD, *1991-1992 Pocketbook of Pediatric Antimicrobial Therapy*, 9th ed., Baltimore, MD: Williams & Wilkins, 1991.

Physician's Desk Reference, 46th ed, Oradell, NJ: Medical Economics Books, 1993.

Report of the Committee on Infectious Diseases, American Academy of Pediatrics, 22nd ed, 1991.

Semla TP, Beizer JL, and Higbee MD, *Geriatric Dosage Handbook*, Hudson, OH: Lexi-Comp Inc, 1993.

Taketomo CK, Hodding JH, and Kraus DM, *Pediatric Dosage Handbook*, 2nd ed, Hudson, OH: Lexi-Comp Inc, 1993.

Trissel L, *Handbook of Injectionable Drugs*, 6th ed, Bethesda, MD: American Society of Hospital Pharmacists, 1992.

United States Pharmacopeia Dispensing Information (USP DI), Rockville, MD: United States Pharmacopeial Convention, Inc, 1993.

ALPHABETICAL LISTING
OF DRUGS

ALPHABETICAL LISTING OF DRUGS

A-200™ Pyrinate [OTC] *see* pyrethrins *on page 408*

A and D™ Ointment [OTC] *see* vitamin A and vitamin D *on page 497*

A-ase *see* asparaginase *on page 34*

Abbokinase® Injection *see* urokinase *on page 488*

Abbott HIVAB HIV-1 EIA *see* diagnostic aids (*in vitro*), blood *on page 137*

Abbott HIVAG-1 *see* diagnostic aids (*in vitro*), blood *on page 137*

Abbott HTLV III Confirmatory EIA *see* diagnostic aids (*in vitro*), blood *on page 137*

absorbable cotton *see* cellulose, oxidized *on page 83*

absorbable gelatin sponge *see* gelatin, absorbable *on page 209*

Absorbine® Antifungal [OTC] *see* tolnaftate *on page 471*

Absorbine® Jock Itch [OTC] *see* tolnaftate *on page 471*

Absorbine Jr.® Antifungal [OTC] *see* tolnaftate *on page 471*

Accupril® *see* quinapril hydrochloride *on page 411*

Accusens T® *see* diagnostic aids (*in vitro*), other *on page 138*

Accutane® *see* isotretinoin *on page 260*

acebutolol hydrochloride (a se byoo' toe lole)
Brand Names Sectral®
Therapeutic Category Antiarrhythmic Agent, Class II; Beta-Adrenergic Blocker
Use Treatment of hypertension; ventricular arrhythmias; angina
Usual Dosage Adults: Oral: 400-800 mg/day in 2 divided doses
Dosage Forms Capsule: 200 mg, 400 mg
Fee AC20

Acel-Immune® *see* diphtheria, tetanus toxoids, and acellular pertussis vaccine *on page 154*

Acephen® [OTC] *see* acetaminophen *on this page*

Aceta® [OTC] *see* acetaminophen *on this page*

acetaminophen (a seet a min' oh fen)
Brand Names Acephen® [OTC]; Aceta® [OTC]; Anacin-3® [OTC]; Apacet® [OTC]; Banesin® [OTC]; Dapa® [OTC]; Datril® [OTC]; Dorcol® [OTC]; Feverall™ [OTC]; Genapap® [OTC]; Halenol® [OTC]; Myapap® Drops [OTC]; Neopap® [OTC]; Panadol® [OTC]; Redutemp® [OTC]; Snaplets-FR® Granules [OTC]; Tempra® [OTC]; Tylenol® [OTC]; Uni-Ace® [OTC]
Synonyms APAP; N-acetyl-P-aminophenol; paracetamol
Therapeutic Category Analgesic, Non-Narcotic; Antipyretic
Use Treatment of mild to moderate pain and fever; does not have antirheumatic effects
Usual Dosage Oral:
Children: 10-15 mg/kg/dose every 4-6 hours as needed; do **not** exceed 5 doses in 24 hours
Adults: 325-650 mg every 4-6 hours or 1000 mg 3-4 times/day; do **not** exceed 4 g/day
Dosage Forms
Caplet: 160 mg, 325 mg, 500 mg
Drops: 100 mg/mL (15 mL); 120 mg/2.5 mL (35 mL)
Granules, premeasured packs: 80 mg (32s)
Elixir: 120 mg/5 mL (5 mL, 10 mL, 13.5 mL, 25 mL, 27 mL, 120 mL, 480 mL, 3780 mL); 130 mg/5 mL (12.5 mL, 25 mL); 160 mg/5 mL (5 mL, 10 mL, 20 mL, 120 mL, 240 mL, 500 mL, 3780 mL); 325 mg/5 mL (480 mL, 3780 mL)
Liquid, oral: 160 mg/5 mL (2.5 mL, 5 mL, 60 mL, 120 mL, 240 mL, 480 mL); 500 mg/15 mL (240 mL)

Suppository, rectal: 120 mg, 125 mg, 325 mg, 650 mg
Suspension: 100 mg/mL, 160 mg/mL
Tablet: 325 mg, 500 mg, 650 mg
Tablet, chewable: 80 mg, 160 mg

acetaminophen and aspirin

Brand Names Excedrin®, Extra Strength [OTC]; Gelpirin® [OTC]
Therapeutic Category Analgesic, Non-Narcotic
Use Relief of mild to moderate pain
Usual Dosage Adults: Oral: 1-2 tablets every 2-6 hours as needed for pain
Dosage Forms Tablet: Acetaminophen 125 mg and aspirin 240 mg with caffeine 32 mg;
acetaminophen 250 mg and aspirin 250 mg with caffeine 65 mg

acetaminophen and codeine

Brand Names Capital® and Codeine; CodAphen®; Margesic® No. 3; Phenaphen® With Codeine; Tylenol® With Codeine
Synonyms codeine and acetaminophen
Therapeutic Category Analgesic, Narcotic
Use Relief of mild to moderate pain
Usual Dosage Doses should be adjusted according to severity of pain and response of the patient. Adult doses of 60 mg codeine and higher fail to give commensurate relief of pain but merely prolong analgesia and are associated with an appreciably increased incidence of side effects. Oral:

Children:
   Analgesic: 0.5-1 mg codeine/kg/dose every 4-6 hours
   Acetaminophen: 10-15 mg/kg/dose every 4 hours up to a maximum of 2.6 g/24 hours
      for children <12 years
   3-6 years: 5 mL 3-4 times/day as needed of elixir
   7-12 years: 10 mL 3-4 times/day as needed of elixir
   >12 years: 15 mL every 4 hours as needed of elixir

Adults:
   Antitussive: Based on codeine (15-30 mg/dose) every 4-6 hours
   Analgesic: Based on codeine (30-60 mg/dose) every 4-6 hours
   1-2 tablets every 4 hours to a maximum of 12 tablets/24 hours

Dosage Forms
Capsule:
   #2: Acetaminophen 325 mg and codeine phosphate 15 mg
   #3: Acetaminophen 325 mg and codeine phosphate 30 mg
   #4: Acetaminophen 325 mg and codeine phosphate 60 mg
Elixir: Acetaminophen 120 mg and codeine phosphate 12 mg per 5 mL with alcohol 7%
Suspension, oral, alcohol free: Acetaminophen 120 mg and codeine phosphate 12 mg per 5 mL
Tablet: Acetaminophen 500 mg and codeine phosphate 30 mg; acetaminophen 650 mg and codeine phosphate 30 mg
Tablet:
   #1: Acetaminophen 300 mg and codeine phosphate 7.5 mg
   #2: Acetaminophen 300 mg and codeine phosphate 15 mg
   #3: Acetaminophen 300 mg and codeine phosphate 30 mg
   #4: Acetaminophen 300 mg and codeine phosphate 60 mg

acetaminophen and hydrocodone *see* hydrocodone and acetaminophen *on page 234*

acetaminophen and isometheptene mucate

Brand Names Midrin®
Therapeutic Category Analgesic, Non-Narcotic; Antimigraine Agent
Use Relief of migraine and tension headache
(Continued)

acetaminophen and isometheptene mucate *(Continued)*

Usual Dosage Adults: Oral: 2 capsules at first sign of headache, followed by 1 capsule every 60 minutes until relieved, up to 5 capsules in a 12-hour period

Dosage Forms Capsule: Acetaminophen 326 mg and isometheptene mucate 65 mg with dichloralphenazone 100 mg

acetaminophen and oxycodone *see* oxycodone and acetaminophen *on page 349*

acetaminophen and pentazocine *see* pentazocine compound *on page 364*

acetaminophen and phenyltoloxamine

Brand Names Percogesic® [OTC]
Therapeutic Category Analgesic, Non-Narcotic
Use Relief of mild to moderate pain
Usual Dosage Adults: Oral: 1-2 tablets every 4 hours
Dosage Forms Tablet: Acetaminophen 325 mg and phenyltoloxamine citrate 30 mg

acetaminophen, chlorpheniramine, and pseudoephedrine

Brand Names Sinutab® [OTC]
Therapeutic Category Analgesic, Non-Narcotic; Antihistamine/Decongestant Combination
Use Temporary relief of sinus symptoms
Usual Dosage Adults: Oral: 2 tablets every 6 hours
Dosage Forms Tablet: Acetaminophen 325 mg, chlorpheniramine hydrochloride 2 mg, and pseudoephedrine hydrochloride 30 mg

Acetasol® HC Otic *see* acetic acid, propanediol diacetate, and hydrocortisone *on next page*

acetazolamide (a set a zole' a mide)

Brand Names AK-Zol®; Dazamide®; Diamox®
Therapeutic Category Anticonvulsant, Miscellaneous; Carbonic Anhydrase Inhibitor; Diuretic, Carbonic Anhydrase Inhibitor
Use Lower intraocular pressure to treat glaucoma, also as a diuretic, adjunct treatment of refractory seizure and acute altitude sickness
Usual Dosage
Children:
Glaucoma:
Oral: 8-30 mg/kg/day divided every 6-8 hours
I.M., I.V.: 20-40 mg/kg/day divided every 6 hours
Edema: Oral, I.M., I.V.: 5 mg/kg or 150 mg/m^2 once every day or every other day
Epilepsy: Oral: 8-30 mg/kg/day in 2-4 divided doses, not to exceed 1 g/day
Adults:
Glaucoma:
Oral: 250 mg 1-4 times/day or 500 mg sustained release capsule twice daily
I.M., I.V.: 250-500 mg, may repeat in 2-4 hours
Edema: Oral, I.M., I.V.: 250-375 mg once daily
Epilepsy: Oral: 8-30 mg/kg/day in 1-4 divided doses
Altitude sickness: Oral: 250 mg every 8-12 hours
Dosage Forms
Capsule, sustained release: 500 mg
Injection: 500 mg/5 mL
Tablet: 125 mg, 250 mg

acetic acid
Brand Names VōSol® Otic
Synonyms ethanoic acid
Therapeutic Category Antibacterial, Otic; Antibacterial, Topical
Use Continuous or intermittent irrigation of the bladder; treatment of superficial bacterial infections of the external auditory canal and vagina
Usual Dosage
Irrigation: For continuous irrigation of the urinary bladder with 0.25% acetic acid irrigation, the rate of administration will approximate the rate of urine flow; usually 500-1500 mL/24 hours; for periodic irrigation of an indwelling urinary catheter to maintain patency, approximately 50 mL of 0.25% acetic acid irrigation is required. (Note dosage of an irrigating solution depends on the capacity or surface area of the structure being irrigated.)
Otic: Insert saturated wick, keep moist 24 hours; remove wick and instill 5 drops 3-4 times/day
Dosage Forms Solution:
Irrigation: 0.25% (1000 mL)
Otic: Acetic acid 2% in propylene glycol (15 mL, 30 mL, 60 mL)

acetic acid, propanediol diacetate, and hydrocortisone
Brand Names Acetasol® HC Otic; VōSol® HC Otic
Therapeutic Category Otic Agent, Anti-infective
Use Treatment of superficial infections of the external auditory canal caused by organisms susceptible to the action of the antimicrobial, complicated by inflammation
Usual Dosage Adults: Otic: Instill 4 drops in ear(s) 3-4 times/day
Dosage Forms Solution, otic: Acetic acid 2%, propylene glycol diacetate 3%, and hydrocortisone 1% (10 mL)

acetohexamide (a set oh hex' a mide)
Brand Names Dymelor®
Therapeutic Category Antidiabetic Agent; Hypoglycemic Agent, Oral; Sulfonylurea Agent
Use Adjunct to diet for the management of mild to moderately severe, stable, noninsulin-dependent (type II) diabetes mellitus
Usual Dosage Adults: Oral: 250 mg to 1.5 g/day in 1-2 divided doses
Dosage Forms Tablet: 250 mg, 500 mg

acetohydroxamic acid (a see' toe hye drox am ik)
Brand Names Lithostat®
Synonyms AHA
Therapeutic Category Urinary Tract Product
Use Adjunctive therapy in chronic urea-splitting urinary infection
Usual Dosage Oral:
Children: Initial: 10 mg/kg/day
Adults: 250 mg 3-4 times/day for a total daily dose of 10-15 mg/kg/day
Dosage Forms Tablet: 250 mg

acetophenazine maleate (a set oh fen' a zeen)
Brand Names Tindal®
Therapeutic Category Antipsychotic Agent
Use Management of manifestations of psychotic disorders
Usual Dosage Adults: Oral: 20 mg 3 times/day up to 40-80 mg/day
Hospitalized schizophrenic patients may require doses as high as 400-600 mg/day
Dosage Forms Tablet: 20 mg

acetoxymethylprogesterone see medroxyprogesterone acetate on page 289

acetylcholine chloride (a se teel koe' leen)
Brand Names Miochol®
Therapeutic Category Cholinergic Agent, Ophthalmic; Ophthalmic Agent, Miotic
Use Produce complete miosis in cataract surgery, keratoplasty, iridectomy and other anterior segment surgery where rapid miosis is required
Usual Dosage Adults: 0.5-2 mL of 1% injection (5-20 mg) instilled into anterior chamber before or after securing one or more sutures
Dosage Forms Powder, intraocular: 1:100 [10 mg/mL] (2 mL, 15 mL)

acetylcysteine (a se teel sis' tay een)
Brand Names Mucomyst®; Mucosol®
Synonyms N-acetylcysteine; N-acetyl-L-cysteine
Therapeutic Category Antidote, Acetaminophen; Mucolytic Agent
Use Adjunctive therapy in patients with abnormal or viscid mucous secretions in acute and chronic bronchopulmonary diseases, pulmonary complications of surgery and cystic fibrosis; diagnostic bronchial studies; antidote for acute acetaminophen toxicity
Usual Dosage
Acetaminophen poisoning: Children and Adults: Oral: 140 mg/kg followed by 17 doses of 70 mg/kg every 4 hours or until acetaminophen assay reveals nontoxic levels; repeat dose if emesis occurs within 1 hour of administration

Inhalation: Acetylcysteine 10% and 20% solution (Mucomyst®) (Dilute with water):
Infants: 2 mL of 5% solution until nebulized given 3-4 times/day
Children: 3-5 mL of 5% to 10% solution until nebulized given 3-4 times/day
Adolescents: 5-10 mL of 5% to 10% solution until nebulized given 3-4 times/day
Note: Patients should receive an aerosolized bronchodilator 10-15 minutes prior to acetylcysteine

Meconium Ileus equivalent: Children and Adults: 100-200 mL of 5% to 10% solution by irrigation or orally
Dosage Forms Solution, as sodium: 10% [100 mg/mL] (4 mL, 10 mL, 30 mL); 20% [200 mg/mL] (4 mL, 10 mL, 30 mL, 100 mL)

acetylsalicylic acid see aspirin on page 34
Aches-N-Pain® [OTC] see ibuprofen on page 245
Achromycin® Ophthalmic see tetracycline on page 458
Achromycin® Topical see tetracycline on page 458
Achromycin® V Oral see tetracycline on page 458
aciclovir see acyclovir on next page
Acid Mantle® [OTC] see aluminum acetate on page 14
acidulated phosphate fluoride see fluoride on page 201
Aclovate® Topical see alclometasone dipropionate on page 11
ACT see dactinomycin on page 125
ACT® [OTC] see fluoride on page 201
Actagen® [OTC] see triprolidine and pseudoephedrine on page 482
Actagen-C® see triprolidine, pseudoephedrine, and codeine on page 482
ACTH see corticotropin on page 116
Acthar® see corticotropin on page 116
Acticort® Topical see hydrocortisone on page 236
Actidose-Aqua® [OTC] see charcoal on page 86
Actidose® With Sorbitol [OTC] see charcoal on page 86
Actifed® [OTC] see triprolidine and pseudoephedrine on page 482

Actifed® With Codeine *see* triprolidine, pseudoephedrine, and codeine *on page 482*

Actigall™ *see* ursodiol *on page 489*

Actimmune® *see* interferon gamma-1b *on page 253*

Actinex® Topical *see* masoprocol *on page 286*

actinomycin D *see* dactinomycin *on page 125*

Activase® Injection *see* alteplase, recombinant *on page 14*

activated carbon *see* charcoal *on page 86*

activated charcoal *see* charcoal *on page 86*

activated dimethicone *see* simethicone *on page 431*

activated ergosterol *see* ergocalciferol *on page 173*

activated methylpolysiloxane *see* simethicone *on page 431*

Acular® Ophthalmic *see* ketorolac tromethamine *on page 264*

Acutrim® Precision Release® [OTC] *see* phenylpropanolamine hydrochloride *on page 373*

ACV *see* acyclovir *on this page*

acycloguanosine *see* acyclovir *on this page*

acyclovir (ay sye' kloe ver)
Brand Names Zovirax® Injection; Zovirax® Oral; Zovirax® Topical
Synonyms aciclovir; ACV; acycloguanosine
Therapeutic Category Antiviral Agent, Oral; Antiviral Agent, Parenteral; Antiviral Agent, Topical
Use Treatment of initial and prophylaxis of recurrent mucosal and cutaneous herpes simplex (HSV-1 and HSV-2) infections; herpes simplex encephalitis; herpes zoster; genital herpes infection; and varicella zoster infections in immunocompromised patients

Usual Dosage

Neonates HSV infection: I.V.: 1500 mg/m^2/day divided every 8 hours or 30 mg/kg/day divided every 8 hours for 10-14 days

Children and Adults: I.V.:
   Mucocutaneous HSV infection: 750 mg/m^2/day divided every 8 hours or 15 mg/kg/day divided every 8 hours for 5-10 days
   HSV encephalitis: 1500 mg/m^2/day divided every 8 hours or 30 mg/kg/day divided every 8 hours for 10 days
   Varicella-zoster virus infection: 1500 mg/m^2/day divided every 8 hours or 30 mg/kg/day divided every 8 hours for 5-10 days

Adults:
   Oral: Initial: 200 mg every 4 hours while awake (5 times/day); prophylaxis: 200 mg 3-4 times/day or 400 mg twice daily. Prophylaxis of varicella or herpes zoster in HIV positive patients: 400 mg 5 times/day
   Topical: $\frac{1}{2}$" ribbon of ointment every 3 hours (6 times/day)

Herpes zoster in immunocompromised patients:
   Children: Oral: 250-600 mg/m^2/dose 4-5 times/day
   Adults: Oral: 800 mg every 4 hours (5 times/day) for 7-10 days
   Children and Adults: I.V.: 7.5 mg/kg/dose every 8 hours

Varicella-zoster infections: Oral:
   Children: 10-20 mg/kg/dose (up to 800 mg) 4 times/day
   Adults: 600-800 mg/dose 5 times/day for 7-10 days or 1000 mg every 6 hours for 5 days

Prophylaxis of bone marrow transplant recipients: Children and Adults: I.V.:
   Autologous patients who are HSV seropositive: 150 mg/m^2/dose every 12 hours; with clinical symptoms of herpes simplex: 150 mg/m^2/dose every 8 hours
   Autologous patients who are CMV seropositive: 500 mg/m^2/dose every 8 hours; for clinically symptomatic CMV infection, ganciclovir should be used in place of acyclovir

(Continued)

7

acyclovir *(Continued)*

Dosage Forms
Capsule: 200 mg
Injection: 500 mg (10 mL); 1000 mg (20 mL)
Ointment, topical: 5% [50 mg/g] (3 g, 15 g)
Suspension, oral (banana flavor): 200 mg/5 mL
Tablet: 800 mg

Adagen™ *see* pegademase bovine *on page 359*

Adalat® *see* nifedipine *on page 334*

Adalat® CC *see* nifedipine *on page 334*

adamantanamine hydrochloride *see* amantadine hydrochloride *on page 17*

Adapin® *see* doxepin hydrochloride *on page 160*

Adeflor® Drops *see* vitamin, multiple (pediatric) *on page 499*

Adeflor® Tablet *see* vitamin, multiple (pediatric) *on page 499*

adenine arabinoside *see* vidarabine *on page 495*

Adenocard® *see* adenosine *on this page*

adenosine (a den' oh seen)

Brand Names Adenocard®
Synonyms 9-beta-D-ribofuranosyladenine
Therapeutic Category Antiarrhythmic Agent, Miscellaneous
Use Treatment of paroxysmal supraventricular tachycardia (PSVT). Orphan drug for treatment of brain tumors in conjunction with BCNU.
Usual Dosage
Children: Initial dose: Rapid I.V.: 0.05 mg/kg; if not effective within 2 minutes, increase dose in 0.05 mg/kg increments every 2 minutes to a maximum dose of 0.25 mg/kg or until termination of PSVT; median dose required: 0.15 mg/kg; do not exceed adult doses

Adults: Rapid I.V. push: 6 mg, if the dose is not effective within 1-2 minutes, a rapid I.V. dose of 12 mg may be given; may repeat 12 mg bolus if needed
Dosage Forms Injection, preservative free: 3 mg/mL (2 mL)

Adipex-P® *see* phentermine hydrochloride *on page 371*

Adlone® Injection *see* methylprednisolone *on page 306*

ADR *see* doxorubicin hydrochloride *on page 161*

Adrenalin® Chloride Inhalation Solution [OTC] *see* epinephrine *on page 171*

Adrenalin® Chloride Injection *see* epinephrine *on page 171*

Adrenalin® Chloride Nasal Solution [OTC] *see* epinephrine *on page 171*

adrenaline *see* epinephrine *on page 171*

adrenocorticotropic hormone *see* corticotropin *on page 116*

Adriamycin PFS™ *see* doxorubicin hydrochloride *on page 161*

Adriamycin RDF™ *see* doxorubicin hydrochloride *on page 161*

Adrucil® Injection *see* fluorouracil *on page 202*

adsorbent charcoal *see* charcoal *on page 86*

Adsorbocarpine® Ophthalmic *see* pilocarpine *on page 377*

Adsorbonac® Ophthalmic [OTC] *see* sodium chloride *on page 434*

Advance® *see* diagnostic aids (*in vitro*), urine *on page 139*

Advil® [OTC] *see* ibuprofen *on page 245*

Aeroaid® **[OTC]** *see* thimerosal *on page 464*

AeroBid®-M Oral Aerosol Inhaler *see* flunisolide *on page 199*

AeroBid® Oral Aerosol Inhaler *see* flunisolide *on page 199*

Aerolate® *see* theophylline *on page 460*

Aerolate III® *see* theophylline *on page 460*

Aerolate JR® *see* theophylline *on page 460*

Aerolate SR® S *see* theophylline *on page 460*

Aeroseb-Dex® Topical Aerosol *see* dexamethasone *on page 132*

Aeroseb-HC® Topical *see* hydrocortisone *on page 236*

Aerosporin® Injection *see* polymyxin b sulfate *on page 384*

AeroZoin® [OTC] *see* benzoin *on page 49*

Afrin® Nasal Solution [OTC] *see* oxymetazoline hydrochloride *on page 350*

Afrinol® [OTC] *see* pseudoephedrine *on page 406*

Aftate® [OTC] *see* tolnaftate *on page 471*

AgNO₃ *see* silver nitrate *on page 430*

AHA *see* acetohydroxamic acid *on page 5*

AHF *see* antihemophilic factor *on page 29*

A-hydroCort® Injection *see* hydrocortisone *on page 236*

Akarpine® Ophthalmic *see* pilocarpine *on page 377*

AK-Chlor® Ophthalmic *see* chloramphenicol *on page 88*

AK-Con® Ophthalmic *see* naphazoline hydrochloride *on page 325*

AK-Dex® Ophthalmic *see* dexamethasone *on page 132*

AK-Dilate® Ophthalmic Solution *see* phenylephrine hydrochloride
on page 372

AK-Fluor Injection *see* fluorescein sodium *on page 200*

AK-Homatropine® Ophthalmic *see* homatropine hydrobromide *on page 230*

Akineton® *see* biperiden hydrochloride *on page 54*

AK-Mycin® Ophthalmic *see* erythromycin, topical *on page 176*

AK-Nefrin® Ophthalmic Solution *see* phenylephrine hydrochloride
on page 372

Akne-Mycin® Topical *see* erythromycin, topical *on page 176*

AK-Pentolate® Ophthalmic *see* cyclopentolate hydrochloride *on page 121*

AK-Poly-Bac® Ophthalmic *see* bacitracin and polymyxin b *on page 42*

AK-Pred® Ophthalmic *see* prednisolone *on page 391*

AK-Spore H.C.® Otic *see* neomycin, polymyxin b, and hydrocortisone
on page 329

AK-Spore® Ophthalmic Solution *see* neomycin, polymyxin b, and gramicidin
on page 329

AK-Sulf® Ophthalmic *see* sodium sulfacetamide *on page 439*

AK-Taine® Ophthalmic *see* proparacaine hydrochloride *on page 401*

AK-Tracin® Ophthalmic *see* bacitracin *on page 42*

AK-Trol® Ophthalmic *see* neomycin, polymyxin b, and dexamethasone
on page 328

AK-Zol® *see* acetazolamide *on page 4*

Ala-Cort® Topical *see* hydrocortisone *on page 236*

Ala-Quin® Topical *see* clioquinol and hydrocortisone *on page 106*

Ala-Scalp® Topical *see* hydrocortisone *on page 236*

Ala-Tet® Oral *see* tetracycline *on page 458*

Alazide® *see* hydrochlorothiazide and spironolactone *on page 233*

Alazine® Oral *see* hydralazine hydrochloride *on page 232*

Albalon-A® Ophthalmic *see* naphazoline and antazoline *on page 325*

Albalon® Liquifilm® Ophthalmic *see* naphazoline hydrochloride *on page 325*

Albuminar® *see* albumin human *on this page*

albumin human
Brand Names Albuminar®; Albutein®; Buminate®; Plasbumin®
Synonyms normal human serum albumin; normal serum albumin (human); salt poor albumin
Therapeutic Category Blood Product Derivative; Plasma Volume Expander
Use Plasma volume expansion and maintenance of cardiac output in the treatment of certain types of shock or impending shock
Usual Dosage 5% should be used in hypovolemic patients; 25% should be used in patients in whom fluid and sodium intake must be minimized

Children: Emergency initial dose: 25 g; nonemergencies: 25% to 50% of the adult dose

Adults: Depends on condition of patient, usual adult dose is 25 g; no more than 250 g should be administered within 48 hours
Hypoproteinemia: I.V.: 0.5-1 g/kg/dose; repeat every 1-2 days as calculated to replace ongoing losses
Hypovolemia: I.V.: 0.5-1 g/kg/dose; repeat as needed; maximum dose: 6 g/kg/day
Dosage Forms Injection: 5% [50 mg/mL] (50 mL, 250 mL, 500 mL, 1000 mL); 25% [250 mg/mL] (10 mL, 20 mL, 50 mL, 100 mL)

Albutein® *see* albumin human *on this page*

albuterol (al byoo' ter ole)
Brand Names Proventil®; Ventolin®; Volmax®
Synonyms salbutamol
Therapeutic Category Adrenergic Agonist Agent; Beta-2-Adrenergic Agonist Agent; Bronchodilator
Use Bronchodilator in reversible airway obstruction due to asthma or COPD
Usual Dosage
Oral:
2-6 years: 0.1-0.2 mg/kg/dose 3 times/day; maximum dose not to exceed 12 mg/day (divided doses)
6-12 years: 2 mg/dose 3-4 times/day; maximum dose not to exceed 24 mg/day (divided doses)
>12 years: 2-4 mg/dose 3-4 times/day; maximum dose not to exceed 32 mg/day (divided doses)

Inhalation MDI: 90 µg/spray:
<12 years: 1-2 inhalations 4 times/day using a tube spacer
≥12 years: 1-2 inhalations every 4-6 hours

Exercise-induced bronchospasm: 2 inhalations 15 minutes before exercising

Inhalation: Nebulization: 2.5 mg = 0.5 mL of the 0.5% inhalation solution to be diluted in 1-2.5 mL of NS
<5 years: 1.25-2.5 mg every 4-6 hours as needed
>5 years: 2.5-5 mg every 4-6 hours
Dosage Forms
Aerosol, oral: 90 µg/spray [200 inhalations] (17 g)
Capsules, microfine, for inhalation, as sulfate (Rotacaps®): 200 µg
Solution, inhalation, as sulfate: 0.083% (3 mL); 0.5% (20 mL)

Syrup, as sulfate (strawberry flavor): 2 mg/5 mL (480 mL)
Tablet, as sulfate: 2 mg, 4 mg
Tablet, extended release (Volmax®): 4 mg, 8 mg

Alcaine® Ophthalmic *see* proparacaine hydrochloride *on page 401*

alclometasone dipropionate (al kloe met' a sone)
Brand Names Aclovate® Topical
Therapeutic Category Corticosteroid, Topical (Low Potency)
Use Inflammation of corticosteroid-responsive dermatosis
Usual Dosage Topical: Apply a thin film to the affected area 2-3 times/day
Dosage Forms
Cream: 0.05% (15 g, 45 g)
Ointment, topical: 0.05% (15 g, 45 g)

alcohol, ethyl
Brand Names Lavacol® [OTC]
Synonyms ethanol
Therapeutic Category Intravenous Nutritional Therapy; Pharmaceutical Aid
Use Topical anti-infective; pharmaceutical aid; as an antidote for ethylene glycol overdose; as antidote for methanol overdose
Usual Dosage I.V. doses of 100-125 mg/kg/hour to maintain blood levels of 100 mg/dL are recommended after a loading dose of 0.6 g/kg; maximum dose: 400 mL of a 5% solution within 1 hour
Dosage Forms
Injection, absolute: 2 mL
Liquid, topical, denatured: 70% (473 mL)
Solution, inhalation: 20%, 40%

Alconefrin® Nasal Solution [OTC] *see* phenylephrine hydrochloride *on page 372*

Aldactazide® *see* hydrochlorothiazide and spironolactone *on page 233*

Aldactone® *see* spironolactone *on page 442*

aldesleukin (al des loo' kin)
Brand Names Proleukin®
Synonyms interleukin-2
Therapeutic Category Antineoplastic Agent, Miscellaneous; Biological Response Modulator
Use Primarily investigated in tumors known to have a response to immunotherapy, such as melanoma and renal cell carcinoma; has been used in conjunction with LAK cells, TIL cells, IL-1, and interferon
Usual Dosage Refer to individual protocols
Adults: Metastatic renal cell carcinoma: Treatment consists of two 5-day treatment cycles separated by a rest period; 600,000 units/kg (0.037 mg/kg)/dose administered every 8 hours by a 15-minute I.V. infusion for a total of 14 doses; following 9 days of rest, the schedule is repeated for another 14 doses, maximum: 28 doses/course
Dosage Forms Powder for injection, lyophilized: 22×10^6 units [18 million units/mL- 1.1 mg/mL]

Aldoclor® *see* chlorothiazide and methyldopa *on page 92*

Aldomet® *see* methyldopa *on page 304*

Aldoril® *see* methyldopa and hydrochlorothiazide *on page 305*

Alersule Forte® *see* chlorpheniramine, phenylephrine, and methscopolamine *on page 95*

Aleve® [OTC] *see* naproxen *on page 326*

Alfenta® Injection *see* alfentanil hydrochloride *on this page*

alfentanil hydrochloride (al fen' ta nill)
Brand Names Alfenta® Injection
Therapeutic Category Analgesic, Narcotic
Use Analgesia; analgesia adjunct; anesthetic agent
Usual Dosage Doses should be titrated to appropriate effects; wide range of doses is dependent upon desired degree of analgesia/anesthesia

Children <12 years: Dose not established

Adults: For anesthesia of ≤30 minutes: Initial (induction): 8-20 μg/kg, then 3-5 μg/kg/dose or 0.5-1 μg/kg/minute for maintenance; total dose: 8-40 μg/kg; higher doses used for longer anesthesia required procedures
Dosage Forms Injection, preservative free: 500 μg/mL (2 mL, 5 mL, 10 mL, 20 mL)

Alferon® N *see* interferon alfa-n3 *on page 252*

alglucerase (al glue' cir race)
Brand Names Ceredase® Injection
Synonyms glucocerebrosidase
Therapeutic Category Enzyme, Glucocerebrosidase
Use Orphan drug for treatment of Gaucher's disease
Usual Dosage Usually administered as a 20-60 units/kg I.V. infusion given with a frequency ranging from 3 times/week to once every 2 weeks
Dosage Forms Injection: 10 units/mL (5 mL); 80 units/mL (5 mL)

alimenazine tartrate *see* trimeprazine tartrate *on page 479*

Alkaban-AQ® Injection *see* vinblastine sulfate *on page 495*

Alka-Mints® [OTC] *see* calcium carbonate *on page 65*

Alkeran® *see* melphalan *on page 290*

Allbee® With C [OTC] *see* vitamin B complex with vitamin C *on page 498*

Aller-Chlor® Oral [OTC] *see* chlorpheniramine maleate *on page 94*

Allerest® 12 Hour Capsule [OTC] *see* chlorpheniramine and phenylpropanolamine *on page 93*

Allerest® 12 Hours Nasal Solution [OTC] *see* oxymetazoline hydrochloride *on page 350*

Allerest® Eye Drops [OTC] *see* naphazoline hydrochloride *on page 325*

Allerfrin® [OTC] *see* triprolidine and pseudoephedrine *on page 482*

Allerfrin® w/Codeine *see* triprolidine, pseudoephedrine, and codeine *on page 482*

Allergan® Ear Drops *see* antipyrine and benzocaine *on page 30*

AllerMax® Oral [OTC] *see* diphenhydramine hydrochloride *on page 152*

Allerphed [OTC] *see* triprolidine and pseudoephedrine *on page 482*

allopurinol (al oh pure' i nole)
Brand Names Zyloprim®
Therapeutic Category Uric Acid Lowering Agent; Uricosuric Agent
Use Prevention of attack of gouty arthritis and nephropathy; also used to treat secondary hyperuricemia which may occur during treatment of tumors or leukemia; to prevent recurrent calcium oxalate calculi

ALPHABETICAL LISTING OF DRUGS

Usual Dosage Oral:
Children: 10 mg/kg/day in 2-3 divided doses or 200-300 mg/m^2/day in 2-4 divided doses, maximum: 600 mg/24 hours
Alternative:
<6 years: 150 mg/day in 3 divided doses
6-10 years: 300 mg/day in 2-3 divided doses
Children >10 years and Adults: Daily doses >300 mg should be administered in divided doses
Myeloproliferative neoplastic disorders: 600-800 mg/day in 2-3 divided doses for prevention of acute uric acid nephropathy for 2-3 days starting 1-2 days before chemotherapy
Gout: 200-300 mg/day (mild); 400-600 mg/day (severe)
Maximum dose: 800 mg/day
Dosage Forms Tablet: 100 mg, 300 mg

Alomide® Ophthalmic *see* Iodoxamide tromethamine *on page 276*
Alophen Pills® [OTC] *see* phenolphthalein *on page 370*
alpha$_1$-PI *see* alpha$_1$-proteinase inhibitor (human) *on this page*

alpha$_1$-proteinase inhibitor (human)
Brand Names Prolastin® Injection
Synonyms alpha$_1$-PI
Therapeutic Category Antitrypsin Deficiency Agent
Use Congenital alpha$_1$-antitrypsin deficiency
Usual Dosage Adults: I.V.: 60 mg/kg once weekly
Dosage Forms Injection, preservative free: ≥20 mg alpha$_1$-PI/mL

alpha chymotrypsin *see* chymotrypsin *on page 101*
Alphamin® Injection *see* hydroxocobalamin *on page 240*
Alphamul® [OTC] *see* castor oil *on page 77*
AlphaNine® *see* factor ix complex (human) *on page 189*
Alphatrex® Topical *see* betamethasone *on page 52*
Alpidine® *see* apraclonidine hydrochloride *on page 31*

alprazolam (al pray' zoe lam)
Brand Names Xanax®
Therapeutic Category Antianxiety Agent; Benzodiazepine
Use Treatment of anxiety; adjunct in the treatment of depression; management of panic attacks
Usual Dosage Oral:
Children <18 years: Dose not established
Adults: 0.25-0.5 mg 2-3 times/day, titrate dose upward; maximum: 4 mg/day (anxiety); 10 mg/day (panic attacks)
Dosage Forms Tablet: 0.25 mg, 0.5 mg, 1 mg, 2 mg

alprostadil (al pross' ta dil)
Brand Names Prostin VR Pediatric® Injection
Synonyms PGE$_1$; prostaglandin E$_1$
Therapeutic Category Prostaglandin
Use Temporary maintenance of patency of ductus arteriosus in neonates with ductal-dependent congenital heart disease until surgery can be performed. These defects include cyanotic (eg, pulmonary atresia, pulmonary stenosis, tricuspid atresia, Fallot's tetral-
(Continued)

13

alprostadil *(Continued)*
ogy, transposition of the great vessels) and acyanotic (eg, interruption of aortic arch, co-arctation of aorta, hypoplastic left ventricle) heart disease.

Usual Dosage I.V. continuous infusion into a large vein, or alternatively through an umbilical artery catheter placed at the ductal opening: 0.05-0.1 μg/kg/minute with therapeutic response, rate is reduced to lowest effective dosage; with unsatisfactory dose, rate is increased gradually; maintenance: 0.01-0.4 μg/kg/minute

PGE$_1$ is usually given at an infusion rate of 0.1 μg/kg/minute, but it is often possible to reduce the dosage to $\frac{1}{2}$ or even $\frac{1}{10}$ without losing the therapeutic effect.

Dosage Forms Injection: 500 μg/mL (1 mL)

Altace™ Oral *see* ramipril *on page 416*

alteplase, recombinant (al' te place)
Brand Names Activase® Injection
Synonyms tissue plasminogen activator, recombinant; t-PA
Therapeutic Category Thrombolytic Agent
Use Management of acute myocardial infarction for the lysis of thrombi in coronary arteries; management of acute massive pulmonary embolism (PE) in adults
Usual Dosage
Coronary artery thrombi:
Total dose of 100 mg given as 60 mg over the first hour (of which 6-10 mg is used over first 1-2 minutes), 20 mg over the second hour, and 20 mg over the third hour
Adults <65 kg: Total dose of 1.25 mg/kg given as 0.75 mg/kg over the first hour, 0.25 mg/kg over the second hour, and 0.25 mg/kg over the third hour

Acute pulmonary embolism: 100 mg over 2 hours
Dosage Forms Powder for injection, lyophilized: 20 mg [11.6 million units] (20 mL); 50 mg [29 million units] (50 mL)

ALternaGEL® [OTC] *see* aluminum hydroxide *on next page*

altretamine (al tret' a meen)
Brand Names Hexalen®
Synonyms hexamethylmelamine
Therapeutic Category Antineoplastic Agent, Alkylating Agent
Use Palliative treatment of persistent or recurrent ovarian cancer
Usual Dosage Adults: Oral: 260 mg/m^2/day (4 divided doses after meals and at bedtime) for 14 or 21 consecutive days in a 28-day cycle
Dosage Forms Capsule: 50 mg

Alu-Cap® [OTC] *see* aluminum hydroxide *on next page*
Aludrox® [OTC] *see* aluminum hydroxide and magnesium hydroxide *on page 16*

aluminum acetate
Brand Names Acid Mantle® [OTC]; Bluboro® [OTC]; Boropak®; Domeboro® [OTC]; Pedi-Boro® [OTC]
Synonyms Burow's solution
Therapeutic Category Topical Skin Product
Use Astringent wet dressing for relief of inflammatory conditions of the skin and to reduce weeping that may occur in dermatitis; treatment of superficial infections of the external auditory canal; reduce edema and crusting associated with moist ear canals; used prophylactically against swimmer's ear.

Usual Dosage
Otic: Instill 4-6 drops every 2-3 hours initially then every 4-6 hours until itching or burning subsides
Topical: Soak the affected area in the solution 2-4 times/day for 15-30 minutes or apply wet dressing soaked in the solution 2-4 times/day for 30-minute treatment periods; rewet dressing with solution every few minutes to keep it moist

Dosage Forms
Powder, to make topical solution: 1 packet/pint of water [1:40 solution]
Solution, otic: Aluminum acetate 1:10 with acetic acid 2% (60 mL)
Tablet: 1 tablet/pint [1:40 dilution]

aluminum acetate and acetic acid
Brand Names Otic Domeboro®
Therapeutic Category Otic Agent, Anti-infective
Use Treatment of superficial infections of the external auditory canal
Usual Dosage Otic: Instill 4-6 drops in ear(s) every 2-3 hours
Dosage Forms Solution, otic: Aluminum acetate 10% and acetic acid 2% (60 mL)

aluminum carbonate
Brand Names Basaljel® [OTC]
Therapeutic Category Antacid
Use Hyperacidity; hyperphosphatemia
Usual Dosage Adults: Oral:
Antacid: 2 tablets/capsules or 10 mL of suspension every 2 hours, up to 12 times/day
Hyperphosphatemia: 2 tablets/capsules or 12 mL of suspension with meals

Dosage Forms
Capsule: Equivalent to 500 mg aluminum hydroxide
Suspension: Equivalent to 400 mg/5 mL aluminum hydroxide
Tablet: Equivalent to 500 mg aluminum hydroxide

aluminum chloride hexahydrate
Brand Names Drysol™
Therapeutic Category Topical Skin Product
Use Astringent in the management of hyperhidrosis
Usual Dosage Adults: Topical: Apply at bedtime
Dosage Forms Solution, topical: 20% in SD alcohol 40 (35 mL, 37.5 mL)

aluminum hydroxide
Brand Names ALternaGEL® [OTC]; Alu-Cap® [OTC]; Alu-Tab® [OTC]; Amphojel® [OTC]; Dialume® [OTC]; Nephrox Suspension [OTC]
Therapeutic Category Antacid; Antidote, Hyperphosphatemia
Use Hyperacidity; hyperphosphatemia
Usual Dosage Oral:
Peptic ulcer disease:
Children: 5-15 mL/dose every 3-6 hours or 1 and 3 hours after meals and at bedtime
Adults: 15-45 mL every 3-6 hours or 1 and 3 hours after meals and at bedtime

Prophylaxis against gastrointestinal bleeding:
Infants: 2-5 mL/dose every 1-2 hours
Children: 5-15 mL/dose every 1-2 hours
Adults: 30-60 mL/dose every hour
Titrate to maintain the gastric pH >5

Hyperphosphatemia:
Children: 50 mg to 150 mg/kg/24 hours in divided doses every 4-6 hours, titrate dosage to maintain serum phosphorus within normal range
(Continued)

aluminum hydroxide *(Continued)*

Adults: 500-1800 mg, 3-6 times/day, between meals and at bedtime

Antacid: Adults: 30 mL 1 and 3 hours postprandial and at bedtime

Dosage Forms
Capsule: 475 mg, 500 mg
Gel: 600 mg/5 mL (360 mL)
Suspension, oral: 320 mg/5 mL (500 mL)
Tablet: 300 mg, 500 mg, 600 mg

aluminum hydroxide and magnesium hydroxide

Brand Names Aludrox® [OTC]; Maalox® [OTC]; Maalox® Therapeutic Concentrate [OTC]
Synonyms magnesium hydroxide and aluminum hydroxide
Therapeutic Category Antacid
Use Antacid, hyperphosphatemia in renal failure
Usual Dosage Adults: Oral: 5-10 mL or 1-2 tablets 4-6 times/day, between meals and at bedtime; may be used every hour for severe symptoms
Dosage Forms
Suspension:
  Aludrox®: Aluminum hydroxide 307 mg and magnesium hydroxide 103 mg per 5 mL
  Maalox®: Aluminum hydroxide 225 mg and magnesium hydroxide 200 mg per 5 mL
  High potency (Maalox® TC): Aluminum hydroxide 600 mg and magnesium hydroxide 300 mg per 5 mL
Tablet, chewable (Maalox®): Aluminum hydroxide 600 mg and magnesium hydroxide 300 mg

aluminum hydroxide, magnesium hydroxide, and simethicone

Brand Names Di-Gel® [OTC]; Gelusil® [OTC]; Maalox® Plus [OTC]; Mylanta® [OTC]; Mylanta®-II [OTC]
Therapeutic Category Antacid; Antiflatulent
Use Temporary relief of hyperacidity associated with gas; may also be used for indications associated with other antacids
Usual Dosage Adults: 15-30 mL or 2-4 tablets 4-6 times/day between meals and at bedtime; may be used every hour for severe symptoms
Dosage Forms
Liquid:
  Gelusil®, Mylanta®: Aluminum hydroxide 200 mg, magnesium hydroxide, 200 mg, and simethicone 25 mg per 5 mL
  Maalox® Plus: Aluminum hydroxide 225 mg, magnesium hydroxide 200 mg, and simethicone 25 mg per 5 mL (30 mL, 180 mL)
  Mylanta®-II: Aluminum hydroxide 400 mg, magnesium hydroxide 400 mg, and simethicone 40 mg per 5 mL (150 mL, 360 mL)
Tablet, chewable:
  Mylanta®: Aluminum hydroxide 200 mg, magnesium hydroxide 200 mg, and simethicone 20 mg
  Mylanta®-II: Aluminum hydroxide 400 mg, magnesium hydroxide 400 mg, and simethicone 40 mg

aluminum hydroxide, magnesium trisilicate, sodium bicarbonate and alginic acid

Brand Names Gaviscon® [OTC]
Therapeutic Category Antacid
Use Temporary relief of hyperacidity
Usual Dosage Adults: Oral: Chew 2-4 tablets or 1-2 tablespoonfuls 4 times/day or as directed by physician
Dosage Forms
Liquid: Aluminum hydroxide 160 mg, magnesium trisilicate 40 mg, sodium bicarbonate 140 mg, and sodium alginate 400 mg per 15 mL

Tablet, chewable: Aluminum hydroxide 80 mg, magnesium trisilicate 20 mg, sodium bicarbonate 70 mg, and alginic acid 200 mg

aluminum phosphate
Brand Names Phosphaljel® [OTC]
Therapeutic Category Electrolyte Supplement, Oral
Use Reduce fecal excretion of phosphates
Usual Dosage Adults: Oral: 15-30 mL every 2 hours between meals
Dosage Forms Suspension, oral: 233 mg/5 mL

aluminum sucrose sulfate, basic *see* sucralfate *on page 445*

Alupent® Inhalation Aerosol *see* metaproterenol sulfate *on page 296*

Alupent® Inhalation Solution *see* metaproterenol sulfate *on page 296*

Alupent® Oral *see* metaproterenol sulfate *on page 296*

Alu-Tab® [OTC] *see* aluminum hydroxide *on page 15*

amantadine hydrochloride (a man' ta deen)
Brand Names Symadine®; Symmetrel®
Synonyms adamantanamine hydrochloride
Therapeutic Category Antiparkinson Agent; Antiviral Agent, Oral
Use Symptomatic and adjunct treatment of parkinsonism; also used in prophylaxis and treatment of influenza A viral infection
Usual Dosage
Children:
1-9 years: 4.4-8.8 mg/kg/day in 1-2 divided doses to a maximum of 150 mg/day
9-12 years: 100-200 mg/day in 1-2 divided doses
After first influenza A virus vaccine dose, amantadine prophylaxis may be administered for up to 6 weeks or until 2 weeks after the second dose of vaccine

Adults:
Parkinson's disease: 100 mg twice daily
Influenza A viral infection: 200 mg/day in 1-2 divided doses
Prophylaxis: Minimum 10-day course of therapy following exposure or continue for 2-3 weeks after influenza A virus vaccine is given
Elderly patients should take the drug in 2 daily doses rather than a single dose to avoid adverse neurologic reactions
Dosage Forms
Capsule: 100 mg
Syrup: 50 mg/5 mL (480 mL)

Amaphen® *see* butalbital compound *on page 63*

ambenonium chloride (am be noe' nee um)
Brand Names Mytelase® Caplets®
Therapeutic Category Cholinergic Agent
Use Treatment of myasthenia gravis
Usual Dosage Adults: Oral: 5-25 mg 3-4 times/day
Dosage Forms Tablet: 10 mg

Ambenyl® Cough Syrup *see* bromodiphenhydramine and codeine *on page 58*

Ambien™ *see* zolpidem tartrate *on page 504*

17

amcinonide (am sin' oh nide)
Brand Names Cyclocort® Topical
Therapeutic Category Corticosteroid, Topical (Medium/High Potency)
Use Relief of the inflammatory and pruritic manifestations of corticosteroid-responsive dermatoses
Usual Dosage Adults: Topical: Apply in a thin film 2-3 times/day
Dosage Forms
Cream: 0.1% (15 g, 30 g, 60 g)
Lotion: 0.1% (20 mL, 60 mL)
Ointment, topical: 0.1% (15 g, 30 g, 60 g)

Amcort® Injection see triamcinolone on page 474

Amen® Oral see medroxyprogesterone acetate on page 289

Americaine® [OTC] see benzocaine on page 48

A-methaPred® Injection see methylprednisolone on page 306

amethocaine hydrochloride see tetracaine hydrochloride on page 457

amethopterin see methotrexate on page 301

amfepramone see diethylpropion hydrochloride on page 146

Amgenal® Cough Syrup see bromodiphenhydramine and codeine on page 58

Amicar® see aminocaproic acid on next page

Amidate® Injection see etomidate on page 187

amikacin sulfate (am i kay' sin)
Brand Names Amikin® Injection
Therapeutic Category Antibiotic, Aminoglycoside
Use Treatment of documented gram-negative enteric infection resistant to gentamicin and tobramycin; documented infection of mycobacterial organisms susceptible to amikacin
Usual Dosage I.M., I.V.:
Neonates:
<1200 g, 0-4 weeks: 7.5 mg/kg/dose every 12 hours
Postnatal age <7 days:
1200-2000 g: 7.5 mg/kg/dose every 12 hours
>2000 g: 10 mg/kg/dose every 12 hours
Postnatal age >7 days:
1200-2000 g: 7 mg/kg/dose every 8 hours
>2000 g: 7.5-10 mg/kg/dose every 8 hours
Infants and Children: 15-20 mg/kg/day divided every 8 hours
Adults: 15 mg/kg/day divided every 8-12 hours
Dosage Forms Injection: 50 mg/mL (2 mL); 250 mg/mL (2 mL, 4 mL)

Amikin® Injection see amikacin sulfate on this page

amiloride and hydrochlorothiazide
Brand Names Moduretic®
Synonyms hydrochlorothiazide and amiloride
Therapeutic Category Diuretic, Combination
Use Antikaliuretic diuretic, antihypertensive
Usual Dosage Adults: Oral: Initial: 1 tablet daily, then may be increased to 2 tablets/day if needed; usually given in a single dose
Dosage Forms Tablet: Amiloride hydrochloride 5 mg and hydrochlorothiazide 50 mg

amiloride hydrochloride (a mill' oh ride)
Brand Names Midamor®
Therapeutic Category Diuretic, Potassium Sparing
Use Counteract potassium loss induced by other diuretics in the treatment of hypertension or edematous conditions including CHF, hepatic cirrhosis and hypoaldosteronism; usually used in conjunction with a more potent diuretic such as thiazides or loop diuretics
Usual Dosage Oral:
Children: Although safety and efficacy have not been established by the FDA in children, a dosage of 0.625 mg/kg/day has been used in children weighing 6-20 kg

Adults: 5-10 mg/day (up to 20 mg)
Dosage Forms Tablet: 5 mg

2-amino-6-mercaptopurine *see* thioguanine *on page 464*

aminobenzylpenicillin *see* ampicillin *on page 26*

aminocaproic acid (a mee noe ka proe' ik)
Brand Names Amicar®
Therapeutic Category Hemostatic Agent
Use Treatment of excessive bleeding from fibrinolysis
Usual Dosage In the management of acute bleeding syndromes, oral dosage regimens are the same as the I.V. dosage regimens in adults and children

Chronic bleeding: Oral, I.V.: 5-30 g/day in divided doses at 3- to 6-hour intervals

Acute bleeding syndrome:
Children: Oral, I.V.: 100 mg/kg or 3 g/m^2 during the first hour, followed by continuous infusion at the rate of 33.3 mg/kg/hour or 1 g/m^2/hour; total dosage should not exceed 18 g/m^2/24 hours
Adults:
Oral: For elevated fibrinolytic activity, give 5 g during first hour, followed by 1-1.25 g/hour for approximately 8 hours or until bleeding stops
I.V.: Give 4-5 g in 250 mL of diluent during first hour followed by continuous infusion at the rate of 1-1.25 g/hour in 50 mL of diluent, continue for 8 hours or until bleeding stops
Dosage Forms
Injection: 250 mg/mL (20 mL, 96 mL, 100 mL)
Syrup (raspberry flavor): 250 mg/mL (480 mL)
Tablet: 500 mg

Amino-Cerv™ Vaginal Cream *see* urea *on page 487*

aminoglutethimide (a mee noe gloo teth' i mide)
Brand Names Cytadren®
Therapeutic Category Antiadrenal Agent; Antineoplastic Agent, Adjuvant
Use Suppression of adrenal function in selected patients with Cushing's syndrome; also used successfully in postmenopausal patients with advanced breast carcinoma and in patients with metastatic prostate carcinoma
Usual Dosage Refer to individual protocols
Adults: Oral: 250 mg every 6 hours may be increased to a total of 2 g/day; give in divided doses, 2-3 times/day to reduce incidence of nausea and vomiting
Dosage Forms Tablet: 250 mg

Amino-Opti-E® Oral [OTC] *see* vitamin E *on page 498*

aminophylline (am in off' i lin)
Brand Names Phyllocontin®; Truphylline®
Synonyms theophylline ethylenediamine
Therapeutic Category Antiasthmatic; Bronchodilator; Theophylline Derivative
(Continued)

aminophylline *(Continued)*

Use Bronchodilator in reversible airway obstruction due to asthma or COPD; for neonatal idiopathic apnea/bradycardia spells

Usual Dosage

Neonates: Apnea of prematurity:
Loading dose: 5 mg/kg for one dose
Maintenance: I.V.:
0-24 days: Begin at 2 mg/kg/day divided every 12 hours and titrate to desired levels and effects
>24 days: 3 mg/kg/day divided every 12 hours; increased dosages may be indicated as liver metabolism matures (usually >30 days of life); monitor serum levels to determine appropriate dosages
Theophylline levels should be initially drawn after 3 days of therapy; repeat levels are indicated 3 days after each increase in dosage or weekly if on a stabilized dosage

Treatment of acute bronchospasm:
Loading dose (in patients not currently receiving aminophylline or theophylline): 6 mg/kg given I.V. over 20-30 minutes; administration rate should not exceed 25 mg/minute

Approximate I.V. maintenance dosages are based upon **continuous infusions**; bolus dosing (often used in children <6 months of age) may be determined by multiplying the hourly infusion rate by 24 hours and dividing by the desired number of doses/day
Infants 6 weeks to 6 months: 0.5 mg/kg/hour
Children:
6 months to 1 year: 0.6-0.7 mg/kg/hour
1-9 years: 1-1.2 mg/kg/hour
12-16 years: 0.7 mg/kg/hour
9-12 years and young adult smokers: 0.9 mg/kg/hour
Adults (healthy, nonsmoking): 0.7 mg/kg/hour
Elderly and patients with cor pulmonale with congestive heart failure or liver failure: 0.25 mg/kg/hour
Dosage should be adjusted according to serum level measurements during the first 12- to 24-hour period. Avoid using suppositories due to erratic, unreliable absorption.

Rectal: Adults: 500 mg 3 times/day

Dosage Forms
Injection, I.V.: 25 mg/mL (10 mL, 20 mL)
Liquid, oral: 105 mg/5 mL (240 mL)
Suppository, rectal (Truphylline®): 250 mg, 500 mg
Tablet: 100 mg, 200 mg
Tablet, controlled release [12 hours] (Phyllocontin®): 225 mg

aminosalicylate sodium *(a mee noe sal i sill' ik)*

Brand Names Sodium P.A.S.
Synonyms PAS
Therapeutic Category Antitubercular Agent; Nonsteroidal Anti-Inflammatory Agent (NSAID), Oral
Use Treatment of tuberculosis with combination drugs
Usual Dosage Oral:
Children: 150-300 mg/kg/day in 3-4 equally divided doses
Adults: 150 mg/kg/day in 2-3 equally divided doses (usually 12-14 g/day)
Dosage Forms Tablet: 500 mg

aminosalicylate sodium *see* para-aminosalicylate sodium *on page 356*

5-aminosalicylic acid *see* mesalamine *on page 294*

amiodarone hydrochloride (a mee' oh da rone)
Brand Names Cordarone®
Therapeutic Category Antiarrhythmic Agent, Class III
Use Management of resistant, life-threatening ventricular arrhythmias unresponsive to conventional therapy with less toxic agents; has also been used for treatment of supraventricular arrhythmias unresponsive to conventional therapy
Usual Dosage Children <1 year should be dosed as calculated by body surface area.

Children: Loading dose: 10-15 mg/kg/day or 600-800 mg/1.73 m^2/day for 4-14 days or until adequate control of arrhythmia or prominent adverse effects occur (this loading dose may be given in 1-2 divided doses/day); dosage should then be reduced to 5 mg/kg/day or 200-400 mg/1.73 m^2/day given once daily for several weeks; if arrhythmia does not recur reduce to lowest effective dosage possible; usual daily minimal dose: 2.5 mg/kg; maintenance doses may be given for 5 of 7 days/week.

Adults: Ventricular arrhythmias: 800-1600 mg/day in 1-2 doses for 1-3 weeks, then 600-800 mg/day in 1-2 doses for 1 month; maintenance: 400 mg/day; lower doses are recommended for supraventricular arrhythmias, usually 100-400 mg/day
Dosage Forms Tablet: 200 mg

Ami-Tex LA® *see* guaifenesin and phenylpropanolamine *on page 219*

Amitone® [OTC] *see* calcium carbonate *on page 65*

amitriptyline and chlordiazepoxide
Brand Names Limbitrol®
Synonyms chlordiazepoxide and amitriptyline
Therapeutic Category Antidepressant, Tricyclic; Antipsychotic Agent
Use Treatment of moderate to severe anxiety and/or agitation and depression
Usual Dosage Oral: Initial dose: 3-4 tablets in divided doses; this may be increased to 6 tablets/day as required; some patients respond to smaller doses and can be maintained on 2 tablets
Dosage Forms Tablet:
5-12.5: Amitriptyline hydrochloride 12.5 mg and chlordiazepoxide 5 mg
10-25: Amitriptyline hydrochloride 25 mg and chlordiazepoxide 10 mg

amitriptyline and perphenazine
Brand Names Etrafon®; Triavil®
Synonyms perphenazine and amitriptyline
Therapeutic Category Antidepressant, Tricyclic; Benzodiazepine
Use Treatment of patients with moderate to severe anxiety and depression
Usual Dosage Oral: 1 tablet 2-4 times/day
Dosage Forms Tablet:
2-10: Amitriptyline hydrochloride 10 mg and perphenazine 2 mg
4-10: Amitriptyline hydrochloride 10 mg and perphenazine 4 mg
2-25: Amitriptyline hydrochloride 25 mg and perphenazine 2 mg
4-25: Amitriptyline hydrochloride 25 mg and perphenazine 4 mg
4-50: Amitriptyline hydrochloride 50 mg and perphenazine 4 mg

amitriptyline hydrochloride (a mee trip' ti leen)
Brand Names Elavil®; Endep®; Enovil®
Therapeutic Category Antidepressant, Tricyclic
Use Used in the treatment of various forms of depression, often in conjunction with psychotherapy; as an analgesic for certain chronic and neuropathic pain, migraine prophylaxis
Usual Dosage
Children <12 years: Not recommended

Adolescents: Oral: Initial: 25-50 mg/day; may give in divided doses; increase gradually to 100 mg/day in divided doses
(Continued)

amitriptyline hydrochloride *(Continued)*
Adults:
Oral: 30-100 mg/day single dose at bedtime or in divided doses; dose may be gradually increased up to 300 mg/day; once symptoms are controlled, decrease gradually to lowest effective dose
I.M.: 20-30 mg 4 times/day
Dosage Forms
Injection: 10 mg/mL (10 mL)
Tablet: 10 mg, 25 mg, 50 mg, 75 mg, 100 mg, 150 mg

amlodipine (am loe' di peen)
Brand Names Norvasc®
Therapeutic Category Calcium Channel Blocker
Use Treatment of hypertension and angina
Usual Dosage Oral: Adults: 2.5-10 mg once daily
Dosage Forms Tablet: 2.5 mg, 5 mg, 10 mg

ammonia spirit, aromatic
Brand Names Aromatic Ammonia Aspirols®
Therapeutic Category Respiratory Stimulant
Use Respiratory and circulatory stimulant, treatment of fainting
Usual Dosage Used as "smelling salts" to treat or prevent fainting
Dosage Forms
Inhalant, crushable glass perles: 0.33 mL, 0.4 mL
Solution: 30 mL, 60 mL, 120 mL

ammonium chloride
Therapeutic Category Metabolic Alkalosis Agent; Urinary Acidifying Agent
Use Diuretic or systemic and urinary acidifying agent; treatment of hypochloremic states
Usual Dosage The following equations represent different methods of correction utilizing either the serum HCO_3^-, the serum Cl^- or the base excess

Correction of refractory hypochloremic metabolic alkalosis: Dose mEq = 0.5 (L/kg) x wt (kg) x [serum HCO_3^--24] mEq/L; give $\frac{1}{2}$ to $\frac{2}{3}$ of the calculated dose, then re-evaluate

Correction of hypochloremia: mEq NH_4Cl = 0.2 L/kg x wt x [103 - serum Cl^-] mEq/L, give $\frac{1}{2}$ to $\frac{2}{3}$ of calculated dose, then re-evaluate

Correction of alkalosis: mEq NH_4Cl = 0.3 L/kg x wt (kg) x base excess (mEq/L), give $\frac{1}{2}$ to $\frac{2}{3}$ of calculated dose, then re-evaluate

Children: Oral, I.V.: 75 mg/kg/day in 4 divided doses for urinary acidification; maximum daily dose: 6 g
Adults:
Oral: 2-3 g every 6 hours
I.V.: 1.5 g/dose every 6 hours
Dosage Forms
Injection: 26.75% [5 mEq/mL] (20 mL)
Tablet: 500 mg
Tablet, enteric coated: 500 mg

ammonium lactate *see* lactic acid with ammonium hydroxide *on page 267*
Amnipaque® *see* radiological/contrast media (non-ionic) *on page 415*

amobarbital (am oh bar' bi tal)
Brand Names Amytal®
Synonyms amylobarbitone
Therapeutic Category Barbiturate; Hypnotic; Sedative

Use
Oral: Hypnotic in short-term treatment of insomnia, to reduce anxiety and provide sedation preoperatively
I.M., I.V.: Used to control status epilepticus or acute seizure episodes; also used in catatonic, negativistic, or manic reactions and in "Amytal® Interviewing" for narcoanalysis

Usual Dosage
Children: Oral:
Insomnia: 2 mg/kg or 70 mg/m^2/day in 4 equally divided doses
Hypnotic: 2-3 mg/kg

Adults:
Insomnia: Oral: 65-200 mg at bedtime
Sedation: Oral: 30-50 mg 2-3 times/day
Preanesthetic: Oral: 200 mg 1-2 hours before surgery
Hypnotic:
Oral: 65-200 mg at bedtime
I.M.: 65-500 mg, should not exceed 500 mg
I.V.: 65-500 mg, should not exceed 1000 mg

Dosage Forms
Capsule, as sodium: 65 mg, 200 mg
Powder: 15 g, 30 g
Powder for injection, as sodium: 250 mg, 500 mg
Tablet: 30 mg, 50 mg, 100 mg

amobarbital and secobarbital
Brand Names Tuinal®
Synonyms secobarbital and amobarbital
Therapeutic Category Barbiturate; Hypnotic
Use Short-term treatment of insomnia
Usual Dosage Adults: Oral: 1-2 capsules at bedtime
Dosage Forms Capsule:
100: Amobarbital 50 mg and secobarbital 50 mg
200: Amobarbital 100 mg and secobarbital 100 mg

Amonidrin® [OTC] *see* guaifenesin *on page 217*

amoxapine (a mox' a peen)
Brand Names Asendin®
Therapeutic Category Antidepressant, Tricyclic
Use Treatment of neurotic and endogenous depression and mixed symptoms of anxiety and depression
Usual Dosage Oral (once symptoms are controlled, decrease gradually to lowest effective dose):

Children: Not established in children <16 years

Adolescents: Initial: 25-50 mg/day; increase gradually to 100 mg/day; may give as divided doses or as a single dose at bedtime

Adults: Initial: 25 mg 2-3 times/day, if tolerated, dosage may be increased to 100 mg 2-3 times/day; may be given in a single bedtime dose when dosage <300 mg/day
Maximum daily dose:
Outpatient: 400 mg
Inpatient: 600 mg
Dosage Forms Tablet: 25 mg, 50 mg, 100 mg, 150 mg

amoxicillin and clavulanate potassium *see* amoxicillin and clavulanic acid
on next page

amoxicillin and clavulanic acid (a mox i sill' in & klav yoo lan' ick)
Brand Names Augmentin®
Synonyms amoxicillin and clavulanate potassium
Therapeutic Category Antibiotic, Penicillin
Use Infections caused by susceptible organisms involving the lower respiratory tract, otitis media, sinusitis, skin and skin structure, and urinary tract
Usual Dosage Oral:
Children <40 kg: 20-40 mg (amoxicillin component)/kg/day in divided doses every 8 hours
Children >40 kg and Adults: 250-500 mg every 8 hours; maximum dose: 2 g/day
Dosage Forms
Suspension, oral (banana flavor):
125: Amoxicillin trihydrate 125 mg and clavulanic acid 31.25 mg per 5 mL (75 mL, 150 mL)
250: Amoxicillin trihydrate 250 mg and clavulanic acid 62.5 mg per 5 mL (75 mL, 150 mL)
Tablet:
250: Amoxicillin trihydrate 250 mg and clavulanic acid 125 mg
500: Amoxicillin trihydrate 500 mg and clavulanic acid 125 mg
Tablet, chewable:
125: Amoxicillin trihydrate 125 mg and clavulanic acid 31.25 mg
250: Amoxicillin trihydrate 250 mg and clavulanic acid 62.5 mg

amoxicillin trihydrate (a mox i sill' in)
Brand Names Amoxil®; Biomox®; Polymox®; Trimox®; Wymox®
Synonyms amoxicillin; p-hydroxyampicillin
Therapeutic Category Antibiotic, Penicillin
Use Infections caused by susceptible organisms involving the respiratory tract, otitis media, sinusitis, skin, and urinary tract; prophylaxis of bacterial endocarditis
Usual Dosage Oral:
Children: 25-50 mg/kg/day in divided doses every 8 hours
Uncomplicated gonorrhea: ≥2 years: 50 mg/kg plus probenecid 25 mg/kg in a single dose; do not use this regimen in children <2 years of age, probenecid is contraindicated in this age group
SBE prophylaxis: 50 mg/kg 1 hour before procedure and 25 mg/kg 6 hours later; not to exceed adult dosage
Adults: 250-500 mg every 8 hours; maximum dose: 2-3 g/day
Uncomplicated gonorrhea: 3 g plus probenecid 1 g in a single dose
Endocarditis prophylaxis: 3 g 1 hour before procedure and 1.5 g 6 hours later
Dosage Forms
Capsule: 250 mg, 500 mg
Powder for oral suspension: 125 mg/5 mL (5 mL, 80 mL, 100 mL, 150 mL, 200 mL); 250 mg/5 mL (5 mL, 80 mL, 100 mL, 150 mL, 200 mL)
Powder for oral suspension, drops: 50 mg/mL (15 mL, 30 mL)
Tablet, chewable: 125 mg, 250 mg

Amoxil® *see* amoxicillin trihydrate *on this page*

amoxycillin *see* amoxicillin trihydrate *on this page*

amphetamine sulfate (am fet' a meen)
Synonyms racemic amphetamine sulfate
Therapeutic Category Amphetamine; Central Nervous System Stimulant, Amphetamine
Use Narcolepsy; exogenous obesity; abnormal behavioral syndrome in children (minimal brain dysfunction); attention deficit hyperactive disorder (ADHD)

Usual Dosage Oral:
Narcolepsy:
Children:
6-12 years: 5 mg/day, increase by 5 mg at weekly intervals
> 12 years: 10 mg/day, increase by 10 mg at weekly intervals
Adults: 5-60 mg/day in divided doses

Minimal brain dysfunction: Children:
3-5 years: 2.5 mg/day, increase by 2.5 mg at weekly intervals
>6 years: 5 mg/day, increase by 5 mg at weekly intervals

Short-term adjunct to exogenous obesity: Children > 12 years and Adults: 10 mg or 15 mg long-acting capsule daily, up to 30 mg/day; or 5-30 mg/day in divided doses (immediate release tablets only)

Dosage Forms Tablet: 5 mg, 10 mg

Amphojel® [OTC] *see* aluminum hydroxide *on page 15*

amphotericin B (am foe ter' i sin)

Brand Names Fungizone®
Synonyms ampho
Therapeutic Category Antifungal Agent, Systemic; Antifungal Agent, Topical
Use Treatment of severe systemic infections and meningitis caused by susceptible fungi; fungal peritonitis; irrigant for bladder fungal infections; and topically for cutaneous and mucocutaneous candidal infections
Usual Dosage The minimum dilution for amphotericin B infusions is 0.1 mg/mL for peripheral lines and 1 mg/mL for central lines

Infants and Children:
Test dose: I.V.: 0.1 mg/kg/dose to a maximum of 1 mg; infuse over 30-60 minutes. If the test dose is tolerated, the initial therapeutic dose is 0.25 mg/kg. The daily dose can then be gradually increased, usually in 0.25 mg/kg increments on each subsequent day until the desired daily dose is reached.
Maintenance dose: 0.25-1 mg/kg/day given once daily; infuse over 2-6 hours. Once therapy has been established, amphotericin B can be administered on an every other day basis at 1-1.5 mg/kg/dose.
I.T.: 25-100 µg every 48-72 hours; increase to 500 µg as tolerated

Adults:
Test dose: I.V.: 1 mg infused over 20-30 minutes. Institute therapy with 0.25 mg/kg administered over 2-6 hours; the daily dose can be gradually increased on subsequent days to the desired level.
Maintenance dose: I.V.: 0.25-1 mg/kg/day or 1.5 mg/kg every other day; do not exceed 1.5 mg/kg/day. If the test dose is tolerated, the initial therapeutic dose is 0.25 mg/kg. The daily dose can then be gradually increased, usually in 0.25 mg/kg increments on each subsequent day until the desired daily dose is reached.
Duration of therapy varies with nature of infection: Histoplasmosis, *Cryptococcus*, or blastomycosis may be treated with total dose of 2-4 g
I.T.: 25-300 µg every 48-72 hours; increase to 500 µg to 1 mg as tolerated

Children and Adults:
Bladder irrigation: 50 mg/day in 1 L of sterile water irrigation solution instilled over 24 hours for 2-7 days or until cultures are clear
Dialysate: 1-2 mg/L of peritoneal dialysis fluid either with or without low-dose I.V. amphotericin B (a total dose of 2-10 mg/kg given over 7-14 days)
Topical: Apply to affected areas 2-4 times/day for 1-4 weeks of therapy depending on nature and severity of infection

Dosage Forms
Cream: 3% (20 g)
Lotion: 3% (30 mL)
Ointment, topical: 3% (20 g)
Powder for injection, lyophilized: 50 mg

ampicillin (am pi sill' in)
Brand Names Marcillin®; Omnipen®; Omnipen®-N; Polycillin®; Polycillin-N®; Principen®; Totacillin®; Totacillin®-N
Synonyms aminobenzylpenicillin
Therapeutic Category Antibiotic, Penicillin
Use Treatment of susceptible bacterial infections
Usual Dosage
Neonates: I.M., I.V.:
  Postnatal age <7 days:
    <2000 g: 50 mg/kg/day in 2 divided doses; meningitis: 100 mg/kg/day in 2 divided doses
    >2000 g: 75 mg/kg/day in 3 divided doses; meningitis: 150 mg/kg/day in 3 divided doses
  Postnatal age >7 days:
    <2000 g: 75 mg/kg/day in 3 divided doses; meningitis: 150 mg/kg/day in 3 divided doses
    >2000 g: 100 mg/kg/day in 4 divided doses; meningitis: 200 mg/kg/day in 4 divided doses
Infants and Children:
  Oral: 50-100 mg/kg/day divided every 6 hours; maximum dose: 2-3 g/day
  I.M., I.V.: 100-200 mg/kg/day in 4-6 divided doses; meningitis: 200-400 mg/kg/day in 4-6 divided doses; maximum dose: 12 g/day
Adults:
  Oral: 250-500 mg every 6 hours
  I.M., I.V.: 8-12 g/day in 4-6 divided doses
Dosage Forms
Capsule, as anhydrous: 250 mg, 500 mg
Capsule, as trihydrate: 250 mg, 500 mg
Powder for injection, as sodium: 125 mg, 250 mg, 500 mg, 1 g, 2 g, 10 g
Powder for oral suspension, as trihydrate: 125 mg/5 mL (5 mL unit dose, 80 mL, 100 mL, 150 mL, 200 mL); 250 mg/5 mL (5 mL unit dose, 80 mL, 100 mL, 150 mL, 200 mL); 500 mg/5 mL (5 mL unit dose, 100 mL)
Powder for oral suspension, drops, as trihydrate: 100 mg/mL (20 mL)

ampicillin and probenecid
Brand Names Polycillin-PRB®; Proampacin®
Therapeutic Category Antibiotic, Penicillin
Use Uncomplicated infections caused by susceptible strains of *Neisseria gonorrhoeae* in adults
Usual Dosage Administer the entire contents of bottle as a single one time dose
Dosage Forms Powder for oral suspension: Ampicillin 3.5 g and probenecid 1 g per bottle

ampicillin sodium and sulbactam sodium
Brand Names Unasyn®
Synonyms sulbactam and ampicillin
Therapeutic Category Antibiotic, Penicillin
Use Treatment of susceptible bacterial infections involved with skin and skin structure, intra-abdominal infections, gynecological infections; spectrum is that of ampicillin plus organisms producing beta-lactamases such as *S. aureus, H. influenzae, E. coli, Klebsiella, Acinetobacter, Enterobacter* and anaerobes
Usual Dosage Not FDA approved for children <12 years of age
Unasyn® (ampicillin/sulbactam) is a combination product. Each 3 g vial contains 2 g of ampicillin and 1 g of sulbactam. Sulbactam has very little antibacterial activity by itself, but effectively extends the spectrum of ampicillin to include beta-lactamase producing strains that are resistant to ampicillin alone. Therefore, dosage recommendations for Unasyn® are based on the ampicillin component.

Children: I.M., I.V.: 100-200 mg ampicillin/kg/day divided every 6 hours; maximum dose: 8 g ampicillin/day

Adults: I.M., I.V.: 1-2 g ampicillin every 6-8 hours; maximum dose: 8 g ampicillin/day
Dosage Forms Powder for injection: 1.5 g [ampicillin sodium 1 g and sulbactam sodium 0.5 g]; 3 g [ampicillin sodium 2 g and sulbactam sodium 1 g]

AMPT *see* metyrosine *on page 310*

amrinone lactate (am' ri none)
Brand Names Inocor®
Therapeutic Category Adrenergic Agonist Agent
Use Treatment of low cardiac output states (sepsis, congestive heart failure); adjunctive therapy of pulmonary hypertension; normally prescribed for patients who have not responded well to therapy with digitalis, diuretics, and vasodilators
Usual Dosage Dosage is based on clinical response. **Note:** Dose should not exceed 10 mg/kg/24 hours.
Neonates: 0.75 mg/kg I.V. bolus over 2-3 minutes followed by maintenance infusion 3-5 µg/kg/minute; I.V. bolus may need to be repeated in 30 minutes
Children: 0.75 mg/kg I.V. bolus over 2-3 minutes followed by maintenance infusion 5-10 µg/kg/minute; I.V. bolus may need to be repeated in 30 minutes
Adults: 0.75 mg/kg I.V. bolus over 2-3 minutes followed by maintenance infusion of 5-10 µg/kg/minute
Dosage Forms Injection: 5 mg/mL (20 mL)

Amvisc® Injection *see* sodium hyaluronate *on page 436*

amyl nitrite (am' il nye trato)
Synonyms isoamyl nitrite
Therapeutic Category Vasodilator, Coronary
Use Coronary vasodilator in angina pectoris; an adjunct in treatment of cyanide poisoning; also used to produce changes in the intensity of heart murmurs
Usual Dosage 1-6 inhalations from 1 capsule are usually sufficient to produce the desired effect
Dosage Forms Inhalant, crushable glass perles: 0.3 mL

amylobarbitone *see* amobarbital *on page 22*

Amytal® *see* amobarbital *on page 22*

Anabolin® Injection *see* nandrolone *on page 324*

Anacin® [OTC] *see* aspirin *on page 34*

Anacin-3® [OTC] *see* acetaminophen *on page 2*

Anadrol® *see* oxymetholone *on page 351*

Anafranil® *see* clomipramine hydrochloride *on page 108*

Ana-Kit® *see* insect sting kit *on page 250*

Anamine T.D.® *see* chlorpheniramine and pseudoephedrine *on page 94*

Anaprox® *see* naproxen *on page 326*

Anaspaz® Oral *see* hyoscyamine sulfate *on page 243*

Anatrast® *see* radiological/contrast media (ionic) *on page 413*

Anatuss® [OTC] *see* guaifenesin, phenylpropanolamine, and dextromethorphan *on page 220*

Anbesol® Maximum Strength [OTC] *see* benzocaine *on page 48*

Ancef® *see* cefazolin sodium *on page 79*

Ancobon® *see* flucytosine *on page 198*

Andro-Cyp® Injection *see* testosterone *on page 456*

Andro/Fem® Injection *see* estradiol and testosterone *on page 178*

Androgyn L.A.® Injection *see* estradiol and testosterone *on page 178*

Android® *see* methyltestosterone *on page 307*

Andro® Injection *see* testosterone *on page 456*

Andro-L.A.® Injection *see* testosterone *on page 456*

Androlone®-D Injection *see* nandrolone *on page 324*

Androlone® Injection *see* nandrolone *on page 324*

Andronate® Injection *see* testosterone *on page 456*

Andropository® Injection *see* testosterone *on page 456*

Anectine® Chloride Injection *see* succinylcholine chloride *on page 445*

Anectine® Flo-Pack® *see* succinylcholine chloride *on page 445*

Anergan® Injection *see* promethazine hydrochloride *on page 399*

Anestacon® Topical Solution *see* lidocaine hydrochloride *on page 273*

aneurine hydrochloride *see* thiamine hydrochloride *on page 463*

Anexsia® *see* hydrocodone and acetaminophen *on page 234*

Angio Conray® *see* radiological/contrast media (ionic) *on page 413*

Angiovist® *see* radiological/contrast media (ionic) *on page 413*

Anhydron® *see* cyclothiazide *on page 123*

anisotropine methylbromide (an iss oh troe' peen)
Brand Names Valpin® 50
Therapeutic Category Anticholinergic Agent; Antispasmodic Agent, Gastrointestinal
Use Adjunctive treatment of peptic ulcer
Usual Dosage Adults: Oral: 50 mg 3 times/day
Dosage Forms Tablet: 50 mg

anisoylated plasminogen streptokinase activator complex *see* anistreplase
on this page

anistreplase (a niss' tre place)
Brand Names Eminase®
Synonyms anisoylated plasminogen streptokinase activator complex; APSAC
Therapeutic Category Thrombolytic Agent
Use Management of acute myocardial infarction (AMI) in adults; lysis of thrombi obstructing coronary arteries, reduction of infarct size; and reduction of mortality associated with AMI
Usual Dosage Adults: I.V.: 30 units injected over 2-5 minutes as soon as possible after onset of symptoms
Dosage Forms Powder for injection, lyophilized: 30 units

Anodynos-DHC® *see* hydrocodone and acetaminophen *on page 234*

Anoquan® *see* butalbital compound *on page 63*

Ansaid® Oral *see* flurbiprofen sodium *on page 204*

ansamycin *see* rifabutin *on page 420*

Answer® *see* diagnostic aids (*in vitro*), urine *on page 139*

Answer® Ovulation *see* diagnostic aids (*in vitro*), urine *on page 139*

Answer® Plus *see* diagnostic aids (*in vitro*), urine *on page 139*
Antabuse® *see* disulfiram *on page 156*
Antazoline-V® Ophthalmic *see* naphazoline and antazoline *on page 325*
Anthra-Derm® *see* anthralin *on this page*

anthralin (an' thra lin)
Brand Names Anthra-Derm®; Drithocreme®; Dritho-Scalp®; Lasan™
Synonyms dithranol
Therapeutic Category Antipsoriatic Agent, Topical; Keratolytic Agent
Use Treatment of psoriasis
Usual Dosage Adults: Topical: Apply in a thin film at bedtime
Dosage Forms
Cream: 0.1% (50 g, 65 g); 0.2% (65 g); 0.25% (50 g); 0.4% (65 g); 0.5% (50 g); 1% (50 g, 65 g)
Ointment, topical: 0.1% (42.5 g); 0.25% (42.5 g); 0.4% (60 g); 0.5% (42.5 g); 1% (42.5 g)

AntibiOtic® Otic *see* neomycin, polymyxin b, and hydrocortisone *on page 329*
antidigoxin fab fragments *see* digoxin immune fab (ovine) *on page 148*
antidiuretic hormone *see* vasopressin *on page 492*

antihemophilic factor (an tee hee moe fill' ik)
Brand Names Hemofil® M; Humate-P®; Kōate®-HP; Kōate®-HS; KoGENate®; Mono-clate-P®; Profilate® OSD
Synonyms AHF; factor viii
Therapeutic Category Antihemophilic Agent; Blood Product Derivative
Use Management of hemophilia A in patients whom a deficiency in factor VIII has been demonstrated
Usual Dosage I.V.: Individualize dosage based on coagulation studies performed prior to and during treatment at regular intervals. One AHF unit is the activity present in 1 mL of normal pooled human plasma; dosage should be adjusted to actual vial size currently stocked in the pharmacy.

Hospitalized patients: 20-50 units/kg/dose; may be higher for special circumstances; dose can be given every 12-24 hours and more frequently in special circumstances

Formula to approximate percentage increase in plasma antihemophilic factor:
Units required = desired level increase (desired level - actual level) x plasma volume (mL)
Total blood volume (mL blood/kg) = 70 mL/kg (adults); 80 mL/kg (children).
Plasma volume = total blood volume (mL) x [1 – Hct (in decimals)]
ie, for a 70 kg adult with a Hct = 40% : plasma volume = [70 kg x 70 mL/kg] x [1 – 0.4] = 2940 mL

To calculate number of units of factor VIII needed to increase level to desired range (highly individualized and dependent on patient's condition):
Number of units = desired level increase [desired level – actual level] x plasma volume (in mL)
ie, for a 100% level in the above patient who has an actual level of 20% the number of units needed = [1 (for a 100% level) – 0.2] x 2940 mL = 2352 units
Dosage Forms Injection: Single-dose vials with varied units; 10 mL, 20 mL, 30 mL

antihemophilic factor (porcine) *see* factor viii:c (porcine) *on page 189*

anti-inhibitor coagulant complex
Brand Names Autoplex T®; Feiba VH Immuno®
Therapeutic Category Hemophilic Agent
Use Patients with factor VIII inhibitors who are to undergo surgery or those who are bleeding
(Continued)
29

anti-inhibitor coagulant complex *(Continued)*
Usual Dosage Dosage range: 25-100 factor VIII correctional units per kg depending on the severity of hemorrhage
Dosage Forms Injection:
Autoplex T®, with heparin 2 units: Each bottle is labeled with correctional units of Factor VIII
Feiba VH Immuno®, heparin free: Each bottle is labeled with correctional units of Factor VIII

Antilirium® Injection *see* physostigmine *on page 376*
Antiminth® [OTC] *see* pyrantel pamoate *on page 407*

antipyrine and benzocaine (an tee pye' reen & ben' zoe kane)
Brand Names Allergan® Ear Drops; Auralgan®; Auroto®; Otocalm® Ear
Synonyms benzocaine and antipyrine
Therapeutic Category Otic Agent, Analgesic; Otic Agent, Cerumenolytic
Use Temporary relief of pain and reduction of inflammation associated with acute congestive and serous otitis media, swimmer's ear, otitis externa; facilitates ear wax removal
Usual Dosage Otic: Fill ear canal; moisten cotton pledget, place in external ear, repeat every 1-2 hours until pain and congestion is relieved; for ear wax removal instill drops 3-4 times/day for 2-3 days
Dosage Forms Solution, otic: Antipyrine 5.4% and benzocaine 1.4% (10 mL, 15 mL)

antirabies serum, equine origin
Synonyms ARS
Therapeutic Category Serum
Use Rabies prophylaxis
Usual Dosage I.M.: 1000 units/55 lb in a single dose, infiltrate up to 50% of dose around the wound
Dosage Forms Injection: 125 units/mL (8 mL)

Antispas® Injection *see* dicyclomine hydrochloride *on page 145*

antithrombin III
Brand Names ATnativ®; Thrombate® III
Therapeutic Category Blood Product Derivative
Use Agent for hereditary antithrombin III deficiency
Usual Dosage After first dose of antithrombin III, level should increase to 120% of normal; thereafter maintain at levels >80%. Generally, achieved by administration of maintenance doses once every 24 hours; initially and until patient is stabilized, measure antithrombin III level at least twice daily, thereafter once daily and always immediately before next infusion.

Initial dosage (units) = [desired AT-III level % - baseline AT-III level %] x body weight (kg) divided by 1%/units/kg

Measure antithrombin III preceding and 30 minutes after dose to calculate *in vivo* recovery rate; maintain level within normal range for 2-8 days depending on type of surgery or procedure
Dosage Forms Powder for injection: 500 units (50 mL)

Anti-Tuss® Expectorant [OTC] *see* guaifenesin *on page 217*

antivenin, black widow spider (equine)
Synonyms black widow spider species antivenin *Latrodectus mactans*
Therapeutic Category Antivenin
Use Treat patients with symptoms of black widow spider bites

Usual Dosage

Children <12 years (severe or shock): I.V.: 2.5 mL in 10-50 mL over 15 minutes

Children and Adults: I.M.: 2.5 mL

Dosage Forms Powder for injection: 6000 antivenin units (2.5 mL)

antivenin (crotalidae) polyvalent (kroe tal' ih day)

Synonyms crotaline antivenin, polyvalent; north and south american antisnake-bite serum; snake (pit vipers) antivenin

Therapeutic Category Antivenin

Use Neutralization of the venoms of North and South America Crotalids: rattlesnake, copperhead, cottonmouth, tropical moccasins, fer-de-lance, bushmaster

Usual Dosage Initial intradermal sensitivity test. The entire initial dose of antivenin should be administered as soon as possible to be most effective (within 4 hours after the bite).

Children and Adults: I.V.: Minimal envenomation: 20-40 mL; moderate envenomation: 50-90 mL; severe envenomation: 100-150 mL

Additional doses of antivenin is based on clinical response to the initial dose. If swelling continues to progress, symptoms increase in severity, hypotension occurs, or decrease in hematocrit appears, an additional 10-50 mL should be administered.

For I.V. infusion: 1:1-1:10 dilution of reconstituted antivenin in normal saline or D₅W should be prepared. Infuse the initial 5-10 mL of diluted antivenin over 3-5 minutes monitoring closely for signs of sensitivity reactions.

Dosage Forms Injection: Lyophilized serum, diluent (10 mL); one vacuum vial to yield 10 mL of serum

antivenin (*Micrurus fulvius*)

Synonyms north american coral snake antivenin

Therapeutic Category Antivenin

Use Neutralize the venom of Eastern coral snake and Texas coral snake but not neutralize venom of Arizona or Sonoran coral snake

Usual Dosage I.V.: 3-5 vials by slow injection

Dosage Forms Injection: One vial antivenin and one vial diluent

Antivert® *see* meclizine hydrochloride *on page 288*

Antrizine® *see* meclizine hydrochloride *on page 288*

Anturane® *see* sulfinpyrazone *on page 449*

Anusol® HC-1 Topical [OTC] *see* hydrocortisone *on page 236*

Anusol® HC-2.5% Topical [OTC] *see* hydrocortisone *on page 236*

Anxanil® Oral *see* hydroxyzine *on page 241*

Apacet® [OTC] *see* acetaminophen *on page 2*

APAP *see* acetaminophen *on page 2*

Apatate® [OTC] *see* vitamin B complex *on page 498*

Aphrodyne™ *see* yohimbine hydrochloride *on page 502*

A.P.L.® *see* chorionic gonadotropin *on page 101*

Aplisol® *see* tuberculin tests *on page 484*

APPG *see* penicillin g procaine, aqueous *on page 362*

apraclonidine hydrochloride (a pra kloe' ni deen)

Brand Names Alpidine®; Iopidine®

Therapeutic Category Alpha-2-Adrenergic Agonist Agent, Ophthalmic

Use Prevention and treatment of postsurgical intraocular pressure elevation

Usual Dosage Ophthalmic: Instill 1 drop in operative eye 1 hour prior to laser surgery, second drop in eye upon completion of procedure

Dosage Forms Solution: 1% with benzalkonium chloride 0.01% (0.25 mL)

Apresazide® *see* hydralazine and hydrochlorothiazide *on page 232*

Apresoline® Injection *see* hydralazine hydrochloride *on page 232*

Apresoline® Oral *see* hydralazine hydrochloride *on page 232*

Aprodine® [OTC] *see* triprolidine and pseudoephedrine *on page 482*

Aprodine® w/C *see* triprolidine, pseudoephedrine, and codeine *on page 482*

APSAC *see* anistreplase *on page 28*

Aquacare® Topical [OTC] *see* urea *on page 487*

Aquachloral® Supprettes® *see* chloral hydrate *on page 87*

AquaMEPHYTON® Injection *see* phytonadione *on page 376*

Aquaphor® Antibiotic Topical [OTC] *see* bacitracin and polymyxin b *on page 42*

Aquaphyllin® *see* theophylline *on page 460*

Aquasol A® Injection *see* vitamin A *on page 496*

Aquasol A® Oral [OTC] *see* vitamin A *on page 496*

Aquasol E® Oral [OTC] *see* vitamin E *on page 498*

Aquatag® *see* benzthiazide *on page 50*

AquaTar® [OTC] *see* coal tar *on page 110*

Aquatensen® *see* methyclothiazide *on page 303*

Aquazide-H® *see* hydrochlorothiazide *on page 233*

aqueous procaine penicillin g *see* penicillin g procaine, aqueous *on page 362*

aqueous testosterone *see* testosterone *on page 456*

Ara-A *see* vidarabine *on page 495*

arabinosylcytosine *see* cytarabine hydrochloride *on page 123*

Ara-C *see* cytarabine hydrochloride *on page 123*

Aralen® Phosphate *see* chloroquine phosphate *on page 91*

Aralen® Phosphate With Primaquine Phosphate *see* chloroquine and primaquine *on page 91*

Aramine® *see* metaraminol bitartrate *on page 297*

Arcet® *see* butalbital compound *on page 63*

Arduan® *see* pipecuronium bromide *on page 378*

Aredia™ *see* pamidronate disodium *on page 353*

Arfonad® Injection *see* trimethaphan camsylate *on page 480*

Argesic®-SA *see* salsalate *on page 425*

arginine hydrochloride (ar' ji neen)
Brand Names R-Gene® 10
Therapeutic Category Metabolic Alkalosis Agent
Use Pituitary function test (growth hormone); management of severe, uncompensated, metabolic alkalosis (pH ≥7.55) **after** optimizing therapy with Na⁺ and K⁺ supplements
Usual Dosage I.V.:
Growth hormone reserve test:
Children: 500 mg/kg over 30 minutes
Adults: 300 mL

Note: Arginine hydrochloride should never be used as an alternative to chloride supplementation but used in the patient who is unresponsive to sodium chloride or potassium chloride supplementation.

Metabolic alkalosis: Children and Adults:
Acid required (mEq) =

[0.2 (L/kg) x wt (kg)] x [103 - serum <1⁻] mEq/L **or**
0.3 (L/kg) x wt (kg) x base excess (mEq/L) **or**
0.5 (L/kg) x wt (kg) x [serum HCO_3 - 24] mEq/L
Give $\frac{1}{2}$ to $\frac{2}{3}$ of calculated dose and re-evaluate

Children: 500 mg/kg/dose administered over 30 minutes

Adults: 30 g administered at a constant rate over 30 minutes
Dosage Forms Injection: 10% [100 mg/mL = 950 mOsm/L] (500 mL)

8-arginine vasopressin *see* vasopressin *on page 492*

Argyrol® S.S. 10% [OTC] *see* silver protein, mild *on page 431*

Aristocort® A Topical *see* triamcinolone *on page 474*

Aristocort® Forte Injection *see* triamcinolone *on page 474*

Aristocort® Intralesional Injection *see* triamcinolone *on page 474*

Aristocort® Oral *see* triamcinolone *on page 474*

Aristocort® Topical *see* triamcinolone *on page 474*

Aristospan® Intra-articular Injection *see* triamcinolone *on page 474*

Aristospan® Intralesional Injection *see* triamcinolone *on page 474*

Arlidin® *see* nylidrin hydrochloride *on page 341*

Arm-a-Med® Isoetharine Inhalation Solution *see* isoetharine *on page 257*

Arm-a-Med® Isoproterenol Inhalation Solution *see* isoproterenol *on page 258*

Arm-a-Med® Metaproterenol Inhalation Solution *see* metaproterenol sulfate *on page 296*

Armour® Thyroid *see* thyroid *on page 466*

Aromatic Ammonia Aspirols® *see* ammonia spirit, aromatic *on page 22*

Arrestin® Injection *see* trimethobenzamide hydrochloride *on page 480*

ARS *see* antirabies serum, equine origin *on page 30*

Artane® *see* trihexyphenidyl hydrochloride *on page 478*

Artha-G® *see* salsalate *on page 425*

Arthropan® [OTC] *see* choline salicylate *on page 100*

Articulose-50® Injection *see* prednisolone *on page 391*

Articulose L.A.® Injection *see* triamcinolone *on page 474*

artificial tears
Brand Names Isopto® Plain [OTC]; Isopto® Tears [OTC]; Tearisol® [OTC]
Synonyms polyvinyl alcohol
Therapeutic Category Ophthalmic Agent, Miscellaneous
Use Ophthalmic lubricant; for relief of dry eyes and eye irritation
Usual Dosage Ophthalmic: Use as needed to relieve symptoms, 1-2 drops into eye(s) 3-4 times/day
Dosage Forms Solution: 15 mL with dropper

ASA *see* aspirin *on next page*

A.S.A. [OTC] *see* aspirin *on next page*

5-ASA *see* mesalamine *on page 294*

Asacol® Oral *see* mesalamine *on page 294*

ascorbic acid *(a skor' bik)*
Brand Names Ascorbicap® [OTC]; C-Crystals® [OTC]; Cecon® [OTC]; Cetane® [OTC]; Cevalin® [OTC]; Ce-Vi-Sol® [OTC]; Dull-C® [OTC]; Flavorcee® [OTC]; Vita-C® [OTC]
Synonyms vitamin C
(Continued)

ascorbic acid *(Continued)*
Therapeutic Category Urinary Acidifying Agent; Vitamin, Water Soluble
Use Prevention and treatment of scurvy; urinary acidification; dietary supplementation; prevention and decreasing the severity of colds
Usual Dosage Oral, I.M., I.V., S.C.:

Children:
Scurvy: 100-300 mg/day in divided doses for at least 2 weeks
Urinary acidification: 500 mg every 6-8 hours
Dietary supplement: 35-45 mg

Adults:
Scurvy: 500-1000 mg for at least 2 weeks
Urinary acidification: 4-12 g/day in 3-4 divided doses
Dietary supplement: 50-60 mg/day
Prevention and treatment of cold: 1-3 g/day

Dosage Forms
Capsule, timed release: 500 mg
Crystals: 4 g/teaspoonful (100 g, 500 g); 5 g/teaspoonful (180 g)
Injection: 250 mg/mL (2 mL, 30 mL); 500 mg/mL (2 mL, 50 mL)
Liquid, oral: 35 mg/0.6 mL (50 mL)
Lozenges: 60 mg
Powder: 4 g/teaspoonful (100 g, 500 g)
Solution, oral: 100 mg/mL (50 mL)
Syrup: 500 mg/5 mL (5 mL, 10 mL, 120 mL, 480 mL)
Tablet: 25 mg, 50 mg, 100 mg, 250 mg, 500 mg, 1000 mg
Tablet:
Chewable: 100 mg, 250 mg, 500 mg
Timed release: 500 mg, 1000 mg, 1500 mg

ascorbic acid and ferrous sulfate *see* ferrous sulfate and ascorbic acid *on page 194*

Ascorbicap® [OTC] *see* ascorbic acid *on previous page*

Ascriptin® [OTC] *see* aspirin *on this page*

Asendin® *see* amoxapine *on page 23*

Asmalix® *see* theophylline *on page 460*

ASN-ase *see* asparaginase *on this page*

asparaginase (a spare' a ji nase)
Brand Names Elspar®
Synonyms A-ase; ASN-ase; colaspase
Therapeutic Category Antineoplastic Agent, Miscellaneous
Use Treatment of acute lymphocytic leukemia, lymphoma
Usual Dosage Refer to individual protocols; the manufacturer recommends performing intradermal sensitivity testing before the initial dose

Children and Adults:
I.M. (preferred route): 6000 units/m^2 3 times/week for 3 weeks for combination therapy
I.V.: 1000 units/kg/day for 10 days for combination therapy or 200 units/kg/day for 28 days if combination therapy is inappropriate
Dosage Forms Injection: 10,000 unit vial

Aspergum® [OTC] *see* aspirin *on this page*

aspirin (as' pir in)
Brand Names Anacin® [OTC]; A.S.A. [OTC]; Ascriptin® [OTC]; Aspergum® [OTC]; Bayer® Aspirin [OTC]; Bufferin® [OTC]; Easprin®; Ecotrin® [OTC]; Empirin® [OTC]; Gensan® [OTC]; Measurin® [OTC]; Synalgos® [OTC]; ZORprin®

Synonyms acetylsalicylic acid; ASA

Therapeutic Category Analgesic, Non-Narcotic; Anti-inflammatory Agent; Antiplatelet Agent; Antipyretic; Nonsteroidal Anti-Inflammatory Agent (NSAID), Oral; Salicylate

Use Treatment of mild to moderate pain, inflammation and fever; may be used as a prophylaxis of myocardial infarction and transient ischemic attacks (TIA)

Usual Dosage

Children:

Analgesic and antipyretic: Oral, rectal: 10-15 mg/kg/dose every 4-6 hours

Anti-inflammatory: Oral: Initial: 60-90 mg/kg/day in divided doses; usual maintenance: 80-100 mg/kg/day divided every 6-8 hours; monitor serum concentrations

Kawasaki disease: Oral: 100 mg/kg/day divided every 6 hours; after fever resolves: 8-10 mg/kg/day once daily; monitor serum concentrations

Adults:

Analgesic and antipyretic: Oral, rectal: 325-1000 mg every 4-6 hours up to 4 g/day

Anti-inflammatory: Oral: Initial: 2.4-3.6 g/day in divided doses; usual maintenance: 3.6-5.4 g/day; monitor serum concentrations

Transient ischemic attack: Oral: 1.3 g/day in 2-4 divided doses

Myocardial infarction prophylaxis: 160-325 mg/day

Dosage Forms

Capsule: 356.4 mg and caffeine 30 mg

Suppository, rectal: 60 mg, 120 mg, 125 mg, 130 mg, 195 mg, 200 mg, 300 mg, 325 mg, 600 mg, 650 mg, 1.2 g

Tablet: 65 mg, 75 mg, 81 mg, 325 mg, 500 mg

Tablet: 400 mg and caffeine 32 mg

Tablet:

Buffered: 325 mg and magnesium-aluminum hydroxide 150 mg; 325 mg, magnesium hydroxide 75 mg, aluminum hydroxide 75 mg, buffered with calcium carbonate; 325 mg and magnesium-aluminum hydroxide 75 mg

Chewable, children's: 81 mg

Controlled release: 800 mg

Enteric coated: 325 mg, 500 mg, 650 mg, 975 mg

Gum: 227.5 mg

Timed release: 650 mg

aspirin and codeine

Brand Names Empirin® With Codeine

Synonyms codeine and aspirin

Therapeutic Category Analgesic, Narcotic

Use Relief of mild to moderate pain

Usual Dosage Oral:

Children:

Aspirin: 10 mg/kg/dose every 4 hours

Codeine: 0.5-1 mg/kg/dose every 4 hours

Adults: 1-2 tablets every 4-6 hours as needed for pain

Dosage Forms Tablet:

#2: Aspirin 325 mg and codeine phosphate 15 mg

#3: Aspirin 325 mg and codeine phosphate 30 mg

#4: Aspirin 325 mg and codeine phosphate 60 mg

aspirin and meprobamate

Brand Names Equagesic®

Synonyms meprobamate and aspirin

Therapeutic Category Skeletal Muscle Relaxant, Long Acting

Use Adjunct to treatment of skeletal muscular disease in patients exhibiting tension and/or anxiety

Usual Dosage Oral: 1 tablet 3-4 times/day

Dosage Forms Tablet: Aspirin 325 mg and meprobamate 200 mg

aspirin and pentazocine see pentazocine compound on page 364

astemizole (a stem' mi zole)
Brand Names Hismanal®
Therapeutic Category Antihistamine
Use Perennial and seasonal allergic rhinitis and other allergic symptoms including urticaria
Usual Dosage Oral:
Children:
<6 years: 0.2 mg/kg/day
6-12 years: 5 mg/day

Children >12 years and Adults: 10-30 mg/day; give 30 mg on first day, 20 mg on second day, then 10 mg/day in a single dose
Dosage Forms Tablet: 10 mg

AsthmaHaler® Inhalation Aerosol see epinephrine on page 171
AsthmaNefrin® Inhalation Solution [OTC] see epinephrine on page 171
Astramorph™ PF Injection see morphine sulfate on page 318
Atabrine® see quinacrine hydrochloride on page 410
Atarax® Oral see hydroxyzine on page 241

atenolol (a ten' oh lole)
Brand Names Tenormin®
Therapeutic Category Antianginal Agent; Beta-Adrenergic Blocker
Use Treatment of hypertension, alone or in combination with other agents; also used in management of angina pectoris; selective inhibitor of beta$_1$-adrenergic receptors; post myocardial infarction patients; acute alcohol withdrawal
Usual Dosage
Oral:
Children: 1-2 mg/kg/dose given daily
Adults: 50-100 mg/dose given daily

I.V.: Adults: For early treatment of myocardial infarction: 5 mg slow I.V. over 5 minutes; may repeat in 10 minutes; if both doses are tolerated, may start oral atenolol 50 mg every 12 hours;

Postmyocardial infarction:
Oral: Follow with 100 mg/day or 50 mg twice daily for 6-9 days postmyocardial infarction
I.V.: Administer as soon as possible 5 mg over 5 minutes; follow with 5 mg I.V. 10 minutes later
Dosage Forms
Injection: 0.5 mg/mL (10 mL)
Tablet: 25 mg, 50 mg, 100 mg

atenolol and chlorthalidone
Brand Names Tenoretic®
Therapeutic Category Antihypertensive, Combination
Use Treatment of hypertension with a cardioselective beta blocker and a diuretic
Usual Dosage Adults: Oral: Initial: One (50) tablet once daily, then individualize dose until optimal dose is achieved
Dosage Forms Tablet:
50: Atenolol 50 mg and chlorthalidone 25 mg
100: Atenolol 100 mg and chlorthalidone 25 mg

ATG *see* lymphocyte immune globulin, anti-thymocyte globulin (equine) *on page 280*

Atgam® *see* lymphocyte immune globulin, anti-thymocyte globulin (equine) *on page 280*

Ativan® *see* lorazepam *on page 278*

ATnativ® *see* antithrombin III *on page 30*

Atolone® Oral *see* triamcinolone *on page 474*

atovaquone (a toe' va kwone)
Brand Names Mepron®
Therapeutic Category Antiprotozoal
Use Acute oral treatment of mild to moderate *Pneumocystis carinii* pneumonia (PCP) in patients who are intolerant to co-trimoxazole
Usual Dosage Adults: Oral: 750 mg 3 times/day with food for 21 days
Dosage Forms Tablet, film coated: 250 mg

Atozine® Oral *see* hydroxyzine *on page 241*

atracurium besylate (a tra kyoo' ree um)
Brand Names Tracrium®
Therapeutic Category Neuromuscular Blocker Agent, Nondepolarizing; Skeletal Muscle Relaxant
Use Ease endotracheal intubation as an adjunct to general anesthesia and to relax skeletal muscle during surgery or mechanical ventilation; does not appear to have a cumulative effect on the duration of blockade; does not relieve pain
Usual Dosage I.V.:
Children 1 month to 2 years: 0.3-0.4 mg/kg initially followed by maintenance doses of 0.08-0.1 mg/kg as needed to maintain neuromuscular blockade

Children >2 years to Adults: 0.4-0.5 mg/kg then 0.08-0.1 mg/kg every 20-45 minutes after initial dose to maintain neuromuscular block

Continuous infusion: 0.4-0.8 mg/kg/hour
Dosage Forms Injection: 10 mg/mL (5 mL, 10 mL)

Atromid-S® *see* clofibrate *on page 107*

atropine and diphenoxylate *see* diphenoxylate and atropine *on page 153*

Atropine-Care® Ophthalmic *see* atropine sulfate *on this page*

atropine sulfate (a' troe peen)
Brand Names Atropine-Care® Ophthalmic; Atropisol® Ophthalmic; Isopto® Atropine Ophthalmic; I-Tropine® Ophthalmic
Therapeutic Category Anticholinergic Agent; Anticholinergic Agent, Ophthalmic; Antidote, Organophosphate Poisoning; Antispasmodic Agent, Gastrointestinal; Bronchodilator; Ophthalmic Agent, Mydriatic
Use Preoperative medication to inhibit salivation and secretions; treatment of sinus bradycardia; management of peptic ulcer; treat exercise-induced bronchospasm; antidote for organophosphate pesticide poisoning; used to produce mydriasis and cycloplegia for examination of the retina and optic disk and accurate measurement of refractive errors; uveitis
Usual Dosage
Preanesthesia: I.M., I.V., S.C.:
Infants:
<5 kg: 0.04 mg/kg/dose repeated every 4-6 hours as needed
(Continued)

37

atropine sulfate *(Continued)*

>5 kg: 0.03 mg/kg/dose repeated every 4-6 hours as needed
Children: 0.01 mg/kg/dose up to a maximum of 0.4 mg/dose; repeat every 4-6 hours as needed
Adults: 0.5 mg/dose repeated every 4-6 hours as needed

Bronchodilation:
Children:
Oral: 0.02 mg/kg/dose 3 times/day
Inhalation: 0.03-0.05 mg/kg/dose 3-4 times/day
Adults: Inhalation: 0.025-0.05 mg/kg/dose over 10 minutes, repeated every 4-5 hours as needed

Cardiopulmonary resuscitation (bradycardia): I.T., I.V.:
Infants: 0.02-0.04 mg/kg/dose; repeat every 2-5 minutes, if needed, up to 2-3 times
Children: 0.01-0.02 mg/kg/dose; repeat every 2-5 minutes, if needed, up to 2-3 times; minimum dose should be 0.1 mg (smaller doses may cause paradoxic bradycardia); maximum total dose is 1 mg (2 mg for adolescents)
Adults: 0.5 mg/dose; repeat every 5 minutes, if needed, up to 2-3 times for a maximum total dose of 2 mg

Organophosphate or carbamate poisoning: I.V.:
Children: 0.02-0.05 mg/kg/dose every 10-20 minutes until atropine effect (dry flushed skin, tachycardia, mydriasis, fever) is observed, then every 1-4 hours to maintain atropine effect for at least 24 hours
Children >12 years and Adults: 1-2 mg/dose every 10-20 minutes until atropine effect (see above) is observed, then 1-3 mg/dose every 1-4 hours, as needed to maintain atropine effect for at least 24 hours

Neuromuscular blockade reversal: I.V.:
Before neostigmine: Give 25-30 μg/kg (0.025-0.03 mg/kg) 30 seconds before neostigmine (0.07-0.08 mg/kg)
Before edrophonium: 10 μg/kg (0.01 mg/kg) 30 seconds before edrophonium (1 mg/kg)
Note: May contain benzyl alcohol as a preservative; administration of benzyl alcohol in doses ranging from 99-234 mg/kg has been associated with a fatal gasping syndrome in neonates; clinical signs of this syndrome include metabolic acidosis, hypotension, CNS depression, and cardiovascular collapse

Dosage Forms
Injection: 0.05 mg/mL (5 mL); 0.1 mg/mL (5 mL, 10 mL); 0.3 mg/mL (1 mL, 30 mL); 0.4 mg/mL (1 mL, 20 mL, 30 mL); 0.5 mg/mL (1 mL, 5 mL, 30 mL); 0.8 mg/mL (0.5 mL, 1 mL); 1 mg/mL (1 mL, 10 mL)
Ointment, ophthalmic: 0.5% (3.5 g); 1% (3.5 g)
Solution, ophthalmic: 0.5% (1 mL, 5 mL); 1% (1 mL, 2 mL, 5 mL, 15 mL); 2% (1 mL, 2 mL); 3% (5 mL)
Tablet: 0.4 mg
Tablet, soluble: 0.4 mg, 0.6 mg

Atropisol® Ophthalmic *see* atropine sulfate *on previous page*

Atrovent® Aerosol Inhalation *see* ipratropium bromide *on page 255*

A/T/S® Topical *see* erythromycin, topical *on page 176*

attapulgite *(at a pull' gite)*

Brand Names Children's Kaopectate® [OTC]; Diar-Aid® [OTC]; Diasorb® [OTC]; Kaopectate® Advanced Formula [OTC]; Kaopectate® Maximum Strength Caplets; Rheaban® [OTC]
Therapeutic Category Antidiarrheal
Use Symptomatic treatment of diarrhea
Usual Dosage Oral:
Children:
<3 years: Not recommended

3-6 years: 750 mg/dose up to 2250 mg/24 hours

6-12 years: 1200-1500 mg/dose up to 4500 mg/24 hours

Adults: 1200-1500 mg after each loose bowel movement or every 2 hours; 15-30 mL up to 8 times/day, up to 9000 mg/24 hours

Dosage Forms

Liquid, oral concentrate: 600 mg/15 mL (180 mL, 240 mL, 360 mL, 480 mL); 750 mg/15 mL (120 mL)

Tablet: 750 mg

Tablet, chewable: 300 mg, 600 mg

Attenuvax® *see* measles virus vaccine, live, attenuated *on page 287*

Augmentin® *see* amoxicillin and clavulanic acid *on page 24*

Auralgan® *see* antipyrine and benzocaine *on page 30*

auranofin (au rane' oh fin)
Brand Names Ridaura®

Therapeutic Category Gold Compound

Use Management of active stage of classic or definite rheumatoid arthritis in patients that do not respond to or tolerate other agents; psoriatic arthritis

Usual Dosage Oral:

Children: Initial: 0.1 mg/kg/day divided daily; usual maintenance: 0.15 mg/kg/day in 1-2 divided doses; maximum: 0.2 mg/kg/day in 1-2 divided doses

Adults: 6 mg/day in 1-2 divided doses; after 3 months may be increased to 9 mg/day in 3 divided doses; if still no response after 3 months at 9 mg/day, discontinue drug

Dosage Forms Capsule: 3 mg [gold 29%]

Aureomycin® *see* chlortetracycline hydrochloride *on page 98*

Auro® Ear Drops [OTC] *see* carbamide peroxide *on page 73*

aurothioglucose (aur oh thye oh gloo' kose)
Brand Names Solganal®

Therapeutic Category Gold Compound

Use Adjunctive treatment in adult and juvenile active rheumatoid arthritis; alternative or adjunct in treatment of pemphigus; for psoriatic patients who do not respond to NSAIDs

Usual Dosage I.M. (doses should initially be given at weekly intervals):

Children 6-12 years: Initial: 0.25 mg/kg/dose first week; increment at 0.25 mg/kg/dose increasing with each weekly dose; maintenance: 0.75-1 mg/kg/dose weekly not to exceed 25 mg/dose to a total of 20 doses, then every 2-4 weeks

Adults: 10 mg first week; 25 mg second and third week; then 50 mg/week until 800 mg to 1 g cumulative dose has been given – if improvement occurs without adverse reactions, give 25-50 mg every 2-3 weeks, then every 3-4 weeks

Dosage Forms Suspension, sterile: 50 mg/mL [gold 50%] (10 mL)

Auroto® *see* antipyrine and benzocaine *on page 30*

Autoplex T® *see* anti-inhibitor coagulant complex *on page 29*

AVC™ Vaginal Cream *see* sulfanilamide *on page 448*

AVC™ Vaginal Suppository *see* sulfanilamide *on page 448*

Aveeno® Cleansing Bar [OTC] *see* sulfur and salicylic acid *on page 450*

Aventyl® Hydrochloride *see* nortriptyline hydrochloride *on page 340*

Avitene® *see* microfibrillar collagen hemostat *on page 312*

Axid® *see* nizatidine *on page 337*

Axotal® *see* butalbital compound *on page 63*

Aygestin® *see* norethindrone *on page 338*

Ayr® Nasal [OTC] *see* sodium chloride *on page 434*

azacitidine (ay za sye' ti deen)
Brand Names Mylosar®
Synonyms AZA-CR; 5-azacytidine; 5-AZC; ladakamycin; NSC-102816
Therapeutic Category Antineoplastic Agent, Miscellaneous
Use Refractory acute lymphocytic and myelogenous leukemia
Usual Dosage Refer to individual protocols
Children and Adults: I.V.: 200-300 mg/m^2/day for 5-10 days, repeated at 2- to 3-week intervals
Dosage Forms Injection: 100 mg

AZA-CR *see* azacitidine *on this page*

Azactam® *see* aztreonam *on next page*

5-azacytidine *see* azacitidine *on this page*

azatadine and pseudoephedrine
Brand Names Trinalin®
Synonyms pseudoephedrine and azatadine
Therapeutic Category Antihistamine/Decongestant Combination
Use Perennial and seasonal allergic rhinitis and other allergic symptoms including urticaria
Usual Dosage Adults: Oral: 1-2 mg twice daily
Dosage Forms Tablet: Azatadine maleate 1 mg and pseudoephedrine sulfate 120 mg

azatadine maleate (a za' ta deen)
Brand Names Optimine®
Therapeutic Category Antihistamine
Use Treatment of perennial and seasonal allergic rhinitis and chronic urticaria
Usual Dosage Children >12 years and Adults: Oral: 1-2 mg twice daily
Dosage Forms Tablet: 1 mg

azathioprine (ay za thye' oh preen)
Brand Names Imuran®
Therapeutic Category Immunosuppressant Agent
Use Adjunct with other agents in prevention of rejection of renal transplants; also used in severe rheumatoid arthritis unresponsive to other agents
Usual Dosage Refer to individual protocols
Children and Adults: Renal transplantation: Oral, I.V.: Initial: 3-5 mg/kg/day; maintenance: 1-3 mg/kg/day

Adults: Rheumatoid arthritis: Oral: 1 mg/kg/day for 6-8 weeks; increase by 0.5 mg/kg every 4 weeks until response or up to 2.5 mg/kg/day I.V. dose is equivalent to oral dose
Dosage Forms
Injection, as sodium: 100 mg (20 mL)
Tablet: 50 mg

5-AZC *see* azacitidine *on this page*

Azdone® *see* hydrocodone and aspirin *on page 234*

azidothymidine *see* zidovudine *on page 503*

azithromycin dihydrate (az ith roe mye' sin)
Brand Names Zithromax™
Therapeutic Category Antibiotic, Macrolide
Use Treatment of adult patients (>16 years of age) with mild to moderate infections of susceptible strains in upper and lower respiratory tract, skin and skin structure, and sexually transmitted diseases
Usual Dosage Adults: Oral: 500 mg as a single dose on day 1 followed by 250 mg daily on days 2-5 (1.5 g total); the recommended dose for nongonococcal urethritis and cervicitis due to *C. trachomatis* is a single 1 g dose
Dosage Forms Capsule: 250 mg

Azmacort™ Oral Inhaler *see* triamcinolone *on page 474*

Azo Gantanol® *see* sulfamethoxazole and phenazopyridine *on page 448*

Azo Gantrisin® *see* sulfisoxazole and phenazopyridine *on page 449*

Azolid® *see* phenylbutazone *on page 371*

Azo-Standard® *see* phenazopyridine hydrochloride *on page 368*

Azostix® [OTC] *see* diagnostic aids (*in vitro*), blood *on page 137*

AZT *see* zidovudine *on page 503*

azthreonam *see* aztreonam *on this page*

aztreonam (az' tree oh nam)
Brand Names Azactam®
Synonyms azthreonam
Therapeutic Category Antibiotic, Miscellaneous
Use Treatment of patients with documented multidrug resistant aerobic gram-negative infection in which beta-lactam therapy is contraindicated; used for urinary tract infection, lower respiratory tract infections, septicemia, skin/skin structure infections, intraabdominal infections, and gynecological infections
Usual Dosage
Neonates: I.M., I.V.:
Postnatal age <7 days:
<2000 g: 60 mg/kg/day in 2 divided doses every 12 hours
>2000 g: 90 mg/kg/day in 3 divided doses every 8 hours
Postnatal age >7 days:
<2000 g: 90 mg/kg/day in 3 divided doses every 8 hours
>2000 g: 120 mg/kg/day in 4 divided doses every 6 hours

Children >1 month: I.M., I.V.: 90-120 mg/kg/day divided every 6-8 hours
Cystic fibrosis: 50 mg/kg/dose every 6-8 hours (ie, up to 200 mg/kg/day); maximum: 6-8 g/day

Adults:
Urinary tract infection: I.M., I.V.: 500 mg to 1 g every 8-12 hours
Moderately severe systemic infections: 1 g I.V. or I.M. or 2 g I.V. every 8-12 hours
Severe systemic or life-threatening infections (especially caused by *Pseudomonas aeruginosa*): I.V.: 2 g every 6-8 hours; maximum: 8 g/day
Dosage Forms Powder for injection: 500 mg (15 mL, 100 mL); 1 g (15 mL, 100 mL); 2 g (15 mL, 100 mL)

Azulfidine® *see* sulfasalazine *on page 448*

Azulfidine® EN-tabs® *see* sulfasalazine *on page 448*

Babee® Teething Lotion [OTC] *see* benzocaine *on page 48*

BAC *see* benzalkonium chloride *on page 47*

B-A-C® *see* butalbital compound *on page 63*

bacampicillin hydrochloride (ba kam pi sill' in)
Brand Names Spectrobid®
Synonyms carampicillin hydrochloride
Therapeutic Category Antibiotic, Penicillin
Use Treatment of susceptible bacterial infections involving the urinary tract, skin structure, upper and lower respiratory tract; activity is identical to that of ampicillin
Usual Dosage Oral:
  Children: 25-50 mg/kg/day in divided doses every 12 hours
  Adults: 400-800 mg every 12 hours
Dosage Forms
  Powder for oral suspension: 125 mg/5 mL [chemically equivalent to ampicillin 87.5 mg per 5 mL] (70 mL)
  Tablet: 400 mg [chemically equivalent to ampicillin 280 mg]

Bacid® [OTC] *see* lactobacillus *on page 267*

Baciguent® Topical [OTC] *see* bacitracin *on this page*

Baci-IM® Injection *see* bacitracin *on this page*

bacillus calmette-guérin *see* BCG *on page 44*

bacitracin (bass i tray' sin)
Brand Names AK-Tracin® Ophthalmic; Baciguent® Topical [OTC]; Baci-IM® Injection
Therapeutic Category Antibiotic, Miscellaneous; Antibiotic, Ophthalmic; Antibiotic, Topical
Use Treatment of susceptible bacterial infections; due to toxicity risks, systemic and irrigant uses of bacitracin should be limited to situations where less toxic alternatives would not be effective
Usual Dosage I.M. recommended; **do not administer I.V.**:
  Infants:
    <2.5 kg: 900 units/kg/day in 2-3 divided doses
    >2.5 kg = 1000 units/kg/day in 2-3 divided doses
  Children: 800-1200 units/kg/day divided every 8 hours
  Adults: 10,000-25,000 units/dose every 6 hours; not to exceed 100,000 units/day

  Topical: Apply 1-5 times/day

  Ophthalmic ointment: $1/4$" to $1/2$" ribbon every 3-4 hours to conjunctival sac for acute infections or 2-3 times/day for mild to moderate infections for 7-10 days

  Irrigation, solution: 50-100 units/mL in normal saline, lactated Ringer's, or sterile water for irrigation; soak sponges in solution for topical compresses 1-5 times/day or as needed during surgical procedures
Dosage Forms
  Injection: 50,000 units
  Ointment:
    Ophthalmic: 500 units/g (1 g, 3.5 g, 454 g)
    Topical: 500 units/g (1.5 g, 3.75 g, 15 g, 30 g, 120 g, 454 g)

bacitracin and polymyxin b
Brand Names AK-Poly-Bac® Ophthalmic; Aquaphor® Antibiotic Topical [OTC]; Polysporin® Ophthalmic; Polysporin® Topical
Therapeutic Category Antibiotic, Ophthalmic; Antibiotic, Topical
Use Treatment of superficial infections caused by susceptible organisms
Usual Dosage
  Ophthalmic: Apply $1/2$" ribbon to the affected eye(s) every 3-4 hours
  Topical: Apply to affected area 1-3 times/day; may cover with sterile bandage if needed
Dosage Forms
  Ointment:
    Ophthalmic: Bacitracin 500 units and polymyxin b sulfate 10,000 units per g (3.5 g)

Topical: Bacitracin 500 units and polymyxin b sulfate 10,000 units per g (1/32 oz, 15 g, 30 g)
Powder, topical: Bacitracin 500 units and polymyxin b sulfate 10,000 units per g (10 g)
Spray, topical: Bacitracin 10,000 units and polymyxin b sulfate 200,000 units (90 g)

bacitracin, neomycin, and polymyxin b

Brand Names Medi-Quick® Topical Ointment [OTC]; Mycitracin® Topical [OTC]; Neomixin® Topical; Neosporin® Ophthalmic Ointment; Neosporin® Topical Ointment [OTC]; Ocutricin® Topical Ointment; Septa® Topical Ointment [OTC]; Triple Antibiotic® Topical

Therapeutic Category Antibiotic, Ophthalmic; Antibiotic, Topical

Use Helps prevent infection in minor cuts, scrapes and burns; short-term treatment of superficial external ocular infections caused by susceptible organisms

Usual Dosage Children and Adults:
Ophthalmic ointment: Instill into the conjunctival sac one or more times/day every 3-4 hours for 7-10 days
Topical: Apply 1-3 times/day

Dosage Forms Ointment:
Ophthalmic: Bacitracin 400 units, neomycin sulfate 3.5 mg, and polymyxin b sulfate 10,000 units and per g
Topical: Bacitracin 400 units, neomycin sulfate 3.5 mg, and polymyxin b sulfate 5000 units per g

bacitracin, neomycin, polymyxin b, and hydrocortisone

Brand Names Cortisporin® Ophthalmic Ointment; Cortisporin® Topical Ointment

Therapeutic Category Antibiotic, Ophthalmic; Antibiotic, Otic; Antibiotic, Topical; Corticosteroid, Ophthalmic; Corticosteroid, Otic; Corticosteroid, Topical (Low Potency)

Use Prevention and treatment of susceptible superficial topical infections

Usual Dosage
Ophthalmic ointment: Apply ½" ribbon to inside of lower lid every 3-4 hours until improvement occurs
Topical: Apply sparingly 2-4 times/day

Dosage Forms Ointment:
Ophthalmic: Bacitracin 400 units, neomycin sulfate 3.5 mg, polymyxin b sulfate 10,000 units, and hydrocortisone 10 mg per g (3.5 g)
Topical: Bacitracin 400 units, neomycin sulfate 3.5 mg, polymyxin b sulfate 10,000 units, and hydrocortisone 10 mg per g (15 g)

baclofen (bak' loe fen)

Brand Names Lioresal®

Therapeutic Category Skeletal Muscle Relaxant

Use Treatment of reversible spasticity associated with multiple sclerosis or spinal cord lesions

Usual Dosage Oral:
Children:
2-7 years: Initial: 10-15 mg/24 hours divided every 8 hours; titrate dose every 3 days in increments of 5-15 mg/day to a maximum of 40 mg/day
≥8 years: Maximum: 60 mg/day in 3 divided doses

Adults: 5 mg 3 times/day, may increase 5 mg/dose every 3 days to a maximum of 80 mg/day

May be necessary to reduce dosage in renal impairment

Dosage Forms
Injection, intrathecal: 0.5 mg/mL (20 mL); 2 mg/mL (5 mL)
Tablet: 10 mg, 20 mg

43

ALPHABETICAL LISTING OF DRUGS

Bacticort® Otic *see* neomycin, polymyxin b, and hydrocortisone *on page 329*

Bactocill® Injection *see* oxacillin sodium *on page 347*

Bactocill® Oral *see* oxacillin sodium *on page 347*

BactoShield® Topical [OTC] *see* chlorhexidine gluconate *on page 90*

Bactrim™ *see* co-trimoxazole *on page 118*

Bactrim™ DS *see* co-trimoxazole *on page 118*

Bactroban® Topical *see* mupirocin *on page 319*

Baker's P&S Topical [OTC] *see* phenol *on page 369*

baking soda *see* sodium bicarbonate *on page 434*

BAL *see* dimercaprol *on page 151*

balanced salt solution
Brand Names BSS® Ophthalmic
Therapeutic Category Ophthalmic Agent, Miscellaneous
Use Intraocular irrigating solution; also used to soothe and cleanse the eye in conjunction with hard contact lenses
Usual Dosage Use as needed for foreign body removal, gonioscopy and other general ophthalmic office procedures
Dosage Forms Ophthalmic:
  Drops: 15 mL
  Solution, sterile: 500 mL

Baldex® Ophthalmic *see* dexamethasone *on page 132*

BAL in Oil® *see* dimercaprol *on page 151*

Balnetar® [OTC] *see* coal tar, lanolin, and mineral oil *on page 111*

Bancap® *see* butalbital compound *on page 63*

Bancap HC® *see* hydrocodone and acetaminophen *on page 234*

Banesin® [OTC] *see* acetaminophen *on page 2*

Banophen® Oral [OTC] *see* diphenhydramine hydrochloride *on page 152*

Banthine® *see* methantheline bromide *on page 298*

Barbidonna® *see* hyoscyamine, atropine, scopolamine, and phenobarbital *on page 242*

Barbita® *see* phenobarbital *on page 369*

Baricon® *see* radiological/contrast media (ionic) *on page 413*

barium sulfate *see* radiological/contrast media (ionic) *on page 413*

Barobag® *see* radiological/contrast media (ionic) *on page 413*

Baro-CAT® *see* radiological/contrast media (ionic) *on page 413*

Baroflave® *see* radiological/contrast media (ionic) *on page 413*

Barophen® *see* hyoscyamine, atropine, scopolamine, and phenobarbital *on page 242*

Barosperse® *see* radiological/contrast media (ionic) *on page 413*

Bar-Test® *see* radiological/contrast media (ionic) *on page 413*

Basaljel® [OTC] *see* aluminum carbonate *on page 15*

Bayer® Aspirin [OTC] *see* aspirin *on page 34*

BCG
Brand Names TheraCys™; TICE® BCG
Synonyms bacillus calmette-guérin; bcg, intravesical
Therapeutic Category Biological Response Modulator; Vaccine, Live Bacteria

44

Use BCG vaccine is no longer recommended for adults at high risk for tuberculosis in the United States. BCG vaccination may be considered for infants and children who are skin test-negative to 5 tuberculin units of tuberculin and who cannot be given isoniazid preventive therapy but have close contact with untreated or ineffectively treated active tuberculosis patients or who belong to groups which other control measures have not been successful.

In the United States, tuberculosis control efforts are directed toward early identification, treatment of cases, and preventive therapy with isoniazid.

Usual Dosage Intravesical treatment and prophylaxis for carcinoma *in situ* of the urinary bladder: Begin between 7-14 days after biopsy or transurethral resection. Give a dose of 3 vials of BCG live intravesically under aseptic conditions once weekly for 6 weeks (induction therapy). Each dose (3 reconstituted vials) is further diluted in an additional 50 mL sterile, preservative free saline for a total of 53 mL. A urethral catheter is inserted into the bladder under aseptic conditions, the bladder is drained, and then the 53 mL suspension is instilled slowly by gravity, following which the catheter is withdrawn. If the bladder catheterization has been traumatic, BCG live should not be administered, and there must be a treatment delay of at least 1 week. Resume subsequent treatment; follow the induction therapy by one treatment given 3, 6, 12, 18 and 24 months following the initial treatment.

Dosage Forms Powder for injection, lyophilized:
TheraCys™: 3.4 ±3 x 10^8 CFU equivalent to approximately 27 mg
Tice® BCG: 1-8 x 10^8 CFU equivalent to approximately 50 mg (2 mL)

bcg, intravesical *see* BCG *on previous page*

BCNU *see* carmustine *on page 76*

B-D Glucose® [OTC] *see* glucose, instant *on page 212*

Because® [OTC] *see* nonoxynol 9 *on page 338*

beclomethasone dipropionate (be kloe meth' a sone)

Brand Names Beclovent® Oral Inhaler; Beconase AQ® Nasal Inhaler; Beconase® Nasal Inhaler; Vancenase® AQ Inhaler; Vancenase® Nasal Inhaler; Vanceril® Oral Inhaler

Therapeutic Category Anti-inflammatory Agent; Corticosteroid, Inhalant

Use
Oral inhalation is used for treatment of bronchial asthma in patients who require chronic administration of corticosteroids
Nasal aerosol is used for the symptomatic treatment of seasonal or perennial rhinitis and nasal polyposis

Usual Dosage
Inhalation:
Children 6-12 years: 1-2 inhalations 3-4 times/day, not to exceed 10 inhalations/day
Adults: 2-4 inhalations twice daily, not to exceed 20 inhalations/day

Aerosol inhalation (nasal):
Children 6-12 years: 1 spray each nostril 3 times/day
Adults: 2-4 sprays each nostril twice daily

Aqueous inhalation (nasal): 1-2 sprays each nostril twice daily

Dosage Forms
Inhalation:
Nasal (Beconase®, Vancenase®): 42 μg/inhalation [200 metered doses] (16.8 g)
Oral (Beclovent®, Vanceril®): 42 μg/inhalation [200 metered doses] (16.8 g)
Spray, aqueous, nasal (Beconase AQ®, Vancenase® AQ): 42 μg/inhalation [200 metered doses] (25 g)

Beclovent® Oral Inhaler *see* beclomethasone dipropionate *on this page*

Beconase AQ® Nasal Inhaler *see* beclomethasone dipropionate *on this page*

Beconase® Nasal Inhaler *see* beclomethasone dipropionate *on this page*

Beef NPH Iletin® II *see* insulin preparations *on page 250*

Beef Regular Iletin® II *see* insulin preparations *on page 250*

Beepen-VK® Oral *see* penicillin V potassium *on page 362*

Beesix® *see* pyridoxine hydrochloride *on page 409*

bee sting kit *see* insect sting kit *on page 250*

Belix® Oral [OTC] *see* diphenhydramine hydrochloride *on page 152*

belladonna (bell a don' a)
Therapeutic Category Anticholinergic Agent; Antispasmodic Agent, Gastrointestinal
Use Decrease gastrointestinal activity in functional bowel disorders and to delay gastric emptying as well as decrease gastric secretion
Usual Dosage Adults: Oral: 0.3-1 mL 3-4 times/day
Dosage Forms Tincture: Belladonna alkaloids 27-23 mg/100 mL with alcohol 65% to 70% (120 mL, 480 mL, 3780 mL)

belladonna and opium
Brand Names B&O Supprettes®
Synonyms opium and belladonna
Therapeutic Category Analgesic, Narcotic
Use Relief of moderate to severe pain associated with rectal or bladder tenesmus that may occur in postoperative states and neoplastic situations; pain associated with ureteral spasms not responsive to non-narcotic analgesics and to space intervals between injections of opiates
Usual Dosage Rectal:
Children: Dose not established
Adults: 1 suppository 1-2 times/day, up to 4 doses/day
Dosage Forms Suppository, rectal:
#15A: Belladonna extract 15 mg and powdered opium 30 mg (12s)
#16A: Belladonna extract 15 mg and powdered opium 60 mg (12s)

belladonna, phenobarbital, and ergotamine tartrate
Brand Names Bellergal-S®
Therapeutic Category Ergot Alkaloid
Use Management and treatment of menopausal disorders, gastrointestinal disorders and recurrent throbbing headache
Usual Dosage Oral: 1 tablet each morning and evening
Dosage Forms Tablet, sustained release: l-alkaloids of belladonna 0.2 mg, phenobarbital 40 mg, and ergotamine tartrate 0.6 mg

Bellergal-S® *see* belladonna, phenobarbital, and ergotamine tartrate *on this page*

Bemote® Oral *see* dicyclomine hydrochloride *on page 145*

Bena-D® Injection *see* diphenhydramine hydrochloride *on page 152*

Benadryl® Injection *see* diphenhydramine hydrochloride *on page 152*

Benadryl® Oral [OTC] *see* diphenhydramine hydrochloride *on page 152*

Benadryl® Topical *see* diphenhydramine hydrochloride *on page 152*

Benahist® Injection *see* diphenhydramine hydrochloride *on page 152*

Ben-Aqua® [OTC] *see* benzoyl peroxide *on page 49*

benazepril hydrochloride (ben ay' ze prill)
Brand Names Lotensin®
Therapeutic Category Angiotensin Converting Enzyme (ACE) Inhibitors
Use Treatment of hypertension, either alone or in combination with other antihypertensive agents

Usual Dosage Adults: Oral: 20-40 mg/day as a single dose or 2 divided doses
Dosage Forms Tablet: 5 mg, 10 mg, 20 mg, 40 mg

bendroflumethiazide (ben droe floo meth eye' a zide)
Brand Names Naturetin®
Therapeutic Category Diuretic, Thiazide
Use Management of mild to moderate hypertension, edema associated with congestive heart failure, pregnancy, or nephrotic syndrome; reportedly does not alter serum electrolyte concentrations appreciably at recommended doses
Usual Dosage Oral:
Children: Initial: 0.1-0.4 mg/kg in 1-2 doses; maintenance dose: 0.05-0.1 mg/kg/day in 1-2 doses

Adults: 2.5-20 mg/day or twice daily in divided doses
Dosage Forms Tablet: 5 mg, 10 mg

Benemid® see probenecid on page 394
Benoject® Injection see diphenhydramine hydrochloride on page 152
Benoxyl® see benzoyl peroxide on page 49

bentiromide (ben teer' oh mide)
Brand Names Chymex®
Synonyms BTPABA
Therapeutic Category Diagnostic Agent, Pancreatic Exocrine Insufficiency
Use Screening test for pancreatic exocrine insufficiency
Usual Dosage
Children <12 years: 14 mg/kg followed with 8 oz of water

Children >12 years and Adults: Administer following an overnight fast and morning void, single 500 mg dose and follow with 8 oz of water
Dosage Forms Solution: 500 mg [PABA 170 mg] in propylene glycol 40% (7.5 mL)

Bentyl® Hydrochloride Injection see dicyclomine hydrochloride on page 145
Bentyl® Hydrochloride Oral see dicyclomine hydrochloride on page 145
Benylin® Cough Syrup [OTC] see diphenhydramine hydrochloride on page 152
Benylin DM® [OTC] see dextromethorphan hydrobromide on page 136
Benylin® Expectorant [OTC] see guaifenesin and dextromethorphan on page 218
Benza® [OTC] see benzalkonium chloride on this page
Benzac W® see benzoyl peroxide on page 49

benzalkonium chloride (benz al koe' nee um)
Brand Names Benza® [OTC]; Zephiran® [OTC]
Synonyms BAC
Therapeutic Category Antibacterial, Topical
Use Surface antiseptic and germicidal preservative
Usual Dosage Thoroughly rinse anionic detergents and soaps from the skin or other areas prior to use of solutions because they reduce the antibacterial activity of BAC; to protect metal instruments stored in BAC solution, add crushed Anti-Rust Tablets, 4 tablets per quart, to antiseptic solution, change solution at least once weekly; not to be used for storage of aluminum or zinc instruments, instruments with lenses fastened by cement, lacquered catheters or some synthetic rubber goods
(Continued)
47

benzalkonium chloride *(Continued)*
Dosage Forms
Concentrate, topical: 17% (500 mL, 4000 mL)
Solution, aqueous: 1:750 (60 mL, 120 mL, 240 mL)
Tincture: 1:750 (30 mL, 960 mL)
Tincture, spray: 1:750 (30 g, 180 g)
Tissue: 1:750 (packets)

benzathine benzylpenicillin *see* penicillin g benzathine *on page 360*
benzathine penicillin g *see* penicillin g benzathine *on page 360*
benzazoline hydrochloride *see* tolazoline hydrochloride *on page 471*
Benzedrex® [OTC] *see* propylhexedrine *on page 404*
benzene hexachloride *see* lindane *on page 274*
benzhexol hydrochloride *see* trihexyphenidyl hydrochloride *on page 478*

benzocaine (ben' zoe kane)
Brand Names Americaine® [OTC]; Anbesol® Maximum Strength [OTC]; Babee® Teething Lotion [OTC]; BiCOZENE® [OTC]; Chiggertox® [OTC]; Dermoplast® [OTC]; Foille Plus® [OTC]; Hurricaine®; Orabase®-B [OTC]; Orabase®-O [OTC]; Orajel® Brace-Aid Oral Anesthetic [OTC]; Orajel® Maximum Strength [OTC]; Orajel® Mouth-Aid [OTC]; Rhulicaine® [OTC]; Rid-A-Pain® [OTC]; Solarcaine® [OTC]; Unguentine® [OTC]
Synonyms ethyl aminobenzoate
Therapeutic Category Local Anesthetic, Oral; Local Anesthetic, Topical
Use Local anesthetic
Usual Dosage
Gel, cream, ointment: Topical: Apply a small amount on affected area
Otic: Instill 4-5 drops into external ear every 1-2 hours as needed
Spray: Topical: To affected area as needed
Dosage Forms Topical:
Aerosol: 5% (97.5 mL, 105 mL); 20% (20 g, 60 g, 120 g)
Cream: 5% (30 g, 454 g); 6% (28.4 g)
Liquid: With benzyl benzoate and soft soap (30 mL)
Lotion: 8% (90 mL)
Ointment: 5% (3.5 g, 30 g)

benzocaine and antipyrine *see* antipyrine and benzocaine *on page 30*
benzocaine and cetylpyridinium chloride *see* cetylpyridinium chloride and benzocaine *on page 85*

benzocaine, butyl aminobenzoate, tetracaine, and benzalkonium chloride
Brand Names Cetacaine®
Synonyms tetracaine hydrochloride, benzocaine butyl aminobenzoate and benzalkonium chloride
Therapeutic Category Local Anesthetic, Topical
Use Topical anesthetic to control pain or gagging
Usual Dosage Topical: Apply to affected area for approximately 1 second or less
Dosage Forms Aerosol: Benzocaine 14%, butyl aminobenzoate 2%, tetracaine 2%, and benzalkonium chloride 0.5% (56 g)

benzocaine, gelatin, pectin, and sodium carboxymethylcellulose
Brand Names Orabase® With Benzocaine [OTC]
Therapeutic Category Local Anesthetic, Topical
Use Topical anesthetic and emollient for oral lesions

Usual Dosage Apply 2-4 times/day
Dosage Forms Paste: Benzocaine 20%, gelatin, pectin, and sodium carboxymethylcellulose (15 g, 5 g)

benzoic acid and salicylic acid
Brand Names Whitfield's Ointment [OTC]
Synonyms salicylic acid and benzoic acid
Therapeutic Category Antifungal Agent, Topical
Use Treatment of athlete's foot and ringworm of the scalp
Usual Dosage Topical: Apply 1-4 times/day
Dosage Forms
  Lotion, topical:
    Full strength: Benzoic acid 12% and salicylic acid 6% with isopropyl alcohol 70% (240 mL)
    Half strength: Benzoic acid 6% and salicylic acid 3% with isopropyl alcohol 70% (240 mL)
  Ointment, topical: Benzoic acid 12% and salicylic acid 6% in anhydrous lanolin and petrolatum (30 g, 454 g)

benzoin (ben' zoin)
Brand Names AeroZoin® [OTC]; TinBen® [OTC]; TinCoBen® [OTC]
Synonyms gum benjamin
Therapeutic Category Pharmaceutical Aid; Protectant, Topical
Use Protective application for irritations of the skin; sometimes used in boiling water as steam inhalants for their expectorant and soothing action
Usual Dosage Apply 1-2 times/day
Dosage Forms
  Spray, as compound tincture: 40% (105 mL)
  Tincture: 79% (480 mL)
  Tincture, as compound tincture: 20% (60 mL); 25% (120 mL)

benzonatate (ben zoe' na tate)
Brand Names Tessalon® Perles
Therapeutic Category Antitussive; Local Anesthetic, Oral
Use Symptomatic relief of nonproductive cough
Usual Dosage Oral:
  Children <10 years: 8 mg/kg in 3-6 divided doses
  Children >10 years and Adults: 100 mg 3 times/day up to 600 mg/day
Dosage Forms Capsule: 100 mg

benzoyl peroxide (ben' zoe ill peer ox' ide)
Brand Names Ben-Aqua® [OTC]; Benoxyl®; Benzac W®; Clear By Design® [OTC]; Clearsil® [OTC]; Dermoxyl® [OTC]; Desquam-X®; Dry and Clear® [OTC]; Loroxide® [OTC]; Oxy-5® [OTC]; PanOxyl® [OTC]; PanOxyl®-AQ; Persa-Gel®; pHisoAc- BP® [OTC]; Theroxide®; Vanoxide® [OTC]; Xerac™ BP [OTC]; Zeroxin®
Therapeutic Category Acne Product; Topical Skin Product
Use Adjunctive treatment of mild to moderate acne vulgaris and acne rosacea
Usual Dosage Children >12 years and Adults: Topical: Apply sparingly 1-3 times/day
Dosage Forms
  Cleanser:
    Bar: 5% (120 g); 10% (120 g)
    Liquid: 5% (120 mL, 150 mL, 240 mL); 10% (120 mL, 150 mL)
  Cream: 5% (30 g); 10% (30 g, 45 g)
  Gel: 2.5% (45 g, 60 g, 90 g); 5% (45 g, 60 g, 90 g, 120 g); 10% (45 g, 60 g, 90 g, 120 g)
  Lotion: 5% (30 mL, 42.5 mL, 60 mL); 5.5% (25 mL); 10% (30 mL, 42.5 mL, 60 mL)

benzoyl peroxide and hydrocortisone
Brand Names Vanoxide-HC®
Therapeutic Category Acne Product; Corticosteroid, Topical (Low Potency); Topical Skin Product
Use Treatment of acne vulgaris and oily skin
Usual Dosage Shake well; apply thin film 1-3 times/day, gently massage into skin
Dosage Forms Lotion: Benzoyl peroxide 5% and hydrocortisone alcohol 0.5% (25 mL)

benzphetamine hydrochloride (benz fet' a meen)
Brand Names Didrex®
Therapeutic Category Anorexiant
Use Short-term adjunct in exogenous obesity
Usual Dosage Adults: Oral: 25-50 mg 2-3 times/day, preferably twice daily, midmorning and midafternoon
Dosage Forms Tablet: 25 mg, 50 mg

benzquinamide hydrochloride (benz kwin' a mide)
Brand Names Emete-Con®
Therapeutic Category Antiemetic
Use Antiemetic associated with anesthesia and surgery
Usual Dosage Not recommended for use in children <12 years of age, safety and efficacy have not been established

I.M.: 50 mg (0.5-1 mg/kg) may be repeated in 1 hour, then every 3-4 hours as needed
I.V. (not recommended route): 25 mg (0.2-0.4 mg/kg)
Dosage Forms Injection: 50 mg per vial

benzthiazide (benz thye' a zide)
Brand Names Aquatag®; Exna®; Hydrex®; Marazide®; Proaqua®
Therapeutic Category Diuretic, Thiazide
Use Management of mild to moderate hypertension; treatment of edema in congestive heart failure and nephrotic syndrome
Usual Dosage Adults: Oral: 50-200 mg/day
Dosage Forms Tablet: 50 mg

benztropine mesylate (benz' troe peen)
Brand Names Cogentin®
Therapeutic Category Anticholinergic Agent; Antiparkinson Agent
Use Adjunctive treatment of all forms of parkinsonism; also used in treatment of drug-induced extrapyramidal effects (except tardive dyskinesia) and acute dystonic reactions
Usual Dosage Titrate dose in 0.5 mg increments at 5- to 6-day intervals
Extrapyramidal reaction, drug induced: Oral, I.M., I.V.:
Children >3 years: 0.02-0.05 mg/kg/dose 1-2 times/day
Adults: 1-4 mg/dose 1-2 times/day

Parkinsonism: Oral: 0.5-6 mg/day in 1-2 divided doses; if one dose is greater, give at bedtime
Dosage Forms
Injection: 1 mg/mL (2 mL)
Tablet: 0.5 mg, 1 mg, 2 mg

benzylpenicillin benzathine *see* penicillin g benzathine *on page 360*
benzylpenicillin potassium *see* penicillin g, parenteral *on page 361*
benzylpenicillin sodium *see* penicillin g, parenteral *on page 361*

benzylpenicilloyl-polylysine (ben' zil pen i sill' oil polly lie' seen)
Brand Names Pre-Pen®
Synonyms penicilloyl-polylysine; PPL
Therapeutic Category Diagnostic Agent, Penicillin Allergy Skin Test
Use Adjunct in assessing the risk of administering penicillin (penicillin or benzylpenicillin) in adults with a history of clinical penicillin hypersensitivity
Usual Dosage
Use scratch technique with a 20-gauge needle to make 3-5 mm scratch on epidermis, apply a small drop of solution to scratch, rub in gently with applicator or toothpick.

A positive reaction consists of a pale wheal surrounding the scratch site which develops within 10 minutes and ranges from 5-15 mm or more in diameter.

If the scratch test is negative an intradermal test may be performed.
Intradermal test: Use intradermal test with a tuberculin syringe with a 26- to 30-gauge short bevel needle; a dose of 0.01-0.02 mL is injected intradermally. A control of 0.9% sodium chloride should be injected at least $1\frac{1}{2}$" from the PPL test site. Most skin responses to the intradermal test will develop within 5-15 minutes.
(–) = no reaction or increase in size compared to control
(±) = wheal slightly larger with or without erythematous flare and larger than control site
(+) = itching and increase in size of original bleb may exceed 20 mm in diameter
Dosage Forms Injection: 0.25 mL per ampul

bepridil hydrochloride (be' pri dil)
Brand Names Vascor®
Therapeutic Category Antianginal Agent; Calcium Channel Blocker
Use Treatment of chronic stable angina; only approved indication is hypertension, but may be used for congestive heart failure; doses should not be adjusted for at least 10 days after beginning therapy
Usual Dosage Adults: Oral: Initial: 200 mg/day, then adjust dose until optimal response is achieved; maximum daily dose: 400 mg
Dosage Forms Tablet: 200 mg, 300 mg, 400 mg

beractant (ber akt' ant)
Brand Names Survanta®
Synonyms bovine lung surfactant; natural lung surfactant
Therapeutic Category Lung Surfactant
Use Prevention and treatment of respiratory distress syndrome in premature infants

Prophylactic therapy: Body weight <1250 g in infants at risk for developing or with evidence of surfactant deficiency

Rescue therapy: Treatment of infants with RDS confirmed by x-ray and requiring mechanical ventilation
Usual Dosage Intratracheal:
Prophylactic treatment: Give 4 mL/kg as soon as possible; as many as 4 doses may be administered during the first 48 hours of life, no more frequently than 6 hours apart. The need for additional doses is determined by evidence of continuing respiratory distress; if the infant is still intubated and requiring at least 30% inspired oxygen to maintain a PaO_2 ≤80 torr.

Rescue treatment: Give 4 mL/kg as soon as the diagnosis of RDS is made.
Dosage Forms Suspension: Phospholipids 25 mg/mL, suspended in sodium chloride 0.9% (8 mL)

Berroca® *see* vitamin B complex with vitamin C and folic acid *on page 498*
Berubigen® *see* cyanocobalamin *on page 120*
Beta-2® Inhalation Solution *see* isoetharine *on page 257*

beta-carotene (kare' oh teen)
Brand Names Max-Caro® [OTC]; Provatene® [OTC]; Solatene®
Therapeutic Category Vitamin, Fat Soluble
Use Reduce the severity of photosensitivity reactions in patients with erythropoietic proto-porphyria (EPP)
Usual Dosage Oral:
Children <14 years: 30-150 mg/day
Adults: 30-300 mg/day
Dosage Forms Capsule: 15 mg, 30 mg

Betadine® [OTC] see povidone-iodine on page 389

9-beta-D-ribofuranosyladenine see adenosine on page 8

Betagan® Liquifilm® Ophthalmic see levobunolol hydrochloride on page 270

Betalene® Topical see betamethasone on this page

Betalin®S see thiamine hydrochloride on page 463

betamethasone (bay ta meth' a sone)
Brand Names Alphatrex® Topical; Betalene® Topical; Betatrex® Topical; Beta-Val® Topical; Celestone® Oral; Celestone® Phosphate Injection; Celestone® Soluspan®; Cel-U-Jec® Injection; Diprolene® AF Topical; Diprolene® Topical; Diprosone® Topical; Maxivate® Topical; Psorion® Topical; Selestoject® Injection; Teladar® Topical; Uticort® Topical; Valisone® Topical
Synonyms flubenisolone
Therapeutic Category Anti-inflammatory Agent; Corticosteroid, Systemic; Corticosteroid, Topical (Medium/High Potency)
Use Inflammatory dermatoses such as seborrheic or atopic dermatitis, neurodermatitis, anogenital pruritus, psoriasis, inflammatory phase of xerosis, late phase of allergic dermatitis or irritant dermatitis
Usual Dosage Children and Adults:
I.M.: Betamethasone sodium phosphate and betamethasone acetate: 0.5-9 mg/day ($\frac{1}{3}$ to $\frac{1}{2}$ of oral dose)
Intrabursal, intra-articular: 0.5-2 mL
Oral: 0.6-7.2 mg/day
Topical: Apply thin film 2-4 times/day
Dosage Forms
Base (Celestone®):
Syrup: 0.6 mg/5 mL
Tablet: 0.6 mg
Benzoate (Uticort®):
Cream, emollient base: 0.025% (60 g)
Gel, topical: 0.025% (15 g, 60 g)
Lotion: 0.025% (60 mL)
Dipropionate (Alphatrex®, Diprosone®, Maxivate®, Teladar®):
Aerosol, topical: 0.1% (85 g)
Cream: 0.05% (15 g, 45 g)
Lotion: 0.05% (20 mL, 30 mL, 60 mL)
Ointment, topical: 0.05% (15 g, 45 g)
Dipropionate (Psorion®):
Cream: 0.05% (15 g, 45 g)
Dipropionate, augmented (Diprolene®, Diprolene® AF):
Cream, emollient base: 0.05% (15 g, 45 g)
Gel, topical: 0.05% (15 g, 45 g)
Lotion: 0.05% (30 mL, 60 mL)
Ointment, topical: 0.05% (15 g, 45 g)
Valerate (Betatrex®, Beta-Val®, Valisone®):
Cream: 0.01% (15 g, 60 g); 0.1% (15 g, 45 g, 110 g, 430 g)

Lotion: 0.1% (20 mL, 60 mL)
Ointment, topical: 0.1% (15 g, 45 g)
Powder for compounding: 5 g, 10 g
Sodium phosphate:
Injection: Equivalent to 3 mg/mL (5 mL)
Sodium phosphate and acetate (Celestone® Soluspan®):
Injection, suspension: 6 mg/mL [betamethasone sodium phosphate 3 mg and beta-methasone acetate 3 mg per mL] (5 mL)

betamethasone dipropionate and clotrimazole
Brand Names Lotrisone®
Therapeutic Category Antifungal Agent, Topical; Corticosteroid, Topical (Medium/High Potency)
Use Topical treatment of various dermal fungal infections
Usual Dosage Topical: Apply twice daily
Dosage Forms Cream: Betamethasone dipropionate 0.05% and clotrimazole 1% (15 g, 45 g)

Betapace® Oral *see* sotalol hydrochloride *on page 441*

Betapen®-VK Oral *see* penicillin V potassium *on page 362*

Betaseron® *see* interferon beta-1b *on page 253*

Betatrex® Topical *see* betamethasone *on previous page*

Beta-Val® Topical *see* betamethasone *on previous page*

betaxolol hydrochloride (be tax' oh lol)
Brand Names Betoptic® Ophthalmic; Betoptic® S Ophthalmic; Kerlone® Oral
Therapeutic Category Beta-Adrenergic Blocker; Beta-Adrenergic Blocker, Ophthalmic
Use Treatment of chronic open-angle glaucoma, ocular hypertension; management of hypertension
Usual Dosage Adults:
Ophthalmic: Instill 1 drop twice daily
Oral: 10 mg/day; may increase dose to 20 mg/day after 7-14 days if desired response is not achieved; initial dose in elderly patients: 5 mg/day
Dosage Forms
Solution, ophthalmic (Betoptic®): 0.5% (2.5 mL, 5 mL, 10 mL)
Suspension, ophthalmic (Betoptic® S): 0.25% (2.5 mL, 10 mL, 15 mL)
Tablet (Kerlone®): 10 mg, 20 mg

bethanechol chloride (be than' e kole)
Brand Names Duvoid®; Myotonachol™; Urecholine®
Therapeutic Category Cholinergic Agent
Use Nonobstructive urinary retention and retention due to neurogenic bladder; treatment and prevention of bladder dysfunction caused by phenothiazines; diagnosis of flaccid or atonic neurogenic bladder
Usual Dosage
Children:
Oral:
Abdominal distention or urinary retention: 0.6 mg/kg/day divided 3-4 times/day
Gastroesophageal reflux: 0.1-0.2 mg/kg/dose given 30 minutes to 1 hour before each meal to a maximum of 4 times/day
S.C.: 0.15-0.2 mg/kg/day divided 3-4 times/day

Adults:
Oral: 10-50 mg 2-4 times/day
S.C.: 2.5-5 mg 3-4 times/day, up to 7.5-10 mg every 4 hours for neurogenic bladder
(Continued)

bethanechol chloride *(Continued)*
Dosage Forms
Injection: 5 mg/mL (1 mL)
Tablet: 5 mg, 10 mg, 25 mg, 50 mg

Betoptic® Ophthalmic *see* betaxolol hydrochloride *on previous page*

Betoptic® S Ophthalmic *see* betaxolol hydrochloride *on previous page*

Bexophene® *see* propoxyphene and aspirin *on page 402*

Biamine® *see* thiamine hydrochloride *on page 463*

Biavax®ₗₗ *see* rubella and mumps vaccines, combined *on page 423*

Biaxin™ Filmtabs® *see* clarithromycin *on page 104*

Bicillin® C-R 900/300 Injection *see* penicillin g benzathine and procaine combined *on page 360*

Bicillin® C-R Injection *see* penicillin g benzathine and procaine combined *on page 360*

Bicillin® L-A Injection *see* penicillin g benzathine *on page 360*

Bicitra® *see* sodium citrate and citric acid *on page 435*

BiCNU® *see* carmustine *on page 76*

BiCOZENE® [OTC] *see* benzocaine *on page 48*

Bili-Labstix® [OTC] *see* diagnostic aids (*in vitro*), urine *on page 139*

Bilopaque® *see* radiological/contrast media (ionic) *on page 413*

Biltricide® *see* praziquantel *on page 390*

Biocef *see* cephalexin monohydrate *on page 84*

Biocult-GC® *see* diagnostic aids (*in vitro*), other *on page 138*

Biomox® *see* amoxicillin trihydrate *on page 24*

Bio-Tab® Oral *see* doxycycline *on page 161*

Biozyme-C® *see* collagenase *on page 114*

biperiden hydrochloride (bye per' i den)
Brand Names Akineton®
Therapeutic Category Antiparkinson Agent
Use Treatment of all forms of Parkinsonism including drug induced type (extrapyramidal symptoms)
Usual Dosage Adults:
Parkinsonism: Oral: 2 mg 3-4 times/day

Extrapyramidal:
Oral: 2-6 mg 2-3 times/day
I.M., I.V.: 2 mg every 30 minutes up to 4 doses or 8 mg/day
Dosage Forms
Injection, as lactate: 5 mg/mL (1 mL)
Tablet, as hydrochloride: 2 mg

biphenabid *see* probucol *on page 395*

bisacodyl (bis a koe' dill)
Brand Names Bisacodyl Uniserts®; Bisco-Lax® [OTC]; Carter's Little Pills® [OTC]; Clyso-drast®; Dulcagen® [OTC]; Dulcolax® [OTC]; Fleet® Laxative [OTC]
Therapeutic Category Laxative, Stimulant
Use Treatment of constipation; colonic evacuation prior to procedures or examination
Usual Dosage
Children:
Oral: >6 years: 5-10 mg (0.3 mg/kg) at bedtime or before breakfast

Rectal suppository:
<2 years: 5 mg as a single dose
>2 years: 10 mg
Adults:
Oral: 5-15 mg as single dose (up to 30 mg when complete evacuation of bowel is required)
Rectal suppository: 10 mg as single dose
Tannex:
Enema: 2.5 g in 1000 mL warm water
Barium enema: 2.5-5 g in 1000 mL barium suspension
Do not give >10 g within 72-hour period
Dosage Forms
Enema: 10 mg/30 mL
Powder (Clysodrast®): 1.5 mg with tannic acid 2.5 g per packet (25s, 50s)
Suppository, rectal: 10 mg
Suppository, rectal, pediatric: 5 mg
Tablet, enteric coated: 5 mg

Bisacodyl Uniserts® see bisacodyl *on previous page*

Bisco-Lax® [OTC] see bisacodyl *on previous page*

bishydroxycoumarin see dicumarol *on page 144*

Bismatrol® [OTC] see bismuth *on this page*

bismuth
Brand Names Bismatrol® [OTC]; Devrom® [OTC]; Pepto-Bismol® [OTC]
Synonyms bismuth subgallate; bismuth subsalicylate
Therapeutic Category Antidiarrheal
Use Symptomatic treatment of mild, nonspecific diarrhea
Usual Dosage Oral:
Nonspecific diarrhea: Subsalicylate:
Children: Up to 8 doses/24 hours:
3-6 years: $\frac{1}{3}$ tablet or 5 mL every 30 minutes to 1 hour as needed
6-9 years: $\frac{2}{3}$ tablet or 10 mL every 30 minutes to 1 hour as needed
9-12 years: 1 tablet or 15 mL every 30 minutes to 1 hour as needed
Adults: 2 tablets or 30 mL every 30 minutes to 1 hour as needed up to 8 doses/24 hours
Prevention of traveler's diarrhea: 2.1 g/day or 2 tablets 4 times/day before meals and at bedtime
Subgallate: 1-2 tablets 3 times/day with meals
Dosage Forms
Liquid, as subsalicylate (Pepto-Bismol®, Bismatrol®): 262 mg/15 mL (120 mL, 240 mL, 360 mL, 480 mL); 524 mg/15 mL (120 mL, 240 mL, 360 mL)
Tablet:
Chewable, as subsalicylate (Pepto-Bismol®, Bismatrol®): 262 mg
Chewable, as subgallate (Devrom®): 200 mg

bismuth subgallate see bismuth *on this page*

bismuth subsalicylate see bismuth *on this page*

bisoprolol fumarate (bis oh' proe lol)
Brand Names Zebeta®
Therapeutic Category Beta-Adrenergic Blocker
Use Treatment of hypertension, alone or in combination with other agents
Usual Dosage Adults: Oral: 5 mg once daily, may be increased to 10 mg, and then up to 20 mg once daily, if necessary; may be given without regard to meals
Dosage Forms Tablet: 5 mg, 10 mg

bistropamide *see* tropicamide *on page 484*

bitolterol mesylate (bye tole' ter ole mess' a late)
Brand Names Tornalate®
Therapeutic Category Beta-2-Adrenergic Agonist Agent; Bronchodilator
Use Prevent and treat bronchial asthma and bronchospasm
Usual Dosage Children >12 years and Adults:
Bronchospasm: 2 inhalations at an interval of at least 1-3 minutes, followed by a third inhalation if needed

Prevention of bronchospasm: 2 inhalations every 8 hours
Dosage Forms
Aerosol, oral: 0.8% [370 μg/metered spray, 300 inhalations] 15 mL
Solution, inhalation: 0.2% (10 mL, 30 mL, 60 mL)

Black Draught® [OTC] *see* senna *on page 428*

black widow spider species antivenin *Latrodectus mactans* *see* antivenin, black widow spider (equine) *on page 30*

Blanex® *see* chlorzoxazone *on page 99*

Blenoxane® *see* bleomycin sulfate *on this page*

bleomycin sulfate (blee oh mye' sin)
Brand Names Blenoxane®
Synonyms BLM
Therapeutic Category Antineoplastic Agent, Antibiotic
Use Palliative treatment of squamous cell carcinomas, testicular carcinoma and lymphomas
Usual Dosage Refer to individual protocol
Children and Adults:
Test dose for lymphoma patients: I.M., I.V., S.C.: 1-2 units of bleomycin for the first 2 doses; monitor vital signs every 15 minutes; wait a minimum of 1 hour before administering remainder of dose
I.M., I.V., S.C.: 10-20 units/m^2 (0.25-0.5 units/kg) 1-2 times/week in combination regimens
I.V. continuous infusion: 15-20 units/m^2/day for 4-5 days

Adults: Intracavitary injection for pleural effusion: 15-240 units have been given
Dosage Forms Powder for injection: 15 units

Bleph®-10 Ophthalmic *see* sodium sulfacetamide *on page 439*

Blephamide® Ophthalmic *see* sodium sulfacetamide and prednisolone *on page 439*

BLM *see* bleomycin sulfate *on this page*

Blocadren® Oral *see* timolol maleate *on page 468*

Bluboro® [OTC] *see* aluminum acetate *on page 14*

Bonine® [OTC] *see* meclizine hydrochloride *on page 288*

boric acid
Brand Names Borofax® Topical [OTC]; Dri-Ear® Otic [OTC]; Swim-Ear® Otic [OTC]
Therapeutic Category Pharmaceutical Aid
Use
Ophthalmic: Mild antiseptic used for inflamed eyelids
Topical ointment: Temporary relief of chapped, chafed, or dry skin, diaper rash, abrasions, minor burns, sunburn, insect bites, and other skin irritations

Usual Dosage Apply to lower eyelid 1-2 times/day
Dosage Forms
Ointment:
  Ophthalmic: 5% (3.5 g); 10% (3.5 g)
  Topical: 5% (52.5 g); 10% (28 g)
  Topical (Borofax®): 5% boric acid and lanolin (1³/₄ oz)
Solution, otic: 2.75% with isopropyl alcohol (30 mL)

Borofax® Topical [OTC] *see* boric acid *on previous page*

Boropak® *see* aluminum acetate *on page 14*

B&O Supprettes® *see* belladonna and opium *on page 46*

botulinum toxin type A (bot' yoo lin num)
Brand Names Oculinum®
Therapeutic Category Ophthalmic Agent, Toxin
Use Treatment of strabismus and blepharospasm
Usual Dosage
Strabismus: 1.25-5 units (0.05-0.15 mL) injected into any one muscle

Blepharospasm: 1.25-5 units (0.05-0.15 mL) injected into the orbicularis oculi muscle
Dosage Forms Powder for injection, lyophilized, preservative free: *Clostridium botulinum* Toxin type A 100 units

bovine lung surfactant *see* beractant *on page 51*

BQ® Tablet [OTC] *see* chlorpheniramine, phenylpropanolamine, and acetaminophen *on page 96*

Breonesin® [OTC] *see* guaifenesin *on page 217*

Brethaire® Inhalation Areosol *see* terbutaline sulfate *on page 454*

Brethine® Injection *see* terbutaline sulfate *on page 454*

Brethine® Oral *see* terbutaline sulfate *on page 454*

bretylium tosylate (bre til' ee um toss' a late)
Brand Names Bretylol®
Therapeutic Category Antiarrhythmic Agent, Class III
Use Ventricular tachycardia and fibrillation; also used in the treatment of other serious ventricular arrhythmias resistant to lidocaine
Usual Dosage
Children:
  I.M.: 2-5 mg/kg as a single dose
  I.V.: Initial: 5 mg/kg, then attempt electrical defibrillation; repeat with 10 mg/kg if ventricular fibrillation persists
  Maintenance dose: I.M., I.V.: 5 mg/kg every 6-8 hours
Adults:
  Immediate life-threatening ventricular arrhythmias; ventricular fibrillation; unstable ventricular tachycardia. **Note**: Patients should undergo defibrillation/cardioversion before and after bretylium doses as necessary:
    Initial dose: I.V.: 5 mg/kg (undiluted) over 1 minute; if arrhythmia persists, give 10 mg/kg (undiluted) over 1 minute and repeat as necessary (usually at 15- to 30-minute intervals) up to a total dose of 30 mg/kg
  Other life-threatening ventricular arrhythmias:
    Initial dose: I.M., I.V.: 5-10 mg/kg, may repeat every 1-2 hours if arrhythmia persist; give I.V. dose (diluted) over 10-30 minutes
    Maintenance dose: I.M.: 5-10 mg/kg every 6-8 hours; I.V. (diluted): 5-10 mg/kg every 6 hours; I.V. infusion (diluted): 1-2 mg/minute (little experience with doses >40 mg/kg/day)
(Continued)

bretylium tosylate *(Continued)*
Dosage Forms
Injection: 50 mg/mL (10 mL, 20 mL)
Injection, premixed in D$_5$W: 1 mg/mL (500 mL); 2 mg/mL (250 mL); 4 mg/mL (250 mL, 500 mL)

Bretylol® *see bretylium tosylate on previous page*

Brevibloc® Injection *see esmolol hydrochloride on page 177*

Brevicon® *see ethinyl estradiol and norethindrone on page 183*

Brevital® Sodium *see methohexital sodium on page 301*

Brexin® L.A. *see chlorpheniramine and pseudoephedrine on page 94*

Bricanyl® Injection *see terbutaline sulfate on page 454*

Bricanyl® Oral *see terbutaline sulfate on page 454*

british anti-lewisite *see dimercaprol on page 151*

Brofed® *see brompheniramine and pseudoephedrine on next page*

Bromaline® [OTC] *see brompheniramine and phenylpropanolamine on next page*

Bromanate® [OTC] *see brompheniramine and phenylpropanolamine on next page*

Bromanate DC® *see brompheniramine, phenylpropanolamine, and codeine on page 60*

Bromanyl® Cough Syrup *see bromodiphenhydramine and codeine on this page*

Bromarest® [OTC] *see brompheniramine maleate on next page*

Bromatapp® [OTC] *see brompheniramine and phenylpropanolamine on next page*

Bromfed-PD® *see brompheniramine and pseudoephedrine on next page*

bromocriptine mesylate *(broe moe krip' teen mess' a late)*
Brand Names Parlodel®
Therapeutic Category Antiparkinson Agent; Ergot Alkaloid
Use Treatment of parkinsonism in patients unresponsive or allergic to levodopa; also used in conditions associated with hyperprolactinemia and to suppress lactation
Usual Dosage Oral:
Parkinsonism: 1.25 mg twice daily, increased by 2.5 mg/day in 2- to 4-week intervals (usual dose range: 30-90 mg/day in 3 divided doses)

Hyperprolactinemia and postpartum lactation: 2.5 mg 2-3 times/day
Dosage Forms
Capsule: 5 mg
Tablet: 2.5 mg

bromodiphenhydramine and codeine *(brome oh dye fen hye' dra meen)*
Brand Names Ambenyl® Cough Syrup; Amgenal® Cough Syrup; Bromanyl® Cough Syrup; Bromotuss® w/Codeine Cough Syrup
Synonyms codeine and bromodiphenhydramine
Therapeutic Category Antihistamine; Cough Preparation
Use Relief of upper respiratory symptoms and cough associated with allergies or common cold
Usual Dosage Oral: 5-10 mL every 4-6 hours
Dosage Forms Liquid: Bromodiphenhydramine hydrochloride 12.5 mg and codeine phosphate 10 mg per 5 mL

Bromotuss® w/Codeine Cough Syrup *see* bromodiphenhydramine and codeine *on previous page*

Bromphen DC® w/Codeine *see* brompheniramine, phenylpropanolamine, and codeine *on next page*

Bromphen® Elixir [OTC] *see* brompheniramine maleate *on this page*

brompheniramine and phenylpropanolamine
(brome fen ir' a meen & fen ill proe pa nole' a meen)
Brand Names Bromaline® [OTC]; Bromanate® [OTC]; Bromatapp® [OTC]; Bromphen® Tablet [OTC]; Dimetapp® [OTC]; Dimetapp® Extentabs® [OTC]; E.N.T.®; Myphetapp® [OTC]; Tamine® [OTC]
Synonyms phenylpropanolamine and brompheniramine
Therapeutic Category Antihistamine/Decongestant Combination
Use Temporary relief of nasal congestion, running nose, sneezing, and itchy, watery eyes
Usual Dosage Oral:
Children:
    1-6 months: 1.25 mL 3-4 times/day
    7-24 months: 2.5 mL 3-4 times/day
    2-4 years: 3.75 mL 3-4 times/day
    4-12 years: 5 mL 3-4 times/day

Adults: 5-10 mL 3-4 times/day or 1 tablet twice daily
Dosage Forms
Elixir (grape flavor): Brompheniramine maleate 2 mg and phenylpropanolamine hydrochloride 12.5 mg per 5 mL with alcohol 2.3% (5 mL, 120 mL, 240 mL, 480 mL, 3780 mL)
Tablet: Brompheniramine maleate 4 mg and phenylpropanolamine hydrochloride 25 mg
Tablet, sustained release: Brompheniramine maleate 12 mg and phenylpropanolamine hydrochloride 75 mg

brompheniramine and pseudoephedrine
(brome fen ir' a meen & soo doe e fed' rin)
Brand Names Brofed®; Bromfed-PD®; Dallergy-JR®; Dristan® Allergy [OTC]; ULTRAbrom® PD
Therapeutic Category Antihistamine/Decongestant Combination
Use Temporary relief of symptoms of seasonal and perennial allergic rhinitis, and vasomotor rhinitis, including nasal obstruction
Usual Dosage Oral:
Children 6-12 years: 1 capsule every 12 hours
Children >12 years and Adults: 1 or 2 capsules every 12 hours
Dosage Forms
Caplet: Brompheniramine maleate 4 mg and pseudoephedrine hydrochloride 60 mg
Capsule, timed-release: Brompheniramine maleate 6 mg and pseudoephedrine hydrochloride 60 mg
Elixir: Brompheniramine maleate 4 mg and pseudoephedrine hydrochloride 30 mg

brompheniramine maleate (brome fen ir' a meen mal' ee ate)
Brand Names Bromarest® [OTC]; Bromphen® Elixir [OTC]; Chlorphed® [OTC]; Codimal-A® Injection; Cophene-B® Injection; Dehist® Injection; Diamine T.D.® Oral [OTC]; Dimetane® Oral [OTC]; Histaject® Injection; Nasahist B® Injection; ND-Stat® Injection; Oraminic® II Injection; Sinusol-B® Injection; Veltane® Tablet
Synonyms parabromdylamine
Therapeutic Category Antihistamine
Use Perennial and seasonal allergic rhinitis and other allergic symptoms including urticaria
Usual Dosage
Oral:
    Children:
        <6 years: 0.125 mg/kg/dose given every 6 hours; maximum: 6-8 mg/day
        6-12 years: 2-4 mg every 6-8 hours; maximum: 12-16 mg/day

(Continued)

brompheniramine maleate *(Continued)*

Adults: 4 mg every 4-6 hours or 8 mg of sustained release form every 8-12 hours or 12 mg of sustained release every 12 hours; maximum: 24 mg/day

I.M., I.V., S.C.:
Children <12 years: 0.5 mg/kg/24 hours divided every 6-8 hours
Adults: 5-50 mg every 4-12 hours, maximum: 40 mg/24 hours

Dosage Forms
Elixir: 2 mg/5 mL with alcohol 3% (120 mL, 480 mL, 4000 mL)
Injection: 10 mg/mL (10 mL)
Tablet: 4 mg, 8 mg, 12 mg
Tablet, sustained release: 8 mg, 12 mg

brompheniramine, phenylpropanolamine, and codeine

Brand Names Bromanate DC®; Bromphen DC® w/Codeine; Dimetane®-DC; Myphetane DC®; Poly-Histine CS®
Therapeutic Category Antihistamine/Decongestant Combination; Cough Preparation
Use Relief of coughs and upper respiratory symptoms, including nasal congestion, associated with allergy or the common cold
Usual Dosage Oral:
Children:
2-6 years: 2.5 mL every 4 hours
6-12 years: 5 mL every 4 hours

Children >12 years and Adults: 10 mL every 4 hours
Dosage Forms Liquid: Brompheniramine maleate 2 mg, phenylpropanolamine hydrochloride 12.5 mg, and codeine phosphate 10 mg per 5 mL with alcohol 0.95% (480 mL)

Bromphen® Tablet [OTC] *see* brompheniramine and phenylpropanolamine *on previous page*
Bronchial® *see* theophylline and guaifenesin *on page 461*
Bronitin® Inhalation Aerosol [OTC] *see* epinephrine *on page 171*
Bronkaid® Inhalation Aerosol [OTC] *see* epinephrine *on page 171*
Bronkephrine® Injection *see* ethylnorepinephrine hydrochloride *on page 186*
Bronkodyl® *see* theophylline *on page 460*
Bronkometer® Aerosol *see* isoetharine *on page 257*
Bronkosol® Inhalation Solution *see* isoetharine *on page 257*
BSS® Ophthalmic *see* balanced salt solution *on page 44*
BTPABA *see* bentiromide *on page 47*
Bucet™ *see* butalbital compound *on page 63*
Bucladin®-S Softab® *see* buclizine hydrochloride *on this page*

buclizine hydrochloride (byoo' kli zeen)

Brand Names Bucladin®-S Softab®
Therapeutic Category Antiemetic; Antihistamine
Use Prevention and treatment of motion sickness; symptomatic treatment of vertigo
Usual Dosage Adults: Oral:
Motion sickness (prophylaxis): 50 mg 30 minutes prior to traveling; may repeat 50 mg after 4-6 hours

Vertigo: 50 mg twice daily, up to 150 mg/day
Dosage Forms Tablet: 50 mg

Bufferin® [OTC] *see* aspirin *on page 34*

bumetanide (byoo met' a nide)
Brand Names Bumex®
Therapeutic Category Diuretic, Loop
Use Management of edema secondary to congestive heart failure or hepatic or renal disease including nephrotic syndrome; may also be used alone or in combination with antihypertensives in the treatment of hypertension
Usual Dosage
Children:
<6 months: Dose not established
>6 months:
Oral: Initial: 0.015 mg/kg/dose once daily or every other day; maximum dose: 0.1 mg/kg/day
I.M., I.V.: Dose not established

Adults:
Oral: 0.5-2 mg/dose (maximum: 10 mg/day) 1-2 times/day
I.M., I.V.: 0.5-1 mg/dose (maximum: 10 mg/day)
Dosage Forms
Injection: 0.25 mg/mL (2 mL, 4 mL, 10 mL)
Tablet: 0.5 mg, 1 mg, 2 mg

Bumex® see bumetanide on this page

Buminate® see albumin human on page 10

bupivacaine hydrochloride (byoo piv' a kane)
Brand Names Marcaine®; Sensorcaine®
Therapeutic Category Local Anesthetic, Injectable
Use Local anesthetic (injectable) for peripheral nerve block, infiltration, sympathetic block, caudal or epidural block, retrobulbar block
Usual Dosage Dose varies with procedure, depth of anesthesia, vascularity of tissues, duration of anesthesia and condition of patient

Caudal block (with or without epinephrine):
Children: 1-3.7 mg/kg
Adults: 15-30 mL of 0.25% or 0.5%

Epidural block (other than caudal block):
Children: 1.25 mg/kg/dose
Adults: 10-20 mL of 0.25% or 0.5%

Peripheral nerve block: 5 mL dose of 0.25% or 0.5% (12.5-25 mg); maximum: 2.5 mg/kg (plain); 3 mg/kg (with epinephrine); up to a maximum of 400 mg/day

Sympathetic nerve block: 20-50 mL of 0.25% (no epinephrine) solution
Dosage Forms
Injection: 0.25% [2.5 mg/mL] (10 mL, 20 mL, 30 mL, 50 mL); 0.5% [5 mg/mL] (10 mL, 20 mL, 30 mL, 50 mL); 0.75% [7.5 mg/mL] (2 mL, 10 mL, 20 mL, 30 mL)
Injection, with epinephrine (1:200,000): 0.25% [2.5 mg/mL] (10 mL, 30 mL, 50 mL); 0.5% [5 mg/mL] (1.8 mL, 3 mL, 5 mL, 10 mL, 30 mL, 50 mL); 0.75% [7.5 mg/mL] (30 mL)

Buprenex® see buprenorphine hydrochloride on this page

buprenorphine hydrochloride (byoo pre nor' feen)
Brand Names Buprenex®
Therapeutic Category Analgesic, Narcotic
Use Management of moderate to severe pain
Usual Dosage Adults: I.M., slow I.V.: 0.3-0.6 mg every 6 hours as needed
Dosage Forms Injection: 0.3 mg/mL (1 mL)

bupropion (byoo proe' pee on)
Brand Names Wellbutrin®
Therapeutic Category Antidepressant
Use Treatment of depression
Usual Dosage Adults: Oral: 100 mg 3 times/day; begin at 100 mg twice daily; may increase to a maximum dose of 450 mg/day
Dosage Forms Tablet: 75 mg, 100 mg

Burow's solution *see aluminum acetate on page 14*
BuSpar® *see buspirone hydrochloride on this page*

buspirone hydrochloride (byoo spye' rone)
Brand Names BuSpar®
Therapeutic Category Antianxiety Agent
Use Management of anxiety
Usual Dosage Adults: Oral: 15 mg/day (5 mg 3 times/day); may increase to a maximum of 60 mg/day
Dosage Forms Tablet: 5 mg, 10 mg

busulfan (byoo sul' fan)
Brand Names Myleran®
Therapeutic Category Antineoplastic Agent, Alkylating Agent
Use Chronic myelogenous leukemia and marrow-ablative conditioning regimens prior to bone marrow transplantation
Usual Dosage Refer to individual protocols
Oral:
Children:
Remission induction of chronic myelogenous leukemia: 0.06-0.12 mg/kg/day or 1.8-4.6 mg/m^2/day; titrate dose to maintain leukocyte count about 20,000/mm^3
BMT marrow-ablative conditioning regimen: 1 mg/kg/dose every 6 hours for 16 doses
Adults: Remission induction of chronic myelogenous leukemia: 4-8 mg/day; maintenance dose: controversial, range from 1-4 mg/day to 2 mg/week
Dosage Forms Tablet: 2 mg

butabarbital sodium (byoo ta bar' bi tal)
Brand Names Butalan®; Buticaps®; Butisol Sodium®
Therapeutic Category Barbiturate; Hypnotic; Sedative
Use Sedative, hypnotic
Usual Dosage
Children: Preop: 2-6 mg/kg/dose; maximum: 100 mg
Adults:
Sedative: 15-30 mg 3-4 times/day
Hypnotic: 50-100 mg
Preop: 50-100 mg 1-1½ hours before surgery
Dosage Forms
Capsule: 15 mg, 30 mg
Elixir, with alcohol 7%: 30 mg/5 mL (480 mL, 3780 mL); 33.3 mg/5 mL (480 mL, 3780 mL)
Tablet: 15 mg, 30 mg, 50 mg, 100 mg

Butace® *see butalbital compound on next page*
Butalan® *see butabarbital sodium on this page*
butalbital, acetaminophen, and caffeine *see butalbital compound on next page*

butalbital and acetaminophen *see* butalbital compound *on this page*

butalbital and aspirin *see* butalbital compound *on this page*

butalbital, aspirin, and caffeine *see* butalbital compound *on this page*

butalbital compound (byoo tal' bi tal)
Brand Names Amaphen®; Anoquan®; Arcet®; Axotal®; B-A-C®; Bancap®; Bucet™; Butace®; Endolor®; Esgic®; Esgic-Plus®; Femcet®; Fiorgen PF®; Fioricet®; Fiorinal®; Isocet®; Isollyl Improved®; Lanorinal®; Marnal®; Medigesic®; Phrenilin®; Phrenilin® Forte®; Repan; Sedapap-10®; Tencet™; Tencon®; Triad®; Triaprin®; Two-Dyne®

Synonyms butalbital, acetaminophen, and caffeine; butalbital and acetaminophen; butalbital and aspirin; butalbital, aspirin, and caffeine

Therapeutic Category Analgesic, Non-Narcotic; Barbiturate

Use Relief of the symptomatic complex of tension or muscle contraction headache

Usual Dosage Adults: Oral: 1-2 tablets or capsules every 4 hours; not to exceed 6/day

Dosage Forms
Capsule, with acetaminophen:
Amaphen®, Anoquan®, Butace®, Endolor®, Esgic®, Femcet®, Margesic®, Medigesic®, Repan, Tencet™, Triad®, Two-Dyne®: Butalbital 50 mg, caffeine 40 mg, and acetaminophen 325 mg
Bancap®, Triapin®: Butalbital 50 mg and acetaminophen 325 mg
Phrenilin® Forte®, Tencon®: Butalbital 50 mg and acetaminophen 650 mg
Capsule, with aspirin: (Fiorgen PF®, Fiorinal®, Isollyl Improved®, Lanorinal®, Marnal®): Butalbital 50 mg, caffeine 40 mg, and aspirin 325 mg
Tablet, with acetaminophen:
Arcet®, Esgic®, Fioricet®, Repan: Butalbital 50 mg, caffeine 40 mg, and acetaminophen 325 mg
Bucet™, Sedapap-10®: Butalbital 50 mg and acetaminophen 650 mg
Esgic-Plus®: Butalbital 50 mg, caffeine 40 mg, and acetaminophen 500 mg
Isocet®: Butalbital 50 mg, caffeine 40 mg, and acetaminophen 325 mg
Phrenilin®: Butalbital 50 mg and acetaminophen 325 mg
Tablet, with aspirin:
Axotal®: Butalbital 50 mg and aspirin 650 mg
B-A-C®: Butalbital 50 mg, caffeine 40 mg, and aspirin 650 mg
Fiorinal®, Isollyl Improved®, Lanorinal®, Marnal®: Butalbital 50 mg, caffeine 40 mg, and aspirin 325 mg

butalbital compound and codeine
Brand Names Fiorinal® With Codeine

Synonyms codeine and butalbital compound

Therapeutic Category Analgesic, Narcotic; Barbiturate

Use Mild to moderate pain when sedation is needed

Usual Dosage Oral: 1-2 capsules every 4-6 hours as needed for pain

Dosage Forms Capsule: Butalbital 50 mg, caffeine 40 mg, aspirin 325 mg and codeine phosphate 30 mg

Butazolidin® *see* phenylbutazone *on page 371*

Buticaps® *see* butabarbital sodium *on previous page*

Butisol Sodium® *see* butabarbital sodium *on previous page*

butoconazole nitrate (byoo toe koe' na zole)
Brand Names Femstat®

Therapeutic Category Antifungal Agent, Vaginal

Use Local treatment of vulvovaginal candidiasis

Usual Dosage Adults:
Nonpregnant: 1 applicatorful (~5 g) intravaginally at bedtime for 3 days, may extend for up to 6 days if necessary

(Continued)

butoconazole nitrate *(Continued)*
Pregnant: **Use only during second or third trimesters**
Dosage Forms Cream, vaginal: 2% with applicator (28 g)

butorphanol tartrate (byoo tor' fa nole)
Brand Names Stadol®; Stadol® NS
Therapeutic Category Analgesic, Narcotic
Use Management of moderate to severe pain
Usual Dosage Adults:
 I.M.: 1-4 mg every 3-4 hours as needed
 I.V.: 0.5-2 mg every 3-4 hours as needed
 Nasal: 1 mg (1 spray in one nostril) initially, allow 60-90 minutes to elapse before deciding whether a second 1 mg dose is needed; this 2 dose sequence may be repeated in 3-4 hours if needed
Dosage Forms
 Injection: 1 mg/mL (1 mL); 2 mg/mL (1 mL, 2 mL, 10 mL)
 Nasal spray: 10 mg/mL [14-15 doses] (2.5 mL)

Byclomine® Injection *see* dicyclomine hydrochloride *on page 145*

Bydramine® Cough Syrup [OTC] *see* diphenhydramine hydrochloride *on page 152*

C8-CCK *see* sincalide *on page 432*

Cafatine® *see* ergotamine derivatives *on page 174*

Cafergot® *see* ergotamine derivatives *on page 174*

Cafetrate® *see* ergotamine derivatives *on page 174*

Calan® *see* verapamil hydrochloride *on page 493*

Cal Carb-HD® [OTC] *see* calcium carbonate *on next page*

Calcibind® *see* cellulose sodium phosphate *on page 83*

Calci-Chew™ [OTC] *see* calcium carbonate *on next page*

Calciday-667® [OTC] *see* calcium carbonate *on next page*

calcifediol (kal si fe dye' ole)
Brand Names Calderol®
Synonyms 25-d$_3$; 25-hydroxycholecalciferol; 25-hydroxyvitamin d$_3$
Therapeutic Category Vitamin D Analog
Use Treatment and management of metabolic bone disease associated with chronic renal failure
Usual Dosage Hepatic osteodystrophy: Oral:
 Infants: 5-7 μg/kg/day

 Children and Adults: 20-100 μg/day or every other day; titrate to obtain normal serum calcium/phosphate levels
Dosage Forms Capsule: 20 μg, 50 μg

Calciferol™ Injection *see* ergocalciferol *on page 173*

Calciferol™ Oral *see* ergocalciferol *on page 173*

Calcijex™ *see* calcitriol *on next page*

Calcimar® *see* calcitonin (salmon) *on next page*

Calci-Mix™ [OTC] *see* calcium carbonate *on next page*

Calciparine® Injection *see* heparin *on page 226*

calcitonin (salmon) (kal si toe' nin)
Brand Names Calcimar®; Miacalcin®
Therapeutic Category Antidote, Hypercalcemia
Use Treatment of Paget's disease of bone and as adjunctive therapy for hypercalcemia; also used in postmenopausal osteoporosis
Usual Dosage Dosage for children not established
Hepatic osteodystrophy:
Infants: 5-7 µg/kg/day
Children and Adults: 20-100 µg/kg/day or every other day, titrate to obtain normal serum calcium/phosphate levels
Skin test: 1 unit/0.1 mL intracutaneously
Paget's disease: I.M., S.C.: 100 units/day
Postmenopause osteoporosis: I.M., S.C.: 100 units/day
Hypercalcemia: I.M., S.C.: 4 units/kg every 12 hours, may increase to maximum of 8 units/kg every 6 hours
Dosage Forms Injection:
Calcimar®: 200 units/mL (2 mL)
Miacalcin®: 100 units/mL (1 mL)

calcitriol (kal si trye' ole)
Brand Names Calcijex™; Rocaltrol®
Synonyms 1,25 dihydroxycholecalciferol
Therapeutic Category Vitamin D Analog
Use Management of hypocalcemia in patients on chronic renal dialysis; reduce elevated parathyroid hormone levels
Usual Dosage Individualize dosage to maintain calcium levels of 9-10 mg/dL

Renal failure: Oral:
Children: Initial: 15 ng/kg/day; maintenance: 30-60 ng/kg/day
Adults: 0.25 µg/day or every other day (may require 0.5-1 µg/day)
Unlabeled dose:
Renal failure: I.V.: Adults: 0.5 µg (0.01 µg/kg) 3 times/week; most doses in the range of 0.5-3 µg (0.01-0.05 µg/kg) 3 times/week
Hypoparathyroidism/pseudohypoparathyroidism: Oral:
Children 1-5 years: 0.25-0.75 µg/day
Children >6 years and Adults: 0.5-2 µg/day
Dosage Forms
Capsule: 0.25 µg, 0.5 µg
Injection: 1 µg/mL (1 mL); 2 µg/mL (1 mL)

calcium acetate
Brand Names Phos-Ex®; PhosLo®
Therapeutic Category Calcium Salt
Use Control of hyperphosphatemia in end stage renal failure and does not promote aluminum absorption
Usual Dosage Adults: Oral: 2 tablets with each meal; dosage may be increased to bring serum phosphate value to <6 mg/dL; most patients require 3-4 tablets with each meal
Dosage Forms
Capsule: 500 mg
Tablet: 250 mg, 667 mg, 1000 mg

calcium carbonate
Brand Names Alka-Mints® [OTC]; Amitone® [OTC]; Cal Carb-HD® [OTC]; Calci-Chew™ [OTC]; Calciday-667® [OTC]; Calci-Mix™ [OTC]; Cal-Plus® [OTC]; Caltrate® 600 [OTC]; Caltrate, Jr.® [OTC]; Chooz® [OTC]; Dicarbosil® [OTC]; Equilet® [OTC]; Florical® [OTC]; Gencalc® 600 [OTC]; Mallamint® [OTC]; Nephro-Calci® [OTC]; Os-Cal® 500 [OTC]; Oyst-Cal 500 [OTC]; Oystercal® 500; Rolaids® Calcium Rich [OTC]; Tums® [OTC]; Tums® E-X Extra Strength Tablet [OTC]; Tums® Extra Strength Liquid [OTC]
(Continued)

calcium carbonate *(Continued)*

Therapeutic Category Antacid; Antidote, Hyperphosphatemia; Calcium Salt
Use Antacid and calcium supplement; control of hyperphosphatemia in end stage renal failure and does not promote aluminum absorption
Usual Dosage Dosage is in terms of elemental calcium
Recommended daily allowance (RDA):
<6 months: 360 mg/day
6-12 months: 540 mg/day
1-10 years: 800 mg/day
10-18 years: 1200 mg/day
Adults: 800 mg/day

Hypocalcemia (dose depends on clinical condition and serum calcium level):
Neonates: 50-150 mg/kg/day in 4-6 divided doses; not to exceed 1 g/day
Children: 20-65 mg/kg/day in 4 divided doses
Adults: 1-2 g or more per day
Dosage Forms
Capsule:
Calci-Mix™: 1250 mg
Florical®: 364 mg with sodium fluoride 8.3 mg
Liquid (Tums® Extra Strength): 1000 mg/5 mL (360 mL)
Powder (Cal Carb-HD®): 6.5 g/packet
Suspension, oral: 1.25 g/5 mL
Tablet:
650 mg
Calciday-667®: 667 mg
Os-Cal® 500, Oyst-Cal 500, Oystercal® 500: 1.25 g
Cal-Plus®, Caltrate® 600, Gencalc® 600, Nephro-Calci®: 1.5 g
Chewable:
Alka-Mints®: 850 mg
Amitone®: 350 mg
Caltrate, Jr.®: 750 mg
Calci-Chew™, Os-Cal®: 750 mg
Chooz®, Dicarbosil®, Equilet®, Tums®: 500 mg
Mallamint®: 420 mg
Rolaids® Calcium Rich: 550 mg
Tums® E-X Extra Strength: 750 mg
Florical®: 364 mg with sodium fluoride 8.3 mg

calcium carbonate and simethicone

Brand Names Titralac® Plus Liquid [OTC]
Synonyms simethicone and calcium carbonate
Therapeutic Category Antacid
Use Relief of acid indigestion, heartburn, peptic esophagitis, hiatal hernia, and gas
Usual Dosage Oral: 0.5-2 g 4-6 times/day
Dosage Forms Liquid: Calcium carbonate 500 mg and simethicone 20 mg per 5 mL

calcium chloride

Therapeutic Category Calcium Salt; Electrolyte Supplement, Parenteral
Use Cardiac resuscitation when epinephrine fails to improve myocardial contractions, cardiac disturbances of hyperkalemia, hypocalcemia or calcium channel blocking agent toxicity
Usual Dosage I.V.:
Cardiac arrest in the presence of hyperkalemia or hypocalcemia, magnesium toxicity, or calcium antagonist toxicity:
Infants and Children: 10-20 mg/kg; may repeat in 10 minutes if necessary
Adults: 1.5-4 mg/kg/dose or 2.5-5 mL/dose every 10 minutes

Hypocalcemia:
Infants and Children: 10-20 mg/kg/dose, repeat every 4-6 hours if needed
Adults: 500 mg to 1 g at 1- to 3-day intervals

Exchange transfusion: 0.45 mEq after each 100 mL of blood exchanged I.V.

Hypocalcemia secondary to citrated blood transfusion give 0.45 mEq **elemental** calcium for each 100 mL citrated blood infused

Tetany:
Infants and Children: 10 mg/kg over 5-10 minutes. May repeat after 6 hours or follow with an infusion with a maximum dose of 200 mg/kg/day
Adults: 1 g over 10-30 minutes; may repeat after 6 hours
Dosage Forms Injection: 10% [100 mg/mL] (10 mL)

calcium citrate
Brand Names Citracal® [OTC]
Therapeutic Category Calcium Salt
Use Adjunct in prevention of postmenopausal osteoporosis, treatment and prevention of calcium depletion
Usual Dosage Oral (dosage is in terms of elemental calcium):
Adults: Oral: 1-2 g/day

Recommended daily allowance (RDA):
<6 months: 360 mg/day
6-12 months: 540 mg/day
1-10 years: 800 mg/day
10-18 years: 1200 mg/day
Adults: 800 mg/day
Dosage Forms
Tablet: 950 mg
Tablet, effervescent: 2376 mg

Calcium Disodium Versenate® see edetate calcium disodium *on page 166*

calcium EDTA see edetate calcium disodium *on page 166*

calcium glubionate (gloo bye' oh nate)
Brand Names Neo-Calglucon® [OTC]
Therapeutic Category Calcium Salt
Use Adjunct in prevention of postmenopausal osteoporosis, treatment and prevention of calcium depletion
Usual Dosage Oral (syrup is a hyperosmolar solution; dosage is in terms of calcium glubionate):

Neonatal hypocalcemia: 1200 mg/kg/day in 4-6 divided doses
Maintenance: Infants and Children: 600-2000 mg/kg/day in 4 divided doses up to a maximum of 9 g/day

Adults: 6-18 g/day in divided doses

Recommended daily allowance (RDA):
<6 months: 360 mg/day
6-12 months: 540 mg/day
1-10 years: 800 mg/day
10-18 years: 1200 mg/day
Adults: 800 mg/day
Dosage Forms Syrup: 1.8 g/5 mL (480 mL)

calcium gluceptate (gloo sep' tate)
Therapeutic Category Calcium Salt
Use Cardiac disturbances of hyperkalemia; cardiac resuscitation when epinephrine fails to improve myocardial contractions
Usual Dosage I.V.:
Cardiac resuscitation in the presence of hypocalcemia, hyperkalemia, or calcium channel blocker toxicity:
(Continued)

calcium gluceptate *(Continued)*

Children: 110 mg/kg/dose or 0.5 mL/kg/dose every 10 minutes
Adults: 5 mL every 10 minutes

Hypocalcemia:
Children: 200-500 mg/kg/day divided every 6 hours
Adults: 500 mg to 1.1 g/dose as needed

Exchange transfusion: 0.45 mEq (0.5 mL) after each 100 mL of blood exchanged

After citrated blood administration: Children and Adults: 0.4 mEq/100 mL blood infused

Dosage Forms Injection: 220 mg/mL (5 mL, 50 mL)

calcium gluconate (gloo' koe nate)

Brand Names Kalcinate®
Therapeutic Category Calcium Salt
Use Treatment and prevention of hypocalcemia, treatment of tetany, cardiac disturbances of hyperkalemia, cardiac resuscitation when epinephrine fails to improve myocardial contractions, hypocalcemia, or calcium chemical blocker toxicity
Usual Dosage Dosage is in terms of elemental calcium
Recommended daily allowance (RDA):
<6 months: 360 mg/day
6-12 months: 540 mg/day
1-10 years: 800 mg/day
10-18 years: 1200 mg/day
Adults: 800 mg/day

Calcium gluconate electrolyte requirement in newborn period:
Premature: 200-1000 mg/kg/24 hours
Term:
0-24 hours: 0-500 mg/kg/24 hours
24-48 hours: 200-500 mg/kg/24 hours
48-72 hours: 200-600 mg/kg/24 hours
>3 days: 200-800 mg/kg/24 hours

Hypocalcemia:
I.V.:
Neonates: 200-400 mg/kg/day as a continuous infusion or in 4 divided doses
Infants and Children: 200-1000 mg/kg/day as a continuous infusion or in 4 divided doses
Adults: 2-15 g/24 hours as a continuous infusion or in divided doses
Oral:
Children: 200-500 mg/kg/day divided every 6 hours
Adults: 500 mg to 2 g 2-4 times/day

Calcium antagonist toxicity, magnesium intoxication; cardiac arrest in the presence of hyperkalemia or hypocalcemia: I.V.:
Infants and Children: 100 mg/kg/dose
Adults: 1-3 g

Tetany: I.V.:
Neonates: 100-200 mg/kg/dose, may follow with 500 mg/kg/day in 3-4 divided doses or as an infusion
Infants and Children: 100-200 mg/kg/dose over 5-10 minutes; may repeat after 6 hours or follow with an infusion of 500 mg/kg/day
Adults: 1-3 g may be administered until therapeutic response occurs

Cardiac resuscitation: I.V.:
Infants and Children: 100 mg/kg/dose (1 mL/kg/dose) every 10 minutes
Adults: 500-800 mg/dose (5-8 mL) every 10 minutes

Hypocalcemia secondary to citrated blood infusion; give 0.45 mEq **elemental** calcium for each 100 mL citrated blood infused

Exchange transfusion:
Neonates: 100 mg/100 mL of citrated blood exchanged
Adults: 300 mg/100 mL of citrated blood exchanged

Maintenance electrolyte requirements for total parenteral nutrition: I.V.: Daily requirements: Adults: 10-20 mEq/1000 kcals/24 hours

Dosage Forms
Injection: 10% [100 mg/mL] (10 mL, 50 mL, 100 mL, 200 mL)
Tablet: 500 mg, 650 mg, 975 mg, 1 g

calcium lactate
Therapeutic Category Calcium Salt
Use Adjunct in prevention of postmenopausal osteoporosis, treatment and prevention of calcium depletion
Usual Dosage Oral:
Infants: 400-500 mg/kg/day divided every 4-6 hours
Children: 500 mg/kg/day divided every 6-8 hours; maximum daily dose: 9 g
Adults: 1.5-3 g divided every 8 hours
Dosage Forms Tablet: 325 mg, 650 mg

calcium leucovorin *see* leucovorin calcium *on page 268*

calcium pantothenate *see* pantothenic acid *on page 355*

calcium phosphate, dibasic
Brand Names Posture® [OTC]
Synonyms dicalcium phosphate
Therapeutic Category Calcium Salt
Use Adjunct in prevention of postmenopausal osteoporosis, treatment and prevention of calcium depletion
Usual Dosage Oral:
Children: 45-65 mg/kg/day <pJ[Adults: 1-2 g/day (doses in g of elemental calcium)
Dosage Forms Tablet, sugar free: 1565.2 mg

calcium polycarbophil (pol ee kar' boe fil)
Brand Names Equalactin® Chewablet Tablet [OTC]; Fiberall® Chewable Tablet [OTC]; FiberCon® Tablet [OTC]; Fiber-Lax® Tablet [OTC]; FiberNorm® [OTC]; Mitrolan® Chewable Tablet [OTC]
Therapeutic Category Antidiarrheal; Laxative, Bulk-Producing
Use Treatment of constipation or diarrhea by restoring a more normal moisture level and providing bulk in the patient's intestinal tract; calcium polycarbophil is supplied as the approved substitute whenever a bulk-forming laxative is ordered in a tablet, capsule, wafer, or other oral solid dosage form
Usual Dosage Oral:
Children:
2-6 years: 500 mg 1-2 times/day, up to 1.5 g/day
6-12 years: 500 mg 1-3 times/day, up to 3 g/day

Adults: 1 g 4 times/day, up to 6 g/day
Dosage Forms Tablet:
Sodium free:
Fiber-Lax®, FiberNorm®: 625 mg
FiberCon®: 500 mg
Chewable:
Equalactin®, Mitrolan®: 500 mg
Fiberall®: 1250 mg

69

calcium undecylenate *see* undecylenic acid and derivatives *on page 486*

Caldecort® Anti-Itch Topical Spray *see* hydrocortisone *on page 236*

Caldecort® Topical [OTC] *see* hydrocortisone *on page 236*

Calderol® *see* calcifediol *on page 64*

Caldesene® Topical [OTC] *see* undecylenic acid and derivatives *on page 486*

Calm-X® Oral [OTC] *see* dimenhydrinate *on page 150*

Cal-Plus® [OTC] *see* calcium carbonate *on page 65*

Caltrate® 600 [OTC] *see* calcium carbonate *on page 65*

Caltrate, Jr.® [OTC] *see* calcium carbonate *on page 65*

Cam-ap-es® *see* hydralazine, hydrochlorothiazide, and reserpine *on page 232*

Campho-Phenique® [OTC] *see* camphor and phenol *on this page*

camphor and phenol
Brand Names Campho-Phenique® [OTC]
Therapeutic Category Topical Skin Product
Use relief of pain and for minor infections
Usual Dosage Apply as needed
Dosage Forms Liquid: Camphor 10.8% and phenol 4.7%

camphorated tincture of opium *see* paregoric *on page 357*

camphor, menthol and phenol
Brand Names Sarna [OTC]
Therapeutic Category Topical Skin Product
Use Relief of dry, itching skin
Usual Dosage Topical: Apply as needed for dry skin
Dosage Forms Lotion, topical: Camphor 0.5%, menthol 0.5%, and phenol 0.5% in emollient base (240 mL)

Candida albicans (Monilia) (kan' dee daa al' bee kans mo nill' ya)
Brand Names Dermatophytin-O
Synonyms *Monilia* skin test
Therapeutic Category Diagnostic Agent, Fungus
Use Screen for detection of nonresponsiveness to antigens in immunocompromised individuals
Usual Dosage 0.1 mL intradermally, examine reaction site in 24-48 hours; induration of ≥ 5 mm in diameter is a positive reaction
Dosage Forms Injection:
 Intradermal: 1:100 (5 mL)
 Scratch: 1:10 (5 mL)

Cankaid® Oral [OTC] *see* carbamide peroxide *on page 73*

cantharidin (can thar' e din)
Brand Names Verr-Canth™
Therapeutic Category Keratolytic Agent
Use Removal of ordinary and periungual warts
Usual Dosage Topical: Apply directly to lesion, cover with nonporous tape, remove tape in 24 hours, reapply if necessary
Dosage Forms Liquid: 0.7% in a film-forming vehicle containing acetone, pyroxylin, castor oil and camphor (7.5 mL)

Cantil® *see* mepenzolate bromide *on page 292*
Capastat® Sulfate *see* capreomycin sulfate *on this page*
Capital® and Codeine *see* acetaminophen and codeine *on page 3*
Capitrol® *see* chloroxine *on page 93*
Capoten® *see* captopril *on this page*
Capozide® *see* captopril and hydrochlorothiazide *on this page*

capreomycin sulfate (kap ree oh mye' sin)
Brand Names Capastat® Sulfate
Therapeutic Category Antibiotic, Miscellaneous; Antitubercular Agent
Use In conjunction with at least one other antituberculosis agent in the treatment of tuberculosis
Usual Dosage Adults: I.M.: 15 mg/kg/day up to 1 g/day for 60-120 days
Dosage Forms Injection: 100 mg/mL (10 mL)

capsaicin (kap say' sin)
Brand Names Zostrix-® HP Topical [OTC]; Zostrix® Topical [OTC]
Therapeutic Category Analgesic, Topical; Topical Skin Product
Use
Zostrix®: Temporary relief of pain (neuralgia) following herpes zoster infections
Zostrix-® HP: Relief of neuralgias such as diabetic neuropathy and postsurgical pain
Usual Dosage Children >2 years and Adults: Apply to area up to 3-4 times/day only
Dosage Forms Cream: 0.025% (45 g, 90 g); 0.075% (30 g, 60 g)

captopril (kap' toe pril)
Brand Names Capoten®
Therapeutic Category Angiotensin Converting Enzyme (ACE) Inhibitors
Use Management of hypertension and treatment of congestive heart failure; increase circulation in Raynaud's phenomenon; idiopathic edema
Usual Dosage Note: Dosage must be titrated according to patient's response; use lowest effective dose. Oral:
Neonates: Initial: 0.05-0.1 mg/kg/dose every 8-24 hours; titrate dose up to 0.5 mg/kg/dose given every 6-24 hours
Infants: Initial: 0.15-0.3 mg/kg/dose; titrate dose upward to maximum of 6 mg/kg/day in 1-4 divided doses; usual required dose: 2.5-6 mg/kg/day
Children: Initial: 0.5 mg/kg/dose; titrate upward to maximum of 6 mg/kg/day in 2-4 divided doses
Older Children: Initial: 6.25-12.5 mg/dose every 12-24 hours; titrate upward to maximum of 6 mg/kg/day
Adolescents and Adults: Initial: 12.5-25 mg/dose given every 8-12 hours; increase by 25 mg/dose to maximum of 450 mg/day
Note: Smaller dosages given every 8-12 hours are indicated in patients with renal dysfunction. Renal function and leukocyte count should be carefully monitored during therapy.
Dosage Forms Tablet: 12.5 mg, 25 mg, 50 mg, 100 mg

captopril and hydrochlorothiazide
Brand Names Capozide®
Therapeutic Category Antihypertensive, Combination
Use Management of hypertension and treatment of congestive heart failure
Usual Dosage Adults: Oral:
Hypertension: Initial: 25 mg 2-3 times/day; may increase at 1- to 2-week intervals up to 150 mg 3 times/day (captopril dosages)
(Continued)

captopril and hydrochlorothiazide *(Continued)*

Congestive heart failure: 6.25-25 mg 3 times/day (maximum: 450 mg/day) (captopril dosages)

Dosage Forms Tablet:
25/15: Captopril 25 mg and hydrochlorothiazide 15 mg
25/25: Captopril 25 mg and hydrochlorothiazide 25 mg
50/15: Captopril 50 mg and hydrochlorothiazide 15 mg
50/25: Captopril 50 mg and hydrochlorothiazide 25 mg

Carafate® *see* sucralfate *on page 445*

caramiphen and phenylpropanolamine

Brand Names Ordine AT® Extended Release Capsule; Rescaps-D® S.R. Capsule; Tuss-Allergine® Modified T.D. Capsule; Tuss-Genade® Modified Capsule; Tussogest® Extended Release Capsule; Tuss-Ornade® Liquid; Tuss-Ornade® Spansule®
Synonyms phenylpropanolamine and caramiphen
Therapeutic Category Antihistamine/Decongestant Combination
Use Symptomatic relief of cough and nasal congestion associated with the common cold
Usual Dosage Oral:
Children:
2-6 years: $\frac{1}{2}$ teaspoonful every 4 hours
6-12 years: 1 teaspoonful every 4 hours

Children >12 years and Adults: 1 capsule every 12 hours or 2 teaspoonfuls every 4 hours
Dosage Forms
Capsule, timed release: Caramiphen edisylate 40 mg and phenylpropanolamine hydrochloride 75 mg
Liquid: Caramiphen edisylate 6.7 mg and phenylpropanolamine hydrochloride 12.5 mg per 5 mL

carampicillin hydrochloride *see* bacampicillin hydrochloride *on page 42*

carbachol (kar' ba kole)

Brand Names Isopto® Carbachol Ophthalmic; Miostat® Intraocular
Synonyms carbacholine; carbamylcholine chloride
Therapeutic Category Cholinergic Agent, Ophthalmic; Ophthalmic Agent, Miotic
Use Lower intraocular pressure in the treatment of glaucoma; to cause miosis during surgery
Usual Dosage Adults:
Ophthalmic: Instill 1-2 drops up to 4 times/day
Intraocular: 0.5 mL instilled into anterior chamber before or after securing sutures
Dosage Forms Solution:
Intraocular (Miostat®): 0.01% (1.5 mL)
Topical, ophthalmic (Isopto® Carbachol): 0.75% (15 mL, 30 mL); 1.5% (15 mL, 30 mL); 2.25% (15 mL); 3% (15 mL, 30 mL)

carbacholine *see* carbachol *on this page*

carbamazepine (kar ba maz' e peen)

Brand Names Epitol®; Tegretol®
Therapeutic Category Anticonvulsant, Miscellaneous
Use Prophylaxis of generalized tonic-clonic, partial (especially complex partial), and mixed partial or generalized seizure disorder; may be used to relieve pain in trigeminal neuralgia or diabetic neuropathy; has been used to treat bipolar disorders
Usual Dosage Oral (dosage must be adjusted according to patient's response and serum concentrations):

Children:
> <6 years: Initial: 5 mg/kg/day; dosage may be increased every 5-7 days to 10 mg/kg/day; then up to 20 mg/kg/day if necessary; administer in 2-4 divided doses/day
>
> 6-12 years: Initial: 100 mg twice daily or 10 mg/kg/day in 2 divided doses; increase by 100 mg/day depending upon response; usual maintenance: 15-30 mg/kg/day in 2-4 divided doses/day; maximum: 1000 mg/24 hours

Children >12 years and Adults: 200 mg twice daily to start, increase by 200 mg/day at weekly intervals until therapeutic levels achieved; usual dose: 800-1200 mg/day in 3-4 divided doses; some patients have required up to 1.6-2.4 g/day

Dosage Forms
Suspension, oral (citrus-vanilla flavor): 100 mg/5 mL (450 mL)
Tablet: 200 mg
Tablet, chewable: 100 mg

carbamide see urea on page 487

carbamide peroxide (kar' ba mide per ox' ide)
Brand Names Auro® Ear Drops [OTC]; Cankaid® Oral [OTC]; Debrox® Otic [OTC]; Gly-Oxide® Oral [OTC]; Murine® Ear Drops [OTC]; Orajel® Brace-Aid Rinse [OTC]; Proxigel® Oral [OTC]
Synonyms urea peroxide
Therapeutic Category Anti-infective Agent, Oral; Otic Agent, Cerumenolytic
Use Relief of minor inflammation of gums, oral mucosal surfaces and lips including canker sores and dental irritation; emulsify and disperse ear wax
Usual Dosage Children >12 years and Adults:
Oral: Apply several drops undiluted to affected area of the mouth 4 times/day and at bedtime for up to 7 days, expectorate after 2-3 minutes; as an adjunct to oral hygiene after brushing, swish 10 drops for 2-3 minutes, then expectorate; gel: massage on affected area 4 times/day
Otic: Instill 5-10 drops twice daily for up to 4 days; keep drops in ear for several minutes by keeping head tilted or placing cotton in ear
Dosage Forms
Gel, oral (Proxigel®): 11% (36 g)
Solution:
Oral (Cankaid®, Gly-Oxide®, Orajel® Brace-Aid Rinse): 10% in glycerin (15 mL, 22.5 mL, 30 mL, 60 mL)
Otic (Auro® Ear Drops, Debrox®, Murine® Ear Drops): 6.5% in glycerin (15 mL, 30 mL)

carbamylcholine chloride see carbachol on previous page

carbenicillin (kar ben i sill' in)
Brand Names Geocillin®
Synonyms carindacillin
Therapeutic Category Antibiotic, Penicillin
Use Treatment of serious infections caused by susceptible gram-negative aerobic bacilli or mixed aerobic-anaerobic bacterial infections and/or urinary tract infections
Usual Dosage Oral:
Children: 30-50 mg/kg/day divided every 6 hours; maximum dose: 2-3 g/day
Adults: 1-2 tablets every 6 hours
Dosage Forms Tablet, film coated: 382 mg

carbidopa (kar bi doe' pa)
Brand Names Lodosyn®
Therapeutic Category Antiparkinson Agent
Use Given with levodopa in the treatment of parkinsonism to enable a lower dosage of the latter to be used and a more rapid response to be obtained, and to decrease side-effects; for details of administration and dosage, see Levodopa
(Continued)

carbidopa *(Continued)*
Usual Dosage Adults: Oral: 70-100 mg/day; maximum daily dose: 200 mg
Dosage Forms Tablet: 25 mg

carbidopa and levodopa *see* levodopa and carbidopa *on page 270*

carbinoxamine and pseudoephedrine
(kar bi nox' a meen & soo doe e fed' rin)
Brand Names Carbiset® Tablet; Carbiset-TR® Tablet; Carbodec® Syrup; Carbodec® Tablet; Carbodec TR® Tablet; Cardec-S® Syrup; Rondec® Drops; Rondec® Filmtab®; Rondec® Syrup; Rondec-TR®
Therapeutic Category Antihistamine/Decongestant Combination
Use Perennial and seasonal allergic rhinitis and other allergic symptoms including urticaria
Usual Dosage Oral:
Children:
Drops: 1-18 months: 0.25-1 mL 4 times/day
Syrup:
18 months to 6 years: 2.5 mL 3-4 times/day
>6 years: 5 mL 2-4 times/day
Adults:
Liquid: 5 mL 4 times/day
Tablets: 1 tablet 4 times/day
Dosage Forms
Drops: Carbinoxamine maleate 2 mg and pseudoephedrine hydrochloride 25 mg per mL (30 mL with dropper)
Syrup: Carbinoxamine maleate 4 mg and pseudoephedrine hydrochloride 60 mg per 5 mL (120 mL, 480 mL)
Tablet:
Film-coated: Carbinoxamine maleate 4 mg and pseudoephedrine hydrochloride 60 mg
Sustained release: Carbinoxamine maleate 8 mg and pseudoephedrine hydrochloride 120 mg

carbinoxamine, pseudoephedrine, and dextromethorphan
Brand Names Carbodec DM®; Cardec DM®; Pseudo-Car® DM; Rondamine-DM® Drops; Rondec®-DM; Tussafed® Drops
Therapeutic Category Antihistamine/Decongestant Combination; Cough Preparation
Use Relief of coughs and upper respiratory symptoms, including nasal congestion, associated with allergy or the common cold
Usual Dosage
Infants: Drops:
1-3 months: $\frac{1}{4}$ mL 4 times/day
3-6 months: $\frac{1}{2}$ mL 4 times/day
6-9 months: $\frac{3}{4}$ mL 4 times/day
9-18 months: 1 mL 4 times/day
Children 1$\frac{1}{2}$ to 6 years: Syrup: 2.5 mL 4 times/day
Children >6 years and Adults: Syrup: 5 mL 4 times/day
Dosage Forms
Drops: Carbinoxamine maleate 2 mg, pseudoephedrine hydrochloride 25 mg, and dextromethorphan hydrobromide 4 mg per mL (30 mL)
Syrup: Carbinoxamine maleate 4 mg, pseudoephedrine hydrochloride 60 mg, and dextromethorphan hydrobromide 15 mg per 5 (120 mL, 480 mL, 4000 mL)

Carbiset® Tablet *see* carbinoxamine and pseudoephedrine *on this page*
Carbiset-TR® Tablet *see* carbinoxamine and pseudoephedrine *on this page*
Carbocaine® Injection *see* mepivacaine hydrochloride *on page 293*

Carbodec DM® *see* carbinoxamine, pseudoephedrine, and dextromethorphan *on previous page*

Carbodec® Syrup *see* carbinoxamine and pseudoephedrine *on previous page*

Carbodec® Tablet *see* carbinoxamine and pseudoephedrine *on previous page*

Carbodec TR® Tablet *see* carbinoxamine and pseudoephedrine *on previous page*

carbol-fuchsin solution (kar bol fook' sin)
Synonyms Castellani paint
Therapeutic Category Antifungal Agent, Topical
Use Treatment of superficial mycotic infections
Usual Dosage Topical: Apply to affected area 2-4 times/day
Dosage Forms Solution: Basic fuchsin 0.3%, boric acid 1%, phenol 4.5%, resorcinol 10%, acetone 5%, and alcohol 10%

carbolic acid *see* phenol *on page 369*

carboplatin (kar' boe pla tin)
Brand Names Paraplatin®
Synonyms CBDCA
Therapeutic Category Antineoplastic Agent, Alkylating Agent
Use Ovarian carcinoma, cervical, small cell lung carcinoma, esophagus, testicular, bladder cancer, mesothelioma, pediatric brain tumors
Usual Dosage Refer to individual protocols
 I.V.
 Children:
  Solid tumor: 560 mg/m^2 once every 4 weeks
  Brain tumor: 175 mg/m^2 once weekly for 4 weeks with a 2 week recovery period between courses; dose is then adjusted on platelet count and neutrophil count values
 Adults: Single agent: 360 mg/m^2 once every 4 weeks; dose is then adjusted on platelet count and neutrophil count values
Dosage Forms Powder for injection, lyophilized: 50 mg, 150 mg, 450 mg

carboprost tromethamine (kar' boe prost tro meth' a meen)
Formerly Known As Prostin/15M®
Brand Names Hemabate™
Therapeutic Category Abortifacient; Prostaglandin
Use Termination of pregnancy
Usual Dosage I.M.: 250 μg to start, 250 μg at 1$^1/_2$-hour to 3$^1/_2$-hour intervals depending on uterine response; a 500 μg/dose may be given if uterine response is not adequate after several 250 μg/dose
Dosage Forms Injection: Carboprost 250 μg and tromethamine 83 μg per mL (1 mL)

carbose d *see* carboxymethylcellulose sodium *on this page*

carboxymethylcellulose sodium (kar box ee meth ill sell' yoo lose)
Brand Names Celluvisc® [OTC]
Synonyms carbose d
Therapeutic Category Ophthalmic Agent, Miscellaneous
Use Preservative free artificial tear substitute
Usual Dosage Adults: Oral: 1.5 g 3-4 times/day
Dosage Forms Solution, ophthalmic, preservative free: 1% (0.3 mL)

ALPHABETICAL LISTING OF DRUGS

Cardec DM® *see* carbinoxamine, pseudoephedrine, and dextromethorphan *on page 74*

Cardec-S® Syrup *see* carbinoxamine and pseudoephedrine *on page 74*

Cardene® *see* nicardipine hydrochloride *on page 333*

Cardene® SR *see* nicardipine hydrochloride *on page 333*

Cardilate® *see* erythrityl tetranitrate *on page 174*

Cardio-Green® *see* indocyanine green *on page 249*

Cardioquin® Oral *see* quinidine *on page 411*

Cardizem® CD *see* diltiazem hydrochloride *on page 150*

Cardizem® Injectable *see* diltiazem hydrochloride *on page 150*

Cardizem® SR *see* diltiazem hydrochloride *on page 150*

Cardizem® Tablet *see* diltiazem hydrochloride *on page 150*

Cardura® *see* doxazosin mesylate *on page 160*

carindacillin *see* carbenicillin *on page 73*

carisoprodate *see* carisoprodol *on this page*

carisoprodol (kar eye soe proe' dole)
Brand Names Rela®; Sodol®; Soma®; Soma® Compound; Soprodol®; Soridol®
Synonyms carisoprodate; isobamate
Therapeutic Category Skeletal Muscle Relaxant
Use Skeletal muscle relaxant
Usual Dosage Adults: Oral: 350 mg 3-4 times/day; take last dose at bedtime; compound: 1-2 tablets 4 times/day
Dosage Forms Tablet:
Rela®, Sodol®, Soma®, Soprodol®, Soridol®: 350 mg
Soma® Compound: Carisoprodol 200 mg and aspirin 325 mg

Carmol-HC® Topical *see* urea and hydrocortisone *on page 488*

Carmol® Topical [OTC] *see* urea *on page 487*

carmustine (kar mus' teen)
Brand Names BiCNU®
Synonyms BCNU
Therapeutic Category Antineoplastic Agent, Alkylating Agent (Nitrosourea)
Use Brain tumors, multiple myeloma and Hodgkin's disease and non-Hodgkin's lymphomas, melanoma, lung cancer
Usual Dosage Refer to individual protocols
Children and Adults: I.V. infusion: 75-100 mg/m^2/day for 2 days or 150-200 mg/m^2 every 6 weeks as a single dose or divided into daily injections on 2 successive days; next dose is to be determined based on hematologic response to the previous dose
Dosage Forms Powder for injection: 100 mg/vial packaged with 3 mL of absolute alcohol for use as a sterile diluent

Carnitor® Injection *see* levocarnitine *on page 270*

Carnitor® Oral *see* levocarnitine *on page 270*

carteolol hydrochloride (kar' tee oh lole)
Brand Names Cartrol® Oral; Ocupress® Ophthalmic
Therapeutic Category Beta-Adrenergic Blocker; Beta-Adrenergic Blocker, Ophthalmic
Use Management of hypertension; treatment of increased intraocular pressure

Usual Dosage Adults:
Oral: 2.5 mg as a single daily dose, with a maintenance dose normally 2.5-5 mg once daily
Ophthalmic: 1 drop in eye(s) twice daily
Dosage Forms
Solution, ophthalmic (Ocupress®): 1% (5 mL, 10 mL)
Tablet (Cartrol®): 2.5 mg, 5 mg

Carter's Little Pills® [OTC] see bisacodyl on page 54

Cartrol® Oral see carteolol hydrochloride on previous page

casanthranol and docusate see docusate and casanthranol on page 158

cascara sagrada (kas kar' a)
Therapeutic Category Laxative, Stimulant
Use Temporary relief of constipation; sometimes used with milk of magnesia ("black and white" mixture)
Usual Dosage Note: Cascara sagrada fluid extract is 5 times more potent than cascara sagrada aromatic fluid extract.

Oral (aromatic fluid extract):
Infants: 1.25 mL/day (range: 0.5-1.5 mL) as needed
Children 2-11 years: 2.5 mL/day (range: 1-3 mL) as needed
Children ≥12 years and Adults: 5 mL/day (range: 2-6 mL) as needed at bedtime (1 tablet as needed at bedtime)
Dosage Forms
Liquid, aromatic fluid extract: 5 mL, 120 mL
Tablet: 325 mg

Castellani paint see carbol-fuchsin solution on page 75

castor oil
Brand Names Alphamul® [OTC]; Emulsoil® [OTC]; Fleet® Flavored Castor Oil [OTC]; Neoloid® [OTC]; Purge® [OTC]
Synonyms oleum ricini
Therapeutic Category Laxative, Stimulant
Use Preparation for rectal or bowel examination or surgery; rarely used to relieve constipation; also applied to skin as emollient and protectant
Usual Dosage Oral:
Castor oil:
Infants <2 years: 1-5 mL or 15 mL/m^2/dose as a single dose
Children 2-11 years: 5-15 mL as a single dose
Children ≥12 years and Adults: 15-60 mL as a single dose

Emulsified castor oil:
Infants: 2.5-7.5 mL/dose
Children <2 years: 5-15 mL/dose
Children 2-11 years: 7.5-30 mL/dose
Children ≥12 years and Adults: 30-60 mL/dose
Dosage Forms
Emulsion, oral:
Alphamul®: 60% (90 mL, 3780 mL)
Emulsoil®: 95% (63 mL)
Fleet® Flavored Castor Oil: 67% (45 mL, 90 mL)
Neoloid®: 36.4% (118 mL)
Liquid, oral:
100% (60 mL, 120 mL, 480 mL)
Purge®: 95% (30 mL, 60 mL)

Cataflam® Oral *see* diclofenac *on page 144*

Catapres® Oral *see* clonidine *on page 108*

Catapres-TTS® Transdermal *see* clonidine *on page 108*

Catarase® *see* chymotrypsin *on page 101*

CBDCA *see* carboplatin *on page 75*

CCNU *see* lomustine *on page 277*

C-Crystals® [OTC] *see* ascorbic acid *on page 33*

2-CdA *see* cladribine *on page 104*

CDDP *see* cisplatin *on page 103*

Ceclor® *see* cefaclor *on this page*

Cecon® [OTC] *see* ascorbic acid *on page 33*

CeeNU® Oral *see* lomustine *on page 277*

Ceepryn® [OTC] *see* cetylpyridinium chloride *on page 85*

cefaclor (sef' a klor)
Brand Names Ceclor®
Therapeutic Category Antibiotic, Cephalosporin (Second Generation)
Use Infections caused by susceptible organisms involving the respiratory tract, otitis media, sinusitis, skin and skin structure, bone and joint, and urinary tract and gynecologic as well as septicemia
Usual Dosage Oral:
  Children >1 month: 20-40 mg/kg/day divided every 8-12 hours; maximum dose: 2 g/day (twice daily option is for treatment of otitis media or pharyngitis)
  Adults: 250-500 mg every 8 hours or daily dose can be given in 2 divided doses
Dosage Forms
  Capsule: 250 mg, 500 mg
  Powder for oral suspension (strawberry flavor): 125 mg/5 mL (75 mL, 150 mL); 187 mg/5 mL (50 mL, 100 mL); 250 mg/5 mL (75 mL, 150 mL); 375 mg/5 mL (50 mL, 100 mL)

cefadroxil monohydrate (sef a drox' ill)
Brand Names Duricef®; Ultracef®
Therapeutic Category Antibiotic, Cephalosporin (First Generation)
Use Treatment of susceptible bacterial infections, including those caused by group A beta-hemolytic *Streptococcus*
Usual Dosage Oral:
  Children: 30 mg/kg/day divided twice daily up to a maximum of 2 g/day
  Adults: 1-2 g/day in 2 divided doses
Dosage Forms
  Capsule, as monohydrate: 500 mg
  Powder for oral suspension: 125 mg/5 mL (50 mL, 100 mL); 250 mg/5 mL (50 mL, 100 mL); 500 mg/5 mL (50 mL, 100 mL)
  Tablet, as monohydrate: 1 g

Cefadyl® *see* cephapirin sodium *on page 84*

cefamandole nafate (sef a man' dole)
Brand Names Mandol®
Therapeutic Category Antibiotic, Cephalosporin (Second Generation)
Use Treatment of susceptible bacterial infection; mainly respiratory tract, skin and skin structure, bone and joint, urinary tract and gynecologic as well as septicemia, perioperative prophylaxis

Usual Dosage I.M., I.V.:
Children: 100-150 mg/kg/day in divided doses every 4-6 hours
Adults: 4-12 g/24 hours divided every 4-6 hours 500-1000 mg every 4-8 hours
Dosage Forms Powder for injection: 500 mg (10 mL); 1 g (10 mL, 100 mL); 2 g (20 mL, 100 mL); 10 g (100 mL)

Cefanex® *see* cephalexin monohydrate *on page 84*

cefazolin sodium (sef a' zoe lin)
Brand Names Ancef®; Kefzol®; Zolicef®
Therapeutic Category Antibiotic, Cephalosporin (First Generation)
Use Treatment of gram-positive bacilli and cocci (except enterococcus); some gram-negative bacilli including *E. coli*, *Proteus*, and *Klebsiella* may be susceptible
Usual Dosage I.M., I.V.:
Neonates:
Postnatal age <7 days: 40 mg/kg/day divided every 12 hours
Postnatal age >7 days:
<2000 g: 40 mg/kg/day in 2 divided doses
>2000 g: 60 mg/kg/day in 3 divided doses
Infants and Children: 50-100 mg/kg/day in 3 divided doses; maximum dose: 6 g/day
Adults: 1-2 g every 8 hours
Dosage Forms
Infusion, premixed, in D_5W (frozen) (Ancef®): 500 mg (50 mL); 1 g (50 mL)
Injection (Kefzol®): 500 mg, 1 g
Powder for injection (Ancef®, Zolicef®): 250 mg, 500 mg, 1 g, 5 g, 10 g, 20 g

cefixime (sef ix' eem)
Brand Names Suprax®
Therapeutic Category Antibiotic, Cephalosporin (Third Generation)
Use Treatment of urinary tract infections, otitis media, respiratory infections due to susceptible organisms; documented poor compliance with other oral antimicrobials; outpatient therapy of serious soft tissue or skeletal infections due to susceptible organisms.
Usual Dosage Oral:
Children: 8 mg/kg/day in 1-2 divided doses; maximum dose: 400 mg/day
Children >50 kg or >12 years and Adults: 400 mg/day in 1-2 divided doses
Dosage Forms
Powder for oral suspension (strawberry flavor): 100 mg/5 mL (50 mL, 100 mL)
Tablet, film coated: 200 mg, 400 mg

Cefizox® *see* ceftizoxime sodium *on page 82*

cefmetazole sodium (sef met' a zole)
Brand Names Zefazone®
Therapeutic Category Antibiotic, Cephalosporin (Second Generation)
Use Second generation cephalosporin with an antibacterial spectrum similar to cefoxitin, useful on many aerobic and anaerobic gram-positive and gram-negative bacteria
Usual Dosage Adults: I.V.:
Infections: 2 g every 6-12 hours for 5-14 days
Prophylaxis: 2 g 30-90 minutes before surgery
Dosage Forms Powder for injection: 1 g, 2 g

Cefobid® *see* cefoperazone sodium *on next page*

cefonicid sodium (se fon' i sid)
Brand Names Monocid®
Therapeutic Category Antibiotic, Cephalosporin (Second Generation)
Use Treatment of susceptible bacterial infection; mainly respiratory tract, skin and skin structure, bone and joint, urinary tract and gynecologic as well as septicemia; second generation cephalosporin
Usual Dosage Adults: I.M., I.V.: 1 g every 24 hours
Dosage Forms Powder for injection: 500 mg, 1 g, 10 g

cefoperazone sodium (sef oh per' a zone)
Brand Names Cefobid®
Therapeutic Category Antibiotic, Cephalosporin (Third Generation)
Use Treatment of susceptible bacterial infection; mainly respiratory tract, skin and skin structure, bone and joint, urinary tract and gynecologic as well as septicemia
Usual Dosage I.M., I.V.:
Neonates: 50 mg/kg/dose every 12 hours
Children: 100-150 mg/kg/day divided every 8-12 hours
Adults: 2-4 g/day in divided doses every 12 hours (up to 12 g/day)
Dosage Forms
Injection, premixed (frozen): 1 g (50 mL); 2 g (50 mL)
Powder for infection: 1 g, 2 g

Cefotan® *see cefotetan disodium on this page*

cefotaxime sodium (sef oh taks' eem)
Brand Names Claforan®
Therapeutic Category Antibiotic, Cephalosporin (Third Generation)
Use Treatment of a documented or suspected meningitis due to susceptible organisms; nonpseudomonal gram-negative rod infection in a patient at risk of developing aminoglycoside-induced nephrotoxicity and/or ototoxicity; infection due to an organism whose susceptibilities clearly favor cefotaxime over cefuroxime or an aminoglycoside
Usual Dosage I.M., I.V.:
Neonates:
Postnatal age <7 days: 100 mg/kg/day in 2 divided doses
Postnatal age >7 days:
<1200 g: 100 mg/kg/day divided every 12 hours
>1200 g: 150 mg/kg/day in 3 divided doses

Infants and Children 1 month to 12 years:
<50 kg: 100-200 mg/kg/day in 3-4 divided doses
Meningitis: 200 mg/kg/day in 4 divided doses
>50 kg: Moderate to severe infection: 1-2 g every 6-8 hours; life-threatening infection: 2 g/dose every 4 hours; maximum dose: 12 g/day

Children >12 years and Adults: 1-2 g every 6-8 hours (up to 12 g/day)
Dosage Forms
Infusion, premixed, in D$_5$W (frozen): 1 g (50 mL); 2 g (50 mL)
Powder for injection: 1 g, 2 g, 10 g

cefotetan disodium (sef' oh tee tan)
Brand Names Cefotan®
Therapeutic Category Antibiotic, Cephalosporin (Second Generation)
Use Treatment of susceptible bacterial infection; mainly respiratory tract, skin and skin structure, bone and joint, urinary tract and gynecologic as well as septicemia
Usual Dosage I.M., I.V.:
Children: 40-80 mg/kg/day divided every 12 hours

Adults: 1-6 g/day in divided doses every 12 hours, 1-2 g may be given every 24 hours for urinary tract infection

Dosage Forms Powder for injection: 1 g (10 mL, 100 mL); 2 g (20 mL, 100 mL); 10 g (100 mL)

cefoxitin sodium (se fox' i tin)
Brand Names Mefoxin®
Therapeutic Category Antibiotic, Cephalosporin (Second Generation)
Use Less active against staphylococci and streptococci than first generation cephalo-sporins, but active against anaerobes including *Bacteroides fragilis*; active against gram-negative enteric bacilli including *E. coli*, *Klebsiella*, and *Proteus*
Usual Dosage I.M., I.V.:
Infants >3 months and Children:
Mild-moderate infection: 80-100 mg/kg/day in divided doses every 4-6 hours
Severe infection: 100-160 mg/kg/day in divided doses every 4-6 hours
Maximum dose: 12 g/day

Adults: 1-2 g every 6-8 hours (I.M. injection is painful)
Dosage Forms
Infusion, premixed, in D₅W (frozen): 1 g (50 mL); 2 g (50 mL)
Powder for injection: 1 g, 2 g, 10 g

cefpodoxime proxetil (sef pode ox' eem)
Brand Names Vantin®
Therapeutic Category Antibiotic, Cephalosporin (Second Generation)
Use Infections caused by susceptible organisms involving the respiratory tract, otitis media, sinusitis, skin and skin structure, bone and joint, and urinary tract and gynecologic as well as septicemia
Usual Dosage Oral:
Children >6 months to 12 years: 10 mg/kg/day, divided every 12 hours, for 10 days
Adults: 100-400 mg every 12 hours, for 7-14 days
Dosage Forms
Granules for oral suspension (lemon creme flavor): 50 mg/5 mL (100 mL); 100 mg/5 mL (100 mL)
Tablet, film coated: 100 mg, 200 mg

cefprozil (sef proe' zil)
Brand Names Cefzil™
Therapeutic Category Antibiotic, Cephalosporin (Second Generation)
Use Infections caused by susceptible organisms involving the respiratory tract, otitis media, sinusitis, skin and skin structure, bone and joint, and urinary tract and gynecologic as well as septicemia
Usual Dosage Oral:
Infants and Children >6 months to 12 years: 7.5-15 mg/kg every 12 hours for 10 days
Children >13 years and Adults: 250-500 mg every 12-24 hours for 10 days
Dosage Forms
Powder for oral suspension, as anhydrous: 125 mg/5 mL (50 mL, 75 mL, 100 mL); 250 mg/5 mL (50 mL, 75 mL, 100 mL)
Tablet, as anhydrous: 250 mg, 500 mg

ceftazidime (sef' tay zi deem)
Brand Names Ceptaz™; Fortaz®; Pentacef™; Tazicef®; Tazidime®
Therapeutic Category Antibiotic, Cephalosporin (Third Generation)
Use Treatment of documented susceptible *Pseudomonas aeruginosa* infection; *Pseudomonas* infection in patient at risk of developing aminoglycoside-induced nephrotoxicity and/or ototoxicity; empiric therapy of a febrile, granulocytopenic patient
Usual Dosage
Neonates:
Postnatal age <7 days: 30-50 mg/kg/dose every 12 hours
(Continued)

ceftazidime *(Continued)*
Postnatal age >7 days: 30-50 mg/kg/dose every 8 hours

Infants and Children 1 month to 12 years: 30-50 mg/kg/dose every 8 hours; maximum dose: 6 g/day

Adults: 1-2 g every 8-12 hours (250-500 mg every 12 hours for urinary tract infections)
Dosage Forms
Infusion, premixed (frozen) (Fortaz®): 1 g (50 mL); 2 g (50 mL)
Powder for injection: 500 mg, 1 g, 2 g, 6 g

Ceftin® Oral *see cefuroxime on next page*

ceftizoxime sodium (sef ti zox' eem)
Brand Names Cefizox®
Therapeutic Category Antibiotic, Cephalosporin (Third Generation)
Use Treatment of susceptible bacterial infection; mainly respiratory tract, skin and skin structure, bone and joint, urinary tract and gynecologic as well as septicemia
Usual Dosage I.M., I.V.:
Children ≥6 months: 50 mg/kg every 6-8 hours to 200 mg/kg/day to maximum of 12 g/24 hours

Adults: 1-2 g every 8-12 hours, up to 2 g every 4 hours or 4 g every 8 hours for life-threatening infections
Dosage Forms
Injection, in D_5W (frozen): 1 g (50 mL); 2 g (50 mL)
Powder for injection: 500 mg, 1 g, 2 g, 10 g

ceftriaxone sodium (sef try ax' one)
Brand Names Rocephin®
Therapeutic Category Antibiotic, Cephalosporin (Third Generation)
Use Treatment of documented infection due to susceptible organisms in patients without I.V. line access; documented or suspected infection due to susceptible organisms in home care patients; treatment of documented or suspected gonococcal infection or chancroid; emergency room management of patients at high risk for bacteremia, periorbital or buccal cellulitis, salmonellosis or shigellosis and pneumonia of unestablished etiology (<5 years of age)
Usual Dosage
Neonates: I.M., I.V.:
Postnatal age <7 days: 50 mg/kg/day given every 24 hours
Postnatal age >7 days:
<2000 g: 50 mg/kg/day given every 24 hours
>2000 g: 75 mg/kg/day given every 24 hours

Gonococcal prophylaxis:
LBW neonates: 25-50 mg/kg as a single dose (dose not to exceed 125 mg)
Neonates: 125 mg as a single dose

Neonatal gonococcal ophthalmia: 25-50 mg/kg/day given every 24 hours

Infants and Children: 50-100 mg/kg/day in 1-2 divided doses
Meningitis: 100 mg/kg/day divided every 12 hours; loading dose of 75 mg/kg may be administered at the start of therapy
Chancroid, uncomplicated gonorrhea: I.M.:
<45 kg: 125 mg as a single dose
>45 kg: 250 mg as a single dose

Adults: 1-2 g every 12-24 hours depending on the type and severity of the infection; maximum dose: 4 g/day
Dosage Forms
Infusion, premixed (frozen): 1 g in $D_{3.8}W$ (50 mL); 2 g in $D_{2.4}W$ (50 mL)
Powder for injection: 250 mg, 500 mg, 1 g, 2 g, 10 g

cefuroxime (se fyoor ox' eem)
Brand Names Ceftin® Oral; Kefurox® Injection; Zinacef® Injection
Therapeutic Category Antibiotic, Cephalosporin (Second Generation)
Use Useful in infections caused by staphylococci, group B streptococci, *H. influenzae* (type A and B), *E. coli*, *Enterobacter*, *Salmonella*, and *Klebsiella*; treatment of susceptible infections of the lower respiratory tract, otitis media, urinary tract, skin and soft tissue, bone and joint, sepsis and gonorrhea
Usual Dosage
Neonates: 10-25 mg/kg/dose every 12 hours

Children:
Oral:
<12 years: 125 mg twice daily
>12 years: 250 mg twice daily
I.M., I.V.: 75-150 mg/kg/day divided every 8 hours; maximum dose: 9 g/day

Adults:
Oral: 125-500 mg twice daily, depending on severity of infection
I.M., I.V.: 100-150 mg/kg/day in divided doses every 6-8 hours; maximum: 6 g/24 hours
Dosage Forms
Infusion, premixed (frozen) (Zinacef®): 750 mg (50 mL); 1.5 g (50 mL)
Powder for injection, as sodium (Kefurox®, Zinacef®): 750 mg, 1.5 g, 7.5 g
Tablet, as axetil (Ceftin®): 125 mg, 250 mg, 500 mg

Cefzil™ *see* cefprozil *on page 81*

Celestone® Oral *see* betamethasone *on page 52*

Celestone® Phosphate Injection *see* betamethasone *on page 52*

Celestone® Soluspan® *see* betamethasone *on page 52*

cellulose, oxidized
Brand Names Oxycel®; Surgicel®
Synonyms absorbable cotton
Therapeutic Category Hemostatic Agent
Use Temporary packing for the control of capillary, venous, or small arterial hemorrhage
Usual Dosage Minimal amounts of an appropriate size are laid on the bleeding site
Dosage Forms
Pad (Oxycel®): 3" x 3", 8 ply
Pledget (Oxycel®): 2" x 1" x 1"
Strip:
Oxycel®: 18" x 2", 4 ply; 5" x ½", 4 ply; 36" x ½", 4 ply
Surgicel®: 2" x 14"; 4" x 8"; 2" x 3"; ½" x 2"

cellulose sodium phosphate
Brand Names Calcibind®
Synonyms csp; sodium cellulose phosphate
Therapeutic Category Urinary Tract Product
Use Adjunct to dietary restriction to reduce renal calculi formation in absorptive hypercalciuria type I
Usual Dosage Adults: Oral: 5 g 3 times/day with meals; decrease dose to 5 g with main meal and 2.5 g with each of two other meals when urinary calcium declines to <150 mg/day
Dosage Forms Powder: 2.5 g packets (90s), 300 g bulk pack

Celluvisc® [OTC] *see* carboxymethylcellulose sodium *on page 75*

Celontin® *see* methsuximide *on page 303*

Cel-U-Jec® Injection *see* betamethasone *on page 52*

Cenafed® [OTC] *see* pseudoephedrine *on page 406*
Cenafed® Plus [OTC] *see* triprolidine and pseudoephedrine *on page 482*
Cena-K® *see* potassium chloride *on page 386*
Cenocort® A Injection *see* triamcinolone *on page 474*
Cenocort® Forte Injection *see* triamcinolone *on page 474*
Cenolate® *see* sodium ascorbate *on page 433*
Centrax® *see* prazepam *on page 390*
Cepacol® [OTC] *see* cetylpyridinium chloride *on next page*
Cepacol® Anesthetic Troches [OTC] *see* cetylpyridinium chloride and benzocaine *on next page*

cephalexin monohydrate (sef a lex' in)
Brand Names Biocef; Cefanex®; Keflex®; Keftab®; Zartan
Therapeutic Category Antibiotic, Cephalosporin (First Generation)
Use Treatment of susceptible bacterial infections, including those caused by group A beta-hemolytic *Streptococcus*, *Staphylococcus*, *Klebsiella pneumoniae*, *E. coli*, *Proteus mirabilis*, and *Shigella*
Usual Dosage Oral:
Children: 25-50 mg/kg/day every 6 hours; severe infections: 50-100 mg/kg/day in divided doses every 6 hours; maximum: 3 g/24 hours

Adults: 250-1000 mg every 6 hours
Dosage Forms
Capsule: 250 mg, 500 mg
Powder for oral suspension: 125 mg/5 mL (5 mL unit dose, 60 mL, 100 mL, 200 mL); 250 mg/5 mL (5 mL unit dose, 100 mL, 200 mL)
Suspension, oral, pediatric: 100 mg/mL [5 mg/drop] (10 mL)
Tablet: 250 mg, 500 mg, 1 g
Tablet, as hydrochloride: 250 mg, 500 mg

cephalothin sodium (sef a' loe thin)
Brand Names Keflin® Injection
Therapeutic Category Antibiotic, Cephalosporin (First Generation)
Use Treatment of susceptible bacterial infections, including those caused by group A beta-hemolytic *Streptococcus*
Usual Dosage I.M., I.V.:
Neonates:
Postnatal age <7 days:
<2000 g: 20 mg every 12 hours
>2000 g: 20 mg every 8 hours
Postnatal age >7 days:
<2000 g: 20 mg every 8 hours
>2000 g: 20 mg every 6 hours

Children: 75-125 mg/kg/day divided every 4-6 hours; maximum dose: 10 g in a 24-hour period

Adults: 500 mg to 2 g every 4-6 hours
Dosage Forms
Infusion, in D_5W (frozen): 1 g (50 mL); 2 g (50 mL)
Powder for injection: 1 g, 2 g, 20 g

cephapirin sodium (sef a pye' rin)
Brand Names Cefadyl®
Therapeutic Category Antibiotic, Cephalosporin (First Generation)
Use Treatment of infections when caused by susceptible strains in serious respiratory, genitourinary, gastrointestinal, skin and soft-tissue, bone and joint infections; septicemia; endocarditis

Usual Dosage I.M., I.V.:
Children: 10-20 mg/kg every 6 hours up to 4 g/24 hours
Adults: 1 g every 6 hours up to 12 g/day
Dosage Forms Powder for injection: 500 mg, 1 g, 2 g, 4 g, 20 g

cephradine (sef' ra deen)
Brand Names Velosef®
Therapeutic Category Antibiotic, Cephalosporin (First Generation)
Use Treatment of susceptible bacterial infections, including those caused by group A beta-hemolytic *Streptococcus*
Usual Dosage Oral, I.M., I.V.:
Children ≥9 months: 25-100 mg/kg/day in equally divided doses every 6-12 hours up to 4 g/day
Adults: 2-4 g/day in 4 equally divided doses up to 8 g/day
Dosage Forms
Capsule: 250 mg, 500 mg
Powder for injection: 250 mg, 500 mg, 1 g, 2 g
Powder for oral suspension: 125 mg/5 mL (5 mL, 100 mL, 200 mL); 250 mg/5 mL (5 mL, 100 mL, 200 mL)

Cephulac® *see* lactulose *on page 267*

Ceptaz™ *see* ceftazidime *on page 81*

Ceredase® Injection *see* alglucerase *on page 12*

Cerespan® Oral *see* papaverine hydrochloride *on page 355*

Cerose-DM® [OTC] *see* chlorpheniramine, phenylephrine, and dextromethorphan *on page 95*

Cerubidine® *see* daunorubicin hydrochloride *on page 127*

Cerumenex® Otic *see* triethanolamine polypeptide oleate-condensate *on page 477*

C.E.S. *see* estrogens, conjugated *on page 179*

Cesamet® *see* nabilone *on page 321*

Cetacaine® *see* benzocaine, butyl aminobenzoate, tetracaine, and benzalkonium chloride *on page 48*

Cetacort® Topical *see* hydrocortisone *on page 236*

Cetamide® Ophthalmic *see* sodium sulfacetamide *on page 439*

Cetane® [OTC] *see* ascorbic acid *on page 33*

Cetapred® Ophthalmic *see* sodium sulfacetamide and prednisolone *on page 439*

cetylpyridinium chloride (see' til peer i di' nee um)
Brand Names Ceepryn® [OTC]; Cepacol® [OTC]
Therapeutic Category Local Anesthetic, Topical
Use Temporary relief of sore throat
Dosage Forms
Lozenge: 1:1500 (24s)
Mouthwash: 0.05% and alcohol 14% (180 mL)

cetylpyridinium chloride and benzocaine (see' til peer i di' nee um)
Brand Names Cepacol® Anesthetic Troches [OTC]
Synonyms benzocaine and cetylpyridinium chloride
Therapeutic Category Local Anesthetic, Oral
(Continued)

85

cetylpyridinium chloride and benzocaine *(Continued)*
Use Symptomatic relief of sore throat
Usual Dosage Use as needed for sore throat
Dosage Forms Troche: Cetylpyridinium chloride 1:1500 and benzocaine 10 mg per troche (18s)

Cevalin® [OTC] *see* ascorbic acid *on page 33*

Ce-Vi-Sol® [OTC] *see* ascorbic acid *on page 33*

CG *see* chorionic gonadotropin *on page 101*

Charcoaid® [OTC] *see* charcoal *on this page*

charcoal
Brand Names Actidose-Aqua® [OTC]; Actidose® With Sorbitol [OTC]; Charcoaid® [OTC]; Charcocaps® [OTC]; Liqui-Char® [OTC]; SuperChar® [OTC]
Synonyms activated carbon; activated charcoal; adsorbent charcoal; liquid antidote; medicinal carbon; medicinal charcoal
Therapeutic Category Antidiarrheal; Antidote, Adsorbent; Antiflatulent
Use Emergency treatment in poisoning by drugs and chemicals; repetitive doses for gastric dialysis in uremia to adsorb various waste products
Usual Dosage Oral:
  Acute poisoning: Single dose: Charcoal with sorbitol:
    Children 1-12 years: 1-2 g/kg/dose or 15-30 g or approximately 5-10 times the weight of the ingested poison; 1 g absorbs 100-1000 mg of poison; the use of repeat oral charcoal with sorbitol doses is not recommended. In young children sorbitol should be repeated no more than 1-2 times/day.
    Adults: 30-100 g

  Charcoal in water:
    Single dose:
      Infants <1 year: 1 g/kg
      Children 1-12 years: 15-30 g or 1-2 g/kg
      Adults: 30-100 g or 1-2 g/kg
    Multiple dose:
      Infants <1 year: 1 g/kg every 4-6 hours
      Children 1-12 years: 20-60 g or 1-2 g/kg every 2-6 hours until clinical observations and serum drug concentration have returned to a subtherapeutic range
      Adults: 20-60 g or 1-2 g/kg every 2-6 hours

  Gastric dialysis: Adults: 20-50 g every 6 hours for 1-2 days
Dosage Forms
  Capsule (Charcocaps®): 260 mg
  Liquid, activated:
    Actidose-Aqua®: 12.5 g (60 mL); 25 g (120 mL)
    Liqui-Char®: 12.5 g (60 mL); 15 g (75 mL); 25 g (120 mL); 30 g (120 mL); 50 g (240 mL)
    SuperChar®: 30 g (240 mL)
  Liquid, activated, with propylene glycol: 12.5 g (60 mL); 25 g (120 mL)
  Liquid, activated, with sorbitol:
    Actidose® With Sorbitol: 25 g (120 mL); 50 g (240 mL)
    Charcoaid®: 30 g (150 mL)
    SuperChar®: 30 g (240 mL)
  Powder for suspension, activated:
    15 g, 30 g, 40 g, 120 g, 240 g
    Superchar®: 30 g

Charcocaps® [OTC] *see* charcoal *on this page*

Chealamide® *see* edetate disodium *on page 167*

Chemet® Oral *see* succimer *on page 445*

Chemstrip® 7 [OTC] *see* diagnostic aids (*in vitro*), urine *on page 139*
Chemstrip® 9 [OTC] *see* diagnostic aids (*in vitro*), urine *on page 139*
Chemstrip® bG [OTC] *see* diagnostic aids (*in vitro*), blood *on page 137*
Chemstrip® K [OTC] *see* diagnostic aids (*in vitro*), urine *on page 139*
Chemstrip® uG [OTC] *see* diagnostic aids (*in vitro*), urine *on page 139*
Chemstrip® uGK [OTC] *see* diagnostic aids (*in vitro*), urine *on page 139*
Chenix® *see* chenodiol *on this page*
chenodeoxycholic acid *see* chenodiol *on this page*

chenodiol (kee noe dye' ole)
Brand Names Chenix®
Synonyms chenodeoxycholic acid
Therapeutic Category Bile Acid; Gallstone Dissolution Agent
Use Oral dissolution of cholesterol gallstones in selected patients
Usual Dosage Adults: Oral: 13-16 mg/kg/day in 2 divided doses, starting with 250 mg twice daily the first 2 weeks and increasing by 250 mg/day each week thereafter until the recommended or maximum tolerated dose is achieved
Dosage Forms Tablet, film coated: 250 mg

Cheracol® *see* guaifenesin and codeine *on page 218*
Cheracol® D [OTC] *see* guaifenesin and dextromethorphan *on page 218*
Chibroxin™ Ophthalmic *see* norfloxacin *on page 339*
Chiggertox® [OTC] *see* benzocaine *on page 48*
Children's Hold® [OTC] *see* dextromethorphan hydrobromide *on page 136*
Children's Kaopectate® [OTC] *see* attapulgite *on page 38*
Children's Motrin® *see* ibuprofen *on page 245*
children's vitamins *see* vitamin, multiple (pediatric) *on page 499*
Chlo-Amine® Oral [OTC] *see* chlorpheniramine maleate *on page 94*
Chlorafed® *see* chlorpheniramine and pseudoephedrine *on page 94*
chloral *see* chloral hydrate *on this page*

chloral hydrate (klor' al hye' drate)
Brand Names Aquachloral® Supprettes®; Noctec® Oral
Synonyms chloral; hydrated chloral; trichloroacetaldehyde monohydrate
Therapeutic Category Hypnotic; Sedative
Use Short-term sedative and hypnotic (<2 weeks), sedative/hypnotic for dental and diagnostic procedures; sedative prior to EEG evaluations
Usual Dosage
Neonates: 25 mg/kg/dose for sedation prior to a procedure

Children:
Sedation, anxiety: Oral, rectal: 5-15 mg/kg/dose every 8 hours, maximum: 500 mg/dose
Prior to EEG: Oral, rectal: 20-25 mg/kg/dose, 30-60 minutes prior to EEG; may repeat in 30 minutes to maximum of 100 mg/kg or 2 g total
Hypnotic: Oral, rectal: 20-40 mg/kg/dose up to a maximum of 50 mg/kg/24 hours or 1 g/dose or 2 g/24 hours
Sedation, nonpainful procedure: Oral: 50-75 mg/kg/dose 30-60 minutes prior to procedure; may repeat 30 minutes after initial dose if needed, to a total maximum dose of 120 mg/kg or 1 g total

Adults: Oral, rectal:
Sedation, anxiety: 250 mg 3 times/day
(Continued)
87

chloral hydrate (Continued)
Hypnotic: 500-1000 mg at bedtime or 30 minutes prior to procedure, not to exceed 2 g/24 hours
Dosage Forms
Capsule: 250 mg, 500 mg
Suppository, rectal: 324 mg, 500 mg, 648 mg
Syrup: 250 mg/5 mL (10 mL); 500 mg/5 mL (5 mL, 10 mL, 480 mL)

chlorambucil (klor am' byoo sil)
Brand Names Leukeran®
Therapeutic Category Antineoplastic Agent, Alkylating Agent (Nitrogen Mustard)
Use Management of chronic lymphocytic leukemia, Hodgkin's and non-Hodgkin's lymphoma; macroglobulinemia, polycythemia vera, trophoblastic neoplasms, ovarian neoplasms; management of nephrotic syndrome unresponsive to conventional therapy
Usual Dosage Refer to individual protocols
Oral:
Children and Adults: General short courses: 0.1-0.2 mg/kg/day or 4-8 mg/m^2/day for 2-3 weeks for remission induction, then adjust dose on basis of blood counts; maintenance therapy: 0.03-0.1 mg/kg/day
Nephrotic syndrome: 0.1-0.2 mg/kg/day every day for 5-15 weeks with low-dose prednisone
Chronic lymphocytic leukemia:
Biweekly regimen: Initial: 0.4 mg/kg dose is increased by 0.1 mg/kg every 2 weeks until a response occurs and/or myelosuppression occurs
Monthly regimen: Initial: 0.4 mg/kg, increase dose by 0.2 mg/kg every 4 weeks until a response occurs and/or myelosuppression occurs
Malignant lymphomas:
Non-Hodgkins lymphoma: 0.1 mg/kg/day
Hodgkins: 0.2 mg/kg/day
Dosage Forms Tablet, sugar coated: 2 mg

chloramphenicol (klor am fen' i kole)
Brand Names AK-Chlor® Ophthalmic; Chloromycetin®; Chloroptic® Ophthalmic; Ophthochlor® Ophthalmic
Therapeutic Category Antibiotic, Miscellaneous; Antibiotic, Ophthalmic; Antibiotic, Otic
Use Treatment of serious infections due to organisms resistant to other less toxic antibiotics or when its penetrability into the site of infection is clinically superior to other antibiotics to which the organism is sensitive; useful in infections caused by *Bacteroides*, *H. influenzae*, *Neisseria meningitidis*, *Salmonella*, and *Rickettsia*
Usual Dosage
Neonates: Initial loading dose: Oral, I.V. (I.M. administration is not recommended): 20 mg/kg (the first maintenance dose should be given 12 hours after the loading dose)
Maintenance dose:
Postnatal age 0-4 weeks, <2000 g: 25 mg/kg/day once every 24 hours
Postnatal age 7-28 days, >2000 g: 50 mg/kg/day divided every 12 hours
Meningitis: Infants and Children: Maintenance dose: I.V.: 75-100 mg/kg/day divided every 6 hours
Other infections: Oral, I.V.:
Infants and Children: 50-75 mg/kg/day divided every 6 hours; maximum daily dose: 4 g/day
Adults: 50 mg/kg/day in divided doses every 6 hours; maximum daily dose: 4 g/day
Children and Adults:
Ophthalmic: Instill 1-2 drops or small amount of ointment every 3-6 hours; increase interval between applications after 48 hours
Topical: Gently rub into the affected area 3-4 times/day
Dosage Forms
Capsule: 250 mg
Cream (Chloromycetin®): 1% (30 g)

Ointment, ophthalmic (AK-Chlor®, Chloromycetin®, Chloroptic®): 1% [10 mg/g] (3.5 g)
Powder for injection, as sodium succinate: 1 g
Powder for ophthalmic solution (Chloromycetin®): 25 mg/vial
Solution:
 Ophthalmic (AK-Chlor®, Chloroptic®, Ophthochlor®): 0.5% [5 mg/mL] (2.5 mL, 7.5 mL, 15 mL)
 Otic (Chloromycetin®): 0.5% (15 mL)
Suspension, oral, as palmitate (custard flavor) (Chloromycetin®): 150 mg/5 mL (60 mL)

chloramphenicol and prednisolone
Brand Names Chloroptic-P® Ophthalmic
Therapeutic Category Antibiotic, Ophthalmic; Corticosteroid, Ophthalmic
Use Topical anti-infective and corticosteroid for treatment of ocular infections
Usual Dosage Ophthalmic: Instill 1-2 drops in eye(s) 2-4 times/day
Dosage Forms Ointment, ophthalmic: Chloramphenicol 1% and prednisolone 0.5% (3.5 g)

chloramphenicol, polymyxin b, and hydrocortisone
Brand Names Ophthocort® Ophthalmic
Therapeutic Category Antibiotic, Ophthalmic
Use Topical anti-infective and corticosteroid for treatment of ocular infections
Usual Dosage Apply ½" ribbon every 3-4 hours until improvement occurs
Dosage Forms Solution, ophthalmic: Chloramphenicol 1%, polymyxin b sulfate 10,000 units, and hydrocortisone acetate 0.5% per g (3.75 g)

Chloraseptic® Oral [OTC] *see* phenol *on page 369*

Chlorate® Oral [OTC] *see* chlorpheniramine maleate *on page 94*

chlordiazepoxide (klor dye az e pox' ide)
Brand Names Libritabs®; Librium®; Mitran® Oral; Reposans-10® Oral
Synonyms methaminodiazepoxide hydrochloride
Therapeutic Category Benzodiazepine; Hypnotic; Sedative
Use Management of anxiety and as a preoperative sedative, symptoms of alcohol withdrawal
Usual Dosage
 Children >6 years: Anxiety: Oral, I.M.: 0.5 mg/kg/24 hours divided every 6-8 hours
 Adults:
 Anxiety: Oral: 15-100 mg divided 3-4 times/day
 Severe anxiety: 20-25 mg 3-4 times/day
 Preoperative sedation:
 Oral: 5-10 mg 3-4 times/day, 1-day preop
 I.M.: 50-100 mg 1-hour preop
 Alcohol withdrawal symptoms: Oral, I.V.: 50-100 mg to start, dose may be repeated in 2-4 hours as necessary to a maximum of 300 mg/24 hours
Dosage Forms
 Capsule, as hydrochloride: 5 mg, 10 mg, 25 mg
 Powder for injection, as hydrochloride: 100 mg
 Tablet: 5 mg, 10 mg, 25 mg

chlordiazepoxide and amitriptyline *see* amitriptyline and chlordiazepoxide *on page 21*

chlordiazepoxide and clidinium *see* clidinium and chlordiazepoxide *on page 105*

Chlordine® S.R. *see* chlorpheniramine and pseudoephedrine *on page 94*

Chloresium® [OTC] *see* chlorophyll *on next page*

chlorhexidine gluconate (klor hex' i deen)

Brand Names BactoShield® Topical [OTC]; Dyna-Hex® Topical [OTC]; Exidine® Scrub [OTC]; Hibiclens® Topical [OTC]; Hibistat® Topical [OTC]; Peridex® Oral Rinse

Therapeutic Category Antibiotic, Oral Rinse; Antibiotic, Topical

Use Skin cleanser for surgical scrub, cleanser skin wounds, germicidal hand rinse, and as antibacterial dental rinse

Usual Dosage Oral rinse (Peridex®)

Precede use of solution by flossing and brushing teeth, completely rinse toothpaste from mouth; swish 15 mL undiluted oral rinse around in mouth for 30 seconds, then expectorate. Caution patient not to swallow the medicine; avoid eating for 2-3 hours after treatment. (The cap on bottle of oral rinse is a measure for 15 mL.)

When used as a treatment of gingivitis, the regimen begins with oral prophylaxis. Patient treats mouth with 15 mL chlorhexidine; swish for 30 seconds, then expectorate. This is repeated twice daily (morning and evening). Patient should have a re-evaluation followed by a dental prophylaxis every 6 months.

Dosage Forms

Foam, topical, with isopropyl alcohol 4% (BactoShield®): 4% (180 mL)

Liquid, topical, with isopropyl alcohol 4%:

Dyna-Hex® Skin Cleanser: 2% (120 mL, 240 mL, 480 mL, 960 mL, 4000 mL); 4% (120 mL, 240 mL, 480 mL, 4000 mL)

BactoShield® 2: 2% (960 mL)

BactoShield®, Exidine® Skin Cleanser, Hibiclens® Skin Cleanser: 4% (15 mL, 120 mL, 240 mL, 480 mL, 960 mL, 4000 mL)

Rinse:

Oral (mint flavor) (Peridex®): 0.12% with alcohol 11.6% (480 mL)

Topical (Hibistat® Hand Rinse): 0.5% with isopropyl alcohol 70% (120 mL, 240 mL)

Sponge/Brush (Hibiclens®): 4% with isopropyl alcohol 4% (22 mL)

Wipes (Hibistat®): 0.5% (50s)

2-chlorodeoxyadenosine see cladribine on page 104

chloroethane see ethyl chloride on page 186

Chlorofon-F® see chlorzoxazone on page 99

Chloromycetin® see chloramphenicol on page 88

chlorophylin see chlorophyll on this page

chlorophyll (klor' oh fill)

Brand Names Chloresium® [OTC]; Derifil® [OTC]

Synonyms chlorophylin

Therapeutic Category Gastrointestinal Agent, Miscellaneous; Topical Skin Product

Use Topically promotes normal healing, relieves pain and inflammation, and reduces malodors in wounds, burns, surface ulcers, abrasions and skin irritations; used orally to control fecal and urinary odors in colostomy, ileostomy, or incontinence

Usual Dosage

Oral: 1-2 tablets/day

Topical: Apply generously and cover with gauze, linen, or other appropriate dressing; do not change dressings more often than every 48-72 hours

Dosage Forms

Ointment, topical (Chloresium®): Chlorophyll copper complex 0.5% (30 g, 120 g)

Solution, topical, in isotonic saline (Chloresium®): Chlorophyll copper complex 0.2% (240 mL, 946 mL)

Tablet:

Chloresium®: Chlorophyll copper complex 14 mg

Derifil®: Water soluble chlorophyll: 100 mg

Sodium free, sugar free: 20 mg

chloroprocaine hydrochloride (klor oh proe' kane)
Brand Names Nesacaine®; Nesacaine®-MPF
Therapeutic Category Local Anesthetic, Injectable
Use For infiltration anesthesia and for peripheral and epidural anesthesia
Usual Dosage Dosage varies with anesthetic procedure, the area to be anesthetized, the vascularity of the tissues, depth of anesthesia required, degree of muscle relaxation required, and duration of anesthesia
Dosage Forms Injection:
Preservative free (Nesacaine®-MPF): 2% (30 mL); 3% (30 mL)
With preservative (Nesacaine®): 1% (30 mL); 2% (30 mL)

Chloroptic® Ophthalmic see chloramphenicol on page 88

Chloroptic-P® Ophthalmic see chloramphenicol and prednisolone on page 89

chloroquine and primaquine
Brand Names Aralen® Phosphate With Primaquine Phosphate
Synonyms primaquine and chloroquine
Therapeutic Category Antimalarial Agent
Use Prophylaxis of malaria, regardless of species, in all areas where the disease is endemic
Usual Dosage
Children: For suggested weekly dosage (based on body weight), see table.

Adults: Start at least 1 day before entering the endemic area; take 1 tablet/week on the same day each week; continue for 4-6 weeks after leaving the endemic area
Dosage Forms Tablet: Chloroquine phosphate 500 mg [base 300 mg] and primaquine phosphate 79 mg [base 45 mg]

chloroquine phosphate (klor' oh kwin)
Brand Names Aralen® Phosphate
Therapeutic Category Amebicide; Antimalarial Agent
Use Suppression or chemoprophylaxis of malaria; treatment of uncomplicated or mild-moderate malaria; extraintestinal amebiasis; rheumatoid arthritis
Usual Dosage Oral:
Malaria (excluding resistant *P. falciparum*):
Suppression or prophylaxis in endemic areas (begin 1-2 weeks prior to, and continue for 6-8 weeks after the period of potential exposure):
Children: 5 mg base/kg/dose weekly, up to a maximum of 300 mg/dose
Adults: 300 mg/dose weekly
Treatment:
Children: 10 mg base/kg/dose, up to a maximum of 600 mg base/dose one time, followed by 5 mg base/kg/dose one time after 6 hours, and then daily for 2 days (total dose of 25 mg base/kg).
Adults: 600 mg base/dose one time, followed by 300 mg base/dose one time after 6 hours, and then daily for 2 days

Extraintestinal amebiasis: Dosage expressed in mg base:
Children: 10 mg/kg once daily for 2-3 weeks (up to 300 mg base/day)
Adults: 600 mg base/day for 2 days followed by 300 mg base/day for at least 2-3 weeks

Rheumatoid arthritis: Adults: 150 mg base once daily

Melanoma treatment: Children: 10 mg/kg base/dose (maximum: 600 mg) as a single dose followed by 5 mg/kg base one time after 6 hours, then daily for 2 days
Dosage Forms Tablet: 250 mg [150 mg base]; 500 mg [300 mg base]

chlorothiazide (klor oh thye' a zide)
Brand Names Diurigen®; Diuril®
Therapeutic Category Diuretic, Thiazide
Use Management of mild to moderate hypertension, or edema associated with congestive heart failure, pregnancy, or nephrotic syndrome in patients unable to take oral hydrochlorothiazide, when a thiazide is the diuretic of choice
(Continued)

chlorothiazide *(Continued)*
Usual Dosage I.V. has been limited in infants and children and is generally not recommended

Infants <6 months and patients with pulmonary interstitial edema:
Oral: 20-40 mg/kg/day in 2 divided doses
I.V.: 2-8 mg/kg/day in 2 divided doses

Infants >6 months and Children:
Oral: 20 mg/kg/day in 2 divided doses
I.V.: 4 mg/kg/day

Adults:
Oral: 500-2 g/day divided in 1-2 doses
I.V.: 100-500 mg/day
Dosage Forms
Powder for injection, lyophilized, as sodium: 500 mg
Suspension, oral: 250 mg/5 mL (237 mL)
Tablet: 250 mg, 500 mg

chlorothiazide and methyldopa
Brand Names Aldoclor®
Synonyms methyldopa and chlorothiazide
Therapeutic Category Antihypertensive, Combination
Use Treatment of hypertension
Usual Dosage Oral: 1 tablet 2-3 times/day for first 48 hours, then adjust
Dosage Forms Tablet:
150: Chlorothiazide 150 mg and methyldopa 250 mg
250: Chlorothiazide 250 mg and methyldopa 250 mg

chlorothiazide and reserpine
Brand Names Diupres-250®; Diupres-500®
Synonyms reserpine and chlorothiazide
Therapeutic Category Antihypertensive, Combination
Use Management of hypertension
Usual Dosage Oral: 1-2 tablets 1-2 times/day
Dosage Forms Tablet:
250: Chlorothiazide 250 mg and reserpine 0.125 mg
500: Chlorothiazide 500 mg and reserpine 0.125 mg

chlorotrianisene *(klor oh trye an' i seen)*
Brand Names TACE®
Therapeutic Category Estrogen Derivative; Estrogen Derivative, Oral
Use Treat inoperable prostatic cancer; management of atrophic vaginitis, female hypogonadism, vasomotor symptoms of menopause; prevention of postpartum breast engorgement (no longer recommended because increased risk of thrombophlebitis)
Usual Dosage Adults: Oral:
Prostatic cancer: 12-25 mg/day

Atrophic vaginitis: 12-25 mg/day in 28-day cycles (21 days on and 7 days off)

Female hypogonadism: 12-25 mg for 21 days followed by I.M. progesterone 100 mg or 5 days of oral progestin; next course may begin on days of induced uterine bleeding

Menopause: 12-25 mg for 30 days

Postpartum breast engorgement: 12 mg 4 times/day for 7 days or 72 mg twice daily for 2 days
Dosage Forms Capsule: 12 mg, 25 mg

chloroxine (klor ox' een)
Brand Names Capitrol®
Therapeutic Category Antiseborrheic Agent, Topical; Shampoos
Use Treatment of dandruff or seborrheic dermatitis of the scalp
Usual Dosage Use twice weekly, massage into wet scalp, avoid contact with eyes, lather should remain on the scalp for approximately 3 minutes, then rinsed; application should be repeated and the scalp rinsed thoroughly
Dosage Forms Shampoo: 2% (120 mL)

Chlorphed® [OTC] see brompheniramine maleate on page 59
Chlorphed®-LA Nasal Solution [OTC] see oxymetazoline hydrochloride on page 350

chlorphenesin carbamate (klor fen' e sin car' baa mate)
Brand Names Maolate®
Therapeutic Category Skeletal Muscle Relaxant
Use Adjunctive treatment of discomfort in short-term, acute, painful musculoskeletal conditions
Usual Dosage Adults: Oral: 800 mg 3 times/day, then adjusted to lowest effective dosage, usually 400 mg 4 times/day for up to a maximum of 2 months
Dosage Forms Tablet: 400 mg

chlorpheniramine and acetaminophen
Brand Names Coricidin® [OTC]
Therapeutic Category Analgesic, Non-Narcotic; Antihistamine
Use Symptomatic relief of congestion, headache, aches and pains of colds and flu
Usual Dosage Adults: Oral: 2 tablets every 4 hours, up to 20/day
Dosage Forms Tablet: Chlorpheniramine maleate 2 mg and acetaminophen 325 mg

chlorpheniramine and phenylephrine
Brand Names Dallergy-D®; Decohistine®; Dihistine®; Histor-D® Liquid; Novahistine® Elixir [OTC]; Prehist®; Ru-Tuss® Liquid
Synonyms phenylephrine and chlorpheniramine
Therapeutic Category Antihistamine/Decongestant Combination
Use Temporary relief of nasal congestion and eustachian tube congestion as well as runny nose, sneezing, itching of nose or throat, itchy and watery eyes
Usual Dosage Oral:
Children:
2-5 years: 2.5 mL every 4 hours
6-12 years: 5 mL every 4 hours

Adults: 10 mL every 4 hours
Dosage Forms
Capsule, sustained release: Chlorpheniramine maleate 8 mg and phenylephrine hydrochloride 20 mg
Liquid: Chlorpheniramine maleate 5 mg and phenylephrine hydrochloride 2 mg per 5 mL (120 mL, 480 mL, 4000 mL)

chlorpheniramine and phenylpropanolamine
Brand Names Allerest® 12 Hour Capsule [OTC]; Condrin-LA®; Contac® Maximum Strength [OTC]; CPA TR®; Demazin® [OTC]; Drize®; Genamin® Cold Syrup [OTC]; Myminic® Syrup [OTC]; Oragest SR®; Ornade® Spansule®; Parhist SR®; Resaid®; Rescon Liquid [OTC]; Rhinolar-EX® 12; Ru-Tuss II®; Triaminic-12® [OTC]; Triaminic® Syrup [OTC]; Trind® Liquid [OTC]; Tripalgen® Cold [OTC]; Triphenyl® Syrup [OTC]
Synonyms phenylpropanolamine and chlorpheniramine
Therapeutic Category Antihistamine/Decongestant Combination
(Continued)
93

chlorpheniramine and phenylpropanolamine *(Continued)*

Use Symptomatic relief of nasal congestion, runny nose, sneezing, itchy nose or throat, and itchy or watery eyes due to the common cold or allergic rhinitis

Usual Dosage

Children <12 years: 5 mL every 3-4 hours

Children >12 years and Adults: 1 capsule every 12 hours or 5-10 mL every 3-4 hours

Dosage Forms

Capsule, sustained release: Chlorpheniramine maleate 12 mg and phenylpropanolamine hydrochloride 75 mg

Liquid: Chlorpheniramine maleate 2 mg and phenylpropanolamine hydrochloride 12.5 mg per 5 mL

Syrup: Chlorpheniramine maleate 2 mg and phenylpropanolamine hydrochloride 12.5 mg per 5 mL

Tablet, sustained release: Chlorpheniramine maleate 12 mg and phenylpropanolamine hydrochloride 75 mg

chlorpheniramine and pseudoephedrine

Brand Names Anamine T.D.®; Brexin® L.A.; Chlorafed®; Chlordine® S.R.; Codimal-L.A.®; Colfed-A®; Co-Pyronil® 2 [OTC]; Deconamine® SR; Deconamine® Tablet; Duralex®; Dura-Tap/PD®; Fedahist® Timecaps®; Isoclor® Tablet; Isoclor® Timesules®; Klerist-D®; Kronofed-A-Jr®; Napril® [OTC]; N D Clear®; Novafed® A; Pseudo-Chlor® [OTC]; Pseudo-gest Plus® [OTC]; Rescon; Rescon-ED®; Rescon Jr; Sudafed Plus® Tablet

Synonyms pseudoephedrine and chlorpheniramine

Therapeutic Category Antihistamine/Decongestant Combination

Use Relief of nasal congestion associated with the common cold, hay fever, and other allergies, sinusitis, eustachian tube blockage, and vasomotor and allergic rhinitis

Usual Dosage Oral:

Capsule: One every 12 hours

Tablet: One 3-4 times/day

Dosage Forms

Capsule: Chlorpheniramine maleate 4 mg and pseudoephedrine hydrochloride 60 mg; chlorpheniramine maleate 12 mg and pseudoephedrine hydrochloride 120 mg

Capsule, sustained release: Chlorpheniramine maleate 4 mg and pseudoephedrine hydrochloride 60 mg; chlorpheniramine maleate 8 mg and pseudoephedrine hydrochloride 120 mg

Tablet: Chlorpheniramine maleate 4 mg and pseudoephedrine hydrochloride 60 mg

chlorpheniramine, ephedrine, phenylephrine, and carbetapentane

Brand Names Rentamine®; Rynatuss® Pediatric Suspension; Tri-Tannate Plus®

Therapeutic Category Antihistamine/Decongestant Combination

Use Symptomatic relief of cough

Usual Dosage Children:

<2 years: Titrate dose individually

2-6 years: 2.5-5 mL every 12 hours

>6 years: 5-10 mL every 12 hours

Dosage Forms Liquid: Carbetapentane tannate 30 mg, phenylephrine tannate 5 mg, ephedrine tannate 5 mg, and chlorpheniramine tannate 4 mg per 5 mL

chlorpheniramine maleate *(klor fen ir' a meen mal' ee ate)*

Brand Names Aller-Chlor® Oral [OTC]; Chlo-Amine® Oral [OTC]; Chlorate® Oral [OTC]; Chlor-Pro® Injection; Chlor-Trimeton® Injection; Chlor-Trimeton® Oral [OTC]; Phenetron® Oral; Telachlor® Oral; Teldrin® Oral [OTC]

Therapeutic Category Antihistamine

Use Perennial and seasonal allergic rhinitis and other allergic symptoms including urticaria

Usual Dosage Oral:
Children: 0.35 mg/kg/day in divided doses every 4-6 hours
2-6 years: 1 mg every 4-6 hours
6-12 years: 2 mg every 4-6 hours, not to exceed 12 mg/day

Adults: 4 mg every 4-6 hours, not to exceed 24 mg/day or sustained release 8-12 mg every 12 hours

Dosage Forms
Capsule: 12 mg
Capsule, timed release: 6 mg, 8 mg, 12 mg
Injection: 10 mg/mL (1 mL, 30 mL); 100 mg/mL (10 mL)
Syrup: 2 mg/5 mL (120 mL, 480 mL, 4000 mL)
Tablet: 4 mg, 8 mg, 12 mg
Tablet:
Chewable: 2 mg
Timed release: 8 mg, 12 mg

chlorpheniramine, phenindamine, and phenylpropanolamine

Brand Names Nolamine®
Therapeutic Category Antihistamine/Decongestant Combination
Use Upper respiratory and nasal congestion
Usual Dosage Adults: Oral: 1 tablet every 8-12 hours
Dosage Forms Tablet, timed release: Chlorpheniramine maleate 4 mg, phenindamine tartrate 24 mg, and phenylpropanolamine hydrochloride 50 mg

chlorpheniramine, phenylephrine, and codeine

Brand Names Pediacof®; Pedituss®
Therapeutic Category Antihistamine/Decongestant Combination; Cough Preparation
Use Symptomatic relief of rhinitis, nasal congestion and cough due to colds or allergy
Usual Dosage Children 6 months to 12 years: 1.25-10 mL every 4-6 hours
Dosage Forms Liquid: Chlorpheniramine maleate 0.75 mg, phenylephrine hydrochloride 2.5 mg, and codeine phosphate 5 mg with potassium iodide 75 mg per 5 mL

chlorpheniramine, phenylephrine, and dextromethorphan

Brand Names Cerose-DM® [OTC]
Therapeutic Category Antihistamine/Decongestant Combination; Cough Preparation
Use Temporary relief of cough due to minor throat and bronchial irritation; relieves nasal congestion, runny nose and sneezing
Usual Dosage Adults: Oral: 5-10 mL 4 times/day
Dosage Forms Liquid: Chlorpheniramine maleate 4 mg, phenylephrine hydrochloride 10 mg, and dextromethorphan hydrobromide 15 mg per 5 mL

chlorpheniramine, phenylephrine, and methscopolamine

Brand Names Alersule Forte®; Dallergy®; Extendryl® SR; Histor-D® Timecelles®
Therapeutic Category Antihistamine/Decongestant Combination
Use Relieves nasal congestion, runny nose and sneezing
Usual Dosage Adults: Oral: 1 capsule every 12 hours
Dosage Forms
Capsule, sustained release: Chlorpheniramine maleate 8 mg, phenylephrine hydrochloride 10 mg, and methscopolamine nitrate 2.5 mg
Syrup: Chlorpheniramine maleate 2 mg, phenylephrine hydrochloride 10 mg, and methscopolamine nitrate 0.625 mg per 5 mL

chlorpheniramine, phenylephrine, and phenyltoloxamine

Brand Names Comhist®; Comhist® LA
Therapeutic Category Antihistamine/Decongestant Combination
Use Symptomatic relief of rhinitis and nasal congestion due to colds or allergy
(Continued)

chlorpheniramine, phenylephrine, and phenyltoloxamine
(Continued)
Usual Dosage Oral: 1 capsule every 8-12 hours or 1-2 tablets 3 times/day
Dosage Forms
    Capsule, sustained release (Comhist® LA): Chlorpheniramine maleate 4 mg, phenyleph-
    rine hydrochloride 20 mg, and phenyltoloxamine citrate 50 mg
    Tablet (Comhist®): Chlorpheniramine maleate 2 mg, phenylephrine hydrochloride 10 mg,
    and phenyltoloxamine citrate 25 mg

chlorpheniramine, phenylpropanolamine, and acetaminophen
Brand Names BQ® Tablet [OTC]; Congestant D® [OTC]; Coricidin 'D'® [OTC]; Dapacin®
Cold Capsule [OTC]; Duadacin® Capsule [OTC]; Tylenol® Cold Effervescent Medication
Tablet [OTC]
Therapeutic Category Analgesic, Non-Narcotic; Antihistamine/Decongestant Combina-
tion
Use Symptomatic relief of nasal congestion and headache from colds/sinus congestion
Usual Dosage Adults: Oral: 2 tablets every 4 hours, up to 12 tablets/day
Dosage Forms
    Capsule: Chlorpheniramine maleate 2 mg, phenylpropanolamine hydrochloride 12.5 mg,
    and acetaminophen 325 mg
    Tablet: Chlorpheniramine maleate 2 mg, phenylpropanolamine hydrochloride 12.5 mg, and
    acetaminophen 325 mg

chlorpheniramine, phenylpropanolamine, and dextromethorphan
Brand Names Triaminicol® Multi-Symptom Cold Syrup [OTC]
Therapeutic Category Antihistamine/Decongestant Combination; Cough Preparation
Use Provides relief of runny nose, sneezing, suppresses cough, promotes nasal and sinus
drainage
Usual Dosage
    Children 6-12 years: 5 mL every 4 hours
    Adults: 10 mL every 4 hours
Dosage Forms Liquid: Chlorpheniramine maleate 2 mg, phenylpropanolamine hydrochlo-
ride 12.5 mg, and dextromethorphan hydrobromide 10 mg per 5 mL

chlorpheniramine, phenyltoloxamine, phenylpropanolamine, and phenylephrine
Brand Names Naldecon®; Naldelate®; Nalgest®; Nalspan®; New Decongestant®; Par
Decon®; Quadra-Hist®; Tri-Phen-Chlor®; Uni-Decon®
Therapeutic Category Antihistamine/Decongestant Combination
Use Symptomatic treatment of nasal and eustachian tube congestion associated with si-
nusitis and acute upper respiratory infection; symptomatic relief of perennial and allergic
rhinitis
Usual Dosage Oral:
    Children:
        3-6 months: 0.25 mL (pediatric drops) every 3-4 hours
        6-12 months: 2.5 mL (pediatric syrup) or 0.5 mL (pediatric drops) every 3-4 hours
        1-6 years: 5 mL (pediatric syrup) or 1 mL (pediatric drops) every 3-4 hours
        6-12 years: 2.5 mL (syrup) or 10 mL (pediatric syrup) or $\frac{1}{2}$ tablet every 3-4 hours
    Children >12 years and 5 mL (syrup) or 1 tablet every 3-4 hours
Dosage Forms
    Drops, pediatric: Chlorpheniramine maleate 0.5 mg, phenyltoloxamine citrate 2 mg, phe-
    nylpropanolamine hydrochloride 5 mg, and phenylephrine hydrochloride 1.25 mg per mL
    Syrup: Chlorpheniramine maleate 2.5 mg, phenyltoloxamine citrate 7.5 mg, phenylpro-
    panolamine hydrochloride 20 mg, and phenylephrine hydrochloride 5 mg per 5 mL
    Syrup, pediatric: Chlorpheniramine maleate 0.5 mg, phenyltoloxamine citrate 2 mg, phe-
    nylpropanolamine hydrochloride 5 mg, and phenylephrine hydrochloride 1.25 mg per 5
    mL

Tablet, sustained release: Chlorpheniramine maleate 5 mg, phenyltoloxamine citrate 15 mg, phenylpropanolamine hydrochloride 40 mg, and phenylephrine hydrochloride 10 mg

chlorpheniramine, pseudoephedrine, and codeine
Brand Names Codehist® DH; Decohistine® DH; Dihistine® DH; Novahistine® DH; Phen DH® w/Codeine; Ryna-C® Liquid
Therapeutic Category Antihistamine/Decongestant Combination; Cough Preparation
Use Temporary relief of cough associated with minor throat or bronchial irritation or nasal congestion due to common cold, allergic rhinitis, or sinusitis
Usual Dosage Oral:
Children:
25-50 lb: 1.25-2.50 mL every 4-6 hours, up to 4 doses in 24-hour period
50-90 lb: 2.5-5 mL every 4-6 hours, up to 4 doses in 24-hour period
Adults: 10 mL every 4-6 hours, up to 4 doses in 24-hour period
Dosage Forms Liquid: Chlorpheniramine maleate 2 mg, pseudoephedrine hydrochloride 30 mg, and codeine phosphate 10 mg (120 mL, 480 mL)

chlorpheniramine, pyrilamine, and phenylephrine
Brand Names Rynatan® Pediatric Suspension; Tritan®; Tritann® Pediatric
Therapeutic Category Antihistamine/Decongestant Combination
Use Symptomatic relief of nasal congestion associated with upper respiratory tract condition
Usual Dosage Children:
<2 years: Titrate dose individually
2-6 years: 2.5-5 mL every 12 hours
>6 years: 5-10 mL every 12 hours
Dosage Forms
Liquid: Chlorpheniramine tannate 2 mg, pyrilamine tannate 12.5 mg, and phenylephrine tannate 5 mg per 5 mL
Tablet: Chlorpheniramine tannate 8 mg, pyrilamine maleate 12.5 mg, and phenylephrine tannate 25 mg

Chlor-Pro® Injection *see* chlorpheniramine maleate *on page 94*

chlorpromazine hydrochloride (klor proe' ma zeen)
Brand Names Ormazine; Thorazine®
Therapeutic Category Antiemetic; Antipsychotic Agent; Phenothiazine Derivative
Use Treatment of nausea and vomiting; psychoses; Tourette's syndrome; mania; intractable hiccups (adults); behavioral problems (children)
Usual Dosage
Children >6 months:
Psychosis:
Oral: 0.5-1 mg/kg/dose every 4-6 hours; older children may require 200 mg/day or higher
I.M., I.V.: 0.5-1 mg/kg/dose every 6-8 hours; maximum I.M./I.V. dose for <5 years (22.7 kg) = 40 mg/day; maximum I.M./I.V. for 5-12 years (22.7-45.5 kg) = 75 mg/day
Nausea and vomiting:
Oral: 0.5-1 mg/kg/dose every 4-6 hours as needed
I.M., I.V.: 0.5-1 mg/kg/dose every 6-8 hours; maximum dose: Same as psychosis
Rectal: 1 mg/kg/dose every 6-8 hours as needed
Adults:
Psychosis:
Oral: Range: 30-800 mg/day in 1-4 divided doses, initiate at lower doses and titrate as needed; usual dose is 200 mg/day; some patients may require 1-2 g/day

(Continued)

chlorpromazine hydrochloride *(Continued)*

I.M., I.V.: 25 mg initially, may repeat (25-50 mg) in 1-4 hours, gradually increase to a maximum of 400 mg/dose every 4-6 hours until patient controlled; usual dose 300-800 mg/day

Nausea and vomiting:
Oral: 10-25 mg every 4-6 hours
I.M., I.V.: 25-50 mg every 4-6 hours
Rectal: 50-100 mg every 6-8 hours
Intractable hiccups: Oral, I.M.: 25-50 mg 3-4 times/day

Dosage Forms
Capsule, sustained action: 30 mg, 75 mg, 150 mg, 200 mg, 300 mg
Concentrate, oral: 30 mg/mL (120 mL); 100 mg/mL (60 mL, 240 mL)
Injection: 25 mg/mL (1 mL, 2 mL, 10 mL)
Suppository, rectal, as base: 25 mg, 100 mg
Syrup: 10 mg/5 mL (120 mL)
Tablet: 10 mg, 25 mg, 50 mg, 100 mg, 200 mg

chlorpropamide (klor proe' pa mide)
Brand Names Diabinese®
Therapeutic Category Antidiabetic Agent; Hypoglycemic Agent, Oral; Sulfonylurea Agent
Use Control blood sugar in adult onset, noninsulin-dependent diabetes (type II). Unlabeled use includes: neurogenic diabetes insipidus
Usual Dosage The dosage of chlorpropamide is variable and should be individualized based upon the patient's response.

Adults: Oral: 250 mg once daily; initial dose in elderly patients: 100 mg once daily; subsequent dosages may be increased or decreased by 50-125 mg/day at 3- to 5-day intervals; maximum daily dose: 750 mg
Dosage Forms Tablet: 100 mg, 250 mg

chlorprothixene (klor proe thix' een)
Brand Names Taractan®
Therapeutic Category Antipsychotic Agent; Thioxanthene Derivative
Use Management of psychotic disorders
Usual Dosage
Children >6 years: Oral: 10-25 mg 3-4 times/day

Adults:
Oral: 25-50 mg 3-4 times/day, to be increased as needed; doses exceeding 600 mg/day are rarely required
I.M.: 25-50 mg up to 3-4 times/day
Dosage Forms
Concentrate, oral, as lactate and hydrochloride (fruit flavor): 100 mg/5 mL (480 mL)
Injection, as hydrochloride: 12.5 mg/mL (2 mL)
Tablet: 10 mg, 25 mg, 50 mg, 100 mg

chlortetracyline hydrochloride (klor te tra sye' kleen)
Brand Names Aureomycin®
Therapeutic Category Antibiotic, Ophthalmic; Antibiotic, Tetracycline Derivative
Use Treatment of superficial infections of the skin due to susceptible organisms, also infection prophylaxis in minor skin abrasions
Usual Dosage Apply 1-5 times/day, cover with sterile bandage if needed
Dosage Forms Ointment:
Ophthalmic: 1% [10 mg/g] (3.5 g)
Topical: 3% (14.2 g, 30 g)

chlorthalidone (klor thal' i done)
Brand Names Hygroton®; Thalitone®
Therapeutic Category Diuretic, Miscellaneous
Use Management of mild to moderate hypertension, used alone or in combination with other agents; treatment of edema associated with congestive heart failure, nephrotic syndrome, or pregnancy
Usual Dosage Oral:
  Children: 2 mg/kg 3 times/week
  Adults: 25-100 mg/day or 100 mg 3 times/week
Dosage Forms
  Tablet:
    Hygroton®: 25 mg, 50 mg, 100 mg
    Thalitone®: 15 mg, 25 mg

Chlor-Trimeton® Injection see chlorpheniramine maleate on page 94

Chlor-Trimeton® Oral [OTC] see chlorpheniramine maleate on page 94

chlorzoxazone (klor zox' a zone)
Brand Names Blanex®; Chlorofon-F®; Flexaphen®; Lobac®; Miflex®; Mus-Lac®; Paraflex®; Parafon Forte™ DSC; Pargen Fortified®; Polyflex®; Remular-S®; Skelex®
Therapeutic Category Centrally Acting Muscle Relaxant; Skeletal Muscle Relaxant
Use Symptomatic treatment of muscle spasm and pain associated with acute musculoskeletal conditions
Usual Dosage Oral:
  Children: 20 mg/kg/day or 600 mg/m²/day in 3-4 divided doses
  Adults: 250-500 mg 3-4 times/day up to 750 mg 3-4 times/day
Dosage Forms
  Caplet (Parafon Forte™ DSC): 500 mg
  Capsule (Blanex®, Lobac®, Miflex®, Mus-Lac®, Skelex®): 250 mg with acetaminophen 300 mg
  Tablet:
    Paraflex®: 250 mg
    Chlorofon-F®, Pargen® Fortified, Polyflex: 250 mg with acetaminophen 300 mg

Cholac® see lactulose on page 267

Cholan-HMB® see dehydrocholic acid on page 128

Cholebrine® see radiological/contrast media (ionic) on page 413

cholecalciferol (kole e kal si' fer ole)
Brand Names Delta-D®
Synonyms d₃
Therapeutic Category Vitamin D Analog
Use Dietary supplement, treatment of vitamin D deficiency or prophylaxis of deficiency
Usual Dosage Adults: Oral: 400-1000 units/day
Dosage Forms Tablet: 400 units, 1000 units

Choledyl® see oxtriphylline on page 349

cholera vaccine (kol' er a)
Therapeutic Category Vaccine, Inactivated Bacteria
Use Primary immunization for cholera prophylaxis
Usual Dosage I.M., S.C.:
  Children:
    6 months to 4 years: 0.2 mL with same dosage schedule
(Continued)

cholera vaccine *(Continued)*
5-10 years: 0.3 mL with same dosage schedule

Children >10 years and Adults: 0.5 mL in 2 doses 1 week to 1 month or more apart

Dosage Forms Injection: Suspension of killed *Vibrio cholerae* (Inaba and Ogawa types) 8 units of each serotype per mL (1.5 mL, 20 mL)

cholestyramine resin (koe less' tir a meen)
Brand Names Cholybar®; Questran®; Questran® Light

Therapeutic Category Antilipemic Agent

Use Adjunct in the management of primary hypercholesterolemia; pruritus associated with elevated levels of bile acids; diarrhea associated with excess fecal bile acids; binding toxicologic agents; pseudomembraneous colitis

Usual Dosage Dosages are expressed in terms of anhydrous resin. Oral:
Children: 240 mg/kg/day in 3 divided doses; need to titrate dose depending on indication

Adults: 3-4 g 3-4 times/day to a maximum of 16-32 g/day in 2-4 divided doses

Dosage Forms
Bar, chewable (caramel or raspberry flavor): 4 g (25s)
Powder: 4 g of resin/9 g of powder (9 g, 378 g)
Powder, for oral suspension, with aspartame: 4 g of resin/5 g of powder (5 g, 210 g)

choline magnesium trisalicylate
Brand Names Tricosal®; Trilisate®

Therapeutic Category Analgesic, Non-Narcotic; Anti-inflammatory Agent; Nonsteroidal Anti-Inflammatory Agent (NSAID), Oral; Salicylate

Use Management of osteoarthritis, rheumatoid arthritis, and other arthritides

Usual Dosage Oral (based on total salicylate content):
Children: 30-60 mg/kg/day given in 3-4 divided doses
Adults: 500 mg to 1.5 g 1-3 times/day

Dosage Forms
Liquid: 500 mg/5 mL [choline salicylate 293 mg and magnesium salicylate 362 mg per 5 mL] (237 mL)
Tablet:
   500 mg: Choline salicylate 293 mg and magnesium salicylate 362 mg
   750 mg: Choline salicylate 440 mg and magnesium salicylate 544 mg
   1000 mg: Choline salicylate 587 mg and magnesium salicylate 725 mg

choline salicylate
Brand Names Arthropan® [OTC]

Therapeutic Category Analgesic, Non-Narcotic; Anti-inflammatory Agent; Nonsteroidal Anti-Inflammatory Agent (NSAID), Oral; Salicylate

Use Temporary relief of pain of rheumatoid arthritis, rheumatic fever, osteoarthritis, and other conditions for which oral salicylates are recommended; useful in patients in which there is difficulty in administering doses in a tablet or capsule dosage form, because of the liquid dosage form

Usual Dosage Adults: 5 mL every 3-4 hours, if necessary, but not more than 6 doses in 24 hours

Dosage Forms Liquid (mint flavor): 870 mg/5 mL (240 mL, 480 mL)

choline theophyllinate *see* oxtriphylline *on page 349*

Cholografin® Meglumine *see* radiological/contrast media (ionic) *on page 413*

Choloxin® *see* dextrothyroxine sodium *on page 137*

Cholybar® *see* cholestyramine resin *on this page*

chondroitin sulfate-sodium hyaluronate
(kon droy' tin sul' fate-so' de um hi a lu ron' ate)
Brand Names Viscoat®
Synonyms sodium hyaluronate-chrondroitin sulfate
Therapeutic Category Ophthalmic Agent, Viscoeleastic
Use Surgical aid in anterior segment procedures, protects corneal endothelium and coats intraocular lens thus protecting it
Usual Dosage Carefully introduce into anterior chamber after thoroughly cleaning the chamber with a balanced salt solution
Dosage Forms Solution: Sodium chondroitin 40 mg and sodium hyaluronate 30 mg (0.25, 0.5 mL)

Chooz® [OTC] *see* calcium carbonate *on page 65*

Chorex® *see* chorionic gonadotropin *on this page*

chorionic gonadotropin (kor re on' ik goe nad' oh troe pin)
Brand Names A.P.L.®; Chorex®; Choron®; Corgonject®; Follutein®; Glukor®; Gonic®; Pregnyl®; Profasi® HP
Synonyms CG; HCG
Therapeutic Category Gonadotropin; Ovulation Stimulator
Use Induce ovulation and pregnancy; treatment of hypogonadotropic hypogonadism, prepubertal cryptorchidism
Usual Dosage Children: I.M.:
Prepubertal cryptorchidism: 1000-2000 units/m^2/dose 3 times/week for 3 weeks

Hypogonadotropic hypogonadism: 500-1000 USP units 3 times/week for 3 weeks, followed by the same dose twice weekly for 3 weeks
Dosage Forms Powder for injection: 200 units/mL (10 mL, 25 mL); 500 units/mL (10 mL); 1000 units/mL (10 mL); 2000 units/mL (10 mL)

Choron® *see* chorionic gonadotropin *on this page*

Chromagen® OB [OTC] *see* vitamin, multiple (prenatal) *on page 499*

Chroma-Pak® *see* trace metals *on page 472*

chromium injection *see* trace metals *on page 472*

Chronulac® *see* lactulose *on page 267*

Chymex® *see* bentiromide *on page 47*

Chymodiactin® *see* chymopapain *on this page*

chymopapain (kye' moe pa pane)
Brand Names Chymodiactin®; Discase®
Therapeutic Category Enzyme, Intradiscal; Enzyme, Proteolytic
Use Alternative to surgery in patients with herniated lumbar intervertebral disks
Usual Dosage 2000-4000 units/disk with a maximum cumulative dose not to exceed 8000 units for patients with multiple disk herniations
Dosage Forms Injection: 4000 units [4 nKat]; 10,000 units [10 nKat]

chymotrypsin (kye moe trip' sin)
Brand Names Catarase®; Zolyse®
Synonyms alpha chymotrypsin
Therapeutic Category Enzyme, Ophthalmic
Use Enzymatic zonulysis for intracapsular lens extraction in cataract surgery
Usual Dosage Irrigate area with 1-2 mL containing 150 units
Dosage Forms Powder for ophthalmic solution:
Catarase®: 150 units [1:10,000] (with 2 mL diluent); 300 units [1:5000] (with 2 mL diluent)
Zolyse®: 750 units (with 9 mL diluent)

ALPHABETICAL LISTING OF DRUGS

Cibalith-S® *see* lithium *on page 276*

ciclopirox olamine (sye kloe peer' ox)
Brand Names Loprox®
Therapeutic Category Antifungal Agent, Topical
Use Treatment of tinea pedis, tinea cruris, tinea corporis, cutaneous candidiasis, tinea versi-color
Usual Dosage Children >10 years and Adults: Apply twice daily, gently massage into affected areas; safety and efficacy in children <10 years have not been established
Dosage Forms
Cream, topical: 1% (15 g, 30 g, 90 g)
Lotion: 1% (30 mL)

Ciloxan™ Ophthalmic *see* ciprofloxacin hydrochloride *on this page*

cimetidine (sye met' i deen)
Brand Names Tagamet®
Therapeutic Category Histamine-2 Antagonist
Use Short-term treatment of active duodenal ulcers and benign gastric ulcers; long-term prophylaxis of duodenal ulcer; gastric hypersecretory states; gastroesophageal reflux; prevention of upper gastrointestinal bleeding in critically ill patients
Usual Dosage Oral, I.M., I.V.:
Neonates: 5-10 mg/kg/day in divided doses every 8-12 hours
Infants: 10-20 mg/kg/day divided every 6-12 hours
Children: 20-30 mg/kg/day in divided doses every 6 hours

Patients with an active bleed: Give cimetidine as a continuous infusion

Adults:
Short-term treatment of active ulcers:
Oral: 300 mg 4 times/day or 800 mg at bedtime or 400 mg twice daily for up to 8 weeks
I.M., I.V.: 300 mg every 6 hours or 37.5 mg/hour by continuous infusion; I.V. dosage should be adjusted to maintain an intragastric pH of 5 or greater
Duodenal ulcer prophylaxis: Oral: 400-800 mg at bedtime
Gastric hypersecretory conditions: Oral, I.M., I.V.: 300-600 mg every 6 hours; dosage not to exceed 2.4 g/day
Dosage Forms
Infusion, as hydrochloride, in NS: 300 mg (50 mL)
Injection, as hydrochloride: 150 mg/mL (2 mL, 8 mL)
Liquid, oral, as hydrochloride (mint-peach flavor): 300 mg/5 mL with alcohol 2.8% (5 mL, 240 mL)
Tablet: 200 mg, 300 mg, 400 mg, 800 mg

Cinobac® Pulvules® *see* cinoxacin *on this page*
Cinonide® Injection *see* triamcinolone *on page 474*

cinoxacin (sin ox' a sin)
Brand Names Cinobac® Pulvules®
Therapeutic Category Antibiotic, Quinolone
Use Urinary tract infections
Usual Dosage Children >12 years and Adults: 1 g/day in 2-4 doses
Dosage Forms Capsule: 250 mg, 500 mg

ciprofloxacin hydrochloride (sip roe flox' a sin)
Brand Names Ciloxan™ Ophthalmic; Cipro™ Injection; Cipro™ Oral
Therapeutic Category Antibiotic, Ophthalmic; Antibiotic, Quinolone
Use Treatment of documented or suspected pseudomonal infection in home care patients; documented multi-drug resistant gram-negative organisms; documented infectious diar-

102

rhea due to *Campylobacter jejuni*, *Shigella*, or *Salmonella*; osteomyelitis caused by susceptible organisms in which parenteral therapy is not feasible; used ophthalmically for treatment of corneal ulcers and conjunctivitis due to strains of microorganisms susceptible to ciprofloxacin

Usual Dosage
Children: Oral: 20-30 mg/kg/day in 2 divided doses; maximum dose: 1.5 g/day

Adults:
Oral: 250-750 mg every 12 hours, depending on severity of infection and susceptibility
Ophthalmic: Instill 1-2 drops in eye(s) every 2 hours while awake for 2 days and 1-2 drops every 4 hours while awake for the next 5 days
I.V.: 200-400 mg every 12 hours depending on severity of infection

Dosage Forms
Infusion, in D_5W: 400 mg (200 mL)
Infusion, in NS or D_5W: 200 mg (100 mL)
Injection: 200 mg (20 mL); 400 mg (40 mL)
Solution, ophthalmic: 3.5 mg/mL (2.5 mL, 5 mL)
Tablet: 250 mg, 500 mg, 750 mg

Cipro™ Injection *see* ciprofloxacin hydrochloride *on previous page*

Cipro™ Oral *see* ciprofloxacin hydrochloride *on previous page*

cisapride (sis' a pride)
Brand Names Propulsid®
Therapeutic Category Antiemetic; Cholinergic Agent
Use Symptomatic treatment of patients with nocturnal heartburn due to gastrointestinal reflux disease
Usual Dosage Adults: Oral: 10 mg 4 times daily at least 15 minutes before meals and at bedtime; in some patients the dosage will need to be increased to 20 mg to obtain a satisfactory result
Dosage Forms Tablet: 10 mg

cisplatin (sis' pla tin)
Brand Names Platinol®; Platinol®-AQ
Synonyms CDDP
Therapeutic Category Antineoplastic Agent, Alkylating Agent
Use Management of metastatic testicular or ovarian carcinoma, advanced bladder cancer, osteosarcoma, Hodgkin's and non-Hodgkin's lymphoma, head or neck cancer, cervical cancer, lung cancer, or other tumors; used alone or with other agents
Usual Dosage Refer to individual protocols
Children and Adults:
I.V.: Intermittent dosing schedule: 37-75 mg/m² once every 2-3 weeks or 50-120 mg/m² once every 3-4 weeks
Daily dosing schedule: 15-20 mg/m²/day for 5 days every 3-4 weeks
Dosage Forms
Injection, aqueous: 1 mg/mL (50 mL, 100 mL)
Powder for injection: 10 mg, 50 mg

13-*cis*-retinoic acid *see* isotretinoin *on page 260*

Citracal® [OTC] *see* calcium citrate *on page 67*

citrate of magnesia *see* magnesium citrate *on page 282*

citric acid and d-gluconic acid irrigant *see* citric acid bladder mixture *on this page*

citric acid bladder mixture
Brand Names Renacidin®
Synonyms citric acid and d-gluconic acid irrigant; hemiacidrin
Therapeutic Category Irrigating Solution

(Continued)

citric acid bladder mixture *(Continued)*
Use Preparing solutions for irrigating indwelling urethral catheters; to dissolve or prevent formation of calcifications
Usual Dosage 30-60 mL of 10% (sterile) solution 2-3 times/day by means of a rubber syringe
Dosage Forms
Powder for solution: Citric acid 156-171 g, magnesium hydroxycarbonate 75-87 g, d-gluconic acid 21-30 g, magnesium acid citrate 9-15 g, calcium carbonate 2-6 g (150 g, 300 g)
Solution, irrigation: Citric acid 6.602 g, magnesium hydroxycarbonate 3.177 g, glucono-delta-lactone 0.198 g and benzoic acid 0.023 g per 100 mL (500 mL)

Citro-Nesia™ [OTC] *see* magnesium citrate *on page 282*
citrovorum factor *see* leucovorin calcium *on page 268*
Citrucel® [OTC] *see* methylcellulose *on page 304*
CL-719 *see* gemfibrozil *on page 210*
cla *see* clarithromycin *on this page*

cladribine (kla' dri been)
Brand Names Leustatin™
Synonyms 2-CdA; 2-chlorodeoxyadenosine
Therapeutic Category Antineoplastic Agent, Antimetabolite
Use Hairy cell and chronic lymphocytic leukemias
Usual Dosage Refer to individual protocols
Adults: I.V.: 0.09 mg/kg/day continuous infusion
Dosage Forms Injection, preservative free: 1 mg/mL (10 mL)

Claforan® *see* cefotaxime sodium *on page 80*

clarithromycin (kla rith' roe mye sin)
Brand Names Biaxin™ Filmtabs®
Synonyms cla
Therapeutic Category Antibiotic, Macrolide
Use Against most respiratory pathogens (eg, *S. pyogenes, S. pneumoniae, S. agalactiae, S. viridans, M. catarrhalis, C. trachomatis, Legionella* spp., *Mycoplasma pneumoniae*[, *S. aureus*). Clarithromycin is highly active (MICs ≤0.25 µg/mL) against *H. influenzae*, the combination of clarithromycin and its metabolite demonstrate an additive effect. Additionally, clarithromycin has shown activity against *C. pneumoniae* (including strain TWAR) and *M. avium* infection.
Usual Dosage Usual dose: 250-500 mg every 12 hours for 7-14 days
Upper respiratory tract: 250-500 mg every 12 hours for 10-14 days
Pharyngitis/tonsillitis: 250 mg every 12 hours for 10 days
Acute maxillary sinusitis: 500 mg every 12 hours for 14 days

Lower respiratory tract: 250-500 mg every 12 hours for 7-14 days
Acute exacerbation of chronic bronchitis due to:
S. pneumoniae: 250 mg every 12 hours for 7-14 days
M. catarrhalis: 250 mg every 12 hours for 7-14 days
H. influenzae: 500 mg every 12 hours for 7-14 days
Pneumonia due to:
S. pneumoniae: 250 mg every 12 hours for 7-14 days
M. pneumoniae: 250 mg every 12 hours for 7-14 days

Uncomplicated skin and skin structure: 250 mg every 12 hours for 7-14 days
Dosage Forms Tablet, film coated: 250 mg, 500 mg

Claritin® *see* loratadine *on page 278*

Clear Away® Disc [OTC] *see* salicylic acid *on page 424*

Clearblue® *see* diagnostic aids (*in vitro*), urine *on page 139*

Clear By Design® [OTC] *see* benzoyl peroxide *on page 49*

Clear Eyes® [OTC] *see* naphazoline hydrochloride *on page 325*

Clearplan® Easy *see* diagnostic aids (*in vitro*), urine *on page 139*

Clearsil® [OTC] *see* benzoyl peroxide *on page 49*

clemastine and phenylpropanolamine
Brand Names Tavist-D®
Therapeutic Category Antihistamine/Decongestant Combination
Use Symptomatic relief of allergic rhinitis; pruritus of the eyes, nose or throat, lacrimation and nasal congestion
Usual Dosage Children >12 years and Adults: Oral: 1 tablet every 12 hours
Dosage Forms Tablet: Clemastine fumarate 1.34 mg and phenylpropanolamine hydrochloride 75 mg

clemastine fumarate (klem' as teen fume' a rate)
Brand Names Tavist®; Tavist®-1 [OTC]
Therapeutic Category Antihistamine
Use Perennial and seasonal allergic rhinitis and other allergic symptoms including urticaria
Usual Dosage Oral:
Children:
>   <12 years: 0.67-1.34 mg every 8-12 hours as needed
>   >12 years: 1.34 mg twice daily to 2.68 mg 3 times/day; do not exceed 8.04 mg/day

>   Adults: 1.34 mg twice daily to 2.68 mg 3 times/day; do not exceed 8.04 mg/day

Dosage Forms
Syrup (citrus flavor): 0.67 mg/5 mL with alcohol 5.5% (120 mL)
Tablet: 1.34 mg, 2.68 mg

Cleocin HCl® Oral *see* clindamycin *on this page*

Cleocin Pediatric® Oral *see* clindamycin *on this page*

Cleocin Phosphate® Injection *see* clindamycin *on this page*

Cleocin T® Topical *see* clindamycin *on this page*

Cleocin® Vaginal *see* clindamycin *on this page*

clidinium and chlordiazepoxide (kli di' nee um & klor dye az e pox' ide)
Brand Names Clindex®; Clinoxide®; Clipoxide®; Librax®; Lidox®; Zebrax®
Synonyms chlordiazepoxide and clidinium
Therapeutic Category Antispasmodic Agent, Gastrointestinal
Use Adjunct treatment of peptic ulcer, treatment of irritable bowel syndrome
Usual Dosage Oral: 1-2 capsules 3-4 times/day, before meals or food and at bedtime
Dosage Forms Capsule: Clidinium bromide 2.5 mg and chlordiazepoxide hydrochloride 5 mg

clindamycin (klin da mye' sin)
Brand Names Cleocin HCl® Oral; Cleocin Pediatric® Oral; Cleocin Phosphate® Injection; Cleocin T® Topical; Cleocin® Vaginal
Therapeutic Category Acne Product; Antibiotic, Anaerobic; Antibiotic, Miscellaneous
Use Useful agent against aerobic and anaerobic streptococci (except enterococci), most staphylococci, *Bacteroides* sp. and *Actinomyces*; used topically in treatment of severe acne
(Continued)

clindamycin *(Continued)*

Usual Dosage Avoid in neonates (contains benzyl alcohol)
Neonates: I.M., I.V.:
Postnatal age <7 days:
≤2000 g: 10 mg/kg/day in 2 equally divided doses
>2000 g: 15 mg/kg/day in 3 divided doses
Postnatal age >7 days:
<1200 g: 10 mg/kg/day in 2 equally divided doses
1200-2000 g: 15 mg/kg/day in 3 divided doses
>2000 g: 20 mg/kg/day in 3-4 divided doses
Infants and Children:
Oral: 10-30 mg/kg/day in 3-4 divided doses
I.M., I.V.: 25-40 mg/kg/day in 3-4 divided doses
Children and Adults: Topical: Apply twice daily
Adults:
Oral: 150-450 mg/dose every 6-8 hours; maximum dose: 1.8 g/day
I.M., I.V.: 1.2-1.8 g/day in 2-4 divided doses; maximum dose: 4.8 g/day
Vaginal: One full applicator (100 mg) inserted intravaginally once daily before bedtime
for seven consecutive days

Dosage Forms
Capsule, as hydrochloride: 75 mg, 150 mg, 300 mg
Cream, vaginal: 2% (40 g)
Gel, topical, as phosphate: 1% [10 mg/g] (7.5 g, 30 g)
Granules for oral solution, as palmitate: 75 mg/5 mL (100 mL)
Infusion, as phosphate, in D_5W: 300 mg (50 mL); 600 mg (50 mL)
Injection, as phosphate: 150 mg/mL (2 mL, 4 mL, 6 mL, 50 mL, 60 mL)
Lotion: 1% [10 mg/mL] (60 mL)
Solution, topical, as phosphate: 1% [10 mg/mL] (30 mL, 60 mL, 480 mL)

Clindex® *see* clidinium and chlordiazepoxide *on previous page*

Clinistix® [OTC] *see* diagnostic aids *(in vitro)*, urine *on page 139*

Clinitest® [OTC] *see* diagnostic aids *(in vitro)*, urine *on page 139*

Clinoril® *see* sulindac *on page 450*

Clinoxide® *see* clidinium and chlordiazepoxide *on previous page*

clioquinol (klye oh kwin' ole)

Formerly Known As iodochlorhydroxyquin
Brand Names Vioform® Topical [OTC]
Therapeutic Category Antifungal Agent, Topical
Use Used topically in the treatment of tinea pedis, tinea cruris, and skin infections caused
by dermatophytic fungi (ring worm)
Usual Dosage Children and Adults: Topical: Apply 2-4 times/day; do not use for longer
than 7 days
Dosage Forms
Cream: 3% (30 g)
Ointment, topical: 3% (30 g)

clioquinol and hydrocortisone

Formerly Known As iodochlorhydroxyquin and hydrocortisone
Brand Names Ala-Quin® Topical; Corque® Topical; Cortin® Topical; Hysone® Topical; Lan-
visone® Topical; Pedi-Cort V® Topical; Racet® Topical; UAD® Topical; Vioform-HC® Topi-
cal
Synonyms hydrocortisone and clioquinol
Therapeutic Category Antifungal Agent, Topical; Corticosteroid, Topical (Low Potency)

Use Contact or atopic dermatitis; eczema; neurodermatitis; anogenital pruritus; mycotic dermatoses; moniliasis
Usual Dosage Topical: Apply in a thin film 3-4 times/day
Dosage Forms
Cream: Clioquinol 3% and hydrocortisone 0.5% (15 g, 30 g); clioquinol 3% and hydrocortisone 1% (15 g, 30 g)
Lotion: Clioquinol 0.75% and hydrocortisone 0.25% (120 mL)
Ointment, topical: Clioquinol 3% and hydrocortisone 1% (20 g, 480 g)

Clipoxide® *see* clidinium and chlordiazepoxide *on page 105*

clobetasol dipropionate (kloe bay' ta sol dye pro pee oh' nate)
Brand Names Temovate® Topical
Therapeutic Category Corticosteroid, Topical (Very High Potency)
Use Short-term relief of inflammation of moderate to severe corticosteroid-responsive dermatosis
Usual Dosage Apply twice daily for up to 2 weeks with no more than 50 g/week
Dosage Forms
Cream: 0.05% (15 g, 30 g, 45 g)
Ointment, topical: 0.05% (15 g, 30 g, 45 g)
Scalp application: 0.05% (25 mL, 50 mL)

Clocort® Maximum Strength [OTC] *see* hydrocortisone *on page 236*

clocortolone pivalate (kloe kor' toe lone)
Brand Names Cloderm® Topical
Therapeutic Category Corticosteroid, Topical (Medium Potency)
Use Inflammation of corticosteroid-responsive dermatoses
Usual Dosage Topical: Apply sparingly and gently rub into affected area 1-4 times/day
Dosage Forms Cream: 0.1% (15 g, 45 g)

Cloderm® Topical *see* clocortolone pivalate *on this page*

clofazimine palmitate (kloe fa' zi meen)
Brand Names Lamprene®
Therapeutic Category Antibiotic, Miscellaneous
Use Treatment of dapsone-resistant leprosy; multibacillary dapsone-sensitive leprosy; erythema nodosum leprosum; *Mycobacterium avium* intracellular (MAI) infections
Usual Dosage Oral:
Children: Leprosy: 1 mg/kg/day every 24 hours in combination with dapsone and rifampin
Adults:
Dapsone-resistant leprosy: 50-100 mg/day in combination with one or more antileprosy drugs for 2 years; then alone 50-100 mg/day
Dapsone-sensitive multibacillary leprosy: 50-100 mg/day in combination with two or more antileprosy drugs for at least 2 years and continue until negative skin smears are obtained, then institute single drug therapy with appropriate agent
Erythema nodosum leprosum: 100-200 mg/day for up to 3 months or longer then taper dose to 100 mg/day when possible
MAI: Combination therapy using clofazimine 100 mg 1 or 3 times/day in combination with other antimycobacterial agents
Dosage Forms Capsule: 50 mg, 100 mg

clofibrate (kloe fye' brate)
Brand Names Atromid-S®
Therapeutic Category Antilipemic Agent
Use Adjunct to dietary therapy in the management of hyperlipidemias associated with high triglyceride levels
(Continued)

clofibrate (Continued)

Usual Dosage Adults: Oral: 500 mg 4 times/day
Dosage Forms Capsule: 500 mg

Clomid® *see* clomiphene citrate *on this page*

clomiphene citrate (kloe' mi feen)

Brand Names Clomid®; Milophene®; Serophene®
Therapeutic Category Ovulation Stimulator
Use Treatment of ovulatory failure in patients desiring pregnancy
Usual Dosage Oral: 50 mg/day for 5 days (first course); start the regimen on or about the fifth day of cycle; if ovulation occurs do not increase dosage; if not, increase next course to 100 mg/day for 5 days
Dosage Forms Tablet: 50 mg

clomipramine hydrochloride (kloe mi' pra meen)

Brand Names Anafranil®
Therapeutic Category Antidepressant, Tricyclic
Use Treatment of obsessive-compulsive disorder (OCD)
Usual Dosage Oral:

Children: Initial: 25 mg/day and gradually increase, as tolerated to a maximum of 3 mg/kg or 100 mg, whichever is smaller

Adults: Initial: 25 mg/day and gradually increase, as tolerated to 100 mg/day the first 2 weeks, may then be increased to a total of 250 mg/day
Dosage Forms Capsule: 25 mg, 50 mg, 75 mg

clonazepam (kloe na' ze pam)

Brand Names Klonopin™
Therapeutic Category Anticonvulsant, Benzodiazepine
Use Prophylaxis of absence (petit mal), petit mal variant (Lennox-Gastaut), akinetic, and myoclonic seizures
Usual Dosage Oral:

Children <10 years or 30 kg:
Initial daily dose: 0.01-0.03 mg/kg/day (maximum: 0.05 mg/kg/day) given in 2-3 divided doses; increase by no more than 0.5 mg every third day until seizures are controlled or adverse effects are seen
Maintenance dose: 0.1-0.2 mg/kg/day divided 3 times/day; not to exceed 0.2 mg/kg/day

Adults:
Initial daily dose not to exceed 1.5 mg given in 3 divided doses; may increase by 0.5-1 mg every third day until seizures are controlled or adverse effects seen
Maintenance dose: 0.05-0.2 mg/kg; do not exceed 20 mg/day
Dosage Forms Tablet: 0.5 mg, 1 mg, 2 mg

clonidine (kloe' ni deen)

Brand Names Catapres® Oral; Catapres-TTS® Transdermal
Therapeutic Category Alpha-Adrenergic Agonist
Use Management of mild to moderate hypertension; either used alone or in combination with other antihypertensives; not recommended for first line therapy for hypertension; also used for heroin withdrawal and in smoking cessation therapy; other uses may include prophylaxis of migraines, glaucoma, paralytic ileus, and diabetes associated diarrhea
Usual Dosage Oral:

Children: Initial: 5-10 µg/kg/day in divided doses every 8-12 hours; increase gradually to 5-25 µg/kg/day in divided doses every 6 hours; maximum: 0.9 mg/day

Adults:
Initial dose: 0.1 mg twice daily
Maintenance dose: 0.2-1.2 mg/day in 2-4 divided doses; maximum recommended dose: 2.4 mg/day

Clonidine tolerance test (test of growth hormone release from the pituitary): 0.15 mg/m^2 or 4 μg/kg as a single dose

Transdermal: Initial dose: 0.1 mg/day, increase every 1-2 weeks; maximum: doses exceeding 0.5 mg/day do not increase efficacy

Dosage Forms
Patch, transdermal: 1, 2, and 3 (0.1, 0.2, 0.3 mg/day to 7-day duration)
Tablet, as hydrochloride: 0.1 mg, 0.2 mg, 0.3 mg

clonidine and chlorthalidone
Brand Names Combipres®
Therapeutic Category Antihypertensive, Combination
Use Management of mild to moderate hypertension
Usual Dosage Oral: 1 tablet 1-2 times/day
Dosage Forms Tablet:
0.1: Clonidine 0.1 mg and chlorthalidone 15 mg
0.2: Clonidine 0.2 mg and chlorthalidone 15 mg
0.3: Clonidine 0.3 mg and chlorthalidone 15 mg

Clopra® see metoclopramide on page 308

clorazepate dipotassium (klor az' e pate)
Brand Names Gen-XENE®; Tranxene®
Therapeutic Category Anticonvulsant, Benzodiazepine; Benzodiazepine; Sedative
Use Treatment of generalized anxiety and panic disorders; management of alcohol withdrawal; adjunct anticonvulsant in management of partial seizures
Usual Dosage Oral:
Anticonvulsant:
Children:
<9 years: Dose not established
9-12 years: Anticonvulsant: Initial: 3.75-7.5 mg/dose twice daily; increase dose by 3.75 mg at weekly intervals, not to exceed 60 mg/day in 2-3 divided doses
Children >12 years and Adults: Initial: Up to 7.5 mg/dose 2-3 times/day; increase dose by 7.5 mg at weekly intervals; usual dose: 0.5-1 mg/kg/day; not to exceed 90 mg/day (up to 3 mg/kg/day has been used)
Anxiety: Adults: 7.5-15 mg 2-4 times/day, or given as single dose of 15-22.5 mg at bedtime
Alcohol withdrawal: Adults: Initial: 30 mg, then 15 mg 2-4 times/day on first day; maximum daily dose: 90 mg; gradually decrease dose over subsequent days
Dosage Forms
Capsule: 3.75 mg, 7.5 mg, 15 mg
Tablet: 3.75 mg, 7.5 mg, 15 mg
Tablet, single dose: 11.25 mg, 22.5 mg

clotrimazole (kloe trim' a zole)
Brand Names Gyne-Lotrimin® Vaginal [OTC]; Lotrimin AF® Topical [OTC]; Lotrimin® Topical; Mycelex®-G Topical; Mycelex®-G Vaginal [OTC]; Mycelex® Troche
Therapeutic Category Antifungal Agent, Oral Nonabsorbed; Antifungal Agent, Topical; Antifungal Agent, Vaginal
Use Treatment of susceptible fungal infections, including oropharyngeal candidiasis, dermatophytoses, superficial mycoses, and cutaneous candidiasis, as well as vulvovaginal candidiasis; limited data suggests that the use of clotrimazole troches may be effective for prophylaxis against oropharyngeal candidiasis in neutropenic patients
(Continued)

clotrimazole *(Continued)*
Usual Dosage
Children >3 years and Adults:
Oral: 10 mg troche dissolved slowly 5 times/day
Topical: Apply twice daily

Adults: Vaginal: 100 mg/day for 7 days or 200 mg/day for 3 days or 500 mg single dose or 5 g (= 1 applicatorful) of 1% vaginal cream daily for 7-14 days
Dosage Forms
Cream:
Topical (Lotrimin®, Lotrimin® AF, Mycelex®, Mycelex® OTC) : 1% (15 g, 30 g, 45 g, 90 g)
Vaginal (Gyne-Lotrimin®, Mycelex®-G): 1% (45 g, 90 g)
Lotion (Lotrimin®): 1% (30 mL)
Solution, topical (Lotrimin®, Lotrimin® AF, Mycelex®, Mycelex® OTC): 1% (10 mL, 30 mL)
Tablet, vaginal (Gyne-Lotrimin®, Mycelex®-G): 100 mg (7s); 500 mg (1s)
Troche (Mycelex®): 10 mg
Twin pack (Mycelex®): Tablet 500 mg (1's) and vaginal cream 1% (7 g)

cloxacillin sodium (klox a sill' in)
Brand Names Cloxapen®; Tegopen®
Therapeutic Category Antibiotic, Penicillin
Use Treatment of susceptible bacterial infections, notably penicillinase-producing staphylococci causing respiratory tract, skin and skin structure, bone and joint, urinary tract infections, endocarditis, septicemia, and meningitis
Usual Dosage Oral:
Children >1 month: 50-100 mg/kg/day in divided doses every 6 hours; up to a maximum of 4 g/day

Adults: 250-500 mg every 6 hours
Dosage Forms
Capsule: 250 mg, 500 mg
Powder for oral suspension: 125 mg/5 mL (100 mL, 200 mL)

Cloxapen® *see* cloxacillin sodium *on this page*

clozapine (kloe' za peen)
Brand Names Clozaril®
Therapeutic Category Antipsychotic Agent
Use Management of schizophrenic patients
Usual Dosage Adults: Oral: 25 mg once or twice daily initially and increased, as tolerated to a target dose of 300-450 mg/day, but may require doses as high as 600-900 mg/day
Dosage Forms Tablet: 25 mg, 100 mg

Clozaril® *see* clozapine *on this page*

Clysodrast® *see* bisacodyl *on page 54*

CMV-IGIV *see* cytomegalovirus immune globulin intravenous, human *on page 124*

coal tar
Brand Names AquaTar® [OTC]; Denorex® [OTC]; DHS® Tar [OTC]; Duplex® T [OTC]; Estar® [OTC]; Fototar® [OTC]; Neutrogena® T/Derm; Pentrax® [OTC]; Polytar® [OTC]; psoriGel® [OTC]; T/Gel® [OTC]; Zetar® [OTC]
Synonyms crude coal tar; L.C.D.; pix carbonis
Therapeutic Category Antipsoriatic Agent, Topical; Antiseborrheic Agent, Topical

Use Topically for controlling dandruff, seborrheic dermatitis, or psoriasis

Usual Dosage

Bath: Add appropriate amount to bath water, for adults usually 60-90 mL of a 5% to 20% solution or 15-25 mL of 30% lotion; soak 5-20 minutes, then pat dry; use once daily to 3 days

Shampoo: Rub shampoo onto wet hair and scalp, rinse thoroughly; repeat; leave on 5 minutes; rinse thoroughly; apply twice weekly for the first 2 weeks then once weekly or more often if needed

Skin: Apply to the affected area 1-4 times/day; decrease frequency to 2-3 times/week once condition has been controlled

Scalp psoriasis: Tar oil bath or coal tar solution may be painted sparingly to the lesions 3-12 hours before each shampoo

Psoriasis of the body, arms, legs: Apply at bedtime; if thick scales are present, use product with salicylic acid and apply several times during the day

Dosage Forms

Cream: 1% to 5%

Gel: Coal tar 5%

Lotion: 2.5% to 30%

Lotion: Coal tar 2% to 5%

Shampoo: Coal tar extract 2% with salicylic acid 2% (60 mL)

Shampoo, topical: Coal tar: 0.5% to 5%

Solution:

Coal tar: 2.5%, 5%, 20%

Coal tar extract: 5%

Suspension, coal tar: 30% to 33.3%

coal tar and salicylic acid

Brand Names X-seb® T [OTC]

Therapeutic Category Antipsoriatic Agent, Topical; Antiseborrheic Agent, Topical

Use Seborrheal dermatitis; dandruff

Usual Dosage Shampoo twice weekly

Dosage Forms Shampoo: Coal tar solution 10% and salicylic acid 4% (120 mL)

coal tar, lanolin, and mineral oil

Brand Names Balnetar® [OTC]

Therapeutic Category Antipsoriatic Agent, Topical; Antiseborrheic Agent, Topical

Use Psoriasis; seborrheal dermatitis; atopic dermatitis; eczematoid dermatitis

Usual Dosage Add to bath water, soak for 5-20 minutes then pat dry

Dosage Forms Oil, bath: Water-dispersible emollient tar 2.5%, lanolin fraction, and mineral oil (240 mL)

Cobex® see cyanocobalamin on page 120

cocaine hydrochloride (koe kane')

Therapeutic Category Local Anesthetic, Topical

Use Topical anesthesia for mucous membranes

Usual Dosage Use lowest effective dose; do not exceed 1 mg/kg; patient tolerance, anesthetic technique, vascularity of tissue and area to be anesthetized will determine dose needed

Dosage Forms

Powder: 5 g, 25 g

Solution, topical: 4% [40 mg/mL] (2 mL, 4 mL, 10 mL); 10% [100 mg/mL] (4 mL, 10 mL)

Tablet, soluble, for topical solution: 135 mg

coccidioidin skin test (kox i dee oh' i din)
Brand Names Spherulin®
Therapeutic Category Diagnostic Agent, Fungus
Use Intradermal skin test in diagnosis of coccidioidomycosis; differential diagnosis of this disease from histoplasmosis, sarcoidosis and other mycotic and bacterial infections. The skin test may be negative in severe forms of disease (anergy) or when prolonged periods of time have passed since infection.
Usual Dosage Children and Adults: Intradermally: 0.1 mL of 1:100 or flexor surface of forearm

Positive reaction: Induration of 5 mm or more; erythema without induration is considered negative; read the test at 24 and 48 hours, since some reactions may not be noticeable after 36 hours. A positive reaction indicates present or past infection with *Coccidioides immitis*.

Negative reaction: A negative test means the individual has not been sensitized to coccidioidin or has lost sensitivity
Dosage Forms Injection: 1:10 (0.5 mL); 1:100 (1 mL)

Codafed® Expectorant *see* guaifenesin, pseudoephedrine, and codeine *on page 221*

Codamine® *see* hydrocodone and phenylpropanolamine *on page 235*

Codamine® Pediatric *see* hydrocodone and phenylpropanolamine *on page 235*

CodAphen® *see* acetaminophen and codeine *on page 3*

Codehist® DH *see* chlorpheniramine, pseudoephedrine, and codeine *on page 97*

codeine (koe' deen)
Synonyms methylmorphine
Therapeutic Category Analgesic, Narcotic; Antitussive
Use Treatment of mild to moderate pain; antitussive in lower doses
Usual Dosage Doses should be titrated to appropriate analgesic effect; when changing routes of administration, note that oral dose is $^2/_3$ as effective as parenteral dose

Analgesic: Oral, I.M., S.C.:
   Children: 0.5-1 mg/kg/dose every 4-6 hours as needed; maximum: 60 mg/dose
   Adults: 30 mg/dose; range: 15-60 mg every 4-6 hours as needed

Antitussive: Oral (for nonproductive cough):
   Children: 1-1.5 mg/kg/day in divided doses every 4-6 hours as needed: Alternatively dose according to age:
      2-6 years: 2.5-5 mg every 4-6 hours as needed; maximum: 30 mg/day
      6-12 years: 5-10 mg every 4-6 hours as needed; maximum: 60 mg/day
   Adults: 10-20 mg/dose every 4-6 hours as needed; maximum: 120 mg/day
Dosage Forms
Injection, as phosphate: 30 mg (1 mL, 2 mL); 60 mg (1 mL, 2 mL)
Solution, oral: 15 mg/5 mL
Tablet, as sulfate: 15 mg, 30 mg, 60 mg
Tablet, as phosphate, soluble: 30 mg, 60 mg
Tablet, as sulfate, soluble: 15 mg, 30 mg, 60 mg

codeine and acetaminophen *see* acetaminophen and codeine *on page 3*

codeine and aspirin *see* aspirin and codeine *on page 35*

codeine and bromodiphenhydramine *see* bromodiphenhydramine and codeine *on page 58*

codeine and butalbital compound *see* butalbital compound and codeine *on page 63*

codeine and guaifenesin *see* guaifenesin and codeine *on page 218*

Codiclear® DH *see* hydrocodone and guaifenesin *on page 235*

Codimal-A® Injection *see* brompheniramine maleate *on page 59*

Codimal® Expectorant [OTC] *see* guaifenesin and phenylpropanolamine *on page 219*

Codimal-L.A.® *see* chlorpheniramine and pseudoephedrine *on page 94*

cod liver oil *see* vitamin A and vitamin D *on page 497*

Codoxy® *see* oxycodone and aspirin *on page 350*

Codroxomin® Injection *see* hydroxocobalamin *on page 240*

Cogentin® *see* benztropine mesylate *on page 50*

Co-Gesic® *see* hydrocodone and acetaminophen *on page 234*

Cognex® Oral *see* tacrine hydrochloride *on page 452*

Colace® [OTC] *see* docusate *on page 157*

colaspase *see* asparaginase *on page 34*

Co-Lav® *see* polyethylene glycol-electrolyte solution *on page 383*

Colax® [OTC] *see* docusate and phenolphthalein *on page 158*

ColBENEMID® *see* colchicine and probenecid *on this page*

colchicine (kol' chi seen)

Therapeutic Category Anti-inflammatory Agent; Uricosuric Agent

Use Treat acute gouty arthritis attacks and to prevent recurrences of such attacks; management of familial Mediterranean fever

Usual Dosage
Treatment for acute gouty arthritis:
  Oral: Initial: 0.5-1.2 mg, then 0.5-0.6 mg every 1-2 hours or 1-1.2 mg every 2 hours until relief or GI side effects occur to a maximum total dose of 8 mg, wait 3 days before initiating a second course
  I.V.: Initial: 1-3 mg, then 0.5 mg every 6 hours until response, not to exceed 4 mg/day; following a full course of colchicine (4 mg), wait 7 days before initiating another course of colchicine (by any route)

Prophylaxis of recurrent attacks: Oral:
  <1 attack/year: 0.5 or 0.6 mg/day/dose for 3-4 days/week
  >1 attack/year: 0.5 or 0.6 mg/day/dose
  Severe cases: 1-1.8 mg/day

Dosage Forms
Injection: 0.5 mg/mL (2 mL)
Tablet: 0.5 mg, 0.6 mg

colchicine and probenecid

Brand Names ColBENEMID®; Proben-C®

Synonyms probenecid and colchicine

Therapeutic Category Uricosuric Agent

Use Treatment of chronic gouty arthritis when complicated by frequent, recurrent acute attacks of gout

Usual Dosage Adults: Oral: 1 tablet daily for 1 week, then 1 tablet twice daily thereafter

Dosage Forms Tablet: Colchicine 0.5 mg and probenecid 0.5 g

Colestid® *see* colestipol hydrochloride *on this page*

colestipol hydrochloride (koe les' ti pole)

Brand Names Colestid®

Therapeutic Category Antilipemic Agent

Use Adjunct in the management of primary hypercholesterolemia; to relieve pruritus associated with elevated levels of bile acids, possibly used to decrease plasma half-life of digoxin as an adjunct in the treatment of toxicity

(Continued)

colestipol hydrochloride *(Continued)*
Usual Dosage 15-30 g/day in divided doses 2-4 times/day
Dosage Forms Granules: 5 g packet, 300 g, 500 g

Colfed-A® *see* chlorpheniramine and pseudoephedrine *on page 94*

colfosceril palmitate (kole fos' er il)
Brand Names Exosurf® Neonatal
Synonyms dipalmitoylphosphatidylcholine; DPPC; synthetic lung surfactant
Therapeutic Category Lung Surfactant
Use Neonatal respiratory distress syndrome:
 Prophylactic therapy: Body weight <1350 g in infants at risk for developing RDS; body weight >1350 g in infants with evidence of pulmonary immaturity
 Rescue therapy: Treatment of infants with RDS based on respiratory distress not attributable to any other causes and chest radiographic findings consistent with RDS
Usual Dosage
 Prophylactic treatment: Give 5 mL/kg as soon as possible; the second and third doses should be administered at 12 and 24 hours later to those infants remaining on ventilators
 Rescue treatment: Give 5 mL/kg as soon as the diagnosis of RDS is made; the second 5 mL/kg dose should be administered 12 hours later
Dosage Forms Powder for injection, lyophilized: 108 mg (10 mL)

colistimethate sodium (koe lis ti meth' ate)
Brand Names Coly-Mycin® M Parenteral
Therapeutic Category Antibiotic, Miscellaneous
Use Treatment of infections due to sensitive strains of certain gram-negative bacilli
Usual Dosage Children and Adults: I.M., I.V.: 2.5-5 mg/kg/day in 2-4 divided doses
Dosage Forms Powder for injection, lyophilized: 150 mg

colistin, neomycin, and hydrocortisone
Brand Names Coly-Mycin® S Otic
Therapeutic Category Antibiotic, Miscellaneous; Corticosteroid, Otic; Otic Agent, Anti-infective
Use Treatment of superficial and susceptible bacterial infections of the external auditory canal; for treatment of susceptible bacterial infections of mastoidectomy and fenestration cavities
Usual Dosage Otic:
 Children: 3 drops in affected ear 3-4 times/day
 Adults: 4 drops in affected ear 3-4 times/day
Dosage Forms Suspension, otic: Colistin sulfate 0.3%, neomycin sulfate 0.47%, and hydrocortisone acetate 1% (5 mL, 10 mL)

colistin sulfate (koe lis' tin)
Brand Names Coly-Mycin® S Oral
Synonyms polymyxin e
Therapeutic Category Antibiotic, Miscellaneous; Antidiarrheal
Use Treat diarrhea in infants and children caused by susceptible organisms, especially *E. coli* and *Shigella*
Usual Dosage Children: 5-15 mg/kg/day in 3 divided doses given every 8 hours
Dosage Forms Powder for oral suspension: 25 mg/5 mL (60 mL)

collagenase (kol' la je nase)
Brand Names Biozyme-C®; Santyl®
Therapeutic Category Enzyme, Topical Debridement
Use Promote debridement of necrotic tissue in dermal ulcers and severe burns

Usual Dosage Topical: Apply daily or every other day
Dosage Forms Ointment, topical: 250 units/g (15 g, 30 g)

Collyrium Fresh® Ophthalmic [OTC] *see* tetrahydrozoline hydrochloride *on page 459*

Colocare® [OTC] *see* diagnostic aids (*in vitro*), feces *on page 138*

Color® Ovulation Test *see* diagnostic aids (*in vitro*), urine *on page 139*

ColoScreen [OTC] *see* diagnostic aids (*in vitro*), feces *on page 138*

Colovage® *see* polyethylene glycol-electrolyte solution *on page 383*

Coly-Mycin® M Parenteral *see* colistimethate sodium *on previous page*

Coly-Mycin® S Oral *see* colistin sulfate *on previous page*

Coly-Mycin® S Otic *see* colistin, neomycin, and hydrocortisone *on previous page*

CoLyte® *see* polyethylene glycol-electrolyte solution *on page 383*

Combipres® *see* clonidine and chlorthalidone *on page 109*

Combistix® [OTC] *see* diagnostic aids (*in vitro*), urine *on page 139*

Comfort® Ophthalmic [OTC] *see* naphazoline hydrochloride *on page 325*

Comhist® *see* chlorpheniramine, phenylephrine, and phenyltoloxamine *on page 95*

Comhist® LA *see* chlorpheniramine, phenylephrine, and phenyltoloxamine *on page 95*

Compazine® Injection *see* prochlorperazine *on page 396*

Compazine® Oral *see* prochlorperazine *on page 396*

Compazine® Rectal *see* prochlorperazine *on page 396*

compound E *see* cortisone acetate *on next page*

compound F *see* hydrocortisone *on page 236*

compound S *see* zidovudine *on page 503*

Concentraid® Nasal *see* desmopressin acetate *on page 131*

Conceptrol® [OTC] *see* nonoxynol 9 *on page 338*

Condrin-LA® *see* chlorpheniramine and phenylpropanolamine *on page 93*

Condylox® *see* podofilox *on page 381*

Conex® [OTC] *see* guaifenesin and phenylpropanolamine *on page 219*

Congess® Jr *see* guaifenesin and pseudoephedrine *on page 220*

Congess® Sr *see* guaifenesin and pseudoephedrine *on page 220*

Congestac® *see* guaifenesin and pseudoephedrine *on page 220*

Congestant D® [OTC] *see* chlorpheniramine, phenylpropanolamine, and acetaminophen *on page 96*

Conray® *see* radiological/contrast media (ionic) *on page 413*

Constant-T® *see* theophylline *on page 460*

Constilac® *see* lactulose *on page 267*

Constulose® *see* lactulose *on page 267*

Contac® Cough Formula Liquid [OTC] *see* guaifenesin and dextromethorphan *on page 218*

Contac® Maximum Strength [OTC] *see* chlorpheniramine and phenylpropanolamine *on page 93*

Control® [OTC] *see* phenylpropanolamine hydrochloride *on page 373*

Contuss® *see* guaifenesin, phenylpropanolamine, and phenylephrine *on page 221*

Contuss® XT *see* guaifenesin and phenylpropanolamine *on page 219*

Cophene-B® Injection *see* brompheniramine maleate *on page 59*

Cophene XP® *see* hydrocodone, pseudoephedrine, and guaifenesin *on page 236*

copper injection *see* trace metals *on page 472*

Co-Pyronil® 2 [OTC] *see* chlorpheniramine and pseudoephedrine *on page 94*

Cordarone® *see* amiodarone hydrochloride *on page 21*

Cordran® SP Topical *see* flurandrenolide *on page 204*

Cordran® Topical *see* flurandrenolide *on page 204*

Corgard® *see* nadolol *on page 322*

Corgonject® *see* chorionic gonadotropin *on page 101*

Coricidin® [OTC] *see* chlorpheniramine and acetaminophen *on page 93*

Coricidin 'D'® [OTC] *see* chlorpheniramine, phenylpropanolamine, and acetaminophen *on page 96*

Corque® Topical *see* clioquinol and hydrocortisone *on page 106*

Correctol® [OTC] *see* docusate and phenolphthalein *on page 158*

CortaGel® Topical [OTC] *see* hydrocortisone *on page 236*

Cortaid® Maximum Strength Topical [OTC] *see* hydrocortisone *on page 236*

Cortaid® with Aloe Topical [OTC] *see* hydrocortisone *on page 236*

Cortatrigen® Otic *see* neomycin, polymyxin b, and hydrocortisone *on page 329*

Cort-Dome® Topical *see* hydrocortisone *on page 236*

Cortef® Feminine Itch Topical *see* hydrocortisone *on page 236*

Cortef® Oral *see* hydrocortisone *on page 236*

Cortenema® Rectal *see* hydrocortisone *on page 236*

Corticaine® Topical *see* dibucaine and hydrocortisone *on page 143*

corticotropin (kor ti koe troe' pin)
Brand Names Acthar®; H.P. Acthar® Gel
Synonyms ACTH; adrenocorticotropic hormone
Therapeutic Category Adrenal Corticosteroid
Use Acute exacerbations of multiple sclerosis; diagnostic aid in adrenocortical insufficiency; severe muscle weakness in myasthenia gravis
Usual Dosage
Acute exacerbation of multiple sclerosis: I.M.: 80-120 units/day for 2-3 weeks
Diagnostic purposes:
   I.M., S.C.: 20 units 4 times/day
   I.V.: 10-25 units in 500 mL 5% dextrose in water over 8 hours
Dosage Forms
Injection, repository (H.P. Acthar® Gel): 40 units/mL (1 mL, 5 mL); 80 units/mL (1 mL, 5 mL)
Powder for injection (Acthar®): 25 units, 40 units

Cortifoam® Rectal *see* hydrocortisone *on page 236*

Cortin® Topical *see* clioquinol and hydrocortisone *on page 106*

cortisol *see* hydrocortisone *on page 236*

cortisone acetate (kor' ti sone)
Brand Names Cortone® Acetate Injection; Cortone® Acetate Oral
Synonyms compound E
Therapeutic Category Adrenal Corticosteroid; Anti-inflammatory Agent; Corticosteroid, Systemic

Use Management of adrenocortical insufficiency

Usual Dosage Depends upon the condition being treated and the response of the patient

Children:
  Anti-inflammatory or immunosuppressive:
    Oral: 2.5-10 mg/kg/day or 20-300 mg/m^2/day in divided doses every 6-8 hours
    I.M.: 1-5 mg/kg/day or 14-375 mg/m^2/day in divided doses every 12-24 hours
  Physiologic replacement:
    Oral: 0.5-0.75 mg/kg/day in divided doses every 8 hours
    I.M.: 0.25-0.35 mg/kg/day once daily

Stress coverage for surgery: I.M.: 1 and 2 days before preanesthesia, and 1-3 days after surgery: 50-62.5 mg/m^2/day; 4 days after surgery: 31-50 mg/m^2/day

Adults: Oral, I.M.: 20-300 mg/day

Dosage Forms
Injection: 50 mg/mL (10 mL)
Tablet: 5 mg, 10 mg, 25 mg

Cortisporin® Ophthalmic Ointment *see* bacitracin, neomycin, polymyxin b, and hydrocortisone *on page 43*

Cortisporin® Ophthalmic Suspension *see* neomycin, polymyxin b, and hydrocortisone *on page 329*

Cortisporin® Otic *see* neomycin, polymyxin b, and hydrocortisone *on page 329*

Cortisporin® Topical Cream *see* neomycin, polymyxin b, and hydrocortisone *on page 329*

Cortisporin® Topical Ointment *see* bacitracin, neomycin, polymyxin b, and hydrocortisone *on page 43*

Cortizone®-5 Topical [OTC] *see* hydrocortisone *on page 236*

Cortizone®-10 Topical [OTC] *see* hydrocortisone *on page 236*

Cortone® Acetate Injection *see* cortisone acetate *on previous page*

Cortone® Acetate Oral *see* cortisone acetate *on previous page*

Cortrosyn® Injection *see* cosyntropin *on this page*

Cosmegen® *see* dactinomycin *on page 125*

cosyntropin (koe sin troe' pin)
Brand Names Cortrosyn® Injection
Synonyms synacthen; tetracosactide
Therapeutic Category Adrenal Corticosteroid
Use Diagnostic test to differentiate primary adrenal from secondary (pituitary) adrenocortical insufficiency
Usual Dosage
Adrenocortical insufficiency: I.M., I.V.:
  Neonates: 0.015 mg/kg/dose
  Children <2 years: 0.125 mg injected over 2 minutes
  Children >2 years and Adults: 0.25 mg injected over 2 minutes

When greater cortisol stimulation is needed, an I.V. infusion may be used: I.V. infusion: 0.25 mg administered over 4-8 hours

Congenital adrenal hyperplasia evaluation: 1 mg/m^2/dose up to a maximum of 1 mg
Dosage Forms Powder for injection: 0.25 mg

Cotazym® *see* pancrelipase *on page 354*

Cotazym-S® *see* pancrelipase *on page 354*

Cotrim® *see* co-trimoxazole *on next page*

Cotrim® DS *see* co-trimoxazole *on this page*

co-trimoxazole (koe-trye mox' a zole)
Brand Names Bactrim™; Bactrim™ DS; Cotrim®; Cotrim® DS; Septra®; Septra® DS; Sulfa-methoprim®; Sulfatrim®; Sulfatrim® DS; Uroplus® DS; Uroplus® SS
Synonyms SMX-TMP; sulfamethoxazole and trimethoprim; TMP-SMX; trimethoprim and sul-famethoxazole
Therapeutic Category Antibiotic, Sulfonamide Derivative
Use Oral treatment of urinary tract infections; acute otitis media in children; acute exacerba-tions of chronic bronchitis in adults; prophylaxis of *Pneumocystis carinii* pneumonitis (PCP); I.V. treatment of documented PCP, empiric treatment of highly suspected PCP in immune compromised patients; treatment of documented or suspected shigellosis, ty-phoid fever, or *Nocardia asteroides* infection in patients who are NPO
Usual Dosage Oral, I.V. (dosage recommendations are based on the trimethoprim compo-nent):

Children >2 months:
Mild to moderate infections: 6-12 mg TMP/kg/day in divided doses every 12 hours
Serious infection/*Pneumocystis*: 15-20 mg TMP/kg/day in divided doses every 6 hours
Urinary tract infection prophylaxis: 2 mg TMP/kg/dose daily
Prophylaxis of *Pneumocystis*: 5-10 mg TMP/kg/day or 150 mg TMP/m^2/day in divided doses every 12 hours 3 days/week; dose should not exceed 320 mg trimethoprim and 1600 mg sulfamethoxazole 3 days/week; Mon, Tue, Wed

Adults: Urinary tract infection/chronic bronchitis: 1 double strength tablet every 12 hours for 10-14 days
Dosage Forms The 5:1 ratio (SMX to TMP) remains constant in all dosage forms:
Injection: Sulfamethoxazole 80 mg and trimethoprim 16 mg per mL (5 mL, 10 mL, 20 mL, 30 mL, 50 mL)
Suspension, oral: Sulfamethoxazole 200 mg and trimethoprim 40 mg per 5 mL (20 mL, 100 mL, 150 mL, 200 mL, 480 mL)
Tablet: Sulfamethoxazole 400 mg and trimethoprim 80 mg
Tablet, double strength: Sulfamethoxazole 800 mg and trimethoprim 160 mg

Coumadin® *see* warfarin sodium *on page 500*

CPA TR® *see* chlorpheniramine and phenylpropanolamine *on page 93*

CPM *see* cyclophosphamide *on page 121*

Creon® *see* pancreatin *on page 353*

Creo-Terpin® [OTC] *see* dextromethorphan hydrobromide *on page 136*

Cresylate® *see* m-cresyl acetate *on page 286*

cromoglicic acid *see* cromolyn sodium *on this page*

cromolyn sodium (kroe' moe lin)
Brand Names Gastrocrom® Oral; Intal® Inhalation Capsule; Intal® Nebulizer Solution; Intal® Oral Inhaler; Nasalcrom® Nasal Solution
Synonyms cromoglicic acid; disodium cromoglycate; DSCG
Therapeutic Category Antihistamine, Inhalation; Inhalation, Miscellaneous
Use Adjunct in the prophylactic management of severe bronchial asthma, prevention of acute bronchospasm, prevention of exercise, induced bronchospasm, allergic rhinitis
Usual Dosage
Children:
Inhalation: >2 years: 20 mg 4 times/day
Nebulization solution: >5 years: 2 inhalations 4 times/day by metered spray, or 20 mg 4 times/day (Spinhaler®); taper frequency to the lowest effective level
For prevention of exercise-induced bronchospasm: Single dose of 2 inhalations (aero-sol) or 20 mg (powder inhalation) just prior to exercise

Nasal: >6 years: 1 spray in each nostril 3-4 times/day
Adults:
Inhalation: 20 mg 4 times/day (Spinhaler®), 2 inhalations 4 times/day by metered spray
Nasal: 1 spray in each nostril 3-4 times/day
Systemic mastocytosis: Oral:
Infants up to 2 years of age: 20 mg/kg/day in 4 divided doses, not to exceed 30 mg/kg/day
Children 2-12 years: 100 mg 4 times/day; not to exceed 40 mg/kg/day
Adults: 200 mg 4 times/day
Food allergy and inflammatory bowel disease: Oral:
Children: 100 mg 4 times/day 15-20 minutes before meals, not to exceed 40 mg/kg/day
Adults: 200 mg 4 times/day 15-20 minutes before meal, up to 400 mg 4 times/day
Dosage Forms
Capsule:
Oral (Gastrocrom®): 100 mg
Oral inhalation (Intal®): 20 mg [to be used with Spinhaler® turbo-inhaler]
Inhalation, oral (Intal®): 800 μg/spray (8.1 g)
Solution, for nebulization (Intal®): 10 mg/mL (2 mL)
Solution:
Nasal (Nasalcrom®): 40 mg/mL (13 mL)

crotaline antivenin, polyvalent *see* antivenin (crotalidae) polyvalent *on page 31*

crotamiton (kroe tam' i tonn)
Brand Names Eurax® Topical
Therapeutic Category Antipruritic, Topical; Scabicidal Agent
Use Treatment of scabies and symptomatic treatment of pruritus
Usual Dosage Topical: Scabicide: Children and Adults: Wash thoroughly and scrub away loose scales, then towel dry; apply a thin layer and massage drug onto skin of the entire body from the neck to the toes (with special attention to skin folds, creases, and interdigital spaces). Repeat application in 24 hours. Take a cleansing bath 48 hours after the final application.
Dosage Forms
Cream: 10% (60 g)
Lotion: 10% (60 mL, 454 mL)

crude coal tar *see* coal tar *on page 110*
Cruex® Topical [OTC] *see* undecylenic acid and derivatives *on page 486*
cryptenamine tannates and methyclothiazide *see* methyclothiazide and cryptenamine tannates *on page 303*
crystalline penicillin *see* penicillin g, parenteral *on page 361*
crystal violet *see* gentian violet *on page 211*
Crystamine® *see* cyanocobalamin *on next page*
Crysticillin® A.S. Injection *see* penicillin g procaine, aqueous *on page 362*
Crystodigin® *see* digitoxin *on page 147*
C-Solve-2® Topical *see* erythromycin, topical *on page 176*
csp *see* cellulose sodium phosphate *on page 83*
CS-T® [OTC] *see* diagnostic aids (*in vitro*), feces *on page 138*
CTX *see* cyclophosphamide *on page 121*
Culturette® 10 Minute Group A Strep ID *see* diagnostic aids (*in vitro*), other *on page 138*

ALPHABETICAL LISTING OF DRUGS

Cuprimine® *see* penicillamine *on page 359*

Curretab® Oral *see* medroxyprogesterone acetate *on page 289*

Cutivate™ Topical *see* fluticasone propionate *on page 205*

CYA *see* cyclosporine *on page 122*

cyanocobalamin (sye an oh koe bal' a min)
Brand Names Berubigen®; Cobex®; Crystamine®; Cyanoject®; Cyomin®; Ener-B® [OTC]; Kaybovite-1000®; Redisol®; Rubramin-PC®; Sytobex®
Synonyms vitamin B_{12}
Therapeutic Category Vitamin, Water Soluble
Use Vitamin B_{12} deficiency; increased B_{12} requirements due to pregnancy, thyrotoxicosis, hemorrhage, malignancy, liver or kidney disease
Usual Dosage
Congenital pernicious anemia (if evidence of neurologic involvement): I.M.: 1000 µg/day for at least 2 weeks; maintenance: 50 µg/month

Vitamin B_{12} deficiency: I.M., S.C.: (oral is not recommended due to poor absorption)
Children: 100 µg/day for 10-15 days (total dose of 1-1.5 mg), then once or twice weekly for several months; may taper to 250-1000 µg every month
Adults: 100 µg/day for 6-7 days
Hematologic signs only:
Children: 10-50 µg/day for 5-10 days, then maintenance: 100-250 µg/dose every 2-4 weeks
Adults: 30 µg/day for 5-10 days, followed by 100-200 µg/month

Methylmalonic aciduria: I.M.: 1 mg/day
Dosage Forms
Gel, nasal (Ener-B®): 400 µg/0.1 mL
Injection: 30 µg/mL (30 mL); 100 µg/mL (1 mL, 10 mL, 30 mL); 1000 µg/mL (1 mL, 10 mL, 30 mL)
Tablet [OTC]: 25 µg, 50 µg, 100 µg, 250 µg, 500 µg, 1000 µg

Cyanoject® *see* cyanocobalamin *on this page*

Cyclan® *see* cyclandelate *on this page*

cyclandelate (sye klan' de late)
Brand Names Cyclan®; Cyclospasmol®
Therapeutic Category Vasodilator, Peripheral
Use Adjunctive therapy in peripheral vascular disease and possibly senility
Usual Dosage Oral: 400-800 mg/day in 2-4 divided doses
Dosage Forms
Capsule: 200 mg, 400 mg
Tablet: 200 mg, 400 mg

cyclizine (sye' kli zeen)
Brand Names Marezine® [OTC]
Therapeutic Category Antiemetic; Antihistamine
Use Prevention and treatment of nausea, vomiting and vertigo associated with motion sickness; control of postoperative nausea and vomiting
Usual Dosage
Children 6-12 years:
Oral: 25 mg up to 3 times/day
I.M.: Not recommended

Adults:
Oral: 50 mg taken 30 minutes before departure, may repeat in 4-6 hours if needed, up to 200 mg/day

I.M.: 50 mg every 4-6 hours as needed
Dosage Forms
Injection, as lactate: 50 mg/mL (1 mL)
Tablet, as hydrochloride: 50 mg

cyclobenzaprine hydrochloride (sye kloe ben' za preen)
Brand Names Flexeril®
Therapeutic Category Skeletal Muscle Relaxant
Use Treatment of muscle spasm associated with acute painful musculoskeletal conditions; supportive therapy in tetanus; ineffective in spasticity secondary to chronic neurologic disorders
Usual Dosage Oral:
Children: Dosage has not been established
Adults: 20-40 mg/day in 2-4 divided doses; maximum dose: 60 mg/day
Dosage Forms Tablet: 10 mg

Cyclocort® Topical see amcinonide on page 18

Cyclogyl® Ophthalmic see cyclopentolate hydrochloride on this page

Cyclomydril® Ophthalmic see cyclopentolate and phenylephrine on this page

cyclopentolate and phenylephrine
Brand Names Cyclomydril® Ophthalmic
Synonyms phenylephrine and cyclopentolate
Therapeutic Category Ophthalmic Agent, Mydriatic
Use Induce mydriasis greater than that produced with cyclopentolate HCl alone
Usual Dosage Ophthalmic: Instill 1 drop every 5-10 minutes, not to exceed 3 instillations
Dosage Forms Solution, ophthalmic: Cyclopentolate hydrochloride 0.2% and phenylephrine hydrochloride 1% (2 mL, 5 mL)

cyclopentolate hydrochloride (sye kloe pen' toe late)
Brand Names AK-Pentolate® Ophthalmic; Cyclogyl® Ophthalmic; I-Pentolate® Ophthalmic
Therapeutic Category Anticholinergic Agent, Ophthalmic; Ophthalmic Agent, Mydriatic
Use Diagnostic procedures requiring mydriasis and cycloplegia
Usual Dosage Ophthalmic:
Infants: Instill 1 drop of 0.5% into each eye 5-10 minutes before examination

Children: Instill 1 drop of 0.5%, 1%, or 2% in eye followed by 1 drop of 0.5% or 1% in 5 minutes, if necessary

Adults: Instill 1 drop of 1% followed by another drop in 5 minutes; 2% solution in heavily pigmented iris
Dosage Forms Solution, ophthalmic: 0.5% (2 mL, 5 mL, 15 mL); 1% (2 mL, 5 mL, 15 mL); 2% (2 mL, 5 mL, 15 mL)

cyclophosphamide (sye kloe foss' fa mide)
Brand Names Cytoxan® Injection; Cytoxan® Oral; Neosar® Injection
Synonyms CPM; CTX; CYT
Therapeutic Category Antineoplastic Agent, Alkylating Agent (Nitrogen Mustard)
Use Management of Hodgkin's disease, malignant lymphomas, multiple myeloma, leukemias, mycosis fungoides, neuroblastoma, ovarian carcinoma, breast carcinoma, a variety of other tumors; nephrotic syndrome, lupus erythematosus, severe rheumatoid arthritis, and rheumatoid vasculitis
Usual Dosage Refer to individual protocols
Children with no hematologic problems:
Induction:
Oral: 2-8 mg/kg/day
(Continued)

121

cyclophosphamide *(Continued)*

    I.V.: 10-20 mg/kg/day divided once daily
    Maintenance: Oral: 2-5 mg/kg (50-150 mg/m^2) twice weekly
    Pediatric solid tumors: I.V.: 250-1800 mg/m^2 once daily for 1-5 days every 21-28 days

Adults with no hematologic problems:
  Induction:
    Oral: 1-5 mg/kg/day
    I.V.: 40-50 mg/kg (1.5-1.8 g/m^2) in divided doses over 2-5 days
  Maintenance:
    Oral: 1-5 mg/kg/day
    I.V.: 10-15 mg/kg (350-550 mg/m^2) every 7-10 days or 3-5 mg/kg (110-185 mg/m^2) twice weekly

Children and Adults: I.V.:
  SLE: 500-750 mg/m^2 every month; maximum: 1 g/m^2
  JRA/vasculitis: 10 mg/kg every 2 weeks

BMT conditioning regimen: I.V.: 50 mg/kg/day once daily for 3-4 days

Nephrotic syndrome: Oral: 2-3 mg/kg/day every day for up to 12 weeks when corticosteroids are unsuccessful

Dosage Forms
Powder for injection: 100 mg, 200 mg, 500 mg, 1 g, 2 g
Powder for injection, lyophilized: 100 mg, 200 mg, 500 mg, 1 g, 2 g
Tablet: 25 mg, 50 mg

cycloserine (sye kloe ser' een)

Brand Names Seromycin® Pulvules®
Therapeutic Category Antibiotic, Miscellaneous; Antitubercular Agent
Use Adjunctive treatment in pulmonary or extrapulmonary tuberculosis; treatment of acute urinary tract infections caused by *E. coli* or *Enterobacter* sp when less toxic therapy has failed or is contraindicated
Usual Dosage Oral:
Tuberculosis:
  Children: 10-20 mg/kg/day in 2 divided doses up to 1000 mg/day
  Adults: Initial: 250 mg every 12 hours for 14 days, then give 500 mg to 1 g/day in 2 divided doses

Urinary tract infection: Adults: 250 mg every 12 hours for 14 days
Dosage Forms Capsule: 250 mg

Cyclospasmol® *see* cyclandelate *on page 120*

cyclosporin A *see* cyclosporine *on this page*

cyclosporine (sye' kloe spor een)

Brand Names Sandimmune® Injection; Sandimmune® Oral
Synonyms CYA; cyclosporin A
Therapeutic Category Immunosuppressant Agent
Use Immunosuppressant used with corticosteroids to prevent graft versus host disease in patients with kidney, liver, heart, and bone marrow transplants. Unlabeled use: Rheumatoid arthritis
Usual Dosage Children and Adults:
Oral: Initial: 14-18 mg/kg/dose daily, beginning 4-12 hours prior to organ transplantation; maintenance: 5-10 mg/kg/day
I.V.: Initial: 5-6 mg/kg/day in divided doses every 12-24 hours; patients should be switched to oral cyclosporine as soon as possible
Dosage Forms
Capsule: 25 mg, 100 mg
Injection: 50 mg/mL (5 mL)
Solution, oral: 100 mg/mL (50 mL)

cyclothiazide (sye kloe thye' a zide)
Brand Names Anhydron®
Therapeutic Category Antihypertensive; Diuretic, Thiazide
Use Management of mild to moderate hypertension; treatment of edema in congestive heart failure and nephrotic syndrome
Usual Dosage Adults: Oral: 2 mg/day; up to 2 mg 2-3 times/day
Dosage Forms Tablet: 2 mg

Cycrin® Oral *see* medroxyprogesterone acetate *on page 289*

Cyklokapron® Injection *see* tranexamic acid *on page 473*

Cyklokapron® Oral *see* tranexamic acid *on page 473*

Cylert® *see* pemoline *on page 359*

Cyomin® *see* cyanocobalamin *on page 120*

cyproheptadine hydrochloride (si proe hep' ta deen)
Brand Names Periactin®
Therapeutic Category Antihistamine
Use Perennial and seasonal allergic rhinitis and other allergic symptoms including urticaria
Usual Dosage Oral:
Children: 0.25 mg/kg/day in 2-3 divided doses or
2-6 years: 2 mg every 8-12 hours (not to exceed 12 mg/day)
7-14 years: 4 mg every 8-12 hours (not to exceed 16 mg/day)

Adults: 12-16 mg/day every 8 hours (not to exceed 0.5 mg/kg/day)
Dosage Forms
Syrup: 2 mg/5 mL with alcohol 5% (473 mL)
Tablet: 4 mg

cysteine hydrochloride (sis' te een)
Therapeutic Category Nutritional Supplement
Use Total parenteral nutrition of infants as an additive to meet the I.V. amino acid requirements
Usual Dosage Combine 500 mg of cysteine with 12.5 g of amino acid, then dilute with 50% dextrose
Dosage Forms Injection: 50 mg/mL (10 mL)

Cystografin® *see* radiological/contrast media (ionic) *on page 413*

Cystospaz-M® Oral *see* hyoscyamine sulfate *on page 243*

Cystospaz® Oral *see* hyoscyamine sulfate *on page 243*

CYT *see* cyclophosphamide *on page 121*

Cytadren® *see* aminoglutethimide *on page 19*

cytarabine hydrochloride (sye tare' a been)
Brand Names Cytosar-U®; Tarabine® PFS
Synonyms arabinosylcytosine; Ara-C; cytosine arabinosine hydrochloride
Therapeutic Category Antineoplastic Agent, Antimetabolite
Use In combination regimens for the treatment of leukemias and non-Hodgkin's lymphomas
Usual Dosage Refer to individual protocols
Children and Adults:
Induction remission:
I.T.: 5-75 mg/m^2 once daily for 4 days or 1 every 4 days until CNS
I.V.: 200 mg/m^2/day for 5 days at 2-week intervals; 100-200 mg/m^2/day for 5- to 10-day therapy course or every day until remission given I.V. continuous drip, or in 2-3 divided doses findings normalize

(Continued)

123

cytarabine hydrochloride *(Continued)*

Maintenance remission:
 I.M., S.C.: 1-1.5 mg/kg single dose for maintenance at 1- to 4-week intervals
 I.V.: 70-200 mg/m^2/day for 2-5 days at monthly intervals

High-dose therapies: Doses as high as 1-3 g/m^2 have been used for refractory or second-ary leukemias or refractory non-Hodgkins lymphoma; dosages of 3 g/m^2 every 12 hours for up to 12 doses have been used

Dosage Forms
Injection, preservative free (Tarabine® PFS): 20 mg/mL (5 mL, 50 mL)
Powder for injection (Cytosar-U®): 100 mg, 500 mg, 1 g, 2 g

CytoGam™ *see* cytomegalovirus immune globulin intravenous, human *on this page*

cytomegalovirus immune globulin intravenous, human

(sye toe meg a low vi' rus)
Brand Names CytoGam™
Synonyms CMV-IGIV
Therapeutic Category Immune Globulin
Use Attenuation of primary CMV disease associated with kidney transplantation
Usual Dosage I.V.: Initial: Administer at 15 mg/kg/hour, then increase to 30 mg/kg/hour after 30 minutes if no untoward reactions, then increase to 60 mg/kg/hour after another 30 minutes, volume not to exceed 75 mL/hour
Dosage Forms Powder for injection, lyophilized: 2500 mg ± 250 mg (50 mL)

Cytomel® Oral *see* liothyronine sodium *on page 274*

Cytosar-U® *see* cytarabine hydrochloride *on previous page*

cytosine arabinosine hydrochloride *see* cytarabine hydrochloride *on previous page*

Cytotec® *see* misoprostol *on page 314*

Cytovene® *see* ganciclovir *on page 208*

Cytoxan® Injection *see* cyclophosphamide *on page 121*

Cytoxan® Oral *see* cyclophosphamide *on page 121*

d$_3$ *see* cholecalciferol *on page 99*

25-d$_3$ *see* calcifediol *on page 64*

D-3-mercaptovaline *see* penicillamine *on page 359*

dacarbazine (da kar' ba zeen)

Brand Names DTIC-Dome®
Synonyms DIC; imidazole carboxamide
Therapeutic Category Antineoplastic Agent, Miscellaneous
Use Metastatic malignant melanoma; in combination with other agents, in Hodgkin's disease; has been used for soft tissue sarcomas and neuroblastomas
Usual Dosage Refer to individual protocols
Children: I.V.:

Solid tumors: 200-470 mg/m^2/day over 5 days every 21-28 days

Neuroblastoma: 800-900 mg/m^2 as a single dose every 3-4 weeks in combination therapy

Adults: I.V.:
 Malignant melanoma: 2-4.5 mg/kg/day for 10 days, repeat in 4 weeks or may use 250 mg/m^2/day for 5 days, repeat in 3 weeks
 Hodgkin's disease: 150 mg/m^2/day for 5 days, repeat every 4 weeks or 375 mg/m^2 on day 1, repeat in 15 days of each 28-day cycle in combination with other agents
Dosage Forms Injection: 100 mg (10 mL, 20 mL); 200 mg (20 mL, 30 mL); 500 mg (50 mL)

dactinomycin (dak ti noe mye' sin)
Brand Names Cosmegen®
Synonyms ACT; actinomycin D
Therapeutic Category Antineoplastic Agent, Antibiotic
Use Management, either alone or with other treatment modalities of Wilms' tumor, rhabdomyosarcoma, neuroblastoma, retinoblastoma, Ewing's sarcoma, trophoblastic neoplasms, testicular carcinoma, and other malignancies
Usual Dosage Refer to individual protocols. Dosage should be based on body surface area in obese or edematous patients.

Children >6 months and Adults: I.V.: 15 μg/kg/day or 400-600 μg/m^2/day for 5 days, may repeat every 3-6 weeks; or 2.5 mg/m^2 given in divided doses over 1 week; 0.75-2 mg/m^2 as a single dose given at intervals of 1-4 weeks have been used
Dosage Forms Powder for injection, lyophilized: 0.5 mg

Dairy Ease® [OTC] *see* lactase enzyme *on page 266*

Daisy® 2 *see* diagnostic aids (*in vitro*), urine *on page 139*

Dalalone D.P.® Injection *see* dexamethasone *on page 132*

Dalalone® Injection *see* dexamethasone *on page 132*

Dalalone L.A.® Injection *see* dexamethasone *on page 132*

Dalcaine® Injection *see* lidocaine hydrochloride *on page 273*

Dalgan® *see* dezocine *on page 137*

Dallergy® *see* chlorpheniramine, phenylephrine, and methscopolamine *on page 95*

Dallergy-D® *see* chlorpheniramine and phenylephrine *on page 93*

Dallergy-JR® *see* brompheniramine and pseudoephedrine *on page 59*

Dalmane® *see* flurazepam hydrochloride *on page 204*

***d*-alpha tocopherol** *see* vitamin E *on page 498*

Damason-P® *see* hydrocodone and aspirin *on page 234*

danazol (da' na zole)
Brand Names Danocrine®
Therapeutic Category Androgen
Use Treatment of endometriosis, fibrocystic breast disease, and hereditary angioedema
Usual Dosage Adults: Oral:
Endometriosis: 100-400 mg twice daily
Fibrocystic breast disease: 50-200 mg twice daily for 2-6 months
Hereditary angioedema: 400-600 mg/day in 2-3 divided doses
Dosage Forms Capsule: 50 mg, 100 mg, 200 mg

Danex® [OTC] *see* pyrithione zinc *on page 410*

Danocrine® *see* danazol *on this page*

Dantrium® *see* dantrolene sodium *on this page*

dantrolene sodium (dan' troe leen)
Brand Names Dantrium®
Therapeutic Category Antidote, Malignant Hyperthermia; Hyperthermia, Treatment; Skeletal Muscle Relaxant
Use Treatment of spasticity associated with spinal cord injury, stroke, cerebral palsy, or multiple sclerosis; also used as treatment of malignant hyperthermia
(Continued)

dantrolene sodium *(Continued)*
Usual Dosage
Spasticity: Oral:
Children: Initial: 0.5 mg/kg/dose twice daily, increase frequency to 3-4 times/day at 4- to 7-day intervals, then increase dose by 0.5 mg/kg to a maximum of 3 mg/kg/dose 2-4 times/day up to 400 mg/day
Adults: 25 mg/day to start, increase frequency to 3-4 times/day, then increase dose by 25 mg every 4-7 days to a maximum of 100 mg 2-4 times/day or 400 mg/day

Hyperthermia: Children and Adults:
Oral: 4-8 mg/kg/day in 4 divided doses
I.V.: 1 mg/kg; may repeat dose up to cumulative dose of 10 mg/kg (mean effective dose: 2.5 mg/kg), then switch to oral dosage
Dosage Forms
Capsule: 25 mg, 50 mg, 100 mg
Powder for injection: 20 mg

Dapa® [OTC] *see* acetaminophen *on page 2*
Dapacin® Cold Capsule [OTC] *see* chlorpheniramine, phenylpropanolamine, and acetaminophen *on page 96*

dapiprazole hydrochloride (da' pi pray zole)
Brand Names Rēv-Eyes™
Therapeutic Category Alpha-Adrenergic Blocking Agent, Ophthalmic
Use Treatment of iatrogenically induced mydriasis produced by adrenergic or parasympatholytic agents
Usual Dosage Ophthalmic: Instill 2 drops followed 5 minutes later by an additional 2 drops applied to the conjunctiva
Dosage Forms Powder, lyophilized: 25 mg [0.5% solution when mixed with supplied diluent]

dapsone (dap' sone)
Synonyms DDS; diaminodiphenylsulfone
Therapeutic Category Antibiotic, Sulfone
Use Treatment of leprosy and dermatitis herpetiformis
Usual Dosage Oral:
Children: Leprosy: 1-2 mg/kg/24 hours; maximum: 100 mg/day
Adults:
Leprosy: 50-100 mg/day
Dermatitis herpetiformis: Start at 50 mg/day, increase to 300 mg/day, or higher to achieve full control, reduce dosage to minimum level as soon as possible
Dosage Forms Tablet: 25 mg, 100 mg

Daranide® *see* dichlorphenamide *on page 144*
Daraprim® *see* pyrimethamine *on page 409*
Darbid® *see* isopropamide iodide *on page 258*
Daricon® *see* oxyphencyclimine hydrochloride *on page 351*
Darvocet-N® *see* propoxyphene and acetaminophen *on page 402*
Darvocet-N® 100 *see* propoxyphene and acetaminophen *on page 402*
Darvon® *see* propoxyphene *on page 402*
Darvon® Compound-65 Pulvules® *see* propoxyphene and aspirin *on page 402*
Darvon-N® *see* propoxyphene *on page 402*
Datril® [OTC] *see* acetaminophen *on page 2*

daunorubicin hydrochloride (daw noe roo' bi sin)
Brand Names Cerubidine®
Synonyms daunomycin; DNR; rubidomycin hydrochloride
Therapeutic Category Antineoplastic Agent, Antibiotic
Use In combination with other agents in the treatment of leukemias
Usual Dosage Refer to individual protocols
I.V.:
Children:
Combination therapy: Remission induction for ALL: 25-45 mg/m^2 on day 1 every week for 4 cycles
<2 years or <0.5 m^2: The manufacturer recommends that the dose is based on body weight rather than body surface area

Adults: 30-60 mg/m^2/day for 3-5 days, repeat dose in 3-4 weeks; total cumulative dose should not exceed 400-600 mg/m^2
Single agent induction for AML: 60 mg/m^2/day for 3 days; repeat every 3-4 weeks
Combination therapy induction for AML: 45 mg/m^2/day for 3 days; Subsequent courses: Every day for 2 days
Combination therapy: Remission induction for ALL: 45 mg/m^2 on days 1, 2, and 3
Dosage Forms Powder for injection, lyophilized: 20 mg

Daypro® see oxaprozin on page 348

Dayto Himbin® see yohimbine hydrochloride on page 502

Dazamide® see acetazolamide on page 4

DC 240® Softgel® [OTC] see docusate on page 157

DCF see pentostatin on page 365

DDAVP® Injection see desmopressin acetate on page 131

DDAVP® Nasal see desmopressin acetate on page 131

ddC see zalcitabine on page 502

DDI see didanosine on page 145

DDS see dapsone on previous page

1-deamino-8-d-arginine vasopressin see desmopressin acetate on page 131

Debrisan® Topical [OTC] see dextranomer on page 135

Debrox® Otic [OTC] see carbamide peroxide on page 73

Decadron®-LA Injection see dexamethasone on page 132

Decadron® Oral see dexamethasone on page 132

Decadron® Phosphate Cream see dexamethasone on page 132

Decadron® Phosphate Injection see dexamethasone on page 132

Decadron® Phosphate Nasal Turbinaire® see dexamethasone on page 132

Decadron® Phosphate Ophthalmic see dexamethasone on page 132

Decadron® Phosphate Respihaler® Oral Inhaler see dexamethasone on page 132

Deca-Durabolin® Injection see nandrolone on page 324

Decaject® Injection see dexamethasone on page 132

Decaject-LA® Injection see dexamethasone on page 132

Decaspray® Topical Aerosol see dexamethasone on page 132

Decholin® see dehydrocholic acid on next page

Declomycin® see demeclocycline hydrochloride on page 129

Decofed® Syrup [OTC] see pseudoephedrine on page 406

Decohistine® see chlorpheniramine and phenylephrine on page 93

Decohistine® DH *see* chlorpheniramine, pseudoephedrine, and codeine *on page 97*

Decohistine® Expectorant *see* guaifenesin, pseudoephedrine, and codeine *on page 221*

Deconamine® SR *see* chlorpheniramine and pseudoephedrine *on page 94*

Deconamine® Tablet *see* chlorpheniramine and pseudoephedrine *on page 94*

Deconsal® II *see* guaifenesin and pseudoephedrine *on page 220*

deferoxamine mesylate (de fer ox' a meen)
Brand Names Desferal® Mesylate
Therapeutic Category Antidote, Aluminum Toxicity; Antidote, Iron Toxicity
Use Acute iron intoxication; chronic iron overload secondary to multiple transfusions; diagnostic test for iron overload; used investigationally in the treatment of aluminum accumulation in renal failure; iron overload secondary to congenital anemias; hemochromatosis; removal of corneal rust rings following surgical removal of foreign bodies
Usual Dosage
Children:
Acute iron intoxication:
I.M.: 90 mg/kg/dose every 8 hours; maximum: 6 g/day
I.V.: 15 mg/kg/hour; maximum: 6 g/day
Chronic iron overload:
I.V.: 15 mg/kg/hour
S.C.: 20-40 mg/kg/day over 8-12 hours
Aluminum induced bone disease: 20-40 mg/kg every hemodialysis treatment, frequency dependent on clinical status of the patient
Adults:
Acute iron intoxication:
I.M.: 1 g stat, then 0.5 g every 4 hours for two doses, then 0.5 g every 4-12 hours up to 6 g/day
I.V.: 15 mg/kg/hour; maximum: 6 g/day
Chronic iron overload:
I.M.: 0.5-1 g every day
S.C.: 1-2 g every day over 8-24 hours
Dosage Forms Powder for injection: 500 mg

Degest® 2 Ophthalmic [OTC] *see* naphazoline hydrochloride *on page 325*

Dehist® Injection *see* brompheniramine maleate *on page 59*

dehydrocholic acid (dee hye droe koe' lik)
Brand Names Cholan-HMB®; Decholin®
Therapeutic Category Bile Acid; Laxative, Hydrocholeretic
Use Relief of constipation; adjunct to various biliary tract conditions
Usual Dosage Children >12 years and Adults: 250-500 mg 2-3 times/day after meals up to 1.5 g/day
Dosage Forms Tablet: 250 mg

Dekasol® Injection *see* dexamethasone *on page 132*

Dekasol-L.A.® Injection *see* dexamethasone *on page 132*

Deladumone® Injection *see* estradiol and testosterone *on page 178*

Delatest® Injection *see* testosterone *on page 456*

Delatestryl® Injection *see* testosterone *on page 456*

Delaxin® *see* methocarbamol *on page 300*

Delcort® Topical see hydrocortisone *on page 236*

Delestrogen® Injection see estradiol *on page 178*

Delfen® [OTC] see nonoxynol 9 *on page 338*

Del-Mycin® Topical see erythromycin, topical *on page 176*

Delsym® [OTC] see dextromethorphan hydrobromide *on page 136*

Delta-Cortef® Oral see prednisolone *on page 391*

deltacortisone see prednisone *on page 393*

Delta-D® see cholecalciferol *on page 99*

deltadehydrocortisone see prednisone *on page 393*

deltahydrocortisone see prednisolone *on page 391*

Deltasone® Oral see prednisone *on page 393*

Delta-Tritex® Topical see triamcinolone *on page 474*

Demadex® Injection see torsemide *on page 472*

Demadex® Oral see torsemide *on page 472*

Demazin® [OTC] see chlorpheniramine and phenylpropanolamine *on page 93*

demecarium bromide (dem e kare' ee um)
Brand Names Humorsol® Ophthalmic
Therapeutic Category Cholinergic Agent, Ophthalmic; Ophthalmic Agent, Miotic
Use Management of chronic simple glaucoma, chronic and acute angle-closure glaucoma; counter effects of cycloplegics
Usual Dosage
Children: Instill 1 drop into eyes twice weekly to a maximum dosage of 1 or 2 drops twice daily for up to 4 months

Adults: Instill 1-2 drops into eyes twice weekly to a maximum dosage of 1 or 2 drops twice daily for up to 4 months
Dosage Forms Solution, ophthalmic: 0.125% (5 mL); 0.25% (5 mL)

demeclocycline hydrochloride (dem e kloe sye' kleen)
Brand Names Declomycin®
Synonyms demethylchlortetracycline
Therapeutic Category Antibiotic, Tetracycline Derivative
Use Treatment of susceptible bacterial infections (acne, gonorrhea, pertussis and urinary tract infections) caused by both gram-negative and gram-positive organisms; used when penicillin is contraindicated; the treatment of chronic syndrome of inappropriate secretion of antidiuretic hormone (SIADH)
Usual Dosage
Children ≥8 years: 8-12 mg/kg/day divided every 6-12 hours

Adults: 150 mg 4 times/day or 300 mg twice daily
Uncomplicated gonorrhea: 600 mg stat, 300 mg every 12 hours for 4 days (3 g total)
SIADH: 900-1200 mg/day or 13-15 mg/kg/day divided every 6-8 hours initially, then decrease to 0.6-0.9 g/day
Dosage Forms
Capsule: 150 mg
Tablet: 150 mg, 300 mg

Demerol® Injection see meperidine hydrochloride *on page 292*

Demerol® Oral see meperidine hydrochloride *on page 292*

demethylchlortetracycline see demeclocycline hydrochloride *on this page*

4-demothoxydaunorubicin see idarubicin hydrochloride *on page 245*

ALPHABETICAL LISTING OF DRUGS

Demser® *see* metyrosine *on page 310*

Demulen® *see* ethinyl estradiol and ethynodiol diacetate *on page 182*

Denorex® [OTC] *see* coal tar *on page 110*

deodorized opium tincture *see* opium tincture *on page 345*

2'-deoxycoformycin *see* pentostatin *on page 365*

Depakene® *see* valproic acid and derivatives *on page 490*

Depakote® *see* valproic acid and derivatives *on page 490*

depAndrogyn® Injection *see* estradiol and testosterone *on page 178*

Depen® *see* penicillamine *on page 359*

depGynogen® Injection *see* estradiol *on page 178*

depMedalone® Injection *see* methylprednisolone *on page 306*

Depo®-Estradiol Injection *see* estradiol *on page 178*

Depogen® Injection *see* estradiol *on page 178*

Depoject® Injection *see* methylprednisolone *on page 306*

Depo-Medrol® Injection *see* methylprednisolone *on page 306*

Deponit® Patch *see* nitroglycerin *on page 336*

Depopred® Injection *see* methylprednisolone *on page 306*

Depo-Provera® Injection *see* medroxyprogesterone acetate *on page 289*

Depo-Testadiol® Injection *see* estradiol and testosterone *on page 178*

Depotest® Injection *see* testosterone *on page 456*

Depotestogen® Injection *see* estradiol and testosterone *on page 178*

Depo®-Testosterone Injection *see* testosterone *on page 456*

deprenyl *see* selegiline hydrochloride *on page 428*

Deproist® Expectorant with Codeine *see* guaifenesin, pseudoephedrine, and codeine *on page 221*

Derifil® [OTC] *see* chlorophyll *on page 90*

Dermacomb® Topical *see* nystatin and triamcinolone *on page 342*

Dermacort® Topical *see* hydrocortisone *on page 236*

Dermarest Dricort® Topical *see* hydrocortisone *on page 236*

Derma-Smoothe/FS® Topical *see* fluocinolone acetonide *on page 199*

Dermatophytin® *see* Trichophyton skin test *on page 477*

Dermatophytin-O *see* Candida albicans (Monilia) *on page 70*

Dermolate® Topical [OTC] *see* hydrocortisone *on page 236*

Dermoplast® [OTC] *see* benzocaine *on page 48*

Dermoxyl® [OTC] *see* benzoyl peroxide *on page 49*

Dermtex® HC with Aloe Topical [OTC] *see* hydrocortisone *on page 236*

DES *see* diethylstilbestrol *on page 146*

Desenex® [OTC] *see* tolnaftate *on page 471*

Desferal® Mesylate *see* deferoxamine mesylate *on page 128*

desflurane (des floo' rane)
  Brand Names Suprane®
  Therapeutic Category General Anesthetic
  Use Induction or maintenance of anesthesia for adults in outpatient and inpatient surgery
  Dosage Forms Liquid: 240 mL

desiccated thyroid *see* thyroid *on page 466*

desipramine hydrochloride (dess ip' ra meen)
Brand Names Norpramin®; Pertofrane®
Synonyms desmethylimipramine HCl
Therapeutic Category Antidepressant, Tricyclic
Use Treatment of various forms of depression, often in conjunction with psychotherapy
Usual Dosage Oral (not recommended for use in children <12 years):
Adolescents: Initial: 25-50 mg/day; gradually increase to 100 mg/day in single or divided doses; maximum: 150 mg/day

Adults: Initial: 75 mg/day in divided doses; increase gradually to 150-200 mg/day in divided or single dose; maximum: 300 mg/day
Dosage Forms
Capsule (Pertofrane®): 25 mg, 50 mg
Tablet (Norpramin®): 10 mg, 25 mg, 50 mg, 75 mg, 100 mg, 150 mg

Desitin® Topical [OTC] *see* zinc oxide, cod liver oil, and talc *on page 504*
desmethylimipramine HCl *see* desipramine hydrochloride *on this page*

desmopressin acetate (des moe press' in)
Brand Names Concentraid® Nasal; DDAVP® Injection; DDAVP® Nasal
Synonyms 1-deamino-8-d-arginine vasopressin
Therapeutic Category Antihemophilic Agent; Hemostatic Agent; Vasopressin Analog, Synthetic
Use Treatment of diabetes insipidus and controlling bleeding in certain types of hemophilia
Usual Dosage
Children:
Diabetes insipidus: 3 months to 12 years: Intranasal: Initial: 5 μg/day divided 1-2 times/day; range: 5-30 μg/day divided 1-2 times/day
Hemophilia: >3 months: I.V.: 0.3 μg/kg by slow infusion; may repeat dose if needed
Nocturnal enuresis: ≥6 years: Intranasal: Initial: 20 μg at bedtime; range: 10-40 μg
Adults:
Diabetes insipidus: I.V., S.C.: 2-4 μg/day in 2 divided doses or $^1/_{10}$ of the maintenance intranasal dose; intranasal: 5-40 μg/day 1-3 times/day
Hemophilia: I.V.: 0.3 μg/kg by slow infusion
Dosage Forms
Injection (DDAVP®): 4 μg/mL (1 mL)
Solution, nasal (Concentraid®, DDAVP®): 100 μg/mL (2.5 mL, 5 mL)

Desogen® *see* ethinyl estradiol and desogestrel *on page 182*
desogestrel and ethinyl estradiol *see* ethinyl estradiol and desogestrel *on page 182*

desonide (dess' oh nide)
Brand Names DesOwen® Topical; Tridesilon® Topical
Therapeutic Category Corticosteroid, Topical (Low Potency)
Use Adjunctive therapy for inflammation in acute and chronic corticosteroid responsive dermatosis
Usual Dosage Topical: Apply 2-4 times/day
Dosage Forms
Cream, topical: 0.05% (15 g, 60 g)
Ointment, topical: 0.05% (15 g, 60 g)
Lotion: 0.05% (60 mL, 120 mL)

DesOwen® Topical *see* desonide *on previous page*

desoximetasone (des ox i met' a sone)
Brand Names Topicort®; Topicort®-LP
Therapeutic Category Corticosteroid, Topical (High Potency)
Use Relieve inflammation and pruritic symptoms of corticosteroid-responsive dermatosis
Usual Dosage Topical:
Children: Apply sparingly in a very thin film to affected area 1-2 times/day
Adults: Apply sparingly in a thin film twice daily
Dosage Forms
Cream, topical:
Topicort®: 0.25% (15 g, 60 g, 120 g)
Topicort®-LP: 0.05% (15 g, 60 g)
Gel, topical: 0.05% (15 g, 60 g)
Ointment, topical (Topicort®): 0.25% (15 g, 60 g)

desoxyephedrine hydrochloride *see* methamphetamine hydrochloride *on page 298*

Desoxyn® *see* methamphetamine hydrochloride *on page 298*

desoxyphenobarbital *see* primidone *on page 394*

desoxyribonuclease and fibrinolysin *see* fibrinolysin and desoxyribonuclease *on page 195*

Despec® Capsule *see* guaifenesin and phenylpropanolamine *on page 219*

Despec® Liquid *see* guaifenesin, phenylpropanolamine, and phenylephrine *on page 221*

Desquam-X® *see* benzoyl peroxide *on page 49*

Desyrel® *see* trazodone hydrochloride *on page 474*

Detussin® Expectorant *see* hydrocodone, pseudoephedrine, and guaifenesin *on page 236*

Devrom® [OTC] *see* bismuth *on page 55*

Dexacen® Injection *see* dexamethasone *on this page*

Dexacen® LA Injection *see* dexamethasone *on this page*

Dexacidin® Ophthalmic *see* neomycin, polymyxin b, and dexamethasone *on page 328*

Dex-A-Diet® [OTC] *see* phenylpropanolamine hydrochloride *on page 373*

dexamethasone (dex a meth' a sone)
Brand Names Aeroseb-Dex® Topical Aerosol; AK-Dex® Ophthalmic; Baldex® Ophthalmic; Dalalone D.P.® Injection; Dalalone® Injection; Dalalone L.A.® Injection; Decadron®-LA Injection; Decadron® Oral; Decadron® Phosphate Cream; Decadron® Phosphate Injection; Decadron® Phosphate Nasal Turbinaire®; Decadron® Phosphate Ophthalmic; Decadron® Phosphate Respihaler® Oral Inhaler; Decaject® Injection; Decaject-LA® Injection; Decaspray® Topical Aerosol; Dekasol® Injection; Dekasol-L.A.® Injection; Dexacen® Injection; Dexacen® LA Injection; Dexasone® Injection; Dexasone® L.A. Injection; Dexone® Injection; Dexone® LA Injection; Dexone® Tablet; Hexadrol® Phosphate Injection; Hexadrol® Tablet; Maxidex® Ophthalmic; Solurex® Injection; Solurex L.A.® Injection
Therapeutic Category Antiemetic; Anti-inflammatory Agent; Corticosteroid, Inhalant; Corticosteroid, Ophthalmic; Corticosteroid, Systemic; Corticosteroid, Topical (Low Potency)
Use Systemically and locally for chronic inflammation, allergic, hematologic, neoplastic, and autoimmune diseases; may be used in management of cerebral edema, septic shock, and as a diagnostic agent
Usual Dosage
Children:
Antiemetic (prior to chemotherapy): 10 mg/m^2/dose for first dose then 5 mg/m^2/dose every 6 hours as needed

Physiologic replacement: Oral, I.M., I.V.: 0.03-0.15 mg/kg/day or 0.6-0.75 mg/m²/day in divided doses every 6-12 hours

Extubation or airway edema: Oral, I.M., I.V.: 0.5-1 mg/kg/day in divided doses every 6 hours beginning 24 hours prior to extubation and continuing for 4-6 doses afterwards

Ophthalmic: Instill 3-4 times/day

Cerebral edema: Loading dose: 1-2 mg/kg/dose as a single dose; maintenance: 1 mg/kg/day (maximum: 16 mg/day) in divided doses every 4-6 hours

Bacterial meningitis in infants and children >2 months: I.V.: 0.6 mg/kg/day in 4 divided doses for the first 4 days of antibiotic treatment; start dexamethasone at the time of the first dose of antibiotic

Adults:

Anti-inflammatory: Oral, I.M., I.V.: 0.75-9 mg/day in divided doses every 6-12 hours

Cerebral edema: I.V. 10 mg stat, 4 mg I.M./I.V. every 6 hours until response is maximized, then switch to oral regimen, then taper off if appropriate

Diagnosis for Cushing's syndrome: Oral: 1 mg at 11 PM, draw blood at 8 AM

ANLL protocol: I.V.: 2 mg/m²/dose every 8 hours for 12 doses

Dosage Forms

Acetate:

Injection:

Dalalone L.A.®, Decadron®-LA, Decaject-LA®, Dexasone® L.A., Dexone® LA, Solurex L.A.®: 8 mg/mL (1 mL, 5 mL)

Dalalone D.P.®: 16 mg/mL (1 mL, 5 mL)

Base:

Aerosol, topical:

Aeroseb-Dex®: 0.01% (58 g)

Decaspray®: 0.04% (25 g)

Elixir (Decadron®, Hexadrol®): 0.5 mg/5 mL (5 mL, 20 mL, 100 mL, 120 mL, 240 mL, 500 mL)

Solution, oral: 0.5 mg/5 mL (5 mL, 20 mL, 500 mL)

Solution, oral concentrate: 0.5 mg/0.5 mL (30 mL)

Suspension, ophthalmic (Maxidex®): 0.1% (5 mL, 15 mL)

Tablet (Decadron®, Dexone®, Hexadrol®): 0.25 mg, 0.5 mg, 0.75 mg, 1 mg, 1.5 mg, 2 mg, 4 mg, 6 mg

Therapeutic pack: Six 1.5 mg tablets and eight 0.75 mg tablets

Sodium Phosphate:

Aerosol, nasal (Decadron® Phosphate Turbinaire®): 84 µg/activation [170 metered doses] (12.6 g)

Aerosol, oral (Decadron® Phosphate Respihaler®): 84 µg/activation [170 metered doses] (12.6 g)

Cream (Decadron® Phosphate): 0.1% (15 g, 30 g)

Injection:

Dalalone®, Decadron® Phosphate, Decaject®, Dexasone®, Hexadrol® Phosphate, Solurex®: 4 mg/mL (1 mL, 2 mL, 2.5 mL, 5 mL, 10 mL, 30 mL)

Hexadrol® Phosphate: 10 mg/mL (1 mL, 10 mL); 20 mg/mL (5 mL)

Decadron® Phosphate: 24 mg/mL (5 mL, 10 mL)

Ointment, ophthalmic (AK-Dex®, Baldex®, Decadron® Phosphate, Maxidex®): 0.05% (3.5 g)

Solution, ophthalmic (AK-Dex®, Baldex®, Decadron® Phosphate, Dexotic®, I-Methasone®): 0.1% (5 mL)

dexamethasone and neomycin *see* neomycin and dexamethasone on page 327

dexamethasone and tobramycin *see* tobramycin and dexamethasone on page 470

Dexasone® Injection *see* dexamethasone *on page 132*

Dexasone® L.A. Injection *see* dexamethasone *on page 132*

Dexasporin® Ophthalmic *see* neomycin, polymyxin b, and dexamethasone *on page 328*

Dexatrim® [OTC] *see* phenylpropanolamine hydrochloride *on page 373*

dexbrompheniramine and pseudoephedrine (dex brom fen eer' a meen)
Brand Names Disobrom® [OTC]; Disophrol® Chrontabs® [OTC]; Drixoral® [OTC]; Histro-drix® [OTC]; Par-Drix® [OTC]; Resporal® [OTC]
Synonyms pseudoephedrine and dexbrompheniramine
Therapeutic Category Antihistamine/Decongestant Combination
Use Relief of symptoms of upper respiratory mucosal congestion in seasonal and perennial nasal allergies, acute rhinitis, rhinosinusitis and eustachian tube blockage
Usual Dosage Children >12 years and Adults: Oral: 1 tablet every 12 hours, may require 1 tablet every 8 hours
Dosage Forms Tablet, timed release: Dexbrompheniramine maleate 6 mg and pseudoephedrine sulfate 120 mg

Dexchlor® *see* dexchlorpheniramine maleate *on this page*

dexchlorpheniramine maleate (dex klor fen eer' a meen)
Brand Names Dexchlor®; Poladex®; Polaramine®; Polargen®
Therapeutic Category Antihistamine
Use Perennial and seasonal allergic rhinitis and other allergic symptoms including urticaria
Usual Dosage Oral:
Children:
2-5 years: 0.5 mg every 4-6 hours
6-11 years: 1 mg every 4-6 hours or 4 mg timed release at bedtime

Adults: 2 mg every 4-6 hours or 4-6 mg timed release at bedtime or 8-10 hours
Dosage Forms
Syrup (orange flavor): 2 mg/5 mL with alcohol 6% (480 mL)
Tablet: 2 mg
Tablet, sustained action: 4 mg, 6 mg

Dexedrine® *see* dextroamphetamine sulfate *on next page*

Dexone® Injection *see* dexamethasone *on page 132*

Dexone® LA Injection *see* dexamethasone *on page 132*

Dexone® Tablet *see* dexamethasone *on page 132*

dexpanthenol (dex pan' the nole)
Brand Names Ilopan-Choline® Oral; Ilopan® Injection; Panthoderm® Cream [OTC]
Synonyms pantothenyl alcohol
Therapeutic Category Gastrointestinal Agent, Stimulant
Use Prophylactic use to minimize paralytic ileus, treatment of postoperative distention
Usual Dosage Adults: Oral: 2-3 tablets 3 times/day
Prevention of postoperative ileus: I.M.: 250-500 mg stat, repeat in 2 hours, followed by doses every 6 hours until danger passes

Paralyzed ileus: I.M.: 500 mg stat, repeat in 2 hours, followed by doses every 6 hours, if needed
Dosage Forms
Cream: 2% (30 g, 60 g)
Injection (Ilopan®): 250 mg/mL (2 mL, 10 mL, 30 mL)
Tablet (Ilopan-Choline®): 50 mg with choline bitartrate 25 mg

dextran
Brand Names Gentran®; LMD®; Macrodex®; Rheomacrodex®
Synonyms dextran 40; dextran 70; dextran 75; dextran, high molecular weight; dextran, low molecular weight
Therapeutic Category Plasma Volume Expander
Use Blood volume expander used in treatment of shock or impending shock when blood or blood products are not available
Usual Dosage I.V.:
Children: Total dose should not be >20 mL/kg during first 24 hours

Adults: 500-1000 mL at rate of 20-40 mL/minute
Dosage Forms Injection:
High molecular weight:
6% dextran 75 in dextrose 5% (500 mL)
Gentran®: 6% dextran 75 in sodium chloride 0.9% (500 mL)
Gentran®, Macrodex®: 6% dextran 70 in sodium chloride 0.9% (500 mL)
Macrodex®: 6% dextran 70 in dextrose 5% (500 mL)

Low molecular weight: Gentran®, LMD®, Rheomacrodex®:
10% dextran 40 in dextrose 5% (500 mL)
10% dextran 40 in sodium chloride 0.9% (500 mL)

dextran 1
Brand Names Promit®
Therapeutic Category Plasma Volume Expander
Use Prophylaxis of serious anaphylactic reactions to I.V. infusion of dextran
Usual Dosage I.V. (time between dextran 1 and dextran solution should not exceed 15 minutes):
Children: 0.3 mL/kg 1-2 minutes before I.V. infusion of dextran
Adults: 20 mL 1-2 minutes before I.V. infusion of dextran
Dosage Forms Injection: 150 mg/mL (20 mL)

dextran 40 *see dextran on this page*

dextran 70 *see dextran on this page*

dextran 75 *see dextran on this page*

dextran, high molecular weight *see dextran on this page*

dextran, low molecular weight *see dextran on this page*

dextranomer (dex tran' oh mer)
Brand Names Debrisan® Topical [OTC]
Therapeutic Category Topical Skin Product
Use Clean exudative wounds; no controlled studies have found dextranomer to be more effective than conventional therapy
Usual Dosage Topical: Apply to affected area once or twice daily
Dosage Forms
Beads: 4 g, 25 g, 60 g, 120 g
Paste: 10 g foil packets

dextroamphetamine sulfate (dex troe am fet' a meen)
Brand Names Dexedrine®; Ferndex®
Therapeutic Category Amphetamine; Anorexiant; Central Nervous System Stimulant, Amphetamine
Use Narcolepsy; abnormal behavioral syndrome in children; exogenous obesity
Usual Dosage Oral:
Children:
Narcolepsy: 6-12 years: Initial: 5 mg/day, may increase at 5 mg increments in weekly intervals until side effects appear; maximum dose: 60 mg/day
(Continued)

135

dextroamphetamine sulfate *(Continued)*

Attention deficit disorder:

> 3-5 years: Initial: 2.5 mg/day given every morning; increase by 2.5 mg/day in weekly intervals until optimal response is obtained, usual range is 0.1-0.5 mg/kg/dose every morning with maximum of 40 mg/day

> ≥6 years: 5 mg once or twice daily; increase in increments of 5 mg/day at weekly intervals until optimal response is reached, usual range is 0.1-0.5 mg/kg/dose every morning (5-20 mg/day) with maximum of 40 mg/day

Adults:

> Narcolepsy: Initial: 10 mg/day, may increase at 10 mg increments in weekly intervals until side effects appear; maximum: 60 mg/day

> Exogenous obesity: 5-30 mg/day in divided doses of 5-10 mg 30-60 minutes before meals

Dosage Forms

Capsule, sustained release: 5 mg, 10 mg, 15 mg

Elixir (orange flavor): 5 mg/5 mL (480 mL)

Tablet: 5 mg, 10 mg

dextromethorphan and guaifenesin *see* guaifenesin and dextromethorphan on page 218

dextromethorphan hydrobromide (dex troe meth or' fan)

Brand Names Benylin DM® [OTC]; Children's Hold® [OTC]; Creo-Terpin® [OTC]; Delsym® [OTC]; Drixoral® Cough Liquid Caps [OTC]; Hold® DM [OTC]; Pertussin® CS [OTC]; Pertussin® ES [OTC]; Robitussin® Cough Calmers [OTC]; Robitussin® Pediatric [OTC]; Scot-Tussin DM® Cough Chasers [OTC]; St. Joseph® Cough Suppressant [OTC]; Sucrets® Cough Calmers [OTC]; Suppress® [OTC]; Trocal® [OTC]; Vicks Formula 44® [OTC]; Vicks Formula 44® Pediatric Formula [OTC]

Therapeutic Category Antitussive

Use Symptomatic relief of coughs caused by minor viral upper respiratory tract infections or inhaled irritants; most effective for a chronic nonproductive cough

Usual Dosage Oral:

Children:

> 2-5 years: 2.5-5 mg every 4 hours or 7.5 mg every 6-8 hours; extended release is 50 mg twice daily

> 6-11 years: 5-10 mg every 4 hours or 15 mg every 6-8 hours; extended release is 30 mg twice daily

Adults: 10-20 mg every 4 hours or 30 mg every 6-8 hours; extended release is 60 mg twice daily

Dosage Forms

Capsule (Drixoral® Cough Liquid Caps): 30 mg

Liquid:

> Pertussin® CS: 3.5 mg/5 mL (120 mL)

> Robitussin® Pediatric, St. Joseph® Cough Suppressant: 7.5 mg/5 mL (60 mL, 120 mL, 240 mL)

> Pertussin® ES, Vicks Formula 44®: 15 mg/5 mL (120 mL, 240 mL)

Liquid, sustained release, as polistirex (Delsym®): 30 mg/5 mL (89 mL)

Lozenges:

> Scot-Tussin DM® Cough Chasers: 2.5 mg

> Children's Hold®, Hold® DM, Robitussin® Cough Calmers, Sucrets® Cough Calmers: 5 mg

> Suppress®, Trocal®: 7.5 mg

Syrup:

> Benylin DM®: 10 mg/5 mL (120 mL, 3780 mL)

> Vicks Formula 44® Pediatric Formula: 15 mg/15 mL (120 mL)

dextropropoxyphene *see* propoxyphene on page 402

dextrose, levulose and phosphoric acid *see* phosphorated carbohydrate solution *on page 375*

Dextrostix® [OTC] *see* diagnostic aids (*in vitro*), blood *on this page*

dextrothyroxine sodium (dex troe thye rox' een)
Brand Names Choloxin®
Therapeutic Category Antilipemic Agent
Use Reduction of elevated serum cholesterol
Usual Dosage Oral:
Children: 0.1 mg/kg/day
Adults: 1-2 mg/day, up to 8 mg/day
Dosage Forms Tablet: 1 mg, 2 mg, 4 mg, 6 mg

Dey-Dose® Isoproterenol Inhalation Solution *see* isoproterenol *on page 258*

Dey-Dose® Metaproterenol Inhalation Solution *see* metaproterenol sulfate *on page 296*

Dey-Drop® Ophthalmic Solution *see* silver nitrate *on page 430*

Dey-Lute® Isoetharine Inhalation Solution *see* isoetharine *on page 257*

dezocine (dez' oh seen)
Brand Names Dalgan®
Therapeutic Category Analgesic, Narcotic
Use Relief of moderate to severe postoperative, acute renal and ureteral colic, and cancer pain
Usual Dosage Adults:
I.M.: Initial: 5-20 mg; may be repeated every 3-6 hours as needed; maximum: 120 mg/day
I.V.: Initial: 2.5-10 mg; may be repeated every 2-4 hours as needed
Dosage Forms Injection, single-dose vial: 5 mg/mL (2 mL); 10 mg/mL (2 mL); 15 mg/mL (2 mL)

DFMO *see* eflornithine hydrochloride *on page 168*

DFP *see* isoflurophate *on page 257*

DHAD *see* mitoxantrone hydrochloride *on page 315*

D.H.E. 45® Injection *see* dihydroergotamine mesylate *on page 149*

DHPG sodium *see* ganciclovir *on page 208*

DHS® Tar [OTC] *see* coal tar *on page 110*

DHS Zinc® [OTC] *see* pyrithione zinc *on page 410*

DHT™ *see* dihydrotachysterol *on page 149*

Diaβeta® *see* glyburide *on page 213*

Diabinese® *see* chlorpropamide *on page 98*

diagnostic aids (*in vitro*), blood
Brand Names Abbott HIVAB HIV-1 EIA; Abbott HIVAG-1; Abbott HTLV III Confirmatory EIA; Azostix® [OTC]; Chemstrip® bG [OTC]; Dextrostix® [OTC]; Diascan-S® [OTC]; Glucostix® [OTC]; MicroTrak® HSV 1/HSV 2 Culture Identification/Typing Test; Mono-Diff®; Mono-Lisa®; Monospot®; Monosticon®; Monosticon® Dri-Dot®; Mono-Sure®; Mono-Test®; Recombigen® HIV-1 LA; Rheumanosticon® Dri-Dot®; Rubacell® II; Rubazyme®; Sickledex™; TPM® Test; Tracer bG® [OTC]; Virogen® Rubella Microlatex®; Virogen® Rubella Slide Test; Visidex® II [OTC]
Synonyms diagnostic test for blood urea nitrogen in blood; diagnostic test for glucose in blood; diagnostic test for infectious mononucleosis; diagnostic test for rheumatoid factor;
(Continued)

diagnostic aids (*in vitro*), blood *(Continued)*

diagnostic test for sickle cell anemia; diagnostic test for toxoplasmosis; diagnostic test for virus (blood)

Dosage Forms

Diagnostic test for glucose in blood:
Chemstrip bG®
Dextrostix®
Diascan-S®
Tracer bG®
Glucostix®
Visidex® II

Diagnostic test for blood urea nitrogen in blood: Azostix®

Diagnostic test for infectious mononucleosis:
Mono-Diff®
Mono-Lisa®
Monospot®
Monosticon®
Monosticon® Dri-Dot®
Mono-Sure®
Mono-Test®

Diagnostic test for rheumatoid factor: Rheumanosticon® Dri-Dot®

Diagnostic test for sickle cell anemia: Sickledex™

Diagnostic test for toxoplasmosis: TPM® Test

Diagnostic test for virus:
Abbott HIVAB HIV-1 EIA
Abbott HIVAG-1
Abbott HTLV I EIA
Abbott HTLV III Confirmatory EIA
MicroTrak® HSV 1/HSV 2 Culture Identification/Typing Test
Recombigen® HIV-1 LA
Rubacell® II
Rubazyme®
Virogen® Rotatest®
Virogen® Rubella Microlatex®
Virogen® Rubella Slide Test

diagnostic aids (*in vitro*), feces

Brand Names Colocare® [OTC]; ColoScreen [OTC]; CS-T® [OTC]; Early Detector® [OTC]; EZ-Detect® [OTC]; Hema-Chek® [OTC]; Hematest® [OTC]; Hemoccult® II [OTC]; Hemoccult® Slides; Rotalex®; Virogen® Rotatest®

Synonyms diagnostic test for virus (feces); diagnostic tests for occult blood (feces)

Dosage Forms

Diagnostic tests for occult blood:
Colocare®
CS-T®
Early Detector®
EZ-Detect®
Hemocult® II

Diagnostic test for virus:
Rotalex®
Virogen® Rotatest®

diagnostic aids (*in vitro*), other

Brand Names Accusens T®; Biocult-GC®; Culturette® 10 Minute Group A Strep ID; Gastroccult®; Gonodecten®; Gonozyme®; Isocult® for *Neisseria gonorrhoeae*; Isocult® for *Staphylococcus aureus*; Isocult® for *Trichomonas vaginalis*; Isocult® Throat Streptococci; Lung Check®; *Neisseria gonorrhoeae*; RapidTest® Strep; Respiracult-Strep®; Respiralex®; Streptonase-B®; Strepto-Sac®; Virogen® Herpes Slide Test

Synonyms diagnostic test for gonorrhea; diagnostic test for occult blood (gastric contents); diagnostic test for precancerous lung cells; diagnostic test for *Staphylococcus*; diagnostic test for *Streptococcus*; diagnostic test for *Trichomonas*; diagnostic test for virus (other); taste function test

Dosage Forms
Diagnostic test for gonorrhea:
Biocult-GC®
Gonodecten®
Gonozyme®
Isocult® for *Neisseria gonorrhoeae*
MicroTrak® *Neisseria gonorrhoeae*
Diagnostic test for precancerous lung cells: Lung Check®
Diagnostic test for occult blood (gastric contents): Gastrocult®
Diagnostic test for *Staphylococcus*: Isocult® for *Staphylococcus aureus*
Culturette® 10 Minute Group A Strep ID
Diagnostic test for *Streptococcus*:
Isocult® Throat Streptococci
RapidTest® Strep
Respiracult-Strep®
Respiralex®
Streptonase-B®
Strepto-Sac®
Taste function test: Accusens T®
Diagnostic test for *Trichomonas*: Isocult® for *Trichomonas vaginalis*
Diagnostic test for virus: Virogen® Herpes Slide Test

diagnostic aids (*in vitro*), urine
Brand Names Advance®; Answer®; Answer® Ovulation; Answer® Plus; Bili-Labstix® [OTC]; Chemstrip® 7 [OTC]; Chemstrip® 9 [OTC]; Chemstrip® K [OTC]; Chemstrip® uG [OTC]; Chemstrip® uGK [OTC]; Clearblue®; Clearplan® Easy; Clinistix® [OTC]; Clinitest® [OTC]; Color® Ovulation Test; Combistix® [OTC]; Daisy® 2; Diastix® [OTC]; e.p.t.® Stick; Fact Plus®; First Response®; Fortel® Home Ovulation; Hema-Combistix® [OTC]; Hemastix® [OTC]; Ictotest® [OTC]; Isocult® for Bacteriuria; Isocult® for *Pseudomonas aeruginosa*; Keto-Diastix® [OTC]; Ketostix® [OTC]; Labstix® [OTC]; Microstix-3®; Multistix® [OTC]; Nimbus®; Nimbus® II; OvuKIT® Acetest® [OTC]; OvuQUICK®; Pregnosis®; Pregnospia® II; Pregnosticon® Dri-Dot®; RAMP® Urine hCG; Tes-Tape® [OTC]; UCG-Slide® Test; Uricult®; Uristix®

Synonyms diagnostic test for acetone, bilirubin, blood, glucose, pH and protein in urine; diagnostic test for acetone, blood, glucose, pH, and protein in urine; diagnostic test for acetone in urine; diagnostic test for bilirubin in the urine; diagnostic test for blood, glucose, pH, and protein in urine; diagnostic test for blood in urine; diagnostic test for glucose and ketones in urine; diagnostic test for glucose and protein in urine; diagnostic test for glucose in urine; diagnostic test for glucose, pH, and protein in urine; diagnostic test for multiple determinations in urine; diagnostic test for *Pseudomonas*; ovulation tests; pregnancy tests

Dosage Forms
Diagnostic test for acetone, bilirubin, blood, glucose, pH and protein in urine: Bili-Labstix®
Diagnostic test for bilirubin in the urine: Ictotest®
Diagnostic test for acetone, blood, glucose, pH, and protein in urine: Labstix®
Diagnostic test for acetone in urine: Acetest®, Chemstrip® K, Ketostix®
Diagnostic test for bacteriuria:
Microstix-3®
Uricult®
Isocult® for Bacteriuria
Diagnostic test for blood, glucose, pH, and protein in urine: Hema-Combistix [OTC]
Diagnostic test for blood in urine: Hemastix®
Diagnostic test for glucose and protein in urine: Uristix®
Diagnostic test for glucose and ketones in urine; Keto-Diastix®
Diagnostic test for glucose in urine:
Chemstrip® uG
(Continued)

139

diagnostic aids (*in vitro*), urine *(Continued)*

Clinistix®
Clinitest®
Diastix®
Tes-Tape®
Diagnostic test for glucose, pH, and protein in urine: Combistix®
Diagnostic test for multiple determinations in urine:
Chemstrip® 7
Chemstrip® 9
Chemstrip® uGK
Hema-Combistix®
Multistix®
Ovulation tests:
Answer® Ovulation
Clearplan® Easy
Color® Ovulation Test
First Response®
Fortel® Home Ovulation
OvuKIT®
OvuQUICK®
Pregnancy tests:
Advance®
Answer®
Answer® Plus
Clearblue®
Daisy® 2
e.p.t.® Stick
Fact Plus®
First Response®
Pregnosis®
Pregnosticon® Dri-Dot®
UCG-Slide® Test
Nimbus®
Nimbus® II
Pregnospia® II
RAMP® Urine hCG
Diagnostic test for *Pseudomonas*:
Isocult® for *Pseudomonas aeruginosa*

diagnostic test for acetone, bilirubin, blood, glucose, pH and protein in urine *see* diagnostic aids (*in vitro*), urine *on previous page*

diagnostic test for acetone, blood, glucose, pH, and protein in urine *see* diagnostic aids (*in vitro*), urine *on previous page*

diagnostic test for acetone in urine *see* diagnostic aids (*in vitro*), urine *on previous page*

diagnostic test for bilirubin in the urine *see* diagnostic aids (*in vitro*), urine *on previous page*

diagnostic test for blood, glucose, pH, and protein in urine *see* diagnostic aids (*in vitro*), urine *on previous page*

diagnostic test for blood in urine *see* diagnostic aids (*in vitro*), urine *on previous page*

diagnostic test for blood urea nitrogen in blood *see* diagnostic aids (*in vitro*), blood *on page 137*

diagnostic test for glucose and ketones in urine *see* diagnostic aids (*in vitro*), urine *on previous page*

diagnostic test for glucose and protein in urine *see* diagnostic aids (*in vitro*), urine *on page 139*

diagnostic test for glucose in blood *see* diagnostic aids (*in vitro*), blood *on page 137*

diagnostic test for glucose in urine *see* diagnostic aids (*in vitro*), urine *on page 139*

diagnostic test for glucose, pH, and protein in urine *see* diagnostic aids (*in vitro*), urine *on page 139*

diagnostic test for gonorrhea *see* diagnostic aids (*in vitro*), other *on page 138*

diagnostic test for infectious mononucleosis *see* diagnostic aids (*in vitro*), blood *on page 137*

diagnostic test for multiple determinations in urine *see* diagnostic aids (*in vitro*), urine *on page 139*

diagnostic test for occult blood (gastric contents) *see* diagnostic aids (*in vitro*), other *on page 138*

diagnostic test for precancerous lung cells *see* diagnostic aids (*in vitro*), other *on page 138*

diagnostic test for *Pseudomonas* *see* diagnostic aids (*in vitro*), urine *on page 139*

diagnostic test for rheumatoid factor *see* diagnostic aids (*in vitro*), blood *on page 137*

diagnostic test for sickle cell anemia *see* diagnostic aids (*in vitro*), blood *on page 137*

diagnostic test for *Staphylococcus* *see* diagnostic aids (*in vitro*), other *on page 138*

diagnostic test for *Streptococcus* *see* diagnostic aids (*in vitro*), other *on page 138*

diagnostic test for toxoplasmosis *see* diagnostic aids (*in vitro*), blood *on page 137*

diagnostic test for *Trichomonas* *see* diagnostic aids (*in vitro*), other *on page 138*

diagnostic test for virus (blood) *see* diagnostic aids (*in vitro*), blood *on page 137*

diagnostic test for virus (feces) *see* diagnostic aids (*in vitro*), feces *on page 138*

diagnostic test for virus (other) *see* diagnostic aids (*in vitro*), other *on page 138*

diagnostic tests for occult blood (feces) *see* diagnostic aids (*in vitro*), feces *on page 138*

Dialose® [OTC] *see* docusate *on page 157*

Dialose® Plus Capsule [OTC] *see* docusate and casanthranol *on page 158*

Dialose® Plus Tablet [OTC] *see* docusate and phenolphthalein *on page 158*

Dialume® [OTC] *see* aluminum hydroxide *on page 15*

Diamine T.D.® Oral [OTC] *see* brompheniramine maleate *on page 59*

diaminodiphenylsulfone *see* dapsone *on page 126*

Diamox® *see* acetazolamide *on page 4*

Diaparene® [OTC] *see* methylbenzethonium chloride *on page 304*

Diapid® Nasal Spray *see* lypressin *on page 280*

Diaqua® *see* hydrochlorothiazide *on page 233*

ALPHABETICAL LISTING OF DRUGS

Diar-Aid® [OTC] *see* attapulgite *on page 38*

Diascan-S® [OTC] *see* diagnostic aids (*in vitro*), blood *on page 137*

Diasorb® [OTC] *see* attapulgite *on page 38*

Diastix® [OTC] *see* diagnostic aids (*in vitro*), urine *on page 139*

diatrizoate meglumine *see* radiological/contrast media (ionic) *on page 413*

diatrizoate meglumine and diatrizoate sodium *see* radiological/contrast media (ionic) *on page 413*

diatrizoate meglumine and iodipamide meglumine *see* radiological/contrast media (ionic) *on page 413*

diatrizoate sodium *see* radiological/contrast media (ionic) *on page 413*

diazepam (dye az' e pam)
Brand Names Valium® Injection; Valium® Oral; Valrelease® Oral; Zetran® Injection
Therapeutic Category Antianxiety Agent; Anticonvulsant, Benzodiazepine; Benzodiazepine; Sedative
Use Management of general anxiety disorders, panic disorders, and to provide preoperative sedation, light anesthesia, and amnesia; treatment of status epilepticus, alcohol withdrawal symptoms; used as a skeletal muscle relaxant
Usual Dosage
Neonates: I.V.: Status epilepticus: 0.5-1 mg/kg/dose every 15-30 minutes for 2-3 doses
Children:
Sedation or muscle relaxation or anxiety:
Oral: 0.12-0.8 mg/kg/day in divided doses every 6-8 hours
I.M., I.V.: 0.04-0.3 mg/kg/dose every 2-4 hours to a maximum of 0.6 mg/kg within an 8-hour period if needed
Status epilepticus: I.V.:
Infants 30 days to 5 years: 0.05-0.3 mg/kg/dose given over 2-3 minutes, every 15-30 minutes to a maximum total dose of 5 mg; repeat in 2-4 hours as needed or 0.2-0.5 mg/dose every 2-5 minutes to a maximum total dose of 5 mg
>5 years: 0.05-0.3 mg/kg/dose given over 2-3 minutes, every 15-30 minutes to a maximum total dose of 10 mg; repeat in 2-4 hours as needed or 1 mg/dose every 2-5 minutes to a maximum of 10 mg;
Adults:
Anxiety:
Oral: 2-10 mg 2-4 times/day
I.M., I.V.: 2-10 mg, may repeat in 3-4 hours if needed
Skeletal muscle relaxation:
Oral: 2-10 mg 2-4 times/day
I.M., I.V.: 5-10 mg, may repeat in 2-4 hours
Status epilepticus: I.V.: 0.2-0.5 mg/kg/dose every 15-30 minutes for 2-3 doses; maximum dose: 30 mg
Dosage Forms
Capsule, sustained release (Valrelease®): 15 mg
Injection: 5 mg/mL (1 mL, 2 mL, 5 mL, 10 mL)
Solution, oral (wintergreen-spice flavor): 5 mg/5 mL (5 mL, 10 mL, 500 mL)
Solution, oral concentrate: 5 mg/mL (30 mL)
Tablet: 2 mg, 5 mg, 10 mg

diazoxide (dye az ox' ide)
Brand Names Hyperstat® I.V.; Proglycem® Oral
Therapeutic Category Antihypertensive; Antihypoglycemic Agent
Use
Oral: Hypoglycemia related to islet cell adenoma, carcinoma, hyperplasia, or adenomatosis, nesidioblastosis, leucine sensitivity, or extrapancreatic malignancy
I.V.: Emergency lowering of blood pressure

Usual Dosage
Hyperinsulinemic hypoglycemia: Oral:
  Newborns and Infants: 8-15 mg/kg/day in divided doses every 8-12 hours
  Children and Adults: 3-8 mg/kg/day in divided doses every 8-12 hours

Hypertension: Children and Adults: I.V.: 1-3 mg/kg (maximum: 150 mg in a single injection); repeat dose in 5-15 minutes until blood pressure adequately reduced; repeat administration every 4-24 hours; monitor blood pressure closely

Dosage Forms
Capsule (Proglycem®): 50 mg
Injection (Hyperstat®): 15 mg/mL (1 mL, 20 mL)
Suspension, oral (chocolate-mint flavor) (Proglycem®): 50 mg/mL (30 mL)

Dibent® Injection *see* dicyclomine hydrochloride *on page 145*

Dibenzyline® *see* phenoxybenzamine hydrochloride *on page 370*

dibucaine (dye' byoo kane)
Brand Names Nupercainal® Topical [OTC]
Therapeutic Category Local Anesthetic, Topical
Use Fast, temporary relief of pain and itching due to hemorrhoids, minor burns, other minor skin conditions
Usual Dosage Children and Adults:
  Rectal: Hemorrhoids: Insert ointment into rectum using a rectal applicator; administer each morning, evening, and after each bowel movement
  Topical: Apply gently to the affected areas; no more than 30 g for adults or 7.5 g for children should be used in any 24-hour period
Dosage Forms
Cream: 0.5% (45 g)
Ointment, topical: 1% (30 g, 60 g)

dibucaine and hydrocortisone
Brand Names Corticaine® Topical
Synonyms hydrocortisone and dibucaine
Therapeutic Category Corticosteroid, Topical (Low Potency); Local Anesthetic, Topical
Use Relief of the inflammatory and pruritic manifestations of corticosteroid-responsive dermatoses and for external anal itching
Usual Dosage Topical: Apply to affected areas 2-4 times/day
Dosage Forms Cream: Dibucaine 5% and hydrocortisone 5%

DIC *see* dacarbazine *on page 124*

dicalcium phosphate *see* calcium phosphate, dibasic *on page 69*

Dicarbosil® [OTC] *see* calcium carbonate *on page 65*

dichlorodifluoromethane and trichloromonofluoromethane
(dye klor oh dye floo or oh meth' ane & tri klor oh mon oh floo or meth' ane
Brand Names Fluori-Methane® Topical Spray
Therapeutic Category Analgesic, Topical
Use Management of myofascial pain, restricted motion, muscle pain; control of pain associated with injections
Usual Dosage Topical: Apply to area from approximately 12" away
Dosage Forms Spray, topical: Dichlorodifluoromethane 15% and trichloromonofluoromethane 85%

dichlorotetrafluoroethane and ethyl chloride *see* ethyl chloride and
dichlorotetrafluoroethane *on page 186*

143

dichlorphenamide (dye klor fen' a mide)
Brand Names Daranide®
Synonyms diclofenamide
Therapeutic Category Carbonic Anhydrase Inhibitor; Diuretic, Carbonic Anhydrase Inhibitor
Use Adjunct in treatment of open-angle glaucoma and perioperative treatment for angle-closure glaucoma
Usual Dosage Adults: Oral: 100-200 mg to start followed by 100 mg every 12 hours until desired response is obtained; maintenance dose: 25-50 mg 1-3 times/day
Dosage Forms Tablet: 50 mg

dichysterol *see* dihydrotachysterol *on page 149*

diclofenac (dye kloe' fen ak)
Brand Names Cataflam® Oral; Voltaren® Ophthalmic; Voltaren® Oral
Therapeutic Category Analgesic, Non-Narcotic; Anti-inflammatory Agent; Nonsteroidal Anti-Inflammatory Agent (NSAID), Ophthalmic; Nonsteroidal Anti-Inflammatory Agent (NSAID), Oral
Use Acute and chronic treatment of rheumatoid arthritis, ankylosing spondylitis, and osteoarthritis; also used for juvenile rheumatoid arthritis, gout, dysmenorrhea, and pain relief; ophthalmic solution for postoperative inflammation after cataract extraction
Usual Dosage Adults:
Oral:
Analgesia (Cataflam®): Starting dose: 50 mg 3 times/day
Rheumatoid arthritis: 150-200 mg/day in 2-4 divided doses
Osteoarthritis: 100-150 mg/day in 2-3 divided doses
Ankylosing spondylitis: 100-125 mg/day in 4-5 divided doses
Ophthalmic: Instill 1 drop into affected eye 4 times/day beginning 24 hours after cataract surgery and continuing for 2 weeks
Dosage Forms
Solution, ophthalmic, as sodium (Voltaren®): 0.1% (2.5 mL, 5 mL)
Tablet, enteric coated, as sodium (Voltaren®): 25 mg, 50 mg, 75 mg
Tablet, as potassium (Cataflam®): 50 mg

diclofenamide *see* dichlorphenamide *on this page*

dicloxacillin sodium (dye klox a sill' in)
Brand Names Dycill®; Dynapen®; Pathocil®
Therapeutic Category Antibiotic, Penicillin
Use Treatment of systemic infections such as pneumonia, skin and soft tissue infections and follow-up therapy for osteomyelitis caused by penicillinase-producing staphylococci
Usual Dosage Oral:
Children <40 kg: 12.5-50 mg/kg/day divided every 6 hours; doses of 50-100 mg/kg/day in divided doses every 6 hours have been used for follow-up therapy of osteomyelitis

Children >40 kg and Adults: 125-500 mg every 6 hours
Dosage Forms
Capsule: 125 mg, 250 mg, 500 mg
Powder for oral suspension: 62.5 mg/5 mL (80 mL, 100 mL, 200 mL)

dicumarol (dye koo' ma role)
Synonyms bishydroxycoumarin
Therapeutic Category Anticoagulant
Use Prophylaxis and treatment of thromboembolic disorders
Usual Dosage Adults: Oral: 25-200 mg/day based on prothrombin time (PT) determinations
Dosage Forms Tablet: 25 mg, 50 mg, 100 mg

dicyclomine hydrochloride (dye sye' kloe meen)
Brand Names Antispas® Injection; Bemote® Oral; Bentyl® Hydrochloride Injection; Bentyl® Hydrochloride Oral; Byclomine® Injection; Dibent® Injection; Dilomine® Injection; Di-Spaz® Injection; Di-Spaz® Oral; Neoquess® Injection; Or-Tyl® Injection; Spasmoject® Injection
Synonyms dicycloverine hydrochloride
Therapeutic Category Antispasmodic Agent, Gastrointestinal
Use Treatment of functional disturbances of GI motility such as irritable bowel syndrome
Usual Dosage
Oral:
Infants >6 months: 5 mg/dose 3-4 times/day
Children: 10 mg/dose 3-4 times/day
Adults: Begin with 80 mg/day in 4 equally divided doses, then increase up to 160 mg/day
I.M. **(should not be used I.V.)**: 80 mg/day in 4 divided doses (20 mg/dose)
Dosage Forms
Capsule: 10 mg, 20 mg
Injection: 10 mg/mL (2 mL, 10 mL)
Syrup: 10 mg/5 mL (118 mL, 473 mL, 946 mL)
Tablet: 20 mg

dicycloverine hydrochloride *see* dicyclomine hydrochloride *on this page*

didanosine (dye dan' oh seen)
Brand Names Videx® Oral
Synonyms DDI
Therapeutic Category Antiviral Agent, Oral
Use Advanced HIV infection in patients who are intolerant of zidovudine therapy or who have demonstrated significant clinical or immunologic deterioration during zidovudine therapy
Usual Dosage Administer on an empty stomach
Children (dosing is based on body surface area (m^2)):
<0.4: 25 mg tablets twice daily or 31 mg powder twice daily
0.5-0.7: 50 mg tablets twice daily or 62 mg powder twice daily
0.8-1: 75 mg tablets twice daily or 94 mg powder twice daily
1.1-1.4: 100 mg tablets twice daily or 125 mg powder twice daily

Adults: Dosing is based on patient weight:
35-49 kg: 125 mg tablets twice daily or 167 mg buffered powder twice daily
50-74 kg: 200 mg tablets twice daily or 250 mg buffered powder twice daily
≥75 mg: 300 mg tablets twice daily or 375 mg buffered powder twice daily

Note: Children >1 year and Adults should receive 2 tablets per dose and children <1 year should receive 1 tablet per dose for adequate buffering and absorption; tablets should be chewed
Dosage Forms
Powder for oral solution:
Buffered (single dose packet): 100 mg, 167 mg, 250 mg, 375 mg
Pediatric: 2 g, 4 g
Tablet, buffered, chewable (mint flavor): 25 mg, 50 mg, 100 mg, 150 mg

dideoxycytidine *see* zalcitabine *on page 502*
Didrex® *see* benzphetamine hydrochloride *on page 50*
Didronel® I.V. *see* etidronate disodium *on page 187*
Didronel® Oral *see* etidronate disodium *on page 187*

dienestrol (dye en ess' trole)
Brand Names DV® Vaginal Cream; Ortho® Dienestrol Vaginal
Therapeutic Category Estrogen Derivative
Use Symptomatic management of atrophic vaginitis in postmenopausal women
(Continued)
145

dienestrol *(Continued)*

Usual Dosage Adults: Vaginal: 1-2 applicatorfuls/day for 2 weeks and then ½ of that dose for 2 weeks; maintenance dose: 1 applicatorful 1-3 times/week for 3 weeks each month
Dosage Forms Cream, vaginal: 0.01% (30 g, 78 g)

diethylpropion hydrochloride (dye eth il proe' pee on)

Brand Names Tenuate®; Tepanil®
Synonyms amfepramone
Therapeutic Category Anorexiant
Use Short-term adjunct in exogenous obesity
Usual Dosage Adults: Oral: 25 mg 3 times/day before meals or food or 75 mg controlled release tablet at midmorning
Dosage Forms
Tablet: 25 mg
Tablet, controlled release: 75 mg

diethylstilbestrol (dye eth il stil bess' trole)

Brand Names Stilphostrol® Injection; Stilphostrol® Oral
Synonyms DES; stilbestrol
Therapeutic Category Estrogen Derivative
Use Management of severe vasomotor symptoms of menopause, for estrogen replacement, and for palliative treatment of inoperable metastatic prostatic carcinoma
Usual Dosage Adults:
Hypogonadism and ovarian failure: Oral: 0.2-0.5 mg/day

Menopausal symptoms: Oral: 0.1-2 mg/day for 3 weeks and then off 1 week

Postmenopausal breast carcinoma: Oral: 15 mg/day

Prostate carcinoma: Oral: 1-3 mg/day

Prostatic cancer: I.V.: 0.5 g to start, then 1 g every 2-5 days followed by 0.25-0.5 g 1-2 times/week as maintenance

Diphosphate:
Oral: 50 mg 3 times/day; increase up to 200 mg or more 3 times/day
I.V.: Give 0.5 g, dissolved in 250 mL of saline or D_5W, administer slowly the first 10-15 minutes then adjust rate so that the entire amount is given in 1 hour
Dosage Forms
Injection, as diphosphate sodium (Stilphostrol®): 0.25 g (5 mL)
Tablet: 1 mg, 2.5 mg, 5 mg
Tablet (Stilphostrol®): 50 mg

difenoxin and atropine (dye fen ox' in)

Brand Names Motofen®
Therapeutic Category Antidiarrheal
Use Treatment of diarrhea
Usual Dosage Adults: Oral: Initial: 2 tablets, then 1 tablet after each loose stool; 1 tablet every 3-4 hours, up to 8 tablets in a 24-hour period; if no improvement after 48 hours, continued administration is not indicated
Dosage Forms Tablet: Difenoxin hydrochloride 1 mg and atropine sulfate 0.025 mg

diflorasone diacetate (dye flor' a sone)

Brand Names Florone® E Topical; Florone® Topical; Maxiflor® Topical; Psorcon™ Topical
Therapeutic Category Corticosteroid, Topical (High Potency)
Use Relieve inflammation and pruritic symptoms of corticosteroid-responsive dermatosis
Usual Dosage Topical:
Cream: Apply 2-4 times/day

Ointment: Apply sparingly 1-3 times/day
Dosage Forms
Cream: 0.05% (15 g, 30 g, 60 g)
Ointment, topical: 0.05% (15 g, 30 g, 60 g)

Diflucan® Injection *see* fluconazole *on page 198*
Diflucan® Oral *see* fluconazole *on page 198*

diflunisal (dye floo' ni sal)
Brand Names Dolobid®
Therapeutic Category Analgesic, Non-Narcotic; Anti-inflammatory Agent; Nonsteroidal Anti-Inflammatory Agent (NSAID), Oral
Use Management of inflammatory disorders usually including rheumatoid arthritis and osteoarthritis; can be used as an analgesic for treatment of mild to moderate pain
Usual Dosage Adults: Oral:
Pain: Initial: 500-1000 mg followed by 250-500 mg every 8-12 hours
Inflammatory condition: 500-1000 mg/day in 2 divided doses
Dosage Forms Tablet: 250 mg, 500 mg

Di-Gel® [OTC] *see* aluminum hydroxide, magnesium hydroxide, and simethicone *on page 16*
Digibind® *see* digoxin immune fab (ovine) *on next page*

digitoxin (di ji tox' in)
Brand Names Crystodigin®
Therapeutic Category Antiarrhythmic Agent, Miscellaneous; Cardiac Glycoside
Use Congestive heart failure; atrial fibrillation; atrial flutter; paroxysmal atrial tachycardia; and cardiogenic shock
Usual Dosage
Children: The doses are very individualized; the maintenance range after neonatal period, the recommended digitalizing dose is as follows:
<1 year: 0.045 mg/kg
1-2 years: 0.04 mg/kg
2 years: 0.03 mg/kg which is equivalent to 0.75 mg/mm^2
Maintenance: Approximately $^1/_{10}$ of the digitalizing dose
Adults:
Rapid oral loading dose: Initial: 0.6 mg followed by 0.4 mg and then 0.2 mg at intervals of 4-6 hours
Slow oral loading dose: 0.2 mg twice daily for a period of 4 days followed by a maintenance dose
Maintenance: 0.05-0.3 mg/day
Most common dose: 0.15 mg/day
Dosage Forms Tablet: 0.05 mg, 0.1 mg, 0.15 mg, 0.2 mg

digoxin (di jox' in)
Brand Names Lanoxicaps®; Lanoxin®
Therapeutic Category Antiarrhythmic Agent, Miscellaneous; Cardiac Glycoside
Use Treatment of congestive heart failure; slows the ventricular rate in tachyarrhythmias such as atrial fibrillation, atrial flutter, supraventricular tachycardia, paroxysmal atrial tachycardia, cardiogenic shock
Usual Dosage See table *on next page*
Dosage Forms
Capsule: 50 μg, 100 μg, 200 μg
Elixir, pediatric (lime flavor): 50 μg/mL with alcohol 10% (60 mL)
Injection: 250 μg/mL (1 mL, 2 mL)
Injection, pediatric: 100 μg/mL (1 mL)
Tablet: 125 μg, 250 μg, 500 μg
(Continued)

147

digoxin (Continued)

Dosage Recommendations for Digoxin*

Age	Total Digitalizing Dose† (µg/kg)		Daily Maintenance Dose‡ (µg/kg)	
	P.O.	I.V. or I.M.	P.O.	I.V. or I.M.
Preterm infant	20–30	15–25	5–7.5	4–6
Full term infant	25–35	20–30	6–10	5–8
1 mo–2 y	35–60	30–50	10–15	7.5–12
2–5 y	30–40	25–35	7.5–10	6–9
5–10 y	20–35	15–30	5–10	4–8
>10 y	10–15	8–12	2.5–5	2–3
Adult	0.75–1.5 mg	0.5–1 mg	0.125–0.5 mg	0.1–0.4 mg

*Based on lean body weight and normal renal function for age. Decrease dose in patients with ↓ renal function.
†Give one–half of the total digitalizing dose (TDD) in the initial dose, then give one–quarter of the TDD in each of two subsequent doses at 8–12 hour intervals. Obtain ECG 6 hours after each dose to assess potential toxicity.
‡Divided every 12 hours in infants and children <10 years old. Given once daily to children >10 years and adults.

digoxin immune fab (ovine)

Brand Names Digibind®
Synonyms antidigoxin fab fragments
Therapeutic Category Antidote, Digoxin
Use Treatment of potentially life-threatening digoxin or digitoxin intoxication in carefully selected patients
Usual Dosage To determine the dose of digoxin immune Fab, first determine the total body load of digoxin (TBL) as follows (using either an approximation of the amount ingested or a postdistribution serum digoxin concentration):

TBL of digoxin (in mg) = C (in ng/mL) x 5.6 x body weight (in kg)/1000 or TBL = mg of digoxin ingested (as tablets or elixir) x 0.8; C = postdistribution digoxin concentration

Dose of digoxin immune Fab (in mg) I.V. = TBL x 66.7 or dose of digoxin immune Fab (in number of 40 mg vials) = [C of digoxin (in ng/mL) x body weight (in kg)]/100
Dosage Forms Powder for injection, lyophilized: 40 mg

Dihistine® *see* chlorpheniramine and phenylephrine *on page 93*

Dihistine® DH *see* chlorpheniramine, pseudoephedrine, and codeine *on page 97*

Dihistine® Expectorant *see* guaifenesin, pseudoephedrine, and codeine *on page 221*

dihydrocodeine compound (dye hye droe koe' deen)

Brand Names Synalgos®-DC
Therapeutic Category Analgesic, Narcotic
Use Management of mild to moderate pain that requires relaxation
Usual Dosage Adults: Oral: 1-2 capsules every 4-6 hours as needed for pain
Dosage Forms Capsule: Dihydrocodeine bitartrate 16 mg, aspirin 356.4 mg, and caffeine 30 mg

dihydroergotamine mesylate (dye hye droe er got' a meen)
Brand Names D.H.E. 45® Injection
Therapeutic Category Ergot Alkaloid
Use To abort or prevent vascular headaches
Usual Dosage
I.M.: 1 mg at first sign of headache; 1 mg every 6 hours for 2 doses (not to exceed 6 mg in 24 hours)
I.V.: Up to 2 mg for faster effects
Dosage Forms Injection: 1 mg/mL (1 mL)

dihydroergotoxine see ergoloid mesylates on page 173

dihydrohydroxycodeinone see oxycodone hydrochloride on page 350

dihydromorphinone see hydromorphone hydrochloride on page 239

dihydrotachysterol (dye hye droe tak iss' ter ole)
Brand Names DHT™; Hytakerol®
Synonyms dichysterol
Therapeutic Category Vitamin D Analog
Use Treatment of hypocalcemia associated with hypoparathyroidism; prophylaxis of hypocalcemic tetany following thyroid surgery
Usual Dosage Oral:
Hypoparathyroidism:
Neonates: 0.05-0.1 mg/day
Infants and young Children: 0.1-0.5 mg/day
Older Children and Adults: 0.5-1 mg/day

Nutritional rickets: 0.5 mg as a single dose or 13-50 μg/day until healing occurs

Renal osteodystrophy: 0.6-6 mg/24 hours; maintenance: 0.25-0.6 mg/24 hours adjusted as necessary to achieve normal serum calcium levels and promote bone healing
Dosage Forms
Capsule: 0.125 mg
Solution:
Concentrate: 0.2 mg/mL (30 mL)
Oral: 0.2 mg/5 mL (500 mL)
Oral, in oil: 0.25 mg/mL (15 mL)
Tablet: 0.125 mg, 0.2 mg, 0.4 mg

dihydroxyaluminum sodium carbonate (dye hye drox' i a loo' mi num)
Brand Names Rolaids® [OTC]
Therapeutic Category Antacid
Use Symptomatic relief of upset stomach associated with hyperacidity
Usual Dosage Oral: Chew 1-2 tablets as needed
Dosage Forms Tablet, chewable: 334 mg

1,25 dihydroxycholecalciferol see calcitriol on page 65

dihydroxypropyl theophylline see dyphylline on page 165

diiodohydroxyquin see iodoquinol on page 254

diisopropyl fluorophosphate see isoflurophate on page 257

Dilacor™ XR see diltiazem hydrochloride on next page

Dilantin® see phenytoin on page 374

Dilantin® With Phenobarbital see phenytoin with phenobarbital on page 375

Dilatrate®-SR see isosorbide dinitrate on page 259

Dilaudid-HP® Injection see hydromorphone hydrochloride on page 239

Dilaudid® Injection *see* hydromorphone hydrochloride *on page 239*
Dilaudid® Oral *see* hydromorphone hydrochloride *on page 239*
Dilaudid® Suppository *see* hydromorphone hydrochloride *on page 239*
Dilocaine® Injection *see* lidocaine hydrochloride *on page 273*
Dilomine® Injection *see* dicyclomine hydrochloride *on page 145*
Dilor® *see* dyphylline *on page 165*

diltiazem hydrochloride (dil tye' a zem)

Brand Names Cardizem® CD; Cardizem® Injectable; Cardizem® SR; Cardizem® Tablet; Dilacor™ XR
Therapeutic Category Antianginal Agent; Calcium Channel Blocker
Use
Cardizem® CD capsule: Hypertension (alone or in combination); chronic stable angina or angina from coronary artery spasm
Cardizem® injection: Atrial fibrillation or atrial flutter; paroxysmal supraventricular tachycardias (PSVT)
Cardizem® SR capsule, Dilacor™ XR capsule: Hypertension (alone or in combination)
Cardizem® tablet: Chronic stable angina or angina from coronary artery spasm
Usual Dosage Adults:
Oral: 30-120 mg 3-4 times/day; dosage should be increased gradually, at 1- to 2-day intervals until optimum response is obtained; usual maintenance dose is usually 240-360 mg/day
Sustained-release capsules (SR): Initial dose of 60-120 mg twice daily
Sustained-release capsules (CD, XR): 180-300 mg once daily
I.V.: Initial 0.25 mg/kg as a bolus over 2 minutes, then continuous infusion of 5-15 mg/hour for up to 24 hours
Dosage Forms
Capsule, sustained release:
Cardizem® CD: 120 mg, 180 mg, 240 mg, 300 mg
Cardizem® SR: 60 mg, 90 mg, 120 mg
Dilacor™ XR: 180 mg, 240 mg
Injection (Cardizem®): 5 mg/mL (5 mL, 10 mL)
Tablet (Cardizem®): 30 mg, 60 mg, 90 mg, 120 mg

dimenhydrinate (dye men hye' dri nate)

Brand Names Calm-X® Oral [OTC]; Dimetabs® Oral; Dinate® Injection; Dommanate® Injection; Dramamine® Injection; Dramamine® Oral [OTC]; Dramilin® Injection; Dramoject® Injection; Dymenate® Injection; Hydrate® Injection; Marmine® Injection; Marmine® Oral [OTC]; Nico-Vert® Oral; Tega-Vert® Oral; TripTone® Caplets® [OTC]; Wehamine® Injection
Therapeutic Category Antiemetic; Antihistamine
Use Treatment and prevention of nausea, vertigo, and vomiting associated with motion sickness
Usual Dosage
Children: Oral, I.M.:
2-5 years: 12.5-25 mg every 6-8 hours, maximum: 75 mg/day
6-12 years: 25-50 mg every 6-8 hours, maximum: 75 mg/day
or
Alternately: 5 mg/kg/day in 4 divided doses, not to exceed 300 mg/day

Adults: Oral, I.M., I.V.: 50-100 mg every 4-6 hours, not to exceed 400 mg/day
Dosage Forms
Capsule: 50 mg
Injection: 50 mg/mL (1 mL, 5 mL, 10 mL)
Liquid: 12.5 mg/4 mL
Tablet: 50 mg
Tablet, chewable: 50 mg

dimercaprol (dye mer kap' role)
Brand Names BAL in Oil®
Synonyms BAL; british anti-lewisite; dithioglycerol
Therapeutic Category Antidote, Arsenic Toxicity; Antidote, Gold Toxicity; Antidote, Lead Toxicity; Antidote, Mercury Toxicity
Use Antidote to gold, arsenic, and mercury poisoning; adjunct to edetate calcium disodium in lead poisoning
Usual Dosage Children and Adults: I.M.:
Mild arsenic and gold poisoning: 2.5 mg/kg/dose every 6 hours for 2 days, then every 12 hours on the third day, and once daily thereafter for 10 days

Severe arsenic and gold poisoning: 3 mg/kg/dose every 4 hours for 2 days then every 6 hours on the third day, then every 12 hours thereafter for 10 days

Mercury poisoning: Initial: 5 mg/kg followed by 2.5 mg/kg/dose 1-2 times/day for 10 days

Lead poisoning (use with edetate calcium disodium):
Mild: 3 mg/kg/dose every 4 hours for 5-7 days
Severe: 4 mg/kg/dose every 4 hours for 5-7 days
Acute encephalopathy: Initial: 4 mg/kg/dose, then every 4 hours
Dosage Forms Injection: 100 mg/mL (3 mL)

Dimetabs® Oral *see* dimenhydrinate *on previous page*

Dimetane®-DC *see* brompheniramine, phenylpropanolamine, and codeine *on page 60*

Dimetane® Oral [OTC] *see* brompheniramine maleate *on page 59*

Dimetapp® [OTC] *see* brompheniramine and phenylpropanolamine *on page 59*

Dimetapp® Extentabs® [OTC] *see* brompheniramine and phenylpropanolamine *on page 59*

dimethoxyphenyl penicillin sodium *see* methicillin sodium *on page 299*

β,β-**dimethylcysteine** *see* penicillamine *on page 359*

dimethyl sulfoxide (dye meth il sul fox' ide)
Brand Names Rimso®-50
Synonyms DMSO
Therapeutic Category Urinary Tract Product
Use Symptomatic relief of interstitial cystitis
Usual Dosage Instill 50 mL directly into bladder and allow to remain for 15 minutes; repeat every 2 weeks until maximum symptomatic relief is obtained
Dosage Forms Solution: 50% [500 mg/mL] (50 mL)

dimethyl tubocurarine iodide *see* metocurine iodide *on page 308*

Dinate® Injection *see* dimenhydrinate *on previous page*

dinoprostone (dye noe prost' one)
Brand Names Prepidil® Vaginal Gel; Prostin E$_2$® Vaginal Suppository
Synonyms PGE$_2$; prostaglandin E$_2$
Therapeutic Category Abortifacient; Prostaglandin
Use Terminate pregnancy from 12th through 28th week of gestation; evacuate uterus in cases of missed abortion or intrauterine fetal death; manage benign hydatidiform mole
Usual Dosage Insert 1 suppository high in vagina, repeat at 3- to 5-hour intervals until abortion occurs up to 240 mg (maximum dose)
Dosage Forms
Gel, vaginal: 0.5 mg in 3 g syringes [each package contains a 10-mm and 20-mm shielded catheter]
(Continued)

dinoprostone *(Continued)*
Suppository, vaginal: 20 mg

Diocto® [OTC] *see* docusate *on page 157*
Diocto C® [OTC] *see* docusate and casanthranol *on page 158*
Diocto-K® [OTC] *see* docusate *on page 157*
Diocto-K Plus® [OTC] *see* docusate and casanthranol *on page 158*
Dioctolose Plus® [OTC] *see* docusate and casanthranol *on page 158*
Dioeze® [OTC] *see* docusate *on page 157*
Dionosil Oily® *see* radiological/contrast media (ionic) *on page 413*
Dioval® Injection *see* estradiol *on page 178*
dipalmitoylphosphatidylcholine *see* colfosceril palmitate *on page 114*
Dipentum® *see* olsalazine sodium *on page 343*
Diphen® Cough [OTC] *see* diphenhydramine hydrochloride *on this page*

diphenhydramine hydrochloride *(dye fen hye' dra meen)*
Brand Names AllerMax® Oral [OTC]; Banophen® Oral [OTC]; Belix® Oral [OTC]; Bena-D® Injection; Benadryl® Injection; Benadryl® Oral [OTC]; Benadryl® Topical; Benahist® Injection; Benoject® Injection; Benylin® Cough Syrup [OTC]; Bydramine® Cough Syrup [OTC]; Diphen® Cough [OTC]; Dormin® Oral [OTC]; Genahist® Oral; Gen-D-phen® Cough Syrup [OTC]; Hydramine® Oral [OTC]; Hydramyn® Syrup [OTC]; Maximum Strength Nytol® [OTC]; Nidryl® Oral [OTC]; Nordryl® Injection; Nordryl® Oral; Nytol® Oral [OTC]; Phendry® Oral [OTC]; Silphen® Cough [OTC]; Sleep-eze 3® Oral [OTC]; Sleepinal® [OTC]; Sominex® Oral [OTC]; Tusstat® Syrup; Twilite® Oral [OTC]; Uni-Bent® Cough Syrup; Wehdryl® Injection
Therapeutic Category Antidote, Hypersensitivity Reactions; Antihistamine; Sedative
Use Symptomatic relief of allergic symptoms caused by histamine release which include nasal allergies and allergic dermatosis; mild nighttime sedation, prevention of motion sickness, as an antitussive has antinauseant and topical anesthetic properties
Usual Dosage
Children: Oral, I.M., I.V.: 5 mg/kg/day or 150 mg/m²/day in divided doses every 6-8 hours, not to exceed 300 mg/day

Adults:
Oral: 25-50 mg every 4-6 hours
I.M., I.V.: 10-50 mg in a single dose every 2-4 hours, not to exceed 400 mg/day
Dosage Forms
Capsule: 25 mg, 50 mg
Cream: 1%, 2%
Elixir: 12.5 mg/5 mL (5 mL, 10 mL, 20 mL, 120 mL, 480 mL, 3780 mL)
Injection: 10 mg/mL (10 mL, 30 mL); 50 mg/mL (1 mL, 10 mL)
Lotion: 1% (75 mL)
Solution, topical spray: 1% (60 mL)
Syrup: 12.5 mg/5 mL (5 mL, 120 mL, 240 mL, 480 mL, 3780 mL)
Tablet: 25 mg, 50 mg

diphenidol hydrochloride *(dye fen' i dole)*
Brand Names Vontrol®
Therapeutic Category Antiemetic
Use Control of nausea and vomiting; peripheral vertigo and associated nausea and vomiting, Ménière's disease and middle and inner ear surgery
Usual Dosage Oral:
Children: 0.88 mg/kg every 4 hours
Adults: 25-50 mg every 4 hours
Dosage Forms Tablet: 25 mg

diphenoxylate and atropine (dye fen ox' i late)
Brand Names Lofene®; Logen®; Lomanate®; Lomodix®; Lomotil®; Lonox®; Low-Quel®
Synonyms atropine and diphenoxylate
Therapeutic Category Antidiarrheal
Use Treatment of diarrhea
Usual Dosage Oral (as diphenoxylate): Initial dose:
Children: 0.3-0.4 mg/kg/day in 2-4 divided doses
  2-5 years: 2 mg 3 times/day
  5-8 years: 2 mg 4 times/day
  8-12 years: 2 mg 5 times/day
  Not recommended for children <2 years of age

Adults: 15-20 mg/day in 3-4 divided doses

Reduce dosage as soon as initial control of symptoms is achieved
Dosage Forms
Solution, oral: Diphenoxylate hydrochloride 2.5 mg and atropine sulfate 0.025 mg per 5 mL (4 mL, 10 mL, 60 mL)
Tablet: Diphenoxylate hydrochloride 2.5 mg and atropine sulfate 0.025 mg

Diphenylan Sodium® *see* phenytoin *on page 374*

diphenylhydantoin *see* phenytoin *on page 374*

diphtheria and tetanus toxoid (dif theer' ee a)
Synonyms DT; tD; tetanus and diphtheria toxoid
Therapeutic Category Toxoid
Use Active immunity against diphtheria and tetanus
Usual Dosage I.M.:
Infants and Children:
  6 weeks to 1 year: Three 0.5 mL doses at least 4 weeks apart; give a reinforcing dose 6-12 months after the third injection
  1-6 years: Give two 0.5 mL doses at least 4 weeks apart; reinforcing dose 6-12 months after second injection; if final dose is given after seventh birthday, use adult preparation
  4-6 years (booster immunization): 0.5 mL; not necessary if all 4 doses were given after fourth birthday – routinely give booster doses at 10-year intervals with the adult preparation

Adults >7 years: 2 primary doses of 0.5 mL each, given at an interval of 4-6 weeks; third (reinforcing) dose of 0.5 mL 6-12 months later; boosters every 10 years
Dosage Forms Injection:
Pediatric use:
  Diphtheria 6.6 Lf units and tetanus 5 Lf units per 0.5 mL (5 mL)
  Diphtheria 10 Lf units and tetanus 5 Lf units per 0.5 mL (0.5 mL, 5 mL)
  Diphtheria 12.5 Lf units and tetanus 5 Lf units per 0.5 mL (5 mL)
  Diphtheria 15 Lf units and tetanus 10 Lf units per 0.5 mL (5 mL)
Adult use:
  Diphtheria 1.5 Lf units and tetanus 5 Lf units per 0.5 mL (0.5 mL, 5 mL)
  Diphtheria 2 Lf units and tetanus 5 Lf units per 0.5 mL (5 mL)
  Diphtheria 2 Lf units and tetanus 10 Lf units per 0.5 mL (5 mL)

diphtheria and tetanus toxoids and pertussis vaccine, adsorbed
Brand Names Tri-Immunol®
Synonyms DPT
Therapeutic Category Toxoid
Use Active immunization of infants and children through 6 years of age (between 2 months and the seventh birthday) against diphtheria, tetanus, and pertussis; recommended for both primary immunization and routine recall; start immunization at once if whooping cough or diphtheria is present in the community
(Continued)

153

diphtheria and tetanus toxoids and pertussis vaccine, adsorbed
(Continued)
Usual Dosage The primary immunization for children 2 months to 6 years of age, ideally beginning at the age of 2-3 months or at 6-week check-up. Administer 0.5 mL I.M. on 3 occasions at 4- to 8-week intervals with a re-enforcing dose administered 1 year after the third injection. The booster doses are given when the child is 4-6 years of age, 0.5 mL I.M.

Dosage Forms Injection:
Diphtheria 6.7 Lf units, tetanus 5 Lf units, and pertussis 4 protective units per 0.5 mL (7.5 mL)
Tri-Immunol®: Diphtheria 12.5 Lf units, tetanus 5 Lf units, and pertussis 4 protective units per 0.5 mL (7.5 mL)

diphtheria, tetanus toxoids, and whole-cell pertussis vaccine and hemophilus b conjugate vaccine
Brand Names Tetramune®
Therapeutic Category Toxoid
Use Active immunization of infants and children through 5 years of age (between 2 months and the sixth birthday) against diphtheria, tetanus, and pertussis and Hemophilus b disease when indications for immunization with DTP vaccine and HIB vaccine coincide
Usual Dosage The primary immunization for children 2 months to 5 years of age, ideally beginning at the age of 2-3 months or at 6-week check-up. Administer 0.5 mL I.M. on 3 occasions at ∼2 month intervals, followed by a fourth 0.5 mL dose at ∼15 months of age
Dosage Forms Injection: 5 mL

diphtheria antitoxin
Therapeutic Category Antitoxin
Use Passive prevention and treatment of diphtheria
Usual Dosage Administer I.M. or slow I.V. infusion: Dosage varies with a range from 20,000 units to 120,000 units
Dosage Forms Injection: 500 units/mL (20 mL, 40 mL)

diphtheria crm$_{197}$ protein conjugate *see* hemophilus b conjugate vaccine
on page 226

diphtheria, tetanus toxoids, and acellular pertussis vaccine
Brand Names Acel-Immune®; Tripedia®
Synonyms DTaP
Therapeutic Category Toxoid
Use Fourth or fifth immunization of children 15 months to 7 years of age (prior to seventh birthday) who have been previously immunized with 3 or 4 doses of whole-cell pertussis DTP vaccine
Dosage Forms Injection:
Acel-Immune®: Diphtheria 7.5 Lf units, tetanus 5 Lf units, and acellular pertussis vaccine 40 μg per 0.5 mL (7.5 mL)
Tripedia®: Diphtheria 6.7 Lf units, tetanus 5 Lf units, and acellular pertussis vaccine 46.8 μg per 0.5 mL (7.5 mL)

diphtheria toxoid conjugate *see* hemophilus b conjugate vaccine
on page 226

dipivalyl epinephrine *see* dipivefrin hydrochloride *on this page*

dipivefrin hydrochloride (dye pi' ve frin)
Brand Names Propine® Ophthalmic
Synonyms dipivalyl epinephrine; DPE
Therapeutic Category Adrenergic Agonist Agent, Ophthalmic; Ophthalmic Agent, Vasoconstrictor

Use Reduce elevated intraocular pressure in chronic open-angle glaucoma; also used to treat ocular hypertension, low tension, and secondary glaucomas
Usual Dosage Adults: Ophthalmic: Initial: 1 drop every 12 hours
Dosage Forms Solution, ophthalmic: 0.1% (5 mL, 10 mL, 15 mL)

Diprivan® Injection *see* propofol *on page 401*
Diprolene® AF Topical *see* betamethasone *on page 52*
Diprolene® Topical *see* betamethasone *on page 52*
dipropylacetic acid *see* valproic acid and derivatives *on page 490*
Diprosone® Topical *see* betamethasone *on page 52*

dipyridamole (dye peer id' a mole)
Brand Names Persantine®
Therapeutic Category Antiplatelet Agent; Vasodilator, Coronary
Use Maintain patency after surgical grafting procedures including coronary artery bypass; with warfarin to decrease thrombosis in patients after artificial heart valve replacement; for chronic management of angina pectoris; with aspirin to prevent coronary artery thrombosis; in combination with aspirin or warfarin to prevent other thromboembolic disorders
Usual Dosage
Children: Oral: 3-6 mg/kg/day in 3 divided doses
Dipyridamole stress test (for evaluation of myocardial perfusion): I.V.: 0.14 mg/kg/minute for a total of 4 minutes
Adults: Oral: 75-400 mg/day in 3-4 divided doses
Dosage Forms
Injection: 10 mg/2 mL
Tablet: 25 mg, 50 mg, 75 mg

Disalcid® *see* salsalate *on page 425*
disalicylic acid *see* salsalate *on page 425*
Disanthrol® [OTC] *see* docusate and casanthranol *on page 158*
Discase® *see* chymopapain *on page 101*
Disobrom® [OTC] *see* dexbrompheniramine and pseudoephedrine *on page 134*
disodium cromoglycate *see* cromolyn sodium *on page 118*
d-isoephedrine hydrochloride *see* pseudoephedrine *on page 406*
Disolan® [OTC] *see* docusate and phenolphthalein *on page 158*
Disonate® [OTC] *see* docusate *on page 157*
Disophrol® Chrontabs® [OTC] *see* dexbrompheniramine and pseudoephedrine *on page 134*

disopyramide phosphate (dye soe peer' a mide)
Brand Names Norpace®
Therapeutic Category Antiarrhythmic Agent, Class Ia
Use Suppression and prevention of unifocal and multifocal premature, ventricular premature complexes, coupled ventricular tachycardia; also effective in the conversion of atrial fibrillation, atrial flutter, and paroxysmal atrial tachycardia to normal sinus rhythm and prevention of the reoccurrence of these arrhythmias after conversion by other methods
Usual Dosage Oral:
Children:
<1 year: 10-30 mg/kg/24 hours in 4 divided doses
1-4 years: 10-20 mg/kg/24 hours in 4 divided doses
4-12 years: 10-15 mg/kg/24 hours in 4 divided doses
12-18 years: 6-15 mg/kg/24 hours in 4 divided doses
(Continued)

disopyramide phosphate *(Continued)*
Adults:
<50 kg: 100 mg every 6 hours or 200 mg every 12 hours (controlled release)
>50 kg: 150 mg every 6 hours or 300 mg every 12 hours (controlled release); if no response, may increase to 200 mg every 6 hours; maximum dose required for patients with severe refractory ventricular tachycardia is 400 mg every 6 hours
Dosage Forms
Capsule: 100 mg, 150 mg
Capsule, sustained action: 100 mg, 150 mg

Disotate® *see* edetate disodium *on page 167*

Di-Spaz® **Injection** *see* dicyclomine hydrochloride *on page 145*

Di-Spaz® **Oral** *see* dicyclomine hydrochloride *on page 145*

Dispos-a-Med® **Isoproterenol Inhalation Solution** *see* isoproterenol *on page 258*

disulfiram *(dye sul' fi ram)*
Brand Names Antabuse®
Therapeutic Category Aldehyde Dehydrogenase Inhibitor Agent; Antialcoholic Agent
Use Management of chronic alcoholics
Usual Dosage Maximum daily dose: 500 mg/day in a single dose for 1-2 weeks; average maintenance dose: 250 mg/day; range: 125-500 mg; duration of therapy is to continue until the patient is fully recovered socially and a basis for permanent self control has been established; maintenance therapy may be required for months or even years
Dosage Forms Tablet: 250 mg, 500 mg

dithioglycerol *see* dimercaprol *on page 151*

dithranol *see* anthralin *on page 29*

Ditropan® *see* oxybutynin chloride *on page 349*

Diucardin® *see* hydroflumethiazide *on page 238*

Diulo® *see* metolazone *on page 309*

Diupres-250® *see* chlorothiazide and reserpine *on page 92*

Diupres-500® *see* chlorothiazide and reserpine *on page 92*

Diurigen® *see* chlorothiazide *on page 91*

Diuril® *see* chlorothiazide *on page 91*

Diutensin® *see* methyclothiazide and cryptenamine tannates *on page 303*

divalproex sodium *see* valproic acid and derivatives *on page 490*

Dizmiss® **[OTC]** *see* meclizine hydrochloride *on page 288*

dl-alpha tocopherol *see* vitamin E *on page 498*

dl-norephedrine hydrochloride *see* phenylpropanolamine hydrochloride *on page 373*

D-mannitol *see* mannitol *on page 285*

4-DMDR *see* idarubicin hydrochloride *on page 245*

D-Med® **Injection** *see* methylprednisolone *on page 306*

DMSO *see* dimethyl sulfoxide *on page 151*

DNR *see* daunorubicin hydrochloride *on page 127*

dobutamine hydrochloride *(doe byoo' ta meen)*
Brand Names Dobutrex® Injection
Therapeutic Category Adrenergic Agonist Agent
Use Short-term management of patients with cardiac decompensation

Usual Dosage I.V. infusion:

Neonates: 2-15 µg/kg/minute, titrate to desired response

Children: 2.5-15 µg/kg/minute, titrate to desired response

Adults: 2.5-15 µg/kg/minute; maximum: 40 µg/kg/minute, titrate to desired response
Dosage Forms Injection: 250 mg (20 mL)

Dobutrex® Injection see dobutamine hydrochloride *on previous page*

Docucal-P® [OTC] see docusate and phenolphthalein *on next page*

docusate (dok' yoo sate)
Brand Names Colace® [OTC]; DC 240® Softgel® [OTC]; Dialose® [OTC]; Diocto® [OTC]; Diocto-K® [OTC]; Dioeze® [OTC]; Disonate® [OTC]; DOK® [OTC]; DOS® Softgel® [OTC]; Doxinate® [OTC]; D-S-S® [OTC]; Kasof® [OTC]; Modane® Soft [OTC]; Pro-Cal-Sof® [OTC]; Pro-Sof® [OTC]; Regulax SS® [OTC]; Regutol® [OTC]; Sulfalax® [OTC]; Surfak® [OTC]

Synonyms doss; dss

Therapeutic Category Laxative, Surfactant; Stool Softener

Use Stool softener in patients who should avoid straining during defecation and constipation associated with hard, dry stools

Usual Dosage Docusate salts are interchangeable; the amount of sodium, calcium, or potassium per dosage unit is clinically insignificant

Infants and Children <3 years: Oral: 10-40 mg/day in 1-4 divided doses

Children: Oral:
3-6 years: 20-60 mg/day in 1-4 divided doses
6-12 years: 40-150 mg/day in 1-4 divided doses

Adolescents and Adults: Oral: 50-500 mg/day in 1-4 divided doses

Older Children and Adults: Rectal: Add 50-100 mg of docusate liquid to enema fluid (saline or water); give as retention or flushing enema

Dosage Forms
Capsule, as calcium:
DC 240® Softgel®, Pro-Cal-Sof®, Sulfalax®: 240 mg
Surfak®: 50 mg, 240 mg
Capsule, as potassium:
Diocto-K®: 100 mg
Kasof®: 240 mg
Capsule, as sodium:
Colace®: 50 mg, 100 mg
Dioeze®: 250 mg
Disonate®: 100 mg, 240 mg
DOK®: 100 mg, 250 mg
DOS® Softgel®: 100 mg, 250 mg
Doxinate®: 250 mg
D-S-S®: 100 mg
Modane® Soft: 100 mg
Pro-Sof®: 100 mg, 250 mg
Regulax SS®: 100 mg, 250 mg
Liquid, as sodium (Diocto®, Colace®, Disonate®, DOK®): 150 mg/15 mL (30 mL, 60 mL, 480 mL)
Solution, oral, as sodium (Doxinate®): 50 mg/mL with alcohol 5% (60 mL, 3780 mL)
Syrup, as sodium:
50 mg/15 mL (15 mL, 30 mL)
Colace®, Diocto®, Disonate®, DOK®, Pro-Sof®: 60 mg/15 mL (240 mL, 480 mL, 3780 mL)
Tablet, as sodium (Dialose®, Regutol®): 100 mg

docusate and casanthranol (dok' yoo sate & ka san' thra nole)
Brand Names Dialose® Plus Capsule [OTC]; Diocto C® [OTC]; Diocto-K Plus® [OTC]; Dioctolose Plus® [OTC]; Disanthrol® [OTC]; DSMC Plus® [OTC]; D-S-S Plus® [OTC]; Genasoft® Plus [OTC]; Peri-Colace® [OTC]; Pro-Sof® Plus [OTC]; Regulace® [OTC]
Synonyms casanthranol and docusate; dss with casanthranol
Therapeutic Category Laxative, Surfactant; Stool Softener
Use Treatment of constipation generally associated with dry, hard stools and decreased intestinal motility
Usual Dosage Oral:
Children: 5-15 mL of syrup at bedtime or 1 capsule at bedtime

Adults: 1-2 capsules or 15-30 mL syrup at bedtime, may be increased to 2 capsules or 30 mL twice daily or 3 capsules at bedtime
Dosage Forms
Capsule (Dialose® Plus, Diocto-K Plus®, Dioctolose Plus®, DSMC Plus®): Docusate potassium 100 mg and casanthranol 30 mg
Capsule (Disanthrol®, D-S-S Plus®, Genasoft® Plus, Peri-Colace®, Pro-Sof® Plus, Regulace®): Docusate sodium 100 mg and casanthranol 30 mg
Syrup (Diocto C®, Peri-Colace®): Docusate sodium 60 mg and casanthranol 30 mg per 15 mL (240 mL, 480 mL, 4000 mL)

docusate and phenolphthalein (dok' yoo sate & fee nol thay' leen)
Brand Names Colax® [OTC]; Correctol® [OTC]; Dialose® Plus Tablet [OTC]; Disolan® [OTC]; Docucal-P® [OTC]; Doxidan® [OTC]; Ex-Lax®, Extra Gentle Pills [OTC]; Feen-a-Mint® Pills [OTC]; Femilax® [OTC]; Modane® Plus [OTC]; Phillips'® LaxCaps® [OTC]; Unilax® [OTC]
Therapeutic Category Laxative, Stimulant; Laxative, Surfactant; Stool Softener
Use Management of chronic functional constipation
Usual Dosage Oral:
Children 6-12 years: 1 capsule daily given at bedtime for 2-3 nights until bowel movements are normal

Children >12 years and Adults: 1-2 capsules daily given at bedtime for 2-3 nights until bowel movements are normal
Dosage Forms
Capsule:
Disolan®: Docusate sodium 100 mg and phenolphthalein 65 mg
Docucal-P®, Doxidan®: Docusate calcium 60 mg and phenolphthalein 65 mg
Ex-Lax®, Extra Gentle Pills: Docusate sodium 60 mg and phenolphthalein 65 mg
Phillips'® LaxCaps®: Docusate sodium 83 mg and phenolphthalein 90 mg
Unilax®: Docusate sodium 230 mg and phenolphthalein 130 mg
Tablet:
Colax®, Correctol®, Dialose® Plus, Feen-A-Mint® Pills, Femilax®, Modane® Plus: Docusate sodium 100 mg and phenolphthalein 65 mg

DOK® [OTC] *see* docusate *on previous page*

Doktors® Nasal Solution [OTC] *see* phenylephrine hydrochloride *on page 372*

Dolacet® *see* hydrocodone and acetaminophen *on page 234*

Dolene® *see* propoxyphene *on page 402*

Dolobid® *see* diflunisal *on page 147*

Dolophine® Oral *see* methadone hydrochloride *on page 298*

Domeboro® [OTC] *see* aluminum acetate *on page 14*

Dommanate® Injection *see* dimenhydrinate *on page 150*

Donnamor® Oral *see* hyoscyamine sulfate *on page 243*

Donnapectolin-PG® *see* hyoscyamine, atropine, scopolamine, kaolin, pectin, and opium *on page 243*

Donnapine® *see* hyoscyamine, atropine, scopolamine, and phenobarbital *on page 242*

Donna-Sed® *see* hyoscyamine, atropine, scopolamine, and phenobarbital *on page 242*

Donnatal® *see* hyoscyamine, atropine, scopolamine, and phenobarbital *on page 242*

Donphen® *see* hyoscyamine, atropine, scopolamine, and phenobarbital *on page 242*

dopamine hydrochloride (doe' pa meen)
Brand Names Dopastat® Injection; Intropin® Injection
Therapeutic Category Adrenergic Agonist Agent
Use Adjunct in the treatment of shock which persists after adequate fluid volume replacement; dose-related inotropic and vasopressor effects; stimulates dopaminergic, beta and alpha receptors; increased renal blood flow at low to moderate doses
Usual Dosage I.V. infusion:
Neonates: 1-20 µg/kg/minute continuous infusion, titrate to desired response

Children: 1-20 µg/kg/minute, maximum: 50 µg/kg/minute continuous infusion, titrate to desired response

Adults: 1 µg/kg/minute up to 50 µg/kg/minute, titrate to desired response

If dosages >20-30 µg/kg/minute are needed, a more direct acting pressor may be more beneficial (ie, epinephrine, norepinephrine)

The hemodynamic effects of dopamine are dose-dependent:
Low-dose: 1-5 µg/kg/minute, increased renal blood flow and urine output
Intermediate-dose: 5-15 µg/kg/minute, increased renal blood flow, heart rate, cardiac contractility, and cardiac output
High-dose: >15 µg/kg/minute, alpha-adrenergic effects begin to predominate, vasoconstriction, increased blood pressure
Dosage Forms
Infusion, in D$_5$W: 0.8 mg/mL (250 mL, 500 mL); 1.6 mg/mL (250 mL, 500 mL); 3.2 mg/mL (250 mL, 500 mL)
Injection: 40 mg/mL (5 mL, 10 mL, 20 mL); 80 mg/mL (5 mL, 20 mL); 160 mg/mL (5 mL)

Dopar® *see* levodopa *on page 270*

Dopastat® Injection *see* dopamine hydrochloride *on this page*

Dopram® Injection *see* doxapram hydrochloride *on next page*

Doral® *see* quazepam *on page 410*

Dorcol® [OTC] *see* acetaminophen *on page 2*

Doriden® *see* glutethimide *on page 213*

Dormin® Oral [OTC] *see* diphenhydramine hydrochloride *on page 152*

dornase alfa
Brand Names Pulmozyme®
Synonyms recombinant human deoxyribonuclease I
Therapeutic Category Enzyme
Use Management of cystic fibrosis patients to reduce the frequency of respiratory infections that require parenteral antibiotics, and to improve pulmonary function
Usual Dosage Children >5 years and Adults: Inhalation: 2.5 mg once or twice daily through selected nebulizers in conjunction with a Pulmo-Aide® or a Pari-Proneb® compressor
Dosage Forms Solution, inhalation: 1 mg/mL (2.5 mL)

Doryx® Oral *see* doxycycline *on page 161*

doss *see* docusate *on page 157*

DOS® Softgel® [OTC] *see* docusate *on page 157*

doxacurium chloride (dox a kyoo' rium)
Brand Names Nuromax® Injection
Therapeutic Category Neuromuscular Blocker Agent, Nondepolarizing
Use Doxacurium is indicated for use as an adjunct to general anesthesia. It provides skeletal muscle relaxation during surgery.
Usual Dosage I.V. (in obese patients, use ideal body weight to calculate dosage):
Children >2 years: Initial: 0.03-0.05 mg/kg followed by maintenance doses of 0.005-0.01 mg/kg after 30-45 minutes

Adults: Surgery: 0.05 mg/kg with thiopental/narcotic or 0.025 mg/kg with succinylcholine; maintenance dose: 0.005-0.01 mg/kg after 60-100 minutes
Dosage Forms Injection: 1 mg/mL (5 mL)

doxapram hydrochloride (dox' a pram)
Brand Names Dopram® Injection
Therapeutic Category Central Nervous System Stimulant, Nonamphetamine; Respiratory Stimulant
Use Respiratory and CNS stimulant
Usual Dosage I.V.:
Neonatal apnea (apnea of prematurity):
Initial: 0.5 mg/kg/hour
Maintenance: 0.5-2.5 mg/kg/hour, titrated to the lowest rate at which apnea is controlled

Adults: Respiratory depression following anesthesia:
Initial: 0.5-1 mg/kg; may repeat at 5-minute intervals; maximum total dose: 2 mg/kg; single doses should not exceed 1.5 mg/kg
I.V. infusion: Initial: 5 mg/minute until adequate response or adverse effects seen; decrease to 1-3 mg/minute; usual total dose: 0.5-4 mg/kg; maximum: 300 mg
Dosage Forms Injection: 20 mg/mL (20 mL)

doxazosin mesylate (dox ay' zoe sin)
Brand Names Cardura®
Therapeutic Category Alpha-Adrenergic Blocking Agent, Oral
Use Treatment of hypertension
Usual Dosage Adults: Oral: 1 mg once daily, may be increased to 2 mg once daily thereafter up to 16 mg if needed
Dosage Forms Tablet: 1 mg, 2 mg, 4 mg, 8 mg

doxepin hydrochloride (dox' e pin)
Brand Names Adapin®; Sinequan®
Therapeutic Category Antianxiety Agent; Antidepressant, Tricyclic
Use Treatment of various forms of depression, usually in conjunction with psychotherapy; treatment of anxiety disorders; analgesic for certain chronic and neuropathic pain
Usual Dosage Oral:
Adolescents: Initial: 25-50 mg/day in single or divided doses; gradually increase to 100 mg/day

Adults: Initial: 30-150 mg/day at bedtime or in 2-3 divided doses; may increase up to 300 mg/day; single dose should not exceed 150 mg; select patients may respond to 25-50 mg/day
Dosage Forms
Capsule: 10 mg, 25 mg, 50 mg, 75 mg, 100 mg, 150 mg
Concentrate, oral: 10 mg/mL (120 mL)

Doxidan® [OTC] *see* docusate and phenolphthalein *on page 158*
Doxinate® [OTC] *see* docusate *on page 157*

doxorubicin hydrochloride (dox oh roo' bi sin)
Brand Names Adriamycin PFS™; Adriamycin RDF™; Rubex®
Synonyms ADR; hydroxydaunomycin hydrochloride
Therapeutic Category Antineoplastic Agent, Antibiotic
Use Treatment of various solid tumors including ovarian, breast and bladder, various lymphomas and leukemias, soft tissue sarcomas, neuroblastoma, osteosarcoma
Usual Dosage Refer to individual protocols
  I.V.: Patient's ideal weight should be used to calculate body surface area):
  Children: 35-75 mg/m^2 as a single dose, repeat every 21 days; or 20 mg/m^2 once weekly
  Adults: 60-75 mg/m^2 as a single dose, repeat every 21 days or other dosage regimens like 20-30 mg/m^2/day for 2-3 days, repeat in 4 weeks or 20 mg/m^2 once weekly
    The lower dose regimen should be given to patients with decreased bone marrow reserve, prior therapy or marrow infiltration with malignant cells
Dosage Forms
  Injection:
    Aqueous, with NS: 2 mg/mL (5 mL, 10 mL, 25 mL)
    Preservative free: 2 mg/mL (5 mL, 10 mL, 25 mL, 100 mL)
  Powder for injection, lyophilized: 10 mg, 20 mg, 50 mg, 100 mg
  Powder for injection, lyophilized, rapid dissolution formula: 10 mg, 20 mg, 50 mg, 150 mg

Doxychel® Injection *see* doxycycline *on this page*
Doxychel® Oral *see* doxycycline *on this page*

doxycycline (dox i sye' kleen)
Brand Names Bio-Tab® Oral; Doryx® Oral; Doxychel® Injection; Doxychel® Oral; Doxy® Oral; Monodox® Oral; Vibramycin® Injection; Vibramycin® Oral; Vibra-Tabs®
Synonyms doxycycline hyclate; doxycycline monohydrate
Therapeutic Category Antibiotic, Tetracycline Derivative
Use Principally in the treatment of infections caused by susceptible *Rickettsia*, *Chlamydia*, and *Mycoplasma* along with uncommon susceptible gram-negative and gram-positive organisms
Usual Dosage Oral, I.V.:
  Children ≥8 years: 2-4 mg/kg/day in 1-2 divided doses, not to exceed 200 mg/day
  Adults: 100-200 mg/day in 1-2 divided doses
Dosage Forms
  Capsule, as hyclate:
    Doxychel®, Monodox®, Vibramycin®: 50 mg
    Doxy®, Doxychel®, Monodox®, Vibramycin®: 100 mg
  Capsule, coated pellets, as hyclate (Doryx®): 100 mg
  Powder for injection, as hyclate (Doxy®, Doxychel®, Vibramycin® IV): 100 mg, 200 mg
  Powder for oral suspension, as monohydrate (raspberry flavor) (Vibramycin®): 25 mg/5 mL (60 mL)
  Syrup, as calcium (raspberry-apple flavor) (Vibramycin®): 50 mg/5 mL (30 mL, 473 mL)
  Tablet, as hyclate
    Doxychel®: 50 mg
    Bio-Tab®, Doxychel®, Vibra-Tabs®: 100 mg

doxycycline hyclate *see* doxycycline *on this page*
doxycycline monohydrate *see* doxycycline *on this page*
Doxy® Oral *see* doxycycline *on this page*
DPA *see* valproic acid and derivatives *on page 490*

DPE *see* dipivefrin hydrochloride *on page 154*

d-penicillamine *see* penicillamine *on page 359*

DPH *see* phenytoin *on page 374*

DPPC *see* colfosceril palmitate *on page 114*

DPT *see* diphtheria and tetanus toxoids and pertussis vaccine, adsorbed
   on page 153

Dramamine® II [OTC] *see* meclizine hydrochloride *on page 288*

Dramamine® Injection *see* dimenhydrinate *on page 150*

Dramamine® Oral [OTC] *see* dimenhydrinate *on page 150*

Dramilin® Injection *see* dimenhydrinate *on page 150*

Dramoject® Injection *see* dimenhydrinate *on page 150*

Dri-Ear® Otic [OTC] *see* boric acid *on page 56*

Drisdol® Oral *see* ergocalciferol *on page 173*

Dristan® Allergy [OTC] *see* brompheniramine and pseudoephedrine
   on page 59

Dristan® Long Lasting Nasal Solution [OTC] *see* oxymetazoline hydrochloride
   on page 350

Drithocreme® *see* anthralin *on page 29*

Dritho-Scalp® *see* anthralin *on page 29*

Drixoral® [OTC] *see* dexbrompheniramine and pseudoephedrine *on page 134*

Drixoral® Cough Liquid Caps [OTC] *see* dextromethorphan hydrobromide
   on page 136

Drixoral® Non-Drowsy [OTC] *see* pseudoephedrine *on page 406*

Drize® *see* chlorpheniramine and phenylpropanolamine *on page 93*

dronabinol (droe nab' i nol)
Brand Names Marinol®
Synonyms tetrahydrocannabinol; THC
Therapeutic Category Antiemetic
Use When conventional antiemetics fail to relieve the nausea and vomiting associated with
   cancer chemotherapy
Usual Dosage Oral:
   Children: NCI protocol recommends 5 mg/m^2 starting 6-8 hours before chemotherapy and
      every 4-6 hours after to be continued for 12 hours after chemotherapy is discontinued
   Adults: 5 mg/m^2 1-3 hours before chemotherapy, then give 5 mg/m^2/dose every 2-4 hours
      after chemotherapy for a total of 4-6 doses/day; dose may be increased up to a maxi-
      mum of 15 mg/m^2/dose if needed (dosage may be increased by 2.5 mg/m^2 increments)
Dosage Forms Capsule: 2.5 mg, 5 mg, 10 mg

droperidol (droe per' i dole)
Brand Names Inapsine®
Therapeutic Category Antiemetic; Antipsychotic Agent
Use Tranquilizer and antiemetic in surgical and diagnostic procedures; antiemetic for can-
   cer chemotherapy; preoperative medication
Usual Dosage Titrate carefully to desired effect
   Children 2-12 years:
      Premedication: I.M.: 0.088-0.165 mg/kg; smaller doses may be sufficient for control of
         nausea or vomiting
      Adjunct to general anesthesia: I.V. induction: 0.088-0.165 mg/kg
      Nausea and vomiting: I.M., I.V.: 0.05-0.06 mg/kg/dose every 4-6 hours as needed

Adults:
    Premedication: I.M., I.V.: 2.5-10 mg 30 minutes to 1 hour preoperatively
    Adjunct to general anesthesia: I.V. induction: 0.22-0.275 mg/kg; maintenance: 1.25-2.5 mg/dose
    Alone in diagnostic procedures: I.M.: Initial: 2.5-10 mg 30 minutes to 1 hour before; then 1.25-2.5 mg if needed
    Nausea and vomiting: I.M., I.V.: 2.5-5 mg/dose every 3-4 hours as needed
Dosage Forms Injection: 2.5 mg/mL (1 mL, 2 mL, 5 mL, 10 mL)

droperidol and fentanyl (droe per' i dole & fen' ta nil)
Brand Names Innovar®
Synonyms fentanyl and droperidol
Therapeutic Category Analgesic, Narcotic
Use Produce and maintain analgesia and sedation during diagnostic or surgical procedures (neuroleptanalgesia and neuroleptanesthesia); adjunct to general anesthesia
Usual Dosage
Children:
    Premedication: I.M.: 0.03 mL/kg 30-60 minutes prior to surgery
    Adjunct to general anesthesia: I.V.: Total dose: 0.05 mL/kg as slow infusion (1 mL/1-2 minutes) until sleep occurs

Adults:
    Premedication: I.M.: 0.5-2 mL 30-60 minutes prior to surgery
    Adjunct to general anesthesia: I.V.: 0.09-0.11 mL/kg as slow infusion (1 mL/1-2 minutes) until sleep occurs
Dosage Forms Injection: Droperidol 2.5 mg and fentanyl 50 μg per mL (2 mL, 5 mL)

Drotic® Otic *see* neomycin, polymyxin b, and hydrocortisone *on page 329*

Dry and Clear® [OTC] *see* benzoyl peroxide *on page 49*

Drysol™ *see* aluminum chloride hexahydrate *on page 15*

DSCG *see* cromolyn sodium *on page 118*

DSMC Plus® [OTC] *see* docusate and casanthranol *on page 158*

D-sorbitol *see* sorbitol *on page 441*

dss *see* docusate *on page 157*

D-S-S® [OTC] *see* docusate *on page 157*

D-S-S Plus® [OTC] *see* docusate and casanthranol *on page 158*

dss with casanthranol *see* docusate and casanthranol *on page 158*

DT *see* diphtheria and tetanus toxoid *on page 153*

DTaP *see* diphtheria, tetanus toxoids, and acellular pertussis vaccine *on page 154*

DTIC-Dome® *see* dacarbazine *on page 124*

DTO *see* opium tincture *on page 345*

d-tubocurarine chloride *see* tubocurarine chloride *on page 484*

Duadacin® Capsule [OTC] *see* chlorpheniramine, phenylpropanolamine, and acetaminophen *on page 96*

Dulcagen® [OTC] *see* bisacodyl *on page 54*

Dulcolax® [OTC] *see* bisacodyl *on page 54*

Dull-C® [OTC] *see* ascorbic acid *on page 33*

DuoCet™ *see* hydrocodone and acetaminophen *on page 234*

Duo-Cyp® Injection *see* estradiol and testosterone *on page 178*

Duofilm® Solution *see* salicylic acid and lactic acid *on page 424*

Duo-Medihaler® Aerosol *see* isoproterenol and phenylephrine *on page 259*

Duo-Trach® Injection *see* lidocaine hydrochloride *on page 273*

Duotrate® *see* pentaerythritol tetranitrate *on page 363*

Duphalac® *see* lactulose *on page 267*

Duplex® T [OTC] *see* coal tar *on page 110*

Durabolin® Injection *see* nandrolone *on page 324*

Duradyne DHC® *see* hydrocodone and acetaminophen *on page 234*

Dura-Estrin® Injection *see* estradiol *on page 178*

Duragen® Injection *see* estradiol *on page 178*

Duragesic™ Transdermal *see* fentanyl citrate *on page 192*

Dura-Gest® *see* guaifenesin, phenylpropanolamine, and phenylephrine *on page 221*

Duralex® *see* chlorpheniramine and pseudoephedrine *on page 94*

Duralone® Injection *see* methylprednisolone *on page 306*

Duralutin® Injection *see* hydroxyprogesterone caproate *on page 240*

Duramorph® Injection *see* morphine sulfate *on page 318*

Duranest® Injection *see* etidocaine hydrochloride *on page 187*

Dura-Tap/PD® *see* chlorpheniramine and pseudoephedrine *on page 94*

Duratest® Injection *see* testosterone *on page 456*

Duratestrin® Injection *see* estradiol and testosterone *on page 178*

Durathate® Injection *see* testosterone *on page 456*

Duration® Nasal Solution [OTC] *see* oxymetazoline hydrochloride *on page 350*

Dura-Vent® *see* guaifenesin and phenylpropanolamine *on page 219*

Duricef® *see* cefadroxil monohydrate *on page 78*

Durrax® Oral *see* hydroxyzine *on page 241*

Duvoid® *see* bethanechol chloride *on page 53*

DV® Vaginal Cream *see* dienestrol *on page 145*

d-xylose

Brand Names Xylo-Pfan® [OTC]
Synonyms wood sugar
Therapeutic Category Diagnostic Agent, Intestinal Absorption
Use For evaluating intestinal absorption and diagnosing malabsorptive states
Usual Dosage Oral:

Infants and young Children: 500 mg/kg as a 5% to 10% aqueous solution

Children: 5 g is dissolved in 250 mL water; additional fluids are permitted and are encouraged for children

Adults: 25 g dissolved in 200-300 mL water followed with an additional 200-400 mL water **or** 5 g dissolved in 200-300 mL water followed by an additional 200-400 mL water
Dosage Forms Powder for oral solution: 25 g

Dyazide® *see* hydrochlorothiazide and triamterene *on page 234*

Dycill® *see* dicloxacillin sodium *on page 144*

Dyclone® *see* dyclonine hydrochloride *on next page*

dyclonine hydrochloride (dye' kloe neen)
Brand Names Dyclone®; Sucrets® [OTC]
Therapeutic Category Local Anesthetic, Oral
Use As a local anesthetic prior to laryngoscopy, bronchoscopy, or endotracheal intubation; use topically for temporary relief of pain associated with oral mucosa, skin, episiotomy, or anogenital lesions
Usual Dosage Children and Adults: Topical solution:
Mouth sores: 5-10 mL of 0.5% or 1% to oral mucosa (swab or swish and then spit) 3-4 times/day as needed; maximum single dose: 200 mg (40 mL of 0.5% solution or 20 mL of 1% solution)

Bronchoscopy: Use 2 mL of the 1% solution or 4 mL of the 0.5% solution sprayed onto the larynx and trachea every 5 minutes until the reflex has been abolished

Children >3 years and Adults: Lozenge: Dissolve 1 in mouth slowly every 2 hours
Dosage Forms
Lozenges: 1.2 mg, 3 mg
Solution, topical: 0.5% (30 mL); 1% (30 mL)

Dyflex® *see* dyphylline *on this page*

dyflos *see* isoflurophate *on page 257*

Dymelor® *see* acetohexamide *on page 5*

Dymenate® Injection *see* dimenhydrinate *on page 150*

Dynacin® Oral *see* minocycline hydrochloride *on page 314*

DynaCirc® *see* isradipine *on page 260*

Dyna-Hex® Topical [OTC] *see* chlorhexidine gluconate *on page 90*

Dynapen® *see* dicloxacillin sodium *on page 144*

dyphylline (dye' fi lin)
Brand Names Dilor®; Dyflex®; Lufyllin®; Neothylline®
Synonyms dihydroxypropyl theophylline
Therapeutic Category Bronchodilator; Theophylline Derivative
Use Bronchodilator in reversible airway obstruction due to asthma or COPD
Usual Dosage
Children: I.M.: 4.4-6.6 mg/kg/day in divided doses

Adults:
Oral: Up to 15 mg/kg 4 times/day, individualize dosage
I.M.: 250-500 mg, do not exceed total dosage of 15 mg/kg every 6 hours
Dosage Forms
Elixir:
Lufyllin®: 100 mg/15 mL with alcohol 20% (473 mL, 3780 mL)
Dilor®: 160 mg/15 mL with alcohol 18% (473 mL)
Injection (Dilor®, Lufyllin®): 250 mg/mL (2 mL)
Tablet (Dilor®, Dyflex®, Lufyllin®, Neothylline®): 200 mg, 400 mg

Dyrenium® *see* triamterene *on page 476*

Early Detector® [OTC] *see* diagnostic aids (*in vitro*), feces *on page 138*

Easprin® *see* aspirin *on page 34*

echothiophate iodide (ek oh thye' oh fate)
Brand Names Phospholine Iodide® Ophthalmic
Synonyms ecostigmine iodide
Therapeutic Category Ophthalmic Agent, Miotic
Use Reverse toxic CNS effects caused by anticholinergic drugs; used as miotic in treatment of glaucoma
(Continued)

echothiophate iodide *(Continued)*
Usual Dosage Adults: Ophthalmic: Glaucoma: Instill 1 drop twice daily into eyes with one dose just prior to bedtime; some patients have been treated with 1 dose/day or every other day. Use lowest concentration and frequency which gives satisfactory response, with a maximum dose of 0.125% once daily, although more intensive therapy may be used for short periods of time

Dosage Forms Powder for reconstitution, ophthalmic: 1.5 mg [0.03%] (5 mL); 3 mg [0.06%] (5 mL); 6.25 mg [0.125%] (5 mL); 12.5 mg [0.25%] (5 mL)

econazole nitrate (e kone' a zole)
Brand Names Spectazole™ Topical
Therapeutic Category Antifungal Agent, Topical
Use Topical treatment of tinea pedis, tinea cruris, tinea corporis, tinea versicolor, and cutaneous candidiasis
Usual Dosage Children and Adults: Topical: Apply a sufficient amount to cover affected areas once daily; for cutaneous candidiasis: apply twice daily; candidal infections and tinea cruris, versicolor, and corporis should be treated for 2 weeks and tinea pedis for 1 month; occasionally, longer treatment periods may be required
Dosage Forms Cream: 1% (15 g, 30 g, 85 g)

Econopred® Ophthalmic *see prednisolone on page 391*

Econopred® Plus Ophthalmic *see prednisolone on page 391*

ecostigmine iodide *see echothiophate iodide on previous page*

Ecotrin® [OTC] *see aspirin on page 34*

edathamil disodium *see edetate disodium on next page*

Edecrin® Oral *see ethacrynic acid on page 180*

Edecrin® Sodium Injection *see ethacrynic acid on page 180*

edetate calcium disodium (ed' e tate)
Brand Names Calcium Disodium Versenate®
Synonyms calcium EDTA
Therapeutic Category Antidote, Lead Toxicity
Use Treatment of acute and chronic lead poisoning; also used as an aid in the diagnosis of lead poisoning
Usual Dosage
Children:
Diagnosis of lead poisoning: Mobilization test: (Asymptomatic patients or lead levels <55 µg/dL): (**Note:** Urine is collected for 24 hours after first EDTA dose and analyzed for lead content; if the ratio of µg of lead in urine to mg calcium EDTA given is >1, then test is considered positive): Children: 500 mg/m² (maximum: 1 g/dose) I.M. or I.V. over 1 hour **or** 2 doses of 500 mg/m² at 12-hour intervals
Asymptomatic lead poisoning: (Blood lead concentration >55 µg/dL or blood lead concentrations of 25-55 µg/dL with blood erythrocyte protoporphyrin concentrations of ≥35 µg/dL with positive mobilization test) or symptomatic lead poisoning without encephalopathy with lead level <100 µg/dL: 1 g/m²/day I.M./I.V. in divided doses every 8-12 hours for 3-5 days (usually 5 days); maximum: 1 g/24 hours or 50 mg/kg/day
Symptomatic lead poisoning with encephalopathy with lead level >100 µg/dL (treatment with calcium EDTA and dimercaprol is preferred): 250 mg/m² I.M. or intermittent I.V. infusion 4 hours after dimercaprol, then at 4-hour intervals thereafter for 5 days (1.5 g/m²/day); dose (1.5 g/m²/day) can also be given as a single I.V. continuous infusion over 12-24 hours/day for 5 days; maximum: 1 g/24 hours or 75 mg/kg/day
Note: Course of therapy may be repeated in 2-3 weeks until blood lead level is normal
Adults: I.M., I.V.:
Diagnosis of lead poisoning: 500 mg/m² (maximum: 1 g/dose) over 1 hour

Treatment: 2 g/day or 1.5 g/m²/day in divided doses every 12-24 hours for 5 days; may repeat course one time after at least 2 days (usually after 2 weeks)

Dosage Forms Injection: 200 mg/mL (5 mL)

edetate disodium (ed' e tate)

Brand Names Chealamide®; Disotate®; Endrate®

Synonyms edathamil disodium; EDTA; sodium edetate

Therapeutic Category Antidote, Hypercalcemia; Chelating Agent, Parenteral

Use Emergency treatment of hypercalcemia; control digitalis-induced cardiac dysrhythmias (ventricular arrhythmias)

Usual Dosage I.V.:

Hypercalcemia:

Children: 40-70 mg/kg slow infusion over 3-4 hours

Adults: 50 mg/kg/day over 3 or more hours

Dysrhythmias: Children and Adults: 15 mg/kg/hour up to 60 mg/kg/day

Dosage Forms Injection: 150 mg/mL (20 mL)

edrophonium chloride (ed roe foe' nee um)

Brand Names Enlon® Injection; Reversol® Injection; Tensilon® Injection

Therapeutic Category Antidote, Neuromuscular Blocking Agent; Cholinergic Agent; Diagnostic Agent, Myasthenia Gravis

Use Diagnosis and differentiation of myasthenia gravis; to reverse nondepolarizing neuromuscular blockers; treatment of paroxysmal atrial tachycardia; a curare antagonist, also used for curare overdose to treat respiratory depression, reverses neuromuscular block produced by curare

Usual Dosage

Infants: I.V.: Initial: 0.1 mg, followed by 0.4 mg if no response; total dose = 0.5 mg

Children:

Diagnosis: Initial: 0.04 mg/kg followed by 0.16 mg/kg if no response, to a maximum total dose of 5 mg for children ≤34 kg, or 10 mg for children >34 kg

Titration of oral anticholinesterase therapy: 0.04 mg/kg once; if strength improves, an increase in neostigmine or pyridostigmine dose is indicated

Adults:

Diagnosis: I.V.: 2 mg test dose administered over 15-30 seconds; 8 mg given 45 seconds later if no response is seen. Test dose may be repeated after 30 minutes.

Titration of oral anticholinesterase therapy: 1-2 mg given 1 hour after oral dose of anticholinesterase; if strength improves, an increase in neostigmine or pyridostigmine dose is indicated

Differentiation of cholinergic from myasthenic crisis: I.V.: 1 mg, may repeat after 1 minute (**Note:** Intubation and controlled ventilation may be required if patient has cholinergic crises.)

Reversal of nondepolarizing neuromuscular blocking agents (neostigmine with atropine usually preferred): I.V.: 10 mg, may repeat every 5-10 minutes up to 40 mg

Termination of paroxysmal atrial tachycardia: I.V.: 5-10 mg

Dosage Forms Injection: 10 mg/mL (1 mL, 10 mL, 15 mL)

EDTA *see* edetate disodium *on this page*

E.E.S.® Oral *see* erythromycin *on page 175*

Effer-K™ *see* potassium bicarbonate and potassium citrate, effervescent *on page 386*

Effer-Syllium® [OTC] *see* psyllium *on page 407*

Effexor® *see* venlafaxine *on page 493*

eflornithine hydrochloride (ee flor' ni theen)
Brand Names Ornidyl® Injection
Synonyms DFMO
Therapeutic Category Antiprotozoal
Use Treatment of meningoencephalitic stage of *Trypanosoma brucei gambiense* infection (sleeping sickness)
Usual Dosage I.V. infusion: 100 mg/kg/dose given every 6 hours (over 45 minutes) for 14 days
Dosage Forms Injection, concentrate: 200 mg/mL (100 mL)

Efodine® [OTC] *see* povidone-iodine *on page 389*

Efudex® Topical *see* fluorouracil *on page 202*

EHDP *see* etidronate disodium *on page 187*

Elase-Chloromycetin® Topical *see* fibrinolysin and desoxyribonuclease *on page 195*

Elase® Topical *see* fibrinolysin and desoxyribonuclease *on page 195*

Elavil® *see* amitriptyline hydrochloride *on page 21*

Eldecort® Topical *see* hydrocortisone *on page 236*

Eldepryl® *see* selegiline hydrochloride *on page 428*

Eldopaque Forte® Topical *see* hydroquinone *on page 239*

Eldopaque® Topical [OTC] *see* hydroquinone *on page 239*

Eldoquin® Forte® Topical *see* hydroquinone *on page 239*

Eldoquin® Topical [OTC] *see* hydroquinone *on page 239*

electrolyte lavage solution *see* polyethylene glycol-electrolyte solution *on page 383*

Elimite™ Cream *see* permethrin *on page 366*

Elixicon® *see* theophylline *on page 460*

Elixophyllin® *see* theophylline *on page 460*

Elixophyllin® SR *see* theophylline *on page 460*

Elocon® Topical *see* mometasone furoate *on page 316*

E-Lor® *see* propoxyphene and acetaminophen *on page 402*

Elspar® *see* asparaginase *on page 34*

Emcyt® *see* estramustine phosphate sodium *on page 179*

Emete-Con® *see* benzquinamide hydrochloride *on page 50*

Emetrol® [OTC] *see* phosphorated carbohydrate solution *on page 375*

Emgel™ Topical *see* erythromycin, topical *on page 176*

Eminase® *see* anistreplase *on page 28*

Emko® [OTC] *see* nonoxynol 9 *on page 338*

EMLA® Topical *see* lidocaine and prilocaine *on page 273*

Empirin® [OTC] *see* aspirin *on page 34*

Empirin® With Codeine *see* aspirin and codeine *on page 35*

Emulsoil® [OTC] *see* castor oil *on page 77*

E-Mycin® Oral *see* erythromycin *on page 175*

enalapril (e nal' a pril)
Brand Names Vasotec® I.V.; Vasotec® Oral
Synonyms enalaprilat
Therapeutic Category Angiotensin Converting Enzyme (ACE) Inhibitors

Use Management of mild to severe hypertension and congestive heart failure

Usual Dosage Use lower listed initial dose in patients with hyponatremia, hypovolemia, severe congestive heart failure, decreased renal function, or in those receiving diuretics

Children:
> Investigational initial oral doses of enalapril of 0.1 mg/kg/day increasing over 2 weeks to 0.12-0.43 mg/kg/day have been used to treat severe congestive heart failure in infants (n=8)
> Investigational I.V. doses of enalaprilat of 5-10 μg/kg/dose administered every 8-24 hours (as determined by blood pressure readings) have been used for the treatment of neonatal hypertension (n=10); monitor patients carefully; select patients may require higher doses

Adults:
> Oral: **Enalapril**: 2.5-5 mg/day then increase as required, usually 10-40 mg/day in 1-2 divided doses
> I.V.: **Enalaprilat**: 0.625-1.25 mg/dose, given over 5 minutes every 6 hours

Dosage Forms
Injection, as enalaprilat: 1.25 mg/mL (1 mL, 2 mL)
Tablet, as maleate: 2.5 mg, 5 mg, 10 mg, 20 mg

enalapril and hydrochlorothiazide
Brand Names Vaseretic® 10-25
Therapeutic Category Antihypertensive, Combination
Use Treatment of hypertension
Usual Dosage Dose is individualized
Dosage Forms Tablet: Enalapril maleate 10 mg and hydrochlorothiazide 25 mg

enalaprilat *see* enalapril *on previous page*

encainide hydrochloride (en kay' nide)
Brand Names Enkaid®
Therapeutic Category Antiarrhythmic Agent, Class Ic
Use Ventricular arrhythmias; supraventricular arrhythmias
Usual Dosage Adults: Oral: 25 mg every 8 hours; may increase to 35 mg every 8 hours after 3-5 days if needed; increase to 50 mg every 8 hours in another 3-5 days if response is not achieved
Dosage Forms Capsule: 25 mg, 35 mg, 50 mg

Encare® [OTC] *see* nonoxynol 9 *on page 338*

Endep® *see* amitriptyline hydrochloride *on page 21*

End Lice® [OTC] *see* pyrethrins *on page 408*

Endolor® *see* butalbital compound *on page 63*

Endrate® *see* edetate disodium *on page 167*

Enduron® *see* methyclothiazide *on page 303*

Enduronyl® *see* methyclothiazide and deserpidine *on page 303*

Enduronyl® Forte *see* methyclothiazide and deserpidine *on page 303*

Enecat® *see* radiological/contrast media (ionic) *on page 413*

Ener-B® [OTC] *see* cyanocobalamin *on page 120*

enflurane (en' floo rane)
Brand Names Ethrane®
Therapeutic Category General Anesthetic
Use General induction and maintenance of anesthesia (inhalation)
(Continued)

enflurane *(Continued)*
Usual Dosage 0.5% to 3%
Dosage Forms Liquid: 125 mL, 250 mL

Engerix-B® *see* hepatitis b vaccine *on page 228*
Enisyl® [OTC] *see* l-lysine hydrochloride *on page 276*
Enkaid® *see* encainide hydrochloride *on previous page*
Enlon® Injection *see* edrophonium chloride *on page 167*
Enomine® *see* guaifenesin, phenylpropanolamine, and phenylephrine *on page 221*
Enovid® *see* mestranol and norethynodrel *on page 296*
Enovil® *see* amitriptyline hydrochloride *on page 21*

enoxacin (en ox' a sin)
Brand Names Penetrex™ Oral
Therapeutic Category Antibiotic, Quinolone
Use Complicated and uncomplicated urinary tract infections caused by susceptible gram-negative and gram-positive bacteria
Usual Dosage Adults: Oral: 400 mg twice daily
Dosage Forms Tablet: 200 mg, 400 mg

enoxaparin sodium (e nox ah pair' in)
Brand Names Lovenox® Injection
Therapeutic Category Anticoagulant
Use Prophylaxis and treatment of thromboembolic disorders (deep vein thrombosis)
Usual Dosage Adults: S.C.: 30 mg twice daily
Dosage Forms Injection, preservative free: 30 mg/0.3 mL

E.N.T.® *see* brompheniramine and phenylpropanolamine *on page 59*
Entex® *see* guaifenesin, phenylpropanolamine, and phenylephrine *on page 221*
Entex® LA *see* guaifenesin and phenylpropanolamine *on page 219*
Entex® PSE *see* guaifenesin and pseudoephedrine *on page 220*
Entolase® *see* pancrelipase *on page 354*
Entrobar® *see* radiological/contrast media (ionic) *on page 413*
Enulose® *see* lactulose *on page 267*
Enzone® *see* pramoxine and hydrocortisone *on page 389*
EPEG *see* etoposide *on page 188*

ephedrine sulfate (e fed' rin)
Brand Names Kondon's Nasal® [OTC]; Pretz-D® [OTC]; Vicks Vatronol® [OTC]
Therapeutic Category Adrenergic Agonist Agent
Use Bronchial asthma; nasal congestion; acute bronchospasm; acute hypotensive states
Usual Dosage
Children: Oral, I.V., S.C.: 3 mg/kg/day or 100 mg/m^2/day divided into 4-6 doses
Adults:
Oral: 25-50 mg every 3-4 hours as needed
I.M., I.V., S.C.: 25-50 mg
Dosage Forms
Capsule: 25 mg, 50 mg
Drops (Vicks Vatronol®): 0.5% (30 mL)
Injection: 25 mg/mL (1 mL); 50 mg/mL (1 mL, 10 mL)
Jelly (Kondon's Nasal®): 1% (20 g)

Spray (Pretz-D®): 0.25% (15 mL)

ephedrine, theophylline and phenobarbital *see* theophylline, ephedrine, and phenobarbital *on page 462*

Epi-C® *see* radiological/contrast media (ionic) *on page 413*

Epifrin® Ophthalmic *see* epinephrine *on this page*

E-Pilo-x® Ophthalmic *see* pilocarpine and epinephrine *on page 377*

Epinal® Ophthalmic *see* epinephrine *on this page*

epinephrine (ep i nef' rin)
Brand Names Adrenalin® Chloride Inhalation Solution [OTC]; Adrenalin® Chloride Injection; Adrenalin® Chloride Nasal Solution [OTC]; AsthmaHaler® Inhalation Aerosol; AsthmaNefrin® Inhalation Solution [OTC]; Bronitin® Inhalation Aerosol [OTC]; Bronkaid® Inhalation Aerosol [OTC]; Epifrin® Ophthalmic; Epinal® Ophthalmic; EpiPen® Injector; EpiPen® Jr Injector; Eppy/N® Ophthalmic; Glaucon® Ophthalmic; Medihaler-Epi® Inhalation Aerosol [OTC]; microNefrin® Inhalation Solution [OTC]; Nephron® Inhalation Solution [OTC]; Primatene® Inhalation Aerosol [OTC]; S-2® Inhalation Solution [OTC]; Sus-Phrine® Injection; Vaponefrin® Inhalation Solution [OTC]

Synonyms adrenaline; racemic epinephrine
Therapeutic Category Adrenergic Agonist Agent; Antidote, Hypersensitivity Reactions; Bronchodilator
Use Bronchospasms; anaphylactic reactions; cardiac arrest; management of open-angle (chronic simple) glaucoma
Usual Dosage
Neonates: Cardiac arrest: I.V. or intratracheal: 0.01-0.03 mg/kg (0.1-0.3 mL/kg 1:10,000 solution) every 3-5 minutes as needed

Children:
Bronchodilator: S.C.: 10 µg/kg (single doses not to exceed 0.5 mg); Injection suspension (1:200): 0.005 mL/kg/dose to a maximum of 0.15 mL every 8-12 hours
Cardiac arrest: I.V. or intratracheal: 0.01 mg/kg (0.1 mL/kg) of 1:10,000 solution (to maximum 5 mL) every 3-5 minutes as needed; infusion rate 0.1-4 µg/kg/minute.
Refractory hypotension (refractory to dopamine/dobutamine): Start infusion 0.1 µg/kg/minute, titrate to desired effect
Hypersensitivity reaction: S.C.: 0.01 mg/kg every 15 minutes for 2 doses then every 4 hours as needed (single doses not to exceed 0.5 mg)
Nebulization (racemic epinephrine):
<10 kg: 2 mL of 1:8 dilution over 15 minutes every 1-4 hours
10-15 kg: 2 mL of 1:6 dilution over 15 minutes every 1-4 hours
15-20 kg: 2 mL of 1:4 dilution over 15 minutes every 1-4 hours
>20 kg: 2 mL of 1:3 dilution over 15 minutes every 1-4 hours

Adults:
Bronchodilator:
I.M., S.C.: 0.1-0.5 mg every 10-15 minutes
I.V.: 0.1-0.25 mg (single dose maximum 1 mg)
Cardiac arrest: I.V., intracardiac: 0.1-1 mg every 5 minutes as needed; intratracheal: 1 mg
Hypersensitivity reaction: I.M., S.C.: 0.2-0.5 mg every 20 minutes to 4 hours (single dose maximum 1 mg)
Ophthalmic: Instill 1-2 drops in eye(s) once or twice daily
Dosage Forms
Aerosol, oral:
Bitartrate (AsthmaHaler®, Bronitin®, Medihaler-Epi®, Primatene® Suspension): 0.3 mg/spray [epinephrine base 0.16 mg/spray] (10 mL, 15 mL, 22.5 mL)
Bronkaid®: 0.5% (10 mL, 15 mL, 22.5 mL)
Primatene®: 0.2 mg/spray (15 mL, 22.5 mL)
(Continued)

epinephrine *(Continued)*

Auto-injector:
   EpiPen®: Delivers 0.3 mg I.M. of epinephrine 1:1000 (2 mL)
   EpiPen® Jr.: Delivers 0.15 mg I.M. of epinephrine 1:2000 (2 mL)
Solution:
   Inhalation:
      Adrenalin®: 1% [10 mg/mL, 1:100] (7.5 mL)
      AsthmaNefrin®, microNefrin®, Nephron®: Racepinephrine 2% [epinephrine base 1.125%] (7.5 mL, 15 mL, 30 mL)
      Vaponefrin®: Racepinephrine 2% [epinephrine base 1%] (15 mL, 30 mL)
   Injection:
      Adrenalin®: 0.01 mg/mL [1:100,000] (5 mL); 0.1 mg/mL [1:10,000] (3 mL, 10 mL); 1 mg/mL [1:1000] (1 mL, 2 mL, 30 mL)
      Suspension (Sus-Phrine®): 5 mg/mL [1:200] (0.3 mL, 5 mL)
      Nasal (Adrenalin®): 0.1% [1 mg/mL, 1:1000] (30 mL)
      Ophthalmic, as borate (Epinal®, Eppy/N®): 0.5% (7.5 mL); 1% (7.5 mL); 2% (7.5 mL)
      Ophthalmic, as hydrochloride (Epifrin®, Glaucon®): 0.1% (1 mL, 30 mL); 0.25% (15 mL); 0.5% (15 mL); 1% (1 mL, 10 mL, 15 mL); 2% (10 mL, 15 mL)
      Topical (Adrenalin®): 0.1% [1 mg/mL, 1:1000] (30 mL, 10 mL)

EpiPen® Injector *see* epinephrine *on previous page*

EpiPen® Jr Injector *see* epinephrine *on previous page*

Epitol® *see* carbamazepine *on page 72*

E.P. Mycin® Oral *see* oxytetracycline hydrochloride *on page 352*

EPO *see* epoetin alfa *on this page*

epoetin alfa (e poe' e tin al fa)

Brand Names Epogen®; Procrit®
Synonyms EPO; erythropoietin; rHuEPO-α
Therapeutic Category Recombinant Human Erythropoietin
Use Treatment of anemia associated with chronic renal failure; anemia related to therapy with AZT-treated HIV-infected patients; anemia of prematurity
Usual Dosage
   In patients on dialysis epoetin alfa usually has been administered as an I.V. bolus 3 times/week. While the administration is independent of the dialysis procedure, it may be administered into the venous line at the end of the dialysis procedure to obviate the need for additional venous access; in patients with CRF not on dialysis, epoetin alfa may be given either as an I.V. or S.C. injection.

   AZT-treated HIV-infected patients: I.V., S.C.: Initial: 100 units/kg/dose 3 times/week for 8 weeks; after 8 weeks of therapy the dose can be adjusted by 50-100 units/kg increments 3 times/week to a maximum dose of 300 units/kg 3 times/week; if the hematocrit exceeds 40%, the dose should be discontinued until the hematocrit drops to 36%

   Anemia of prematurity: S.C.: 25-100 units/kg/dose 3 times/week
Dosage Forms Injection, preservative free: 2000 units (1 mL); 3000 units (1 mL); 4000 units (1 mL); 10,000 units (1 mL)

Epogen® *see* epoetin alfa *on this page*

Eppy/N® Ophthalmic *see* epinephrine *on previous page*

epsom salts *see* magnesium sulfate *on page 283*

EPT *see* teniposide *on page 453*

e.p.t.® Stick *see* diagnostic aids (*in vitro*), urine *on page 139*

Equagesic® *see* aspirin and meprobamate *on page 35*

Equalactin® Chewablet Tablet [OTC] *see* calcium polycarbophil *on page 69*

Equanil® *see* meprobamate *on page 293*
Equilet® [OTC] *see* calcium carbonate *on page 65*
Ercaf® *see* ergotamine derivatives *on next page*
Ergamisol® *see* levamisole hydrochloride *on page 269*

ergocalciferol (er goe kal sif' e role)
Brand Names Calciferol™ Injection; Calciferol™ Oral; Drisdol® Oral
Synonyms activated ergosterol; viosterol; vitamin D₂
Therapeutic Category Vitamin D Analog
Use Refractory rickets; hypophosphatemia; hypoparathyroidism
Usual Dosage
Dietary supplementation: Oral:
Premature infants: 10-20 μg/day (400-800 units), up to 750 μg/day (30,000 units)
Infants and healthy Children: 10 μg/day (400 units)

Renal failure: Oral:
Children: 0.1-1 mg/day (4000-40,000 units)
Adults: 0.5 mg/day (20,000 units)

Hypoparathyroidism: Oral:
Children: 1.25-5 mg/day (50,000-200,000 units) and calcium supplements
Adults: 625 μg-5 mg/day (25,000-200,000 units) and calcium supplements

Vitamin D-dependent rickets: Oral:
Children: 75-125 μg/day (3000-5000 units)
Adults: 250 μg-1.5 mg/day (10,000-60,000 units)

Nutritional rickets and osteomalacia:
Oral:
Children and Adults (with normal absorption): 25 μg/day (1000 units)
Children with malabsorption: 250-625 μg/day (10,000-25,000 units)
I.M.: Adults: 250 μg/day
Dosage Forms
Capsule (Drisdol®): 50,000 units [1.25 mg]
Injection (Calciferol™): 500,000 units/mL [12.5 mg/mL] (1 mL)
Liquid (Calciferol™, Drisdol®): 8000 units/mL [200 μg/mL] (60 mL)
Tablet (Calciferol™): 50,000 units [1.25 mg]

ergoloid mesylates (er' goe loyd mess' i lates)
Brand Names Germinal®; Hydergine®; Hydergine® LC; Hydro-Ergoloid®; Niloric®
Synonyms dihydroergotoxine; hydrogenated ergot alkaloids
Therapeutic Category Ergot Alkaloid
Use Treatment of cerebrovascular insufficiency in primary progressive dementia, Alzheimer's dementia, and senile onset
Usual Dosage Adults: Oral: 1 mg 3 times/day up to 4.5-12 mg/day; up to 6 months of therapy may be necessary
Dosage Forms
Capsule, liquid (Hydergine® LC): 1 mg
Liquid (Hydergine®): 1 mg/mL (100 mL)
Tablet:
Oral:
0.5 mg
Gerimal®, Hydergine®: 1 mg
Sublingual:
Gerimal®, Hydergine®: 0.5 mg
Gerimal®, Hydergine®, Niloric®: 1 mg

ergometrine maleate *see* ergonovine maleate *on next page*

ergonovine maleate (er goe noe' veen)
Brand Names Ergotrate® Maleate
Synonyms ergometrine maleate
Therapeutic Category Ergot Alkaloid
Use Prevention and treatment of postpartum and postabortion hemorrhage caused by uterine atony or subinvolution
Usual Dosage Adults:
Oral: 1-2 tablets every 6-12 hours for usually 48 hours
I.M.: 0.2 mg, repeat dose in 2-4 hours as needed
Dosage Forms Injection: 0.2 mg/mL (1 mL)

Ergostat® *see* ergotamine derivatives *on this page*

ergotamine derivatives (er got' a meen)
Brand Names Cafatine®; Cafergot®; Cafetrate®; Ercaf®; Ergostat®; Medihaler Ergotamine™; Wigraine®
Therapeutic Category Adrenergic Blocking Agent; Ergot Alkaloid
Use Vascular headache, such as migraine or cluster
Usual Dosage
Older Children and Adolescents: Oral: 1 tablet at onset of attack; then 1 tablet every 30 minutes as needed, up to a maximum of 3 tablets per attack
Adults:
Oral (Cafergot®): 2 tablets at onset of attack; then 1 tablet every 30 minutes as needed; maximum: 6 tablets per attack; do not exceed 10 tablets/week
Rectal (Cafergot® suppositories, Wigraine® suppositories, Cafatine-PB® suppositories): 1 at first sign of an attack; follow with second dose after 1 hour, if needed; maximum dose: 2 per attack; do not exceed 5/week
Oral (Ergostat®): 1 tablet under tongue at first sign, then 1 tablet every 30 minutes, 3 tablets/24 hours, 5 tablets/week
Dosage Forms
Aerosol, oral (Medihaler Ergotamine™): Ergotamine tartrate 360 µg/metered spray [62.5 doses] (2.5 mL)
Suppository, rectal (Cafatine®, Cafergot®, Cafetrate®, Wigraine®): Ergotamine tartrate 2 mg and caffeine 100 mg (12s)
Tablet (Cafergot®, Ercaf®, Wigraine®): Ergotamine tartrate 1 mg and caffeine 100 mg
Tablet, sublingual (Ergostat®): Ergotamine tartrate 2 mg

Ergotrate® Maleate *see* ergonovine maleate *on this page*
Erycette® Topical *see* erythromycin, topical *on page 176*
Eryc® Oral *see* erythromycin *on next page*
EryDerm® Topical *see* erythromycin, topical *on page 176*
Erygel® Topical *see* erythromycin, topical *on page 176*
Erymax® Topical *see* erythromycin, topical *on page 176*
EryPed® Oral *see* erythromycin *on next page*
Ery-sol® Topical *see* erythromycin, topical *on page 176*
Ery-Tab® Oral *see* erythromycin *on next page*

erythrityl tetranitrate (e ri' thri till te tra nye' trate)
Brand Names Cardilate®
Therapeutic Category Antianginal Agent; Nitrate; Vasodilator, Coronary
Use Prophylaxis and long-term treatment of frequent or recurrent anginal pain and reduced exercise tolerance associated with angina pectoris
Usual Dosage Adults: Oral: 5 mg under the tongue or in the buccal pouch 3 times/day or 10 mg before meals or food, chewed 3 times/day, increasing in 2-3 days if needed
Dosage Forms Tablet, oral or sublingual: 10 mg

Erythrocin® Oral *see* erythromycin *on this page*

erythromycin (er ith roe mye' sin)
Brand Names E.E.S.® Oral; E-Mycin® Oral; Eryc® Oral; EryPed® Oral; Ery-Tab® Oral; Erythrocin® Oral; Ilosone® Oral; PCE® Oral; Wyamycin® S Oral
Synonyms erythromycin base; erythromycin estolate; erythromycin ethylsuccinate; erythromycin gluceptate; erythromycin lactobionate; erythromycin stearate
Therapeutic Category Antibiotic, Macrolide; Antibiotic, Ophthalmic
Use Treatment of susceptible bacterial infections including *M. pneumoniae*, *Legionella* pneumonia, Lyme disease, diphtheria, pertussis, chancroid, *Chlamydia*, and *Campylobacter* gastroenteritis; used in conjunction with neomycin for decontaminating the bowel
Usual Dosage
Neonates:
Oral:
Postnatal age <7 days: 20 mg/kg/day in divided doses every 12 hours
Postnatal age >7 days, <1200 g: 20 mg/kg/day in divided doses every 12 hours; ≥1200 g: 30 mg/kg/day in divided doses every 8 hours
Prophylaxis of neonatal gonococcal or chlamydial conjunctivitis: 0.5-1 cm ribbon of ointment should be instilled into each conjunctival sac

Infants and Children:
Oral: Do not exceed 2 g/day
Base and ethylsuccinate: 30-50 mg/kg/day divided every 6-8 hours
Estolate: 30-50 mg/kg/day divided every 8-12 hours
Stearate: 20-40 mg/kg/day divided every 6 hours
Pre-op bowel preparation: 20 mg/kg erythromycin base at 1, 2, and 11 PM on the day before surgery combined with mechanical cleansing of the large intestine and oral neomycin
I.V.: Lactobionate: 20-40 mg/kg/day divided every 6 hours, not to exceed 4 g/day

Adults:
Oral:
Base: 333 mg every 8 hours
Estolate, stearate or base: 250-500 mg every 6-12 hours
Ethylsuccinate: 400-800 mg every 6-12 hours
Pre-op bowel preparation: 1 g erythromycin base at 1, 2, and 11 PM on the day before surgery combined with mechanical cleansing of the large intestine and oral neomycin
I.V.: 15-20 mg/kg/day divided every 6 hours or given as a continuous infusion over 24 hours
Dosage Forms
Erythromycin base:
Capsule, delayed release: 250 mg
Capsule, delayed release, enteric coated pellets (Eryc®): 250 mg
Tablet, delayed release: 333 mg
Tablet, enteric coated (E-Mycin®, Ery-Tab®, E-Base®): 250 mg, 333 mg, 500 mg
Tablet, film coated: 250 mg, 500 mg
Tablet, polymer coated particles (PCE®): 333 mg, 500 mg

Erythromycin estolate:
Capsule (Ilosone® Pulvules®): 250 mg
Suspension, oral (Ilosone®): 125 mg/5 mL (480 mL); 250 mg/mL (480 mL)
Tablet (Ilosone®): 500 mg

Erythromycin ethylsuccinate:
Granules for oral suspension (EryPed®): 400 mg/5 mL (60 mL, 100 mL, 200 mL)
Powder for oral suspension (E.E.S.®): 200 mg/5 mL (100 mL, 200 mL)
Suspension, oral (E.E.S.®, EryPed®): 200 mg/5 mL (5 mL, 100 mL, 200 mL, 480 mL); 400 mg/5 mL (5 mL, 60 mL, 100 mL, 200 mL, 480 mL)
Suspension, oral [drops] (EryPed®): 100 mg/2.5 mL (50 mL)
Tablet (E.E.S.®): 400 mg
(Continued)

erythromycin *(Continued)*

    Tablet, chewable (EryPed®): 200 mg

    Erythromycin gluceptate:
      Injection: 1000 mg (30 mL)

    Erythromycin lactobionate:
      Powder for injection: 500 mg, 1000 mg

    Erythromycin stearate:
      Tablet, film coated (Eramycin®, Erythrocin®, Wyamycin® S): 250 mg, 500 mg

erythromycin and sulfisoxazole (er ith roe mye' sin & sul fi sox' a zole)

Brand Names Eryzole® Oral; Pediazole® Oral

Synonyms sulfisoxazole and erythromycin

Therapeutic Category Antibiotic, Macrolide; Antibiotic, Sulfonamide Derivative

Use Treatment of susceptible bacterial infections of the upper and lower respiratory tract; otitis media in children caused by susceptible strains of *Haemophilus influenzae*; and other infections in patients allergic to penicillin

Usual Dosage Dosage recommendation is based on the product's erythromycin content. Oral:

    Children ≥2 months: 40-50 mg/kg/day of erythromycin in divided doses every 6-8 hours; not to exceed 2 g erythromycin or 6 g sulfisoxazole/day or approximately 1.25 mL/kg/day divided every 6-8 hours

    Adults: 400 mg erythromycin and 1200 mg sulfisoxazole every 6 hours

Dosage Forms Suspension, oral: Erythromycin ethylsuccinate 200 mg and sulfisoxazole acetyl 600 mg per 5 mL (100 mL, 150 mL, 200 mL)

erythromycin base *see* erythromycin *on previous page*

erythromycin estolate *see* erythromycin *on previous page*

erythromycin ethylsuccinate *see* erythromycin *on previous page*

erythromycin gluceptate *see* erythromycin *on previous page*

erythromycin lactobionate *see* erythromycin *on previous page*

erythromycin stearate *see* erythromycin *on previous page*

erythromycin, topical

Brand Names AK-Mycin® Ophthalmic; Akne-Mycin® Topical; A/T/S® Topical; C-Solve-2® Topical; Del-Mycin® Topical; Emgel™ Topical; Erycette® Topical; EryDerm® Topical; Erygel® Topical; Erymax® Topical; Ery-sol® Topical; E-Solve-2® Topical; ETS-2%® Topical; Ilotycin® Ophthalmic; Staticin® Topical; T-Stat® Topical

Therapeutic Category Acne Product; Antibiotic, Topical

Use Topical treatment of acne vulgaris

Usual Dosage Children and Adults:

    Ophthalmic: Instill one or more times daily depending on the severity of the infection

    Topical: Apply 2% solution over the affected area twice daily after the skin has been thoroughly washed and patted dry

Dosage Forms

    Gel (A/T/S®, Emgel™, Erygel®): 2% [20 mg/g] (27 g, 30 g, 60 g)

    Ointment:

      Ophthalmic (Ilotycin®, AK-Mycin®): 0.5% [5 mg/g] (1 g, 3.5 g, 3.75 g)

      Topical (Akne-Mycin®): 2% [20 mg/g] (25 g)

    Solution, topical:

      Staticin®: 1.5% [15 mg/mL] (60 mL)

      Akne-mycin®, A/T/S®, C-Solve-2®, Del-Mycin®, Eryderm™, Ery-sol®, E-Solve®, ETS-2%®, T-Stat®: 2% [20 mg/mL] (60 mL, 66 mL, 120 mL)

    Swab (Erycette®): 2% [20 mg/mL] (60s)

erythropoietin *see* epoetin alfa *on page 172*

Eryzole® Oral *see* erythromycin and sulfisoxazole *on previous page*

eserine salicylate *see* physostigmine *on page 376*

Esgic® *see* butalbital compound *on page 63*

Esgic-Plus® *see* butalbital compound *on page 63*

Esidrix® *see* hydrochlorothiazide *on page 233*

Eskalith® *see* lithium *on page 276*

esmolol hydrochloride (ess' moe lol)

Brand Names Brevibloc® Injection
Therapeutic Category Antiarrhythmic Agent, Class II; Beta-Adrenergic Blocker
Use Supraventricular tachycardia (primarily to control ventricular rate) and hypertension (especially perioperatively)
Usual Dosage Must be adjusted to individual response and tolerance
    Children: An extremely limited amount of information regarding esmolol use in pediatric patients is currently available. Some centers have utilized doses of 100-500 μg/kg given over 1 minute for control of supraventricular tachycardias. Loading doses of 500 μg/kg/minute over 1 minute with maximal doses of 50-250 μg/kg/minute (mean 173) have been used in addition to nitroprusside in a small number of patients (7 patients; 7-19 years of age; median 13 years) to treat postoperative hypertension after coarctation of aorta repair.
    Adults: I.V.: Loading dose: 500 μg/kg over 1 minute; follow with a 50 μg/kg/minute infusion for 4 minutes; if response is inadequate, rebolus with another 500 μg/kg loading dose over 1 minute, and increase the maintenance infusion to 100 μg/kg/minute. Repeat this process until a therapeutic effect has been achieved or to a maximum recommended maintenance dose of 200 μg/kg/minute. Usual dosage range: 50-200 μg/kg/minute with average dose = 100 μg/kg/minute.
Dosage Forms Injection: 10 mg/mL (10 mL); 250 mg/mL (10 mL)

E-Solve-2® Topical *see* erythromycin, topical *on previous page*

Esoterica® Facial Topical [OTC] *see* hydroquinone *on page 239*

Esoterica® Regular Topical [OTC] *see* hydroquinone *on page 239*

Esoterica® Sensitive Skin Formula [OTC] *see* hydroquinone *on page 239*

Esoterica® Topical Sunscreen [OTC] *see* hydroquinone *on page 239*

Espotabs® [OTC] *see* phenolphthalein *on page 370*

Estar® [OTC] *see* coal tar *on page 110*

estazolam (ess ta' zoe lam)

Brand Names ProSom™
Therapeutic Category Benzodiazepine; Hypnotic; Sedative
Use Short-term management of insomnia
Usual Dosage Adults: Oral: 1 mg at bedtime, some patients may require 2 mg
Dosage Forms Tablet: 1 mg, 2 mg

Estinyl® *see* ethinyl estradiol *on page 182*

Estivin® II Ophthalmic [OTC] *see* naphazoline hydrochloride *on page 325*

Estrace® Oral *see* estradiol *on next page*

Estraderm® Transdermal *see* estradiol *on next page*

Estra-D® Injection *see* estradiol *on next page*

estradiol (ess tra dye' ole)

Brand Names Delestrogen® Injection; depGynogen® Injection; Depo®-Estradiol Injection; Depogen® Injection; Dioval® Injection; Dura-Estrin® Injection; Duragen® Injection; Estrace® Oral; Estraderm® Transdermal; Estra-D® Injection; Estra-L® Injection; Estro-Cyp® Injection; Estroject-L.A.® Injection; Gynogen L.A.® Injection; Valergen® Injection

Synonyms estradiol cypionate; estradiol valerate

Therapeutic Category Estrogen Derivative

Use Treatment of atrophic vaginitis, atrophic dystrophy of vulva, menopausal symptoms, female hypogonadism, ovariectomy, primary ovarian failure, inoperable breast cancer, inoperable prostatic cancer, mild to severe vasomotor symptoms associated with menopause; prevention of postmenopausal osteoporosis

Usual Dosage Adults (all dosage needs to be adjusted based upon the patient's response):

Male: Prostate cancer: Valerate:
I.M.: ≥30 mg or more every 1-2 weeks
Oral: 1-2 mg 3 times/day

Female:
Hypogonadism:
Oral: 1-2 mg/day in a cyclic regimen for 3 weeks on drug, then 1 week off drug
I.M.: Cypionate: 1.5-2 mg/month; valerate: 10-20 mg/month
Transdermal: 0.05 mg patch initially (titrate dosage to response) applied twice weekly in a cyclic regimen, for 3 weeks on drug and 1 week off drug
Atrophic vaginitis, kraurosis vulvae: Vaginal: Insert 2-4 g/day for 2 weeks then gradually reduce to $^1/_2$ the initial dose for 2 weeks followed by a maintenance dose of 1 g 1-3 times/week
Moderate to severe vasomotor symptoms: I.M.:
Cypionate: 1-5 mg every 3-4 months
Valerate: 10-20 mg every 4 weeks
Postpartum breast engorgement: I.M.: Valerate: 10-25 mg at end of first stage of labor

Dosage Forms
Cream, vaginal (Estrace®): 0.1 mg/g (42.5 g)
Injection, as cypionate (depGynogen®, Depo®-Estradiol, Depogen®, Dura-Estrin®, Estra-D®, Estro-Cyp®, Estroject-L.A.®): 5 mg/mL (5 mL, 10 mL)
Injection, as valerate:
Delestrogen®, Valergen®: 10 mg/mL (5 mL, 10 mL); 20 mg/mL (1 mL, 5 mL, 10 mL); 40 mg/mL (5 mL, 10 mL)
Dioval®, Duragen®, Estra-L®, Gynogen L.A.®: 20 mg/mL (10 mL); 40 mg/mL (10 mL)
Tablet, micronized (Estrace®): 1 mg, 2 mg
Transdermal system (Estraderm®):
0.05 mg/24 hours [10 cm²], total estradiol 4 mg
0.1 mg/24 hours [20 cm²], total estradiol 8 mg

estradiol and testosterone (ess tra dye' ole & tess toss' ter one)

Brand Names Andro/Fem® Injection; Androgyn L.A.® Injection; Deladumone® Injection; depAndrogyn® Injection; Depo-Testadiol® Injection; Depotestogen® Injection; Duo-Cyp® Injection; Duratestrin® Injection; Estra-Testrin® Injection; Valertest No.1® Injection

Synonyms testosterone and estradiol

Therapeutic Category Estrogen and Androgen Combination

Use Vasomotor symptoms associated with menopause; postpartum breast engorgement

Usual Dosage Dose is individualized

Dosage Forms Injection:
Andro/Fem®, depAndrogyn®, Depo-Testadiol®, Depotestogen®, Duo-Cyp®, Duratestrin®: Estradiol cypionate 2 mg and testosterone cypionate 50 mg per mL in cottonseed oil (1 mL, 10 mL)
Androgyn L.A.®, Deladumone®, Estra-Testrin®, Valertest No.1®: Estradiol valerate 4 mg and testosterone enanthate 90 mg per mL in sesame oil (5 mL, 10 mL)

estradiol cypionate *see* estradiol *on previous page*

estradiol valerate *see* estradiol *on previous page*

Estradurin® *see* polyestradiol phosphate *on page 383*

Estra-L® Injection *see* estradiol *on previous page*

estramustine phosphate sodium (ess tra muss' teen)
Brand Names Emcyt®
Therapeutic Category Antineoplastic Agent, Hormone (Estrogen/Nitrogen Mustard)
Use Palliative treatment of prostatic carcinoma
Usual Dosage Refer to individual protocols
  Oral: 1 capsule for each 22 lb/day, in 3-4 divided doses
Dosage Forms Capsule: 140 mg

Estratab® *see* estrogens, esterified *on this page*

Estratest H.S.® Oral *see* estrogens with methyltestosterone *on next page*

Estratest® Oral *see* estrogens with methyltestosterone *on next page*

Estra-Testrin® Injection *see* estradiol and testosterone *on previous page*

Estro-Cyp® Injection *see* estradiol *on previous page*

estrogenic substance aqueous *see* estrone *on next page*

estrogens, conjugated (ess' troe jenz)
Brand Names Premarin® Injection; Premarin® Oral; Premarin® Vaginal
Synonyms C.E.S.
Therapeutic Category Estrogen Derivative
Use Atrophic vaginitis; hypogonadism; primary ovarian failure; vasomotor symptoms of menopause; prostatic carcinoma; osteoporosis prophylactic
Usual Dosage Adults:
  Male: Prostate cancer: Oral: 1.25-2.5 mg 3 times/day
  Female:
    Hypogonadism: Oral: 2.5-7.5 mg/day for 20 days, off 10 days and repeat until menses occur
    Abnormal uterine bleeding:
      Oral: 2.5-5 mg/day for 7-10 days; then decrease to 1.25 mg/day for 2 weeks
      I.V.: 25 mg every 6-12 hours until bleeding stops
    Moderate to severe vasomotor symptoms: Oral: 0.625-1.25 mg/day
    Postpartum breast engorgement: Oral: 3.75 mg every 4 hours for 5 doses, then 1.25 mg every 4 hours for 5 days
    Atrophic vaginitis, kraurosis vulvae: Vaginal: 2-4 g instilled/day 3 weeks on and 1 week off
Dosage Forms
  Cream, vaginal: 0.625 mg/g (42.5 g)
  Injection: 25 mg (5 mL)
  Tablet: 0.3 mg, 0.625 mg, 0.9 mg, 1.25 mg, 2.5 mg

estrogens, esterified
Brand Names Estratab®; Menest®
Therapeutic Category Estrogen Derivative
Use Atrophic vaginitis; hypogonadism; primary ovarian failure; vasomotor symptoms of menopause; prostatic carcinoma; osteoporosis prophylactic
Usual Dosage Adults: Oral:
  Male: Prostate cancer: 1.25-2.5 mg 3 times/day

  Female:
    Hypogonadism: 2.5-7.5 mg/day for 20 days, off 10 days and repeat until menses occur
(Continued)

estrogens, esterified *(Continued)*
Moderate to severe vasomotor symptoms: 0.3-1.25 mg/day
Dosage Forms Tablet: 0.3 mg, 0.625 mg, 1.25 mg, 2.5 mg

estrogens with methyltestosterone
Brand Names Estratest H.S.® Oral; Estratest® Oral; Premarin® With Methyltestosterone Oral
Therapeutic Category Estrogen and Androgen Combination
Use Atrophic vaginitis; hypogonadism; primary ovarian failure; vasomotor symptoms of menopause; prostatic carcinoma; osteoporosis prophylactic
Usual Dosage Lowest dose that will control symptoms should be chosen, normally given 3 weeks on and 1 week off
Dosage Forms Tablet:
Estratest®: Esterified estrogen 1.25 mg and methyltestosterone 2.5 mg
Estratest H.S.®: Esterified estrogen 0.625 mg and methyltestosterone 1.25 mg
Premarin® With Methyltestosterone: Conjugated estrogen 0.625 mg and methyltestosterone 5 mg; conjugated estrogen 1.25 mg and methyltestosterone 10 mg

Estroject-L.A.® Injection *see* estradiol *on page 178*

estrone (es' trone)
Brand Names Estronol® Injection; Kestrone® Injection; Theelin® Injection
Synonyms estrogenic substance aqueous
Therapeutic Category Estrogen Derivative
Use Atrophic vaginitis; hypogonadism; primary ovarian failure; vasomotor symptoms of menopause; prostatic carcinoma; osteoporosis prophylactic
Usual Dosage Adults: I.M.:
Vasomotor symptoms, atrophic vaginitis: 0.1-0.5 mg 2-3 times/week
Primary ovarian failure, hypogonadism: 0.1-1 mg/week, up to 2 mg/week
Prostatic carcinoma: 2-4 mg 2-3 times/week
Dosage Forms Injection: 2 mg/mL (10 mL, 30 mL); 5 mg/mL (10 mL)

Estronol® Injection *see* estrone *on this page*

estropipate (ess' troe pih pate)
Brand Names Ogen® Oral; Ogen® Vaginal; Ortho-Est® Oral
Synonyms piperazine estrone sulfate
Therapeutic Category Estrogen Derivative
Use Atrophic vaginitis; hypogonadism; primary ovarian failure; vasomotor symptoms of menopause; prostatic carcinoma; osteoporosis prophylactic
Usual Dosage Adults: Female:
Moderate to severe vasomotor symptoms: Oral: 0.625-5 mg/day
Hypogonadism: Oral: 1.25-7.5 mg/day for 3 weeks followed by an 8- to 10-day rest period
Atrophic vaginitis or kraurosis vulvae: Vaginal: Instill 2-4 g/day 3 weeks on and 1 week off
Dosage Forms
Cream, vaginal: 0.15% [estropipate 1.5 mg/g] (42.5 g tube)
Tablet: 0.625 mg [estropipate 0.75 mg]; 1.25 mg [estropipate 1.5 mg]; 2.5 mg [estropipate 3 mg]; 5 mg [estropipate 6 mg]

Estrovis® *see* quinestrol *on page 411*

ethacrynic acid (eth a krin' ik)
Brand Names Edecrin® Oral; Edecrin® Sodium Injection
Synonyms sodium ethacrynate
Therapeutic Category Diuretic, Loop

Use Management of edema secondary to congestive heart failure; hepatic or renal disease
Usual Dosage
Children:
Oral: 25 mg/day to start, increase by 25 mg/day at intervals of 2-3 days as needed, to a maximum of 3 mg/kg/day
I.V.: 1 mg/kg/dose, (maximum: 50 mg/dose); repeat doses not recommended
Adults:
Oral: 50-100 mg/day increased in increments of 25-50 mg at intervals of several days to a maximum of 400 mg/24 hours
I.V.: 0.5-1 mg/kg/dose (maximum: 50 mg/dose); repeat doses not recommended
Dosage Forms
Powder for injection, as ethacrynate sodium: 50 mg (50 mL)
Tablet: 25 mg, 50 mg

ethambutol hydrochloride (e tham' byoo tole)
Brand Names Myambutol®
Therapeutic Category Antitubercular Agent
Use Treatment of tuberculosis and other mycobacterial diseases in conjunction with other antituberculosis agents
Usual Dosage Oral (not recommended in children <12 years of age):
Children >12 years: 15 mg/kg/day once daily

Adolescents and Adults: 15-25 mg/kg/day once daily, not to exceed 2.5 g/day
Dosage Forms Tablet: 100 mg, 400 mg

Ethamolin® Injection *see* ethanolamine oleate *on this page*
ethanoic acid *see* acetic acid *on page 5*
ethanol *see* alcohol, ethyl *on page 11*

ethanolamine oleate (eth' a nol a meen)
Brand Names Ethamolin® Injection
Therapeutic Category Sclerosing Agent
Use Mild sclerosing agent used for bleeding esophageal varices
Usual Dosage Adults: 1.5-5 mL per varix, up to 20 mL total or 0.4 mL/kg; patients with severe hepatic dysfunction should receive less than recommended maximum dose
Dosage Forms Injection: 5% [50 mg/mL] (2 mL)

Ethaquin® *see* ethaverine hydrochloride *on this page*
Ethatab® *see* ethaverine hydrochloride *on this page*

ethaverine hydrochloride
Brand Names Ethaquin®; Ethatab®; Ethavex-100®; Isovex®
Therapeutic Category Vasodilator
Use Peripheral and cerebral vascular insufficiency associated with arterial spasm
Usual Dosage Adults: Oral: 100 mg three times/daily
Dosage Forms
Capsule (Isovex®): 100 mg
Tablet (Ethaquin®, Ethatab®, Ethavex-100®): 100 mg

Ethavex-100® *see* ethaverine hydrochloride *on this page*

ethchlorvynol (eth klor vi' nole)
Brand Names Placidyl®
Therapeutic Category Hypnotic; Sedative
Use Short-term management of insomnia
(Continued)

ethchlorvynol *(Continued)*
Usual Dosage Oral: 500-1000 mg at bedtime
Dosage Forms Capsule: 200 mg, 500 mg, 750 mg

ethinyl estradiol (eth' in il ess tra dye' ole)
Brand Names Estinyl®
Therapeutic Category Estrogen Derivative
Use Atrophic vaginitis; hypogonadism; primary ovarian failure; vasomotor symptoms of menopause; prostatic carcinoma; osteoporosis prophylactic
Usual Dosage Adults: Oral:
Hypogonadism: 0.05 mg 1-3 times/day for 2 weeks

Prostatic carcinoma: 0.15-2 mg/day

Vasomotor symptoms: 0.02-0.05 mg for 21 days, off 7 days and repeat
Dosage Forms Tablet: 0.02 mg, 0.05 mg, 0.5 mg

ethinyl estradiol and desogestrel (lee' voe nor jess trel)
Brand Names Desogen®; Ortho-Cept™
Synonyms desogestrel and ethinyl estradiol
Therapeutic Category Contraceptive, Oral
Use Prevention of pregnancy
Usual Dosage
Contraception: Oral: 1 tablet daily, beginning on day 5 of menstrual cycle (first day of menstrual flow is day 1). With 21-tablet packages, new dosing cycle begins 7 days after last tablet taken. With 28-tablet packages, dosage is 1 tablet daily without interruption; extra tablets are placebos, If next menstrual period does not begin on schedule, rule out pregnancy before starting new dosing cycle. If menstrual period begins, start new dosing cycle 7 days after last tablet was taken. if all doses have been taken on schedule and 1 menstrual period is missed, continue dosing cycle. If 2 consecutive menstrual periods are missed, pregnancy test is required before new dosing cycle is started.
One dose missed: Take as soon as remembered or take 2 tablets next day
Two doses missed: Take 2 tablets as soon as remembered or 2 tablets next 2 days
Three doses missed: Begin new compact of tablets starting on day 1 of next cycle
Dosage Forms Tablet: Ethinyl estradiol 0.03 mg and desogestrel 0.15 mg (21s, 28s)

ethinyl estradiol and ethynodiol diacetate
(eth' in il ess tra dye' ole & e thye noe dye' ole)
Brand Names Demulen®
Synonyms ethynodiol diacetate and ethinyl estradiol
Therapeutic Category Contraceptive, Oral
Use Prevention of pregnancy; treatment of hypermenorrhea, endometriosis, female hypogonadism
Usual Dosage
For 21-tablet cycle packs, with 21 active tablets (28-day packs have 21 active tablets and 7 inert tablets): Take 1 tablet daily starting on the fifth day of menstrual cycle, with day 1 being the first day of menstruation; begin taking a new cycle pack on the eighth day after taking the last tablet from the previous pack

With 28-tablet packages, dosage is 1 tablet daily without interruption; extra tablets are placebos or contain iron. If next menstrual period does not begin on schedule, rule out pregnancy before starting new dosing cycle. If menstrual period begins, start new dosing cycle 7 days after last tablet was taken. if all doses have been taken on schedule and 1 menstrual period is missed, continue dosing cycle. If 2 consecutive menstrual periods are missed, pregnancy test is required before new dosing cycle is started.

One dose missed: Take as soon as remembered or take 2 tablets next day
Two doses missed: Take 2 tablets as soon as remembered or 2 tablets next 2 days
Three doses missed: Begin new compact of tablets starting on day 1 of next cycle
Dosage Forms Tablet:

1/35: Ethinyl estradiol 0.035 mg and ethynodiol diacetate 1 mg (21s, 28s)
1/50: Ethinyl estradiol 0.05 mg and ethynodiol diacetate 1 mg (21s, 28s)

ethinyl estradiol and fluoxymesterone
(eth i nil ess tra dye' ole & floo ox i mes' te rone)
Brand Names Halodrin®
Synonyms fluoxymesterone and estradiol
Therapeutic Category Androgen; Estrogen Derivative
Use Moderate to severe vasomotor symptoms of menopause, postpartum breast engorgement
Usual Dosage Oral: 1-2 tablets at bedtime given cyclically, 3 weeks on and 1 week off
Dosage Forms Tablet: Ethinyl estradiol 0.02 mg and fluoxymesterone 1 mg

ethinyl estradiol and levonorgestrel
(eth' in il ess tra dye' ole & lee' voe nor jess trel)
Brand Names Levlen®; Nordette®; Tri-Levlen®; Triphasil®
Synonyms levonorgestrel and ethinyl estradiol
Therapeutic Category Contraceptive, Oral
Use Prevention of pregnancy; treatment of hypermenorrhea, endometriosis, female hypogonadism
Usual Dosage
Contraception: Oral: 1 tablet daily, beginning on day 5 of menstrual cycle (first day of menstrual flow is day 1). With 20-tablet and 21-tablet packages, new dosing cycle begins 7 days after last tablet taken. With 28-tablet packages, dosage is 1 tablet daily without interruption; extra tablets are placebos or contain iron. If next menstrual period does not begin on schedule, rule out pregnancy before starting new dosing cycle. If menstrual period begins, start new dosing cycle 7 days after last tablet was taken. if all doses have been taken on schedule and 1 menstrual period is missed, continue dosing cycle. If 2 consecutive menstrual periods are missed, pregnancy test is required before new dosing cycle is started.

Triphasic oral contraceptive: 1 tablet/day in the sequence specified by the manufacturer
Dosage Forms Tablet:
Levlen®, Nordette®: Ethinyl estradiol 0.03 mg and levonorgestrel 0.15 mg (21s, 28s)
Tri-Levlen®, Triphasil®: Phase 1 (6 brown tablets): Ethinyl estradiol 0.03 mg and levonorgestrel 0.05 mg; Phase 2 (5 white tablets): Ethinyl estradiol 0.04 mg and levonorgestrel 0.075 mg; Phase 3 (10 yellow tablets): Ethinyl estradiol 0.03 mg and levonorgestrel 0.125 mg (21s, 28s)

ethinyl estradiol and norethindrone
(eth' in il ess tra dye' ole & nor eth in' drone)
Brand Names Brevicon®; Genora®; Loestrin®; Modicon™; N.E.E.® 1/35; Nelova™; Norcept-E® 1/35; Norethin™ 1/35E; Norinyl® 1+35; Norlestrin®; Ortho-Novum™ 1/35; Ortho-Novum™ 7/7/7; Ortho-Novum™ 10/11; Ovcon®; Tri-Norinyl®
Synonyms norethindrone acetate and ethinyl estradiol
Therapeutic Category Contraceptive, Oral
Use Prevention of pregnancy; treatment of hypermenorrhea, endometriosis, female hypogonadism
Usual Dosage
For 21-tablet cycle packs, with 21 active tablets (28-day packs have 21 active tablets and 7 inert tablets): Take 1 tablet daily starting on the fifth day of menstrual cycle, with day 1 being the first day of menstruation; begin taking a new cycle pack on the eighth day after taking the last tablet from the previous pack

With 28-tablet packages, dosage is 1 tablet daily without interruption; extra tablets are placebos or contain iron. If next menstrual period does not begin on schedule, rule out pregnancy before starting new dosing cycle. If menstrual period begins, start new dosing cycle 7 days after last tablet was taken. if all doses have been taken on schedule and 1

(Continued)
183

ethinyl estradiol and norethindrone *(Continued)*

menstrual period is missed, continue dosing cycle. If 2 consecutive menstrual periods are missed, pregnancy test is required before new dosing cycle is started.

One dose missed: Take as soon as remembered or take 2 tablets next day
Two doses missed: Take 2 tablets as soon as remembered or 2 tablets next 2 days
Three doses missed: Begin new compact of tablets starting on day 1 of next cycle

Biphasic oral contraceptive (Ortho-Novum™ 10/11): 1 color tablet/day for 10 days, then next color tablet for 11 days

Triphasic oral contraceptive (Ortho-Novum™ 7/7/7, Tri-Norinyl®, Triphasil®): 1 tablet/day in the sequence specified by the manufacturer

Dosage Forms Tablet:

Brevicon®, Genora® 0.5/35, Modicon™, Nelova™ 0.5/35E: Ethinyl estradiol 0.035 mg and norethindrone 0.5 mg (21s, 28s)

Loestrin® 1.5/30: Ethinyl estradiol 0.03 mg and norethindrone acetate 1.5 mg (21s)

Loestrin® Fe 1.5/30: Ethinyl estradiol 0.03 mg and norethindrone acetate 1.5 mg with ferrous fumarate 75 mg in 7 inert tablets (28s)

Loestrin® 1/20: Ethinyl estradiol 0.02 mg and norethindrone acetate 1 mg (21s)

Loestrin® Fe 1/20: Ethinyl estradiol 0.02 mg and norethindrone acetate 1 mg with ferrous fumarate 75 mg in 7 inert tablets (28s)

Genora® 1/35, N.E.E.® 1/35, Nelova® 1/35E, Norcept-E® 1/35, Norethin™ 1/35E, Norinyl® 1+35, Ortho-Novum™ 1/35: Ethinyl estradiol 0.035 mg and norethindrone 1 mg (21s, 28s)

Norlestrin® 1/50: Ethinyl estradiol 0.05 mg and norethindrone acetate 1 mg (21s, 28s)

Norlestrin® Fe 1/50: Ethinyl estradiol 0.05 mg and norethindrone acetate 1 mg with ferrous fumarate 75 mg in 7 inert tablets (28s)

Norlestrin® 2.5/50: Ethinyl estradiol 0.05 mg and norethindrone acetate 2.5 mg (21s)

Norlestrin® Fe 2.5/50: Ethinyl estradiol 0.05 mg and norethindrone acetate 2.5 mg with ferrous fumarate 75 mg in 7 inert tablets (28s)

Ortho-Novum™ 7/7/7: Phase 1 (7 white tablets): Ethinyl estradiol 0.035 mg and norethindrone 0.5 mg; Phase 2 (7 light peach tablets): Ethinyl estradiol 0.035 mg and norethindrone 0.75 mg; Phase 3 (7 peach tablets): Ethinyl estradiol 0.035 mg and norethindrone 1 mg (21s, 28s)

Ortho-Novum™ 10/11: Phase 1 (10 white tablets): Ethinyl estradiol 0.035 mg and norethindrone 0.5 mg; Phase 2 (11 dark yellow tablets): Ethinyl estradiol 0.035 mg and norethindrone 1 mg (21s, 28s)

Ovcon® 35: Ethinyl estradiol 0.035 mg and norethindrone 0.4 mg (21s, 28s)

Ovcon® 50: Ethinyl estradiol 0.050 mg and norethindrone 1 mg (21s, 28s)

Tri-Norinyl®: Phase 1 (7 blue tablets): Ethinyl estradiol 0.035 mg and norethindrone 0.5 mg; Phase 2 (9 green tablets): Ethinyl estradiol 0.035 mg and norethindrone 1 mg; Phase 3 (5 blue tablets): Ethinyl estradiol 0.035 mg and norethindrone 0.5 mg (21s, 28s)

ethinyl estradiol and norgestimate

Brand Names Ortho™ Tri-Cyclen®
Synonyms norgestimate and ethinyl estradiol
Therapeutic Category Contraceptive, Oral
Use Prevention of pregnancy
Usual Dosage

Contraception: Oral: 1 tablet daily, beginning on day 5 of menstrual cycle (first day of menstrual flow is day 1). With 21-tablet packages, new dosing cycle begins 7 days after last tablet taken. With 28-tablet packages, dosage is 1 tablet daily without interruption; extra tablets are placebos or contain iron. If next menstrual period does not begin on schedule, rule out pregnancy before starting new dosing cycle. If menstrual period begins, start new dosing cycle 7 days after last tablet was taken. if all doses have been taken on schedule and 1 menstrual period is missed, continue dosing cycle. If 2 consecutive menstrual periods are missed, pregnancy test is required before new dosing cycle is started.

One dose missed: Take as soon as remembered or take 2 tablets next day
Two doses missed: Take 2 tablets as soon as remembered or 2 tablets next 2 days
Three doses missed: Begin new compact of tablets starting on day 1 of next cycle

Triphasic oral contraceptive: 1 tablet/day in the sequence specified by the manufacturer
Dosage Forms Tablet: Phase 1 (7 white tablets): Ethinyl estradiol 0.035 mg and norgesti-

mate 0.18 mg; Phase 2 (5 light blue tablets): Ethinyl estradiol 0.035 mg and norgestimate 0.215 mg; Phase 3 (10 blue tablets): Ethinyl estradiol 0.035 mg and norgestimate 0.25 mg (21s, 28s)

ethinyl estradiol and norgestrel (eth' in il ess tra dye' ole & nor jess' trel)
Brand Names Lo/Ovral®; Ovral®
Synonyms norgestrel and ethinyl estradiol
Therapeutic Category Contraceptive, Oral
Use Prevention of pregnancy; treatment of hypermenorrhea, endometriosis, female hypogonadism
Usual Dosage Contraception: Oral: 1 tablet daily, beginning on day 5 of menstrual cycle (first day of menstrual flow is day 1). With 20-tablet and 21-tablet packages, new dosing cycle begins 7 days after last tablet taken; with 28-tablet packages, dosage is 1 tablet daily without interruption; extra tablets are placebos or contain iron. If next menstrual period does not begin on schedule, rule out pregnancy before starting new dosing cycle; if menstrual period begins, start new dosing cycle 7 days after last tablet was taken; if all doses have been taken on schedule and 1 menstrual period is missed, continue dosing cycle; if two consecutive menstrual periods are missed, pregnancy test is required before new dosing cycle is started.
    One dose missed: Take as soon as remembered or take 2 tablets next day
    Two doses missed: Take 2 tablets as soon as remembered or 2 tablets next 2 days
    Three doses missed: Begin new compact of tablets starting on day 1 of next cycle
Dosage Forms Tablet:
Lo/Ovral®: Ethinyl estradiol 0.03 mg and norgestrel 0.3 mg (21s and 28s)
Ovral®: Ethinyl estradiol 0.05 mg and norgestrel 0.5 mg (21s and 28s)

ethiodized oil *see* radiological/contrast media (ionic) *on page 413*
Ethiodol® *see* radiological/contrast media (ionic) *on page 413*

ethionamide (e thye on am' ide)
Brand Names Trecator®-SC
Therapeutic Category Antitubercular Agent
Use In conjunction with other antituberculosis agents in the treatment of tuberculosis and other mycobacterial diseases
Usual Dosage Oral:
Children: 15-20 mg/kg/day in 2 divided doses, not to exceed 1 g/day
Adults: 500-1000 mg/day in 1-3 divided doses
Dosage Forms Tablet, sugar coated: 250 mg

Ethmozine® *see* moricizine hydrochloride *on page 317*

ethopropazine hydrochloride (eth oh proe' pa zeen)
Brand Names Parsidol®
Therapeutic Category Antiparkinson Agent
Use Treatment of Parkinsonism, drug induced extrapyramidal reactions, and congenital athetosis
Usual Dosage Adults: Oral: 50-600 mg/day
Dosage Forms Tablet: 10 mg, 50 mg

ethosuximide (eth oh sux' i mide)
Brand Names Zarontin®
Therapeutic Category Anticonvulsant, Succinimide
Use Management of absence (petit mal) seizures, myoclonic seizures, and akinetic epilepsy
(Continued)

ethosuximide *(Continued)*
Usual Dosage Oral:
Children 3-6 years: Initial: 250 mg; increment: 250 mg/day at 4- to 7-day intervals; maintenance: 20-40 mg/kg/day; maximum: 1500 mg/day in 2 divided doses

Children >6 years and Adults: Initial: 500 mg/day; maintenance: 20-40 mg/kg/day; increment: 250 mg/day at 4- to 7-day intervals; maximum: 1500 mg/day in 2 divided doses
Dosage Forms
Capsule: 250 mg
Syrup (raspberry flavor): 250 mg/5 mL (473 mL)

ethotoin (eth' o toin)
Brand Names Peganone®
Synonyms ethylphenylhydantoin
Therapeutic Category Anticonvulsant, Hydantoin
Use Generalized tonic-clonic or complex-partial seizures
Usual Dosage Oral:
Children: 250 mg twice daily, up to 250 mg 4 times/day

Adults: 250 mg 4 times/day after meals, may be increased up to 3 g/day in divided doses 4 times/day
Dosage Forms Tablet: 250 mg, 500 mg

ethoxynaphthamido penicillin sodium *see* nafcillin sodium *on page 322*

Ethrane® *see* enflurane *on page 169*

ethyl aminobenzoate *see* benzocaine *on page 48*

ethyl chloride
Synonyms chloroethane
Therapeutic Category Local Anesthetic, Topical
Use Local anesthetic in minor operative procedures and to relieve pain caused by insect stings and burns, and irritation caused by myofascial and visceral pain syndromes
Usual Dosage Dosage varies with use
Dosage Forms Spray: 100 mL, 120 mL

ethyl chloride and dichlorotetrafluoroethane
Brand Names Fluro-Ethyl® Aerosol
Synonyms dichlorotetrafluoroethane and ethyl chloride
Therapeutic Category Local Anesthetic, Topical
Use Topical refrigerant anesthetic to control pain associated with minor surgical procedures, dermabrasion, injections, contusions, and minor strains
Usual Dosage Press gently on side of spray valve allowing the liquid to emerge as a fine mist approximately 2" to 4" from site of application
Dosage Forms Aerosol: Ethyl chloride 25% and dichlorotetrafluoroethane 75% (225 g)

ethylnorepinephrine hydrochloride (eth il nor ep i nef' rin)
Brand Names Bronkephrine® Injection
Therapeutic Category Adrenergic Agonist Agent; Bronchodilator
Use Bronchial asthma and reversible bronchospasm
Usual Dosage I.M., S.C.:
Children: Usually 0.1-0.5 mL
Adults: 0.5-1 mL
Dosage Forms Injection: 2 mg/mL (1 mL)

ethylphenylhydantoin *see* ethotoin *on this page*

ethynodiol diacetate and ethinyl estradiol *see* ethinyl estradiol and ethynodiol diacetate *on page 182*

etidocaine hydrochloride (e ti' doe kane)
Brand Names Duranest® Injection
Therapeutic Category Local Anesthetic, Injectable
Use Infiltration anesthesia; peripheral nerve blocks; central neural blocks
Usual Dosage Varies with procedure; use 1% for peripheral nerve block, central nerve block, lumbar peridural caudal; use 1.5% for maxillary infiltration or inferior alveolar nerve block; use 1% or 1.5% for intra-abdominal or pelvic surgery, lower limb surgery, or caesarean section
Dosage Forms
Injection: 1% [10 mg/mL] (30 mL)
Injection, with epinephrine 1:200,000: 1% [10 mg/mL] (30 mL); 1.5% [15 mg/mL] (20 mL)

etidronate disodium (e ti droe' nate)
Brand Names Didronel® I.V.; Didronel® Oral
Synonyms EHDP; sodium etidronate
Therapeutic Category Antidote, Hypercalcemia; Biphosphonate Derivative
Use Symptomatic treatment of Paget's disease and heterotopic ossification due to spinal cord injury or after total hip replacement, hypercalcemia associated with malignancy
Usual Dosage Adults: Oral:
Paget's disease: 5 mg/kg/day given every day for no more than 6 months; may give 10 mg/kg/day for up to 3 months. Daily dose may be divided if adverse GI effects occur.

Heterotopic ossification with spinal cord injury: 20 mg/kg/day for 2 weeks, then 10 mg/kg/day for 10 weeks (This dosage has been used in children, however, treatment greater than 1 year has been associated with a rachitic syndrome.)

Hypercalcemia associated with malignancy. I.V.. 7.5 mg/kg/day for 3 days
Dosage Forms
Injection: 50 mg/mL (6 mL)
Tablet: 200 mg, 400 mg

etodolac (ee toe doe' lak)
Brand Names Lodine®
Therapeutic Category Analgesic, Non-Narcotic; Anti-inflammatory Agent; Nonsteroidal Anti-Inflammatory Agent (NSAID), Oral
Use Acute and long-term use in the management of signs and symptoms of osteoarthritis and management of pain
Usual Dosage Adults: Oral:
Acute pain: 200-400 mg every 6-8 hours, as needed, not to exceed total daily doses of 1200 mg
Osteoarthritis: Initial: 800-1200 mg/day given in divided doses: 400 mg 2 or 3 times/day; 300 mg 2, 3 or 4 times/day; 200 mg 3 or 4 times/day; total daily dose should not exceed 1200 mg; for patients weighing <60 kg, total daily dose should not exceed 20 mg/kg
Dosage Forms Capsule: 200 mg, 300 mg

etomidate (e tom' i date)
Brand Names Amidate® Injection
Therapeutic Category General Anesthetic
Use Induction of general anesthesia
Usual Dosage Children > 10 years and Adults: I.V.: 0.2-0.6 mg/kg over period of 30-60 seconds
Dosage Forms Injection: 2 mg/mL (10 mL, 20 mL)

etoposide (e toe poe' side)
Brand Names VePesid® Injection; VePesid® Oral
Synonyms EPEG; VP-16
Therapeutic Category Antineoplastic Agent, Miotic Inhibitor
Use Treatment of testicular and lung carcinomas, malignant lymphoma, Hodgkin's disease, leukemias, neuroblastoma; etoposide has also been used in the treatment of Ewing's sarcoma, rhabdomyosarcoma, Wilms' tumor and brain tumors
Usual Dosage Refer to individual protocols

Pediatric solid tumors: I.V.: 60-120 mg/m²/day for 3-5 days every 3-6 weeks

Leukemia in children: I.V.: 100-200 mg/m²/day for 5 days

Testicular cancer: I.V.: 50-100 mg/m²/day on days 1-5 or 100 mg/m²/day on days 1, 3 and 5 every 3-4 weeks for 3-4 courses

Small cell lung cancer:
> Oral: Twice the I.V. dose rounded to the nearest 50 mg given once daily if total dose ≤400 mg or in divided doses if >400 mg
> I.V.: 35 mg/m²/day for 4 days or 50 mg/m²/day for 5 days every 3-4 weeks

Dosage Forms
Capsule: 50 mg
Injection: 20 mg/mL (5 mL)

Etrafon® *see* amitriptyline and perphenazine *on page 21*

etretinate (e tret' i nate)
Brand Names Tegison®
Therapeutic Category Antipsoriatic Agent, Systemic
Use Treatment of severe recalcitrant psoriasis in patients intolerant of or unresponsive to standard therapies
Usual Dosage Adults: Oral: Individualized; Initial: 0.75-1 mg/kg/day in divided doses up to 1.5 mg/kg/day; maintenance dose established after 8-10 weeks of therapy 0.5-0.75 mg/kg/day
Dosage Forms Capsule: 10 mg, 25 mg

ETS-2%® Topical *see* erythromycin, topical *on page 176*

Eudal-SR® *see* guaifenesin and pseudoephedrine *on page 220*

Eulexin® *see* flutamide *on page 205*

Eurax® Topical *see* crotamiton *on page 119*

Euthroid® *see* liotrix *on page 275*

Eutron® *see* methyclothiazide and pargyline *on page 303*

Evac-Q-Mag® [OTC] *see* magnesium citrate *on page 282*

Evac-U-Gen® [OTC] *see* phenolphthalein *on page 370*

Evac-U-Lax® [OTC] *see* phenolphthalein *on page 370*

Everone® Injection *see* testosterone *on page 456*

E-Vista® Injection *see* hydroxyzine *on page 241*

Excedrin®, Extra Strength [OTC] *see* acetaminophen and aspirin *on page 3*

Excedrin® IB [OTC] *see* ibuprofen *on page 245*

Exelderm® Topical *see* sulconazole nitrate *on page 446*

Exidine® Scrub [OTC] *see* chlorhexidine gluconate *on page 90*

Ex-Lax® [OTC] *see* phenolphthalein *on page 370*

Ex-Lax®, Extra Gentle Pills [OTC] *see* docusate and phenolphthalein *on page 158*

Exna® *see* benzthiazide *on page 50*

Exosurf® Neonatal *see* colfosceril palmitate *on page 114*

Exsel® Shampoo *see* selenium sulfide *on page 428*

Extendryl® SR *see* chlorpheniramine, phenylephrine, and methscopolamine *on page 95*

Extra Action Cough Syrup [OTC] *see* guaifenesin and dextromethorphan *on page 218*

Eye-Sed® Ophthalmic [OTC] *see* zinc sulfate *on page 504*

Eyesine® Ophthalmic [OTC] *see* tetrahydrozoline hydrochloride *on page 459*

Eye-Zine® Ophthalmic [OTC] *see* tetrahydrozoline hydrochloride *on page 459*

EZ-Detect® [OTC] *see* diagnostic aids (*in vitro*), feces *on page 138*

Ezide® *see* hydrochlorothiazide *on page 233*

F₃T *see* trifluridine *on page 478*

factor viii:c (porcine)

Brand Names Hyate®:C

Synonyms antihemophilic factor (porcine)

Therapeutic Category Hemophilic Agent

Use Treatment of congenital hemophiliacs with antibodies to human factor VIII:C and also for previously nonhemophiliac patients with spontaneously acquired inhibitors to human factor VIII:C; patients with inhibitors who are bleeding or who are to undergo surgery

Usual Dosage

Clinical response should be used to assess efficacy rather than relying upon a particular laboratory value for recovery of factor VIII:C.

Initial dose:

Antibody level to human factor VIII:C <50 BU/mL: Initial: 100-150 porcine units/kg (body weight) is recommended

Antibody level to human factor VIII:C >50 BU/mL: Activity of the antibody to porcine factor VIII:C should be determined; an antiporcine antibody level of >20 BU/mL indicates that the patient is unlikely to benefit from treatment; for lower titers, a dose of 100-150 porcine units/kg is recommended

If a patient has previously been treated with Hyate®:C, this may provide a guide a to his likely response and therefore assist in estimation of the preliminary dose

Subsequent doses: Following administration of the initial dose, if the recovery of factor VIII:C in the patient's plasma is not sufficient, a further higher dose should be administered. If recovery after the second dose is still insufficient a third and higher dose may prove effective

Dosage Forms Powder for injection, lyophilized: 400-700 porcine units to be reconstituted with 20 mL sterile water

factor ix complex (human)

Brand Names AlphaNine®; Konȳne® 80; Mononine®; Profilnine® Heat-Treated; Proplex® SX-T; Proplex® T

Therapeutic Category Antihemophilic Agent; Blood Product Derivative

Use Control bleeding in patients with factor IX deficiency (Hemophilia B or Christmas Disease); prevention/control of bleeding in hemophilia A patients with inhibitors to factor VIII

Usual Dosage Factor IX deficiency (1 unit/kg raises IX levels 1%): Children and Adults: I.V.:

Hospitalized patients: 20-50 units/kg/dose; may be higher in special cases; may be given every 24 hours or more often in special cases

Inhibitor patients: 75-100 units/kg/dose; may be given every 6-12 hours

Dosage Forms Injection:

AlphaNine®: 500 units, 1000 units, 1500 units

Konȳne® 80: 10 mL, 20 mL

(Continued)

factor ix complex (human) *(Continued)*
Mononine®: 250 units, 500 units, 1000 units
Profilnine® Heat-Treated: Single dose vial
Proplex® SX-T: Vial
Proplex® T: Vial

factor viii *see* antihemophilic factor *on page 29*
Fact Plus® *see* diagnostic aids (*in vitro*), urine *on page 139*
Factrel® Injection *see* gonadorelin *on page 215*

famotidine (fa moe' ti deen)
Brand Names Pepcid® I.V.; Pepcid® Oral
Therapeutic Category Histamine-2 Antagonist
Use Therapy and treatment of duodenal ulcer, gastric ulcer, control gastric pH in critically ill patients, symptomatic relief in gastritis, gastroesophageal reflux, active benign ulcer, and pathological hypersecretory conditions
Usual Dosage
Children: Oral, I.V.: Doses of 1-2 mg/kg/day have been used; maximum dose: 40 mg
Adults:
Oral:
Duodenal ulcer, gastric ulcer: 40 mg/day at bedtime for 4-8 weeks
Hypersecretory conditions: Initial: 20 mg every 6 hours, may increase up to 160 mg every 6 hours
GERD: 20 mg twice daily for 6 weeks
I.V.: 20 mg every 12 hours
Dosage Forms
Injection: 10 mg/mL (2 mL, 4 mL)
Powder for oral suspension (cherry-banana-mint flavor): 40 mg/5 mL (50 mL)
Tablet, film coated: 20 mg, 40 mg

Fansidar® *see* sulfadoxine and pyrimethamine *on page 447*
Fastin® *see* phentermine hydrochloride *on page 371*

fat emulsion
Brand Names Intralipid®; Liposyn®
Synonyms intravenous fat emulsion
Therapeutic Category Caloric Agent; Intravenous Nutritional Therapy
Use Source of calories and essential fatty acids for patients requiring parenteral nutrition of extended duration
Usual Dosage Fat emulsion should not exceed 60% of the total daily calories

Premature infants: Initial dose: 0.25-0.5 g/kg/day, increase by 0.25-0.5 g/kg/day to a maximum of 3-4 g/kg/day; maximum rate of infusion: 0.15 g/kg/hour (0.75 mL/kg/hour of 20% solution)

Infants and Children: Initial dose: 0.5-1 g/kg/day, increase by 0.5 g/kg/day to a maximum of 3-4 g/kg/day; maximum rate of infusion: 0.25 g/kg/hour (1.25 mL/kg/hour of 20% solution)

Children and Adults: Fatty acid deficiency: 8% to 10% of total caloric intake; infuse once or twice weekly

Adolescents and Adults: Initial dose: 1 g/kg/day, increase by 0.5-1 g/kg/day to a maximum of 2.5 g/kg/day; maximum rate of infusion: 0.25 g/kg/hour (1.25 mL/kg/hour of 20% solution); do not exceed 50 mL/hour (20%) or 100 mL/hour (10%)

Note: At the onset of therapy, the patient should be observed for any immediate allergic reactions such as dyspnea, cyanosis, and fever. Slower initial rates of infusion may be used for the first 10-15 minutes of the infusion, eg, 0.1 mL/minute of 10% of 0.05 mL/ minute of 20% solution.

Dosage Forms Injection: 10% [100 mg/mL] (100 mL, 250 mL, 500 mL); 20% [200 mg/mL] (100 mL, 250 mL, 500 mL)

5-FC *see* flucytosine *on page 198*

Fedahist® Expectorant [OTC] *see* guaifenesin and pseudoephedrine *on page 220*

Fedahist® Expectorant Pediatric [OTC] *see* guaifenesin and pseudoephedrine *on page 220*

Fedahist® Timecaps® *see* chlorpheniramine and pseudoephedrine *on page 94*

Feen-a-Mint® [OTC] *see* phenolphthalein *on page 370*

Feen-a-Mint® Pills [OTC] *see* docusate and phenolphthalein *on page 158*

Feiba VH Immuno® *see* anti-inhibitor coagulant complex *on page 29*

felbamate (fel' ba mate)

Brand Names Felbatol™

Therapeutic Category Anticonvulsant, Miscellaneous

Use Monotherapy and adjunctive therapy in patients 14 years of age and older with partial and secondarily generalized seizures; adjunctive therapy in children 2 years of age and older who have partial and generalized seizures associated with Lennox-Gastaut syndrome

Usual Dosage

Monotherapy: 1200 mg/day in divided doses 3 or 4 times/day; titrate previously untreated patients under close clinical supervision, increasing the dosage in 600 mg increments every 2 weeks to 2400 mg/day based on clinical response and thereafter to 3600 mg/day if clinically indicated

Conversion to monotherapy: Initiate at 1200 mg/day in divided doses 3 or 4 times/day, reduce the dosage of the concomitant anticonvulsant(s) by 33% at the initiation of felbamate therapy; at week 2, increase the felbamate dosage to 2400 mg/day while reducing the dosage of the other anticonvulsant(s) up to an additional 33% of their original dosage; at week 3, increase the felbamate dosage up to 3600 mg/day and continue to reduce the dosage of the other anticonvulsant(s) as clinically indicated

Adjunctive therapy:
Week 1:
Felbamate: 1200 mg/day initial dose
Concomitant anticonvulsant(s): Reduce original dosage by 20% to 33%
Week 2:
Felbamate: 2400 mg/day (Therapeutic range)
Concomitant anticonvulsant(s): Reduce original dosage by up to an additional 33%
Week 3:
Felbamate: 3600 mg/day (Therapeutic range)
Concomitant anticonvulsant(s): Reduce original dosage as clinically indicated

Dosage Forms

Suspension, oral: 600 mg/5 mL (240 mL, 960 mL)
Tablet: 400 mg, 600 mg

Felbatol™ *see* felbamate *on this page*

Feldene® *see* piroxicam *on page 380*

felodipine (fe loe' di peen)

Brand Names Plendil®

Therapeutic Category Calcium Channel Blocker

Use Management of angina pectoris due to coronary insufficiency, hypertension

(Continued)

felodipine *(Continued)*
Usual Dosage Adults: Oral: 5-10 mg once daily
Dosage Forms Tablet, extended release: 5 mg, 10 mg

Femcet® *see* butalbital compound *on page 63*
Femilax® [OTC] *see* docusate and phenolphthalein *on page 158*
Femiron® [OTC] *see* ferrous fumarate *on next page*
Femstat® *see* butoconazole nitrate *on page 63*
Fenesin™ [OTC] *see* guaifenesin *on page 217*

fenfluramine hydrochloride (fen flure' a meen)
Brand Names Pondimin®
Therapeutic Category Adrenergic Agonist Agent; Anorexiant
Use Short-term adjunct in exogenous obesity
Usual Dosage Adults: Oral: 20 mg 3 times/day before meals or food, up to 40 mg 3 times/day
Dosage Forms Tablet: 20 mg

fenoprofen calcium (fen oh proe' fen)
Brand Names Nalfon®
Therapeutic Category Analgesic, Non-Narcotic; Anti-inflammatory Agent; Nonsteroidal Anti-Inflammatory Agent (NSAID), Oral
Use Symptomatic treatment of acute and chronic rheumatoid arthritis and osteoarthritis; relief of mild to moderate pain
Usual Dosage Oral:
Children: Juvenile arthritis: 900 mg/m^2/day, then increase over 4 weeks to 1.8 g/m^2/day
Adults:
   Arthritis: 300-600 mg 3-4 times/day up to 3.2 g/day
   Pain: 200 mg every 4-6 hours as needed
Dosage Forms
Capsule: 200 mg, 300 mg
Tablet: 600 mg

fentanyl and droperidol *see* droperidol and fentanyl *on page 163*

fentanyl citrate (fen' ta nil sit' rate)
Brand Names Duragesic™ Transdermal; Sublimaze® Injection
Therapeutic Category Analgesic, Narcotic; General Anesthetic
Use Sedation; relief of pain; preoperative medication; adjunct to general or regional anesthesia; management of chronic pain (transdermal product)
Usual Dosage Doses should be titrated to appropriate effects; wide range of doses, dependent upon desired degree of analgesia/anesthesia
Children:
   Sedation for minor procedures/analgesia: I.M., I.V.:
      1-3 years: 2-3 μg/kg/dose; may repeat after 30-60 minutes as required
      3-12 years: 1-2 μg/kg/dose; may repeat at 30- to 60-minute intervals as required.
      Note: Children 18-36 months of age may require 2-3 μg/kg/dose
   Continuous sedation/analgesia: Initial I.V. bolus: 1-2 μg/kg then 1 μg/kg/hour; titrate upward; usual: 1-3 μg/kg/hour
   Transdermal: Not recommended
Children <12 years and Adults:
   Sedation for minor procedures/analgesia: 0.5-1 μg/kg/dose; higher doses are used for major procedures

Preoperative sedation, adjunct to regional anesthesia, postoperative pain: I.M., I.V.: 50-100 μg/dose

Adjunct to general anesthesia: I.M., I.V.: 2-50 μg/kg

General anesthesia without additional anesthetic agents: I.V. 50-100 μg/kg with O_2 and skeletal muscle relaxant

Transdermal: Initial: 25 μg/hour system; if currently receiving opiates, convert to fentanyl equivalent and administer equianalgesic dosage (see package insert for further information)

Dosage Forms

Injection, as citrate: 0.05 mg/mL (2 mL, 5 mL, 10 mL, 20 mL, 50 mL)

Transdermal system: 25 μg/hour [10 cm^2]; 50 μg/hour [20 cm^2]; 75 μg/hour [30 cm^2]; 100 μg/hour [40 cm^2] all available in 5's

Feosol® [OTC] *see* ferrous sulfate *on next page*

Feostat® [OTC] *see* ferrous fumarate *on this page*

Feratab® [OTC] *see* ferrous sulfate *on next page*

Fergon® [OTC] *see* ferrous gluconate *on next page*

Fer-In-Sol® [OTC] *see* ferrous sulfate *on next page*

Fer-Iron® [OTC] *see* ferrous sulfate *on next page*

Ferndex® *see* dextroamphetamine sulfate *on page 135*

Fero-Grad 500® [OTC] *see* ferrous sulfate and ascorbic acid *on next page*

Fero-Gradumet® [OTC] *see* ferrous sulfate *on next page*

Ferospace® [OTC] *see* ferrous sulfate *on next page*

Ferralet® [OTC] *see* ferrous gluconate *on next page*

Ferralyn® Lanacaps® [OTC] *see* ferrous sulfate *on next page*

Ferra-TD® [OTC] *see* ferrous sulfate *on next page*

Ferro-Sequels® [OTC] *see* ferrous fumarate *on this page*

ferrous fumarate (fair' us fyoo' ma rate)

Brand Names Femiron® [OTC]; Feostat® [OTC]; Ferro-Sequels® [OTC]; Fumasorb® [OTC]; Fumerin® [OTC]; Hemocyte® [OTC]; Ircon® [OTC]; Nephro-Fer™ [OTC]; Span-FF® [OTC]

Therapeutic Category Iron Salt

Use Prevention and treatment of iron deficiency anemias

Usual Dosage

Children: 3 mg/kg 3 times/day

Adults: 200 mg 3-4 times/day

Dosage Forms Amount of elemental iron is listed in brackets

Capsule, controlled release (Span-FF®): 325 mg [106 mg]

Drops (Feostat®): 45 mg/0.6 mL [15 mg/0.6 mL] (60 mL)

Suspension, oral (Feostat®): 100 mg/5 mL [33 mg/5 mL] (240 mL)

Tablet:

325 mg [106 mg]

Chewable (chocolate flavor) (Feostat®): 100 mg [33 mg]

Femiron®: 63 mg [20 mg]

Fumerin®: 195 mg [64 mg]

Fumasorb®, Ircon®: 200 mg [66 mg]

Hemocyte®: 324 mg [106 mg]

Nephro-Fer™: 350 mg [115 mg]

Timed release (Ferro-Sequels®): Ferrous fumarate 150 mg [50 mg] and docusate sodium 100 mg

ferrous gluconate (fair' us gloo' koe nate)
Brand Names Fergon® [OTC]; Ferralet® [OTC]; Simron® [OTC]
Therapeutic Category Iron Salt
Use Prevention and treatment of iron deficiency anemias
Usual Dosage Oral (dose expressed in terms of elemental iron):
Iron deficiency anemia: 3-6 Fe mg/kg/day in 3 divided doses

Maintenance:
Preterm infants:
Birthweight <1000 g: 4 Fe mg/kg/day
Birthweight 1000-1500 g: 3 Fe mg/kg/day
Birthweight 1500-2500 g: 2 Fe mg/kg/day
Term Infants and Children: 1-2 Fe mg/kg/day in 3 divided doses, up to a maximum of 18 Fe mg/day
Adults: 60-100 Fe mg/day in 3 divided doses

Dosage Forms Amount of elemental iron is listed in brackets
Capsule, soft gelatin (Simron®): 86 mg [10 mg]
Elixir (Fergon®): 300 mg/5 mL [34 mg/5 mL] with alcohol 7% (480 mL)
Tablet:
300 mg [34 mg]
325 mg [38 mg]
Fergon®, Ferralet®: 320 mg [37 mg]
Sustained release (Ferralet® Slow Release): 320 mg [37 mg]

ferrous sulfate (fair' us sul fate)
Brand Names Feosol® [OTC]; Feratab® [OTC]; Fer-In-Sol® [OTC]; Fer-Iron® [OTC]; Fero-Gradumet® [OTC]; Ferospace® [OTC]; Ferralyn® Lanacaps® [OTC]; Ferra-TD® [OTC]; Mol-Iron® [OTC]; Slow FE® [OTC]
Synonyms FeSO$_4$
Therapeutic Category Iron Salt
Use Prevention and treatment of iron deficiency anemias
Usual Dosage Oral (dose expressed in terms of elemental iron):
Children:
Severe iron deficiency anemia: 4-6 mg Fe/kg/day in 3 divided doses
Mild to moderate iron deficiency anemia: 3 mg Fe/kg/day in 1-2 divided doses
Prophylaxis: 1-2 mg Fe/kg/day up to a maximum of 15 mg/day

Adults: Iron deficiency: 60-100 Fe/kg/day in divided doses
Dosage Forms Amount of elemental iron is listed in brackets
Capsule:
Exsiccated (Fer-In-Sol®): 190 mg [60 mg]
Exsiccated, timed release (Feosol®): 159 mg [50 mg]
Exsiccated, timed release (Ferralyn® Lanacaps®, Ferra-TD®): 250 mg [50 mg]
Ferospace®: 250 mg [50 mg]
Drops, oral:
Fer-In-Sol®: 75 mg/0.6 mL [15 mg/0.6 mL] (50 mL)
Fer-Iron®: 125 mg/mL [25 mg/mL] (50 mL)
Elixir (Feosol®): 220 mg/5 mL [44 mg/5 mL] with alcohol 5% (473 mL, 4000 mL)
Syrup (Fer-In-Sol®): 90 mg/5 mL [18 mg/5 mL] with alcohol 5% (480 mL)
Tablet:
324 mg [65 mg]
Exsiccated (Feosol®) 200 mg [65 mg]
Exsiccated, timed release (Slow FE®): 160 mg [50 mg]
Feratab®: 300 mg [60 mg]
Mol-Iron®: 195 mg [39 mg]
Timed release (Fero-Gradumet®): 525 mg [105 mg]

ferrous sulfate and ascorbic acid
Brand Names Fero-Grad 500® [OTC]
Synonyms ascorbic acid and ferrous sulfate
Therapeutic Category Iron Salt; Vitamin

Use Treatment of iron deficiency in nonpregnant adults; treatment and prevention of iron deficiency in pregnant adults
Usual Dosage Adults: Oral: 1 tablet daily
Dosage Forms Tablet: Ferrous sulfate 525 mg and ascorbic acid 500 mg

ferrous sulfate, ascorbic acid, and vitamin B-complex
Brand Names Iberet®-Liquid [OTC]
Therapeutic Category Iron Salt; Vitamin
Use Conditions of iron deficiency with an increased needed for B-complex vitamins and vitamin C
Usual Dosage Oral:
Children 1-3 years: 5 mL twice daily after meals
Children >4 years and Adults: 10 mL 3 times/day after meals
Dosage Forms Liquid: Ferrous sulfate 78.75 mg, ascorbic acid 375 mg, B_1 4.5 mg, B_2 4.5 mg, B_3 22.5 mg, B_5 7.5 mg, B_6 3.75 mg, B_{12} 18.75 mg all per 15 mL

ferrous sulfate, ascorbic acid, vitamin B-complex, and folic acid
Brand Names Iberet-Folic-500®
Therapeutic Category Iron Salt; Vitamin
Use Treatment of iron deficiency and prevention of concomitant folic acid deficiency where there is an associated deficient intake or increased need for B-complex vitamins
Usual Dosage Adults: Oral: 1 tablet daily
Dosage Forms Tablet, controlled release: Ferrous sulfate 105 mg, ascorbic acid 500 mg, B_1 6 mg, B_2 6 mg, B_3 30 mg, B_5 10 mg, B_6 5 mg, B_{12} 25 μg, Folic acid 800 μg

$FeSO_4$ see ferrous sulfate on previous page

Festal® II see pancrelipase on page 354

Feverall™ [OTC] see acetaminophen on page 2

Fiberall® Chewable Tablet [OTC] see calcium polycarbophil on page 69

Fiberall® Powder [OTC] see psyllium on page 407

Fiberall® Wafer [OTC] see psyllium on page 407

FiberCon® Tablet [OTC] see calcium polycarbophil on page 69

Fiber-Lax® Tablet [OTC] see calcium polycarbophil on page 69

FiberNorm® [OTC] see calcium polycarbophil on page 69

fibrinolysin and desoxyribonuclease
(fye bri noe lye' sin & des oxy ribe oh nuke' lee ase)
Brand Names Elase-Chloromycetin® Topical; Elase® Topical
Synonyms desoxyribonuclease and fibrinolysin
Therapeutic Category Enzyme, Topical Debridement
Use Debriding agent; cervicitis; and irrigating agent in infected wounds
Usual Dosage
Ointment: 2-3 times/day
Wet dressing: 3-4 times/day
Dosage Forms
Ointment, topical:
Elase®: Fibrinolysin 1 unit and desoxyribonuclease 666.6 units per g (10 g, 30 g)
Elase-Chloromycetin®: Fibrinolysin 1 unit and desoxyribonuclease 666.6 units per g with chloramphenicol 10 mg per g (10 g, 30 g)
Powder, dry: Fibrinolysin 25 units and desoxyribonuclease 15,000 units per 30 g

filgrastim (fil gra' stim)
Brand Names Neupogen® Injection
Synonyms G-CSF; granulocyte colony stimulating factor
Therapeutic Category Colony Stimulating Factor
(Continued)
195

filgrastim *(Continued)*
Use Decrease the period of neutropenia and the associated risk of infection in patients with nonmyeloid malignancies receiving myelosuppressive chemotherapeutic regimens associated with a significant incidence of severe neutropenia with fever; it has also been used in AIDS patients on zidovudine and in patients with noncancer chemotherapy-induced neutropenia

Usual Dosage Children and Adults (refer to individual protocols): I.V., S.C.: 5-10 μg/kg/day (approximately 150-300 μg/m^2/day) once daily for up to 14 days until ANC = 10,000/mm^3; dose escalations at 5 μg/kg/day may be required in some individuals when response at 5 μg/kg/day is not adequate; dosages of 0.6-120 μg/kg/day have been used in children ranging in age from 3 months to 18 years

Dosage Forms Injection, preservative free: 300 μg/mL (1 mL, 1.6 mL)

Filibon® [OTC] *see* vitamin, multiple (prenatal) *on page 499*

finasteride (fi nas' teer ide)
Brand Names Proscar® Oral
Therapeutic Category Antiandrogen
Use Early data indicate that finasteride is useful in the treatment of benign prostatic hyperplasia
Usual Dosage Refer to individual protocols
Adults: Benign prostatic hyperplasia: Oral: 5 mg/day as a single dose; clinical responses occur within 12 weeks to 6 months of initiation of therapy; long-term administration is recommended for maximal response
Dosage Forms Tablet, film coated: 5 mg

Fiorgen PF® *see* butalbital compound *on page 63*
Fioricet® *see* butalbital compound *on page 63*
Fiorinal® *see* butalbital compound *on page 63*
Fiorinal® With Codeine *see* butalbital compound and codeine *on page 63*
First Response® *see* diagnostic aids (*in vitro*), urine *on page 139*
fisalamine *see* mesalamine *on page 294*
Flagyl® Oral *see* metronidazole *on page 309*
Flarex® Ophthalmic *see* fluorometholone *on page 202*
Flatulex [OTC] *see* simethicone *on page 431*
Flavorcee® [OTC] *see* ascorbic acid *on page 33*

flavoxate hydrochloride (fla vox' ate)
Brand Names Urispas®
Therapeutic Category Antispasmodic Agent, Urinary
Use Antispasmodic to provide symptomatic relief of dysuria, nocturia, suprapubic pain, urgency, and incontinence
Usual Dosage Children >12 years and Adults: 100-200 mg 3-4 times/day
Dosage Forms Tablet, film coated: 100 mg

Flaxedil® *see* gallamine triethiodide *on page 208*

flecainide acetate (fle kay' nide)
Brand Names Tambocor®
Therapeutic Category Antiarrhythmic Agent, Class Ic
Use Prevention and suppression of documented life-threatening ventricular arrhythmias (ie, sustained ventricular tachycardia); controlling symptomatic, disabling supraventricular tachycardias in patients without structural heart disease

Usual Dosage Oral:
Children: Initial: 3 mg/kg/day in 3 divided doses; usual 3-6 mg/kg/day in 3 divided doses; up to 11 mg/kg/day for uncontrolled patients with subtherapeutic levels

Adults: Initial: 100 mg every 12 hours, increase by 100 mg/day (given in 2 doses/day) every 4 days to maximum of 400 mg/day; for patients receiving 400 mg/day who are not controlled and have trough concentrations <0.6 µg/mL, dosage may be increased to 600 mg/day

Dosage Forms Tablet: 50 mg, 100 mg, 150 mg

Fleet® Babylax® Rectal [OTC] see glycerin on page 214

Fleet® Enema [OTC] see sodium phosphate on page 437

Fleet® Flavored Castor Oil [OTC] see castor oil on page 77

Fleet® Laxative [OTC] see bisacodyl on page 54

Fleet® Phospho®-Soda [OTC] see sodium phosphate on page 437

Flexaphen® see chlorzoxazone on page 99

Flexeril® see cyclobenzaprine hydrochloride on page 121

Flo-Coat® see radiological/contrast media (ionic) on page 413

Florical® [OTC] see calcium carbonate on page 65

Florinef® Acetate see fludrocortisone acetate on page 199

Florone® E Topical see diflorasone diacetate on page 146

Florone® Topical see diflorasone diacetate on page 146

Floropryl® Ophthalmic see isoflurophate on page 257

Florvite® see vitamin, multiple (pediatric) on page 499

flosequinan (floe se' kwi nan)
Brand Names Manoplax®
Therapeutic Category Vasodilator, Peripheral
Use Management of congestive heart failure (CHF) in patients not responding to diuretics, with or without digitalis, who cannot tolerate an angiotensin-converting enzyme (ACE) inhibitor or who have not responded to a regimen including an ACE inhibitor
Usual Dosage Adults: Oral:
Patients not receiving ACE inhibitors: 100 mg administered daily as a single dose in the morning, if tolerated

Patients receiving concomitant ACE inhibitors: Initial: 50 mg once daily in the morning, titrating upward at weekly intervals up to 100 mg once daily up to 150 mg/day
Dosage Forms Tablet, film coated: 50 mg, 75 mg, 100 mg

Floxin® Injection see ofloxacin on page 343

Floxin® Oral see ofloxacin on page 343

floxuridine (flox yoor' i deen)
Brand Names FUDR®
Synonyms fluorodeoxyuridine
Therapeutic Category Antineoplastic Agent, Antimetabolite
Use Palliative management of carcinomas of head, neck, and brain as well as liver, gallbladder, and bile ducts
Usual Dosage Refer to individual protocols
Adults:
Intra-arterial infusion: 0.1-0.6 mg/kg/day for 14 days followed by heparinized saline for 14 days
(Continued)

197

floxuridine *(Continued)*

Investigational: I.V.: 0.5-1 mg/kg/day for 6-15 days
Dosage Forms
Injection, preservative free: 100 mg/mL (5 mL)
Powder for injection: 500 mg (5 mL, 10 mL)

flubenisolone *see* betamethasone *on page 52*

fluconazole (floo koe' na zole)

Brand Names Diflucan® Injection; Diflucan® Oral
Therapeutic Category Antifungal Agent, Systemic
Use Treatment of susceptible fungal infections including oropharyngeal and esophageal candidiasis; treatment of systemic candidal infections including urinary tract infection, peritonitis, and pneumonia; treatment of cryptococcal meningitis
Usual Dosage The daily dose of fluconazole is the same for oral and I.V. administration

Efficacy of fluconazole has not been established in children; a small number of patients from ages 3-13 years have been treated with fluconazole using doses of 3-6 mg/kg/day once daily. Doses as high as 12 mg/kg/day once daily have been used to treat candidiasis in immunocompromised children.

Adult doses of fluconazole: Oral, I.V.: For once daily dosing, see table.

Indication	Day 1	Daily Therapy	Minimum Duration of Therapy
Oropharyngeal candidiasis	200 mg	100 mg	14 d
Esophageal candidiasis	200 mg	100 mg	21 d
Systemic candidiasis	400 mg	200 mg	28 d
Cryptococcal meningitis acute	400 mg	200 mg	10–12 wk after CSF culture becomes negative
relapse	200 mg	200 mg	

Dosage Forms
Injection: 2 mg/mL (100 mL, 200 mL)
Tablet: 50 mg, 100 mg, 200 mg

flucytosine (floo sye' toe seen)

Brand Names Ancobon®
Synonyms 5-FC; 5-flurocytosine
Therapeutic Category Antifungal Agent, Systemic
Use Treatment of susceptible fungal infections, usually strains of *Candida* or *Cryptococcus*
Usual Dosage Children and Adults: Oral: 50-150 mg/kg/day in divided doses every 6 hours
Dosage Forms Capsule: 250 mg, 500 mg

Fludara® *see* fludarabine phosphate *on this page*

fludarabine phosphate (floo dare' a been)

Brand Names Fludara®
Therapeutic Category Antineoplastic Agent, Antimetabolite
Use Treatment of chronic lymphocytic leukemia (B-cell) in patients who have not responded to other alkylating agent regiment
Usual Dosage Refer to individual protocols
Adults: I.V.:

Chronic lymphocytic leukemia: 25 mg/m^2/day over a 30-minute period for 5 days

Non-Hodgkin's lymphoma: Loading dose: 20 mg/m^2 followed by 30 mg/m^2/day for 48 hours

Dosage Forms Powder for injection, lyophilized: 50 mg (6 mL)

fludrocortisone acetate (floo droe kor' ti sone)
Brand Names Florinef® Acetate
Synonyms fluohydrocortisone acetate; 9α-fluorohydrocortisone acetate
Therapeutic Category Mineralocorticoid
Use Addison's disease; partial replacement therapy for adrenal insufficiency and for treatment of salt-losing forms of congenital adrenogenital syndrome
Usual Dosage Oral:
Infants and Children: 0.05-0.1 mg/day
Adults: 0.05-0.2 mg/day
Dosage Forms Tablet: 0.1 mg

Flu-Imune® *see* influenza virus vaccine *on page 249*

Flumadine® Oral *see* rimantadine hydrochloride *on page 421*

flumazenil (floo' may ze nil)
Brand Names Romazicon™ Injection
Therapeutic Category Antidote, Benzodiazepine
Use Benzodiazepine antagonist – reverses sedative effects of benzodiazepines used in general anesthesia; for management of benzodiazepine overdose
Usual Dosage Reversal of conscious sedation or general anesthesia: 0.2 mg (2 mL) administered I.V. over 15 seconds; if desired effect is not achieved after 60 seconds, repeat in 0.2 mg (2 mL) increments every 60 seconds up to a total of 1 mg (10 mL); in event of resedation, repeat doses may be given at 20-minute intervals with no more than 1 mg (10 mL) given at any one time, with a maximum of 3 mg in any 1 hour
Dosage Forms Injection: 0.1 mg/mL (5 mL, 10 mL)

flunisolide (floo niss' oh lide)
Brand Names AeroBid®-M Oral Aerosol Inhaler; AeroBid® Oral Aerosol Inhaler; Nasalide® Nasal Aerosol
Therapeutic Category Anti-inflammatory Agent; Corticosteroid, Inhalant
Use Steroid-dependent asthma; nasal solution is used for seasonal or perennial rhinitis
Usual Dosage
Children:
Oral inhalation: >6 years: 2 inhalations twice daily up to 4 inhalations/day
Nasal: 6-14 years: 1 spray each nostril 2-3 times/day, not to exceed 4 sprays/day each nostril

Adults:
Oral inhalation: 2 inhalations twice daily up to 8 inhalations/day
Nasal: 2 sprays each nostril twice daily; maximum dose: 8 sprays/day in each nostril
Dosage Forms Inhalant:
Nasal (Nasalide®): 25 μg/actuation [200 sprays] (25 mL)
Oral:
AeroBid®: 250 μg/actuation [100 metered doses] (7 g)
AeroBid®-M (menthol flavor): 250 μg/actuation [100 metered doses] (7 g)

fluocinolone acetonide (floo oh sin' oh lone)
Brand Names Derma-Smoothe/FS® Topical; Fluonid® Topical; Flurosyn® Topical; FS Shampoo® Topical; Synalar-HP® Topical; Synalar® Topical; Synemol® Topical
Therapeutic Category Corticosteroid, Topical (Medium Potency)
(Continued)

fluocinolone acetonide *(Continued)*
Use Relief of susceptible inflammatory dermatosis
Usual Dosage Children and Adults: Topical: Apply 2-4 times/day
Dosage Forms
Cream:
Flurosyn®, Synalar®: 0.01% (15 g, 30 g, 60 g, 425 g)
Flurosyn®, Synalar®, Synemol®: 0.025% (15 g, 60 g, 425 g)
Synalar-HP®: 0.2% (12 g)
Ointment, topical (Flurosyn®, Synalar®): 0.025% (15 g, 30 g, 60 g, 425 g)
Oil (Derma-Smoothe/FS®): 0.01% (120 mL)
Shampoo (FS Shampoo®): 0.01% (180 mL)
Solution, topical (Fluonid®, Synalar®): 0.01% (20 mL, 60 mL)

fluocinonide (floo oh sin' oh nide)
Brand Names Fluonex® Topical; Lidex-E® Topical; Lidex® Topical
Therapeutic Category Corticosteroid, Topical (High Potency)
Use Anti-inflammatory, antipruritic, relief of inflammatory and pruritic manifestations
Usual Dosage Children and Adults: Topical: Apply thin layer to affected area 2-4 times/day depending on the severity of the condition
Dosage Forms
Cream:
Anhydrous, emollient (Fluonex®, Lidex®): 0.05% (15 g, 30 g, 60 g, 120 g)
Aqueous, emollient (Lidex-E®): 0.05% (15 g, 30 g, 60 g, 120 g)
Gel, topical (Lidex®): 0.05% (15 g, 30 g, 60 g, 120 g)
Ointment, topical (Lidex®): 0.05% (15 g, 30 g, 60 g, 120 g)
Solution, topical (Lidex®): 0.05% (20 mL, 60 mL)

Fluogen® *see* influenza virus vaccine *on page 249*
fluohydrocortisone acetate *see* fludrocortisone acetate *on previous page*
Fluonex® Topical *see* fluocinonide *on this page*
Fluonid® Topical *see* fluocinolone acetonide *on previous page*
Fluoracaine® Ophthalmic *see* proparacaine and fluorescein *on page 400*

fluorescein sodium (flure' e seen)
Brand Names AK-Fluor Injection; Fluorescite® Injection; Fluorets® Ophthalmic Strips; Fluor-I-Strip®; Fluor-I-Strip-AT®; Fluress® Ophthalmic Solution; Ful-Glo® Ophthalmic Strips; Funduscein® Injection
Synonyms soluble fluorescein
Therapeutic Category Diagnostic Agent, Ophthalmic Dye
Use Demonstrates defects of corneal epithelium; diagnostic aid in ophthalmic angiography
Usual Dosage
Injection: Perform intradermal skin test before use to avoid possible allergic reaction
Children: 3.5 mg/lb (7.5 mg/kg) injected rapidly into antecubital vein
Adults: 500-750 mg injected rapidly into antecubital vein
Strips: Moisten with sterile water or irrigating solution, touch conjunctiva with moistened tip, blink several times after application
Topical solution: Instill 1-2 drops, allow a few seconds for staining, then wash out excess with sterile irrigation solution
Dosage Forms
Injection (AK-Fluor, Fluorescite®, Funduscein®): 10% [100 mg/mL] (5 mL, 10 mL); 25% [250 mg/mL] (2 mL, 3 mL)
Ophthalmic:
Solution:
2% [20 mg/mL] (1 mL, 2 mL, 15 mL)
Fluress®: 0.25% [2.5 mg/mL] with benoxinate 0.4% (5 mL)

Strip:
Ful-Glo®: 0.6 mg
Fluorets®, Fluor-I-Strip-AT®: 1 mg
Fluor-I-Strip®: 9 mg

Fluorescite® Injection *see* fluorescein sodium *on previous page*

Fluorets® Ophthalmic Strips *see* fluorescein sodium *on previous page*

fluoride
Brand Names ACT® [OTC]; Fluorigard® [OTC]; Fluorinse®; Fluoritab®; Flura®; Flura-Drops®; Flura-Loz®; Gel Kam®; Gel-Tin® [OTC]; Karidium®; Karigel®; Karigel®-N; Listermint® with Fluoride [OTC]; Luride®; Luride® Lozi-Tab®; Luride®-SF Lozi-Tab®; Minute-Gel®; Pediaflor®; Pharmaflur®; Phos-Flur®; Point-Two®; Prevident®; Stop® [OTC]
Synonyms acidulated phosphate fluoride; sodium fluoride; stannous fluoride
Therapeutic Category Mineral, Oral; Mineral, Oral Topical
Use Prevention of dental caries
Usual Dosage Oral:
Recommended daily fluoride supplement (2.2 mg of sodium fluoride is equivalent to 1 mg of fluoride ion): See table.

Sodium Fluoride

Fluoride Content of Drinking Water	Daily Dose, Oral (mg)
<0.3 ppm Birth – 2 y	0.25–0.5
2–3 y	0.5
3–12 y	1
0.3–0.7 ppm Birth – 2 y	0.13
2–3 y	0.25
3–12 y	0.25–0.75

Dental rinse or gel:
Children 6-12 years: 5-10 mL rinse or apply to teeth and spit daily after brushing
Adults: 10 mL rinse or apply to teeth and spit daily after brushing
Dosage Forms Fluoride ion content listed in brackets
Drops, oral, as sodium:
Fluoritab®, Flura-Drops®: 0.55 mg/drop [0.25 mg/drop] (22.8 mL, 24 mL)
Karidium®, Luride®: 0.275 mg/drop [0.125 mg/drop] (30 mL, 60 mL)
Pediaflor®: 1.1 mg/mL [0.5 mg/mL] (50 mL)
Gel, topical:
Acidulated phosphate fluoride (Minute-Gel®): 1.23% (480 mL)
Sodium fluoride (Karigel®, Karigel®-N, PreviDent®): 1.1% [0.5%] (24 g, 30 g, 60 g, 120 g, 130 g, 250 g)
Stannous fluoride (Gel Kam®, Gel-Tin®, Stop®): 0.4% [0.1%] (60 g, 65 g, 105 g, 120 g)
Lozenge, as sodium (Flura-Loz®)(raspberry flavor): 2.2 mg [1 mg]
Rinse, topical, as sodium:
ACT®, Fluorigard®: 0.05% [0.02%] (90 mL, 180 mL, 300 mL, 360 mL, 480 mL)
Fluorinse®, Point-Two®: 0.2% [0.09%] (240 mL, 480 mL, 3780 mL)
Listermint® with Fluoride: 0.02% [0.01%] (180 mL, 300 mL, 360 mL, 480 mL, 540 mL, 720 mL, 960 mL, 1740 mL)
Solution, oral, as sodium (Phos-Flur®): 0.44 mg/mL [0.2 mg/mL] (250 mL, 500 mL, 3780 mL)
Tablet, as sodium:
Chewable:
Fluoritab®, Luride® Lozi-Tab®, Pharmaflur®: 1.1 mg [0.5 mg]
(Continued)

fluoride *(Continued)*

Fluoritab®, Karidium®, Luride® Lozi-Tab®, Luride®-SF Lozi-Tab®, Pharmaflur®: 2.2 mg [1 mg]
Flura®, Karidium®: 2.2 mg [1 mg]

Fluorigard® [OTC] *see fluoride on previous page*

Fluori-Methane® Topical Spray *see dichlorodifluoromethane and trichloromonofluoromethane on page 143*

Fluorinse® *see fluoride on previous page*

Fluor-I-Strip® *see fluorescein sodium on page 200*

Fluor-I-Strip-AT® *see fluorescein sodium on page 200*

Fluoritab® *see fluoride on previous page*

fluorodeoxyuridine *see floxuridine on page 197*

9α-fluorohydrocortisone acetate *see fludrocortisone acetate on page 199*

fluorometholone (flure oh meth' oh lone)
Brand Names Flarex® Ophthalmic; Fluor-Op® Ophthalmic; FML® Forte Ophthalmic; FML® Ophthalmic
Therapeutic Category Anti-inflammatory Agent; Corticosteroid, Ophthalmic
Use Inflammatory conditions of the eye, including keratitis, iritis, cyclitis, and conjunctivitis
Usual Dosage Children >2 years and Adults: Ophthalmic: 1-2 drops into conjunctival sac every hour during day, every 2 hours at night until favorable response is obtained, then use 1 drop every 4 hours; in mild or moderate inflammation: 1-2 drops into conjunctival sac 2-4 times/day. Ointment may be applied every 4 hours in severe cases or 1-3 times/day in mild to moderate cases.
Dosage Forms Ophthalmic:
Ointment (FML®): 0.1% (3.5 g)
Suspension:
Flarex®, Fluor-Op®, FML®: 0.1% (5 mL, 10 mL, 15 mL)
FML® Forte: 0.25% (2 mL, 5 mL, 10 mL, 15 mL)

Fluoroplex® Topical *see fluorouracil on this page*

Fluor-Op® Ophthalmic *see fluorometholone on this page*

fluorouracil (flure oh yoor' a sill)
Brand Names Adrucil® Injection; Efudex® Topical; Fluoroplex® Topical
Synonyms 5-fluorouracil; 5-FU
Therapeutic Category Antineoplastic Agent, Antimetabolite
Use Treatment of colon, breast, rectal, gastric, and pancreatic carcinomas; also used topically for management of multiple actinic or solar keratoses and superficial basal cell carcinomas
Usual Dosage Refer to individual protocols
Children and Adults:
I.V.: Initial: 12 mg/kg/day (maximum: 800 mg/day) for 4-5 days; maintenance: 6 mg/kg every other day for 4 doses
Single weekly bolus dose of 15 mg/kg can be administered depending on the patient's reaction to the previous course of treatment; maintenance dose of 5-15 mg/kg/week as a single dose not to exceed 1 g/week
I.V. infusion: 15 mg/kg/day (maximum daily dose: 1 g) has been given by I.V. infusion over 4 hours for 5 days
Oral: 20 mg/kg/day for 5 days every 5 weeks for colorectal carcinoma; 15 mg/kg/week for hepatoma
Topical: 5% cream twice daily
Dosage Forms
Cream, topical:
Efudex®: 5% (25 g)

Fluoroplex®: 1% (30 g)
Injection (Adrucil®): 50 mg/mL (10 mL, 20 mL, 50 mL, 100 mL)
Solution, topical:
Efudex®: 2% (10 mL); 5% (10 mL)
Fluoroplex®: 1% (30 mL)

5-fluorouracil *see* fluorouracil *on previous page*
Fluosol® *see* intravascular perfluorochemical emulsion *on page 253*
fluostigmin *see* isoflurophate *on page 257*
Fluothane® *see* halothane *on page 225*

fluoxetine hydrochloride (floo ox' e teen)
Brand Names Prozac®
Therapeutic Category Antidepressant; Serotonin Antagonist
Use Treatment of major depression
Usual Dosage Oral:
Children <18 years: Dose not established

Adults: 20 mg/day in the morning; may increase after several weeks by 20 mg/day increments; maximum: 80 mg/day; doses >20 mg should be divided into 2 daily doses
   Note: Lower doses of 5 mg/day have been used for initial treatment
Dosage Forms
Capsule: 10 mg, 20 mg
Liquid (mint flavor): 20 mg/5 mL (120 mL)

fluoxymesterone (floo ox i mes' te rone)
Brand Names Halotestin®
Therapeutic Category Androgen
Use Replacement of endogenous testicular hormone; in female used as palliative treatment of breast cancer, postpartum breast engorgement
Usual Dosage Adults: Oral:
Male:
Hypogonadism: 5-20 mg/day
Delayed puberty: 2.5-20 mg/day for 4-6 months

Female:
Breast carcinoma: 10-40 mg/day in divided doses for 1-3 months
Breast engorgement: 2.5 mg after delivery, 5-10 mg/day in divided doses for 4-5 days
Dosage Forms Tablet: 2 mg, 5 mg, 10 mg

fluoxymesterone and estradiol *see* ethinyl estradiol and fluoxymesterone
on page 183

fluphenazine (floo fen' a zeen)
Brand Names Permitil® Oral; Prolixin Decanoate® Injection; Prolixin Enanthate® Injection;
Prolixin® Injection; Prolixin® Oral
Synonyms fluphenazine decanoate; fluphenazine enanthate; fluphenazine hydrochloride
Therapeutic Category Antipsychotic Agent; Phenothiazine Derivative
Use Management of manifestations of psychotic disorders
Usual Dosage Adults:
Oral: 0.5-10 mg/day in divided doses every 6-8 hours; usual maximum dose 20 mg/day
I.M.: 2.5-10 mg/day in divided doses every 6-8 hours; usual maximum dose 10 mg/day
I.M., S.C. (Decanoate®): Oral to I.M., S.C. conversion ratio = 12.5 mg, I.M., S.C. every 3 weeks for every 10 mg of oral fluphenazine
(Continued)

fluphenazine *(Continued)*
Dosage Forms
Concentrate, as hydrochloride:
Permitil®: 5 mg/mL with alcohol 1% (118 mL)
Prolixin®: 5 mg/mL with alcohol 14% (120 mL)
Elixir, as hydrochloride (Prolixin®): 2.5 mg/5 mL with alcohol 14% (60 mL, 473 mL)
Injection, as decanoate (Prolixin Decanoate®): 25 mg/mL (1 mL, 5 mL)
Injection, as enanthate (Prolixin Enanthate®): 25 mg/mL (5 mL)
Injection, as hydrochloride (Prolixin®): 2.5 mg/mL (10 mL)
Tablet, as hydrochloride
Permitil®: 2.5 mg, 5 mg, 10 mg
Prolixin®: 1 mg, 2.5 mg, 5 mg, 10 mg

fluphenazine decanoate *see fluphenazine on previous page*

fluphenazine enanthate *see fluphenazine on previous page*

fluphenazine hydrochloride *see fluphenazine on previous page*

Flura® *see fluoride on page 201*

Flura-Drops® *see fluoride on page 201*

Flura-Loz® *see fluoride on page 201*

flurandrenolide (flure an dren' oh lide)
Brand Names Cordran® SP Topical; Cordran® Topical
Synonyms flurandrenolone
Therapeutic Category Corticosteroid, Topical (Medium Potency)
Use Inflammation of corticosteroid-responsive dermatoses
Usual Dosage
Children:
Ointment or cream: Apply 1-2 times/day
Tape: Apply once daily

Adults: Cream, lotion, ointment: Apply 2-3 times/day
Dosage Forms
Cream, emulsified base (Cordran® SP): 0.025% (30 g, 60 g); 0.05% (15 g, 30 g, 60 g)
Lotion (Cordran®): 0.05% (15 mL, 60 mL)
Ointment, topical (Cordran®): 0.025% (30 g, 60 g); 0.05% (15 g, 30 g, 60 g)
Tape, topical (Cordran®): 4 μg/cm^2 (7.5 cm x 60 cm, 7.5 cm x 200 cm rolls)

flurandrenolone *see flurandrenolide on this page*

flurazepam hydrochloride (flure az' e pam)
Brand Names Dalmane®
Therapeutic Category Benzodiazepine; Hypnotic; Sedative
Use Short-term treatment of insomnia
Usual Dosage Oral:
Children:
<15 years: Dose not established
>15 years: 15 mg at bedtime

Adults: 15-30 mg at bedtime
Dosage Forms Capsule: 15 mg, 30 mg

flurbiprofen sodium (flure bi' proe fen)
Brand Names Ansaid® Oral; Ocufen® Ophthalmic
Therapeutic Category Analgesic, Non-Narcotic; Anti-inflammatory Agent; Nonsteroidal Anti-Inflammatory Agent (NSAID), Ophthalmic
Use For inhibition of intraoperative miosis; acute or long-term treatment of signs of symptoms of rheumatoid arthritis and osteoarthritis; prevention and management of postopera-

ALPHABETICAL LISTING OF DRUGS

tive ocular inflammation and postoperative cystoid macular edema remains to be determined

Usual Dosage
Oral: Rheumatoid arthritis and osteoarthritis: 200-300 mg/day in 2, 3, or 4 divided doses

Ophthalmic: Instill 1 drop every 30 minutes, 2 hours prior to surgery (total of 4 drops to each affected eye)

Dosage Forms
Solution, ophthalmic (Ocufen®): 0.03% (2.5 mL, 5 mL, 10 mL)
Tablet (Ansaid®): 50 mg, 100 mg

Fluress® Ophthalmic Solution see fluorescein sodium on page 200

5-flurocytosine see flucytosine on page 198

Fluro-Ethyl® Aerosol see ethyl chloride and dichlorotetrafluoroethane on page 186

Flurosyn® Topical see fluocinolone acetonide on page 199

flutamide (floo' ta mide)
Brand Names Eulexin®
Therapeutic Category Antiandrogen
Use In combination with LHRH agonistic analogs for the treatment of metastatic prostatic carcinoma
Usual Dosage Oral: 2 capsules every 8 hours
Dosage Forms Capsule: 125 mg

Flutex® Topical see triamcinolone on page 474

fluticasone propionate (floo tik' a sone)
Brand Names Cutivate™ Topical
Therapeutic Category Corticosteroid, Topical (Medium Potency)
Use Relief of inflammation and pruritus associated with corticosteroid-responsive dermatoses
Usual Dosage Apply sparingly in a thin film twice daily
Dosage Forms
Cream: 0.05% (15 g, 30 g, 60 g)
Ointment, topical: 0.005% (15 g, 60 g)

Fluzone® see influenza virus vaccine on page 249

FML® Forte Ophthalmic see fluorometholone on page 202

FML® Ophthalmic see fluorometholone on page 202

Foille Plus® [OTC] see benzocaine on page 48

folacin see folic acid on this page

folate see folic acid on this page

Folbesyn® see vitamin B complex with vitamin C and folic acid on page 498

Folex® Injection see methotrexate on page 301

folic acid
Brand Names Folvite® Injection; Folvite® Oral
Synonyms folacin; folate; pteroylglutamic acid
Therapeutic Category Vitamin, Water Soluble
Use Treatment of megaloblastic and macrocytic anemias due to folate deficiency
(Continued)
205

folic acid *(Continued)*
Usual Dosage Folic acid deficiency:
Infants: 15 μg/kg/dose daily or 50 μg/day

Children: Oral, I.M., I.V., S.C.: 1 mg/day initial dosage; maintenance dose: 1-10 years: 0.1-0.3 mg/day

Children >11 years and Adults: Oral, I.M., I.V., S.C.: 1 mg/day initial dosage; maintenance dose: 0.5 mg/day
Dosage Forms
Injection, as sodium folate: 5 mg/mL (10 mL); 10 mg/mL (10 mL)
    Folvite®: 5 mg/mL (10 mL)
Tablet: 0.1 mg, 0.4 mg, 0.8 mg, 1 mg
    Folvite®: 1 mg

folinic acid *see leucovorin calcium on page 268*

Follutein® *see chorionic gonadotropin on page 101*

Folvite® Injection *see folic acid on previous page*

Folvite® Oral *see folic acid on previous page*

Forane® *see isoflurane on page 257*

5-formyl tetrahydrofolate *see leucovorin calcium on page 268*

Fortaz® *see ceftazidime on page 81*

Fortel® Home Ovulation *see diagnostic aids (in vitro), urine on page 139*

foscarnet *(fos kar' net)*
Brand Names Foscavir® Injection
Synonyms pfa; phosphonoformic acid
Therapeutic Category Antiviral Agent, Parenteral
Use Alternative to ganciclovir for treatment of CMV retinitis and other CMV infections; alternative to acyclovir for treatment of acyclovir-resistant HSV infections
Usual Dosage
Induction treatment: 60 mg/kg 3 times/day for 14-21 days
Maintenance therapy: 90-120 mg/kg/day
Dosage Forms Injection: 24 mg/mL (250 mL, 500 mL)

Foscavir® Injection *see foscarnet on this page*

fosinopril *(foe sin' oh pril)*
Brand Names Monopril®
Therapeutic Category Angiotensin Converting Enzyme (ACE) Inhibitors
Use Treatment of hypertension, either alone or in combination with other antihypertensive agents
Usual Dosage Adults: Oral: 20-40 mg/day
Dosage Forms Tablet: 10 mg, 20 mg

Fostex® [OTC] *see sulfur and salicylic acid on page 450*

Fototar® [OTC] *see coal tar on page 110*

Freezone® Solution [OTC] *see salicylic acid on page 424*

frusemide *see furosemide on next page*

FS Shampoo® Topical *see fluocinolone acetonide on page 199*

5-FU *see fluorouracil on page 202*

FUDR® *see floxuridine on page 197*

Ful-Glo® Ophthalmic Strips *see fluorescein sodium on page 200*

Fulvicin® P/G see griseofulvin on page 217
Fulvicin-U/F® see griseofulvin on page 217
Fumasorb® [OTC] see ferrous fumarate on page 193
Fumerin® [OTC] see ferrous fumarate on page 193
Funduscein® Injection see fluorescein sodium on page 200
Fungizone® see amphotericin B on page 25
Fungoid® Topical see triacetin on page 474
Furacin® Topical see nitrofurazone on page 336
Furadantin® see nitrofurantoin on page 335
Furalan® see nitrofurantoin on page 335
Furan® see nitrofurantoin on page 335
Furanite® see nitrofurantoin on page 335

furazolidone (fur a zoe' li done)
Brand Names Furoxone®
Therapeutic Category Antibiotic, Miscellaneous; Antidiarrheal; Antiprotozoal
Use Treatment of bacterial or protozoal diarrhea and enteritis caused by susceptible organisms: *Giardia lamblia* and *Vibrio cholerae*
Usual Dosage Oral:
Children >1 month: 5-8.8 mg/kg/day in 3-4 divided doses for 7-10 days, not to exceed 400 mg/day
Adults: 100 mg 4 times/day for 7-10 days
Dosage Forms
Liquid: 50 mg/15 mL (60 mL, 473 mL)
Tablet: 100 mg

furazosin see prazosin hydrochloride on page 391

furosemide (fur oh' se mide)
Brand Names Lasix® Injection; Lasix® Oral
Synonyms frusemide
Therapeutic Category Diuretic, Loop
Use Management of edema associated with congestive heart failure and hepatic or renal disease; used alone or in combination with antihypertensives in treatment of hypertension
Usual Dosage
Neonates, premature:
Oral: Bioavailability is poor by this route. Doses of 1-4 mg/kg/dose 1-2 times/day have been used.
I.M., I.V.: 1-2 mg/kg/dose given every 12-24 hours
Children and Infants:
Oral: 2 mg/kg/dose increased in increments of 1 mg/kg/dose with each succeeding dose until a satisfactory effect is achieved to a maximum of 6 mg/kg/dose no more frequently than 6 hours
I.M., I.V.: 1 mg/kg/dose, increasing by each succeeding dose at 1 mg/kg/dose at intervals of 6-12 hours until a satisfactory response up to 6 mg/kg/dose
Adults:
Oral: 20-80 mg/dose initially increased in increments of 20-40 mg/dose at intervals of 6-8 hours; usual maintenance dose interval is twice daily or every day
I.M., I.V.: 20-40 mg/dose, may be repeated in 1-2 hours as needed and increased by 20 mg/dose with each succeeding dose up to 600 mg/day; usual dosing interval: 6-12 hours
Dosage Forms
Injection: 10 mg/mL (2 mL, 4 mL, 5 mL, 6 mL, 8 mL, 10 mL, 12 mL)
Solution, oral: 10 mg/mL (60 mL, 120 mL); 40 mg/5 mL (5 mL, 10 mL, 500 mL)
(Continued)

furosemide *(Continued)*
Tablet: 20 mg, 40 mg, 80 mg

Furoxone® *see* furazolidone *on previous page*

gadopentetate dimeglumine *see* radiological/contrast media (ionic) *on page 413*

gallamine triethiodide (gal' a meen)
Brand Names Flaxedil®
Therapeutic Category Neuromuscular Blocker Agent, Nondepolarizing; Skeletal Muscle Relaxant
Use Produce skeletal muscle relaxation during surgery after general anesthesia has been induced
Usual Dosage I.V.: 1 mg/kg then repeat dose of 0.5-1 mg/kg in 30-40 minutes for prolonged procedures
Dosage Forms Injection: 20 mg/mL (10 mL)

gallium nitrate (gal' ee um)
Brand Names Ganite™
Therapeutic Category Antidote, Hypercalcemia
Use Treatment of clearly symptomatic cancer-related hypercalcemia that has not responded to adequate hydration
Usual Dosage Adults: I.V. infusion: 200 mg/m^2 for 5 consecutive days
Dosage Forms Injection: 25 mg/mL (20 mL)

Gamastan® *see* immune globulin, intramuscular *on page 247*
Gamimune® N *see* immune globulin, intravenous *on page 247*
gamma benzene hexachloride *see* lindane *on page 274*
Gammagard® *see* immune globulin, intravenous *on page 247*
gamma globulin *see* immune globulin, intramuscular *on page 247*
Gammar® *see* immune globulin, intramuscular *on page 247*

ganciclovir (gan sye' kloe vir)
Brand Names Cytovene®
Synonyms DHPG sodium; GCV sodium; nordeoxyguanosine
Therapeutic Category Antiviral Agent, Parenteral
Use CMV retinitis treatment of immunocompromised individuals, including patients with acquired immunodeficiency syndrome; investigational use in treatment of CMV pneumonia in marrow transplant recipients has not been rewarding, promising results have been achieved in AIDS patients and organ transplant recipients with CMV colitis, pneumonitis, and multiorgan involvement
Usual Dosage Slow I.V. infusion

Retinitis: Children >3 months and Adults: Induction therapy: 5 mg/kg/dose every 12 hours for 14-21 days followed by maintenance therapy; maintenance therapy: 5 mg/kg/day as a single daily dose for 7 days/week or 6 mg/kg/day for 5 days/week

Other CMV infections: 5 mg/kg/dose every 12 hours for 14-21 days or 2.5 mg/kg/dose every 8 hours; maintenance therapy: 5 mg/kg/day as a single daily dose for 7 days/week or 6 mg/kg/day for 5 days/week
Dosage Forms Powder for injection, lyophilized: 500 mg (10 mL)

Ganite™ *see* gallium nitrate *on this page*
Gantanol® *see* sulfamethoxazole *on page 448*

Gantrisin® Ophthalmic *see* sulfisoxazole *on page 449*

Gantrisin® Oral *see* sulfisoxazole *on page 449*

Garamycin® Injection *see* gentamicin sulfate *on page 211*

Garamycin® Ophthalmic *see* gentamicin sulfate *on page 211*

Garamycin® Topical *see* gentamicin sulfate *on page 211*

Gastroccult® *see* diagnostic aids (*in vitro*), other *on page 138*

Gastrocrom® Oral *see* cromolyn sodium *on page 118*

Gastrografin® *see* radiological/contrast media (ionic) *on page 413*

Gastrosed™ Oral *see* hyoscyamine sulfate *on page 243*

Gas-X® [OTC] *see* simethicone *on page 431*

Gaviscon® [OTC] *see* aluminum hydroxide, magnesium trisilicate, sodium bicarbonate and alginic acid *on page 16*

G-CSF *see* filgrastim *on page 195*

GCV sodium *see* ganciclovir *on previous page*

Gee Gee® [OTC] *see* guaifenesin *on page 217*

gelatin, absorbable

Brand Names Gelfilm® Ophthalmic; Gelfoam® Topical

Synonyms absorbable gelatin sponge

Therapeutic Category Hemostatic Agent

Use Adjunct to provide hemostasis in surgery; also used in oral and dental surgery; in open prostatic surgery

Usual Dosage Hemostasis: Apply packs or sponges dry or saturated with sodium chloride. When applied dry, hold in place with moderate pressure. When applied wet, squeeze to remove air bubbles. Prostatectomy cones are designed for use with the Foley bag catheter. The powder is applied as a paste prepared by adding approximately 4 mL of sterile saline solution to the powder.

Dosage Forms Gelfoam®

Cones, prostatectomy:
    Size 13 cm (13 cm in diameter) (6s)
    Size 18 cm (18 cm in diameter) (6s)
Packs:
    Size 2 cm (40 cm x 2 cm) (1s)
    Size 6 cm (40 cm x 6 cm) (6s)
Packs, dental:
    Size 2 (10 mm x 20 mm x 7 mm) (15s)
    Size 4 (20 mm x 20 mm x 7 mm) (15s)
Sponges:
    Size 12-3 mm (20 mm x 60 mm x 3 mm) (4s)
    Size 12-7 mm (20 mm x 60 mm x 7 mm) (4s)
    Size 50 (80 mm x 62.5 mm x 10 mm) (4s)
    Size 100 (80 mm x 125 mm x 10 mm) (6s)
    Size 100, compressed (80 mm x 125 mm) (6s)
    Size 200 (80 mm x 250 mm x 10 mm) (6s)

Gelfilm® (sterile)
    Film: 100 mm x 125 mm (1s)
    Ophthalmic: 25 mm x 50 mm (6s)

gelatin, pectin, and methylcellulose

Brand Names Orabase® Plain [OTC]

Therapeutic Category Protectant, Topical

Use Temporary relief from minor oral irritations

Usual Dosage Press small dabs into place until the involved area is coated with a thin film; do not try to spread onto area; may be used as often as needed

Dosage Forms Paste, oral: 5 g, 15 g

Gelfilm® Ophthalmic *see* gelatin, absorbable *on previous page*

Gelfoam® Topical *see* gelatin, absorbable *on previous page*

Gel Kam® *see* fluoride *on page 201*

Gelpirin® [OTC] *see* acetaminophen and aspirin *on page 3*

Gel-Tin® [OTC] *see* fluoride *on page 201*

Gelucast® *see* zinc gelatin *on page 503*

Gelusil® [OTC] *see* aluminum hydroxide, magnesium hydroxide, and simethicone *on page 16*

gemfibrozil (jem fi' broe zil)
Brand Names Lopid®
Synonyms CL-719
Therapeutic Category Antilipemic Agent
Use Hypertriglyceridemia in types IV and V hyperlipidemia; increases HDL cholesterol
Usual Dosage Oral: 1200 mg/day in 2 divided doses, 30 minutes before breakfast and supper
Dosage Forms
Capsule: 300 mg
Tablet, film coated: 600 mg

Genabid® Oral *see* papaverine hydrochloride *on page 355*

Genac® [OTC] *see* triprolidine and pseudoephedrine *on page 482*

Genagesic® *see* propoxyphene and acetaminophen *on page 402*

Genahist® Oral *see* diphenhydramine hydrochloride *on page 152*

Genamin® Cold Syrup [OTC] *see* chlorpheniramine and phenylpropanolamine *on page 93*

Genamin® Expectorant [OTC] *see* guaifenesin and phenylpropanolamine *on page 219*

Genapap® [OTC] *see* acetaminophen *on page 2*

Genapax® Vaginal *see* gentian violet *on next page*

Genasoft® Plus [OTC] *see* docusate and casanthranol *on page 158*

Genaspor® [OTC] *see* tolnaftate *on page 471*

Genatuss® [OTC] *see* guaifenesin *on page 217*

Genatuss DM® [OTC] *see* guaifenesin and dextromethorphan *on page 218*

Gencalc® 600 [OTC] *see* calcium carbonate *on page 65*

Gen-D-phen® Cough Syrup [OTC] *see* diphenhydramine hydrochloride *on page 152*

Gen-K® *see* potassium chloride *on page 386*

Genoptic® Ophthalmic *see* gentamicin sulfate *on next page*

Genoptic® S.O.P. Ophthalmic *see* gentamicin sulfate *on next page*

Genora® *see* ethinyl estradiol and norethindrone *on page 183*

Genpril® [OTC] *see* ibuprofen *on page 245*

Gensan® [OTC] *see* aspirin *on page 34*

Gentab-LA® *see* guaifenesin and phenylpropanolamine *on page 219*

Gentacidin® Ophthalmic *see* gentamicin sulfate *on next page*

Gent-AK® Ophthalmic *see* gentamicin sulfate *on next page*

gentamicin and prednisolone *see* prednisolone and gentamicin *on page 392*

gentamicin sulfate (jen ta mye' sin)

Brand Names Garamycin® Injection; Garamycin® Ophthalmic; Garamycin® Topical; Genoptic® Ophthalmic; Genoptic® S.O.P. Ophthalmic; Gentacidin® Ophthalmic; Gent-AK® Ophthalmic; Gentrasul® Ophthalmic; G-myticin® Topical; Jenamicin® Injection

Therapeutic Category Antibiotic, Aminoglycoside; Antibiotic, Ophthalmic; Antibiotic, Topical

Use Treatment of susceptible bacterial infections, normally gram-negative organisms including *Pseudomonas*, *Proteus*, *Serratia*, and gram-positive *Staphylococcus*; treatment of bone infections, CNS infections, respiratory tract infections, skin and soft tissue infections, as well as abdominal and urinary tract infections, endocarditis, and septicemia

Usual Dosage Dosage should be based on an estimate of ideal body weight

Neonates: I.M., I.V.:
  Postnatal age <7 days:
    <1000 g and <28 weeks GA: 2.5 mg/kg/dose every 24 hours
    <1500 g and <34 weeks GA: 2.5 mg/kg/dose every 18 hours
    >1500 g and >34 weeks GA: 2.5 mg/kg/dose every 12 hours
  Postnatal age >7 days:
    <1200 g: 2.5 mg/kg/dose every 18-24 hours
    >1200 g: 2.5 mg/kg/dose every 8 hours

Newborns: Intrathecal: 1 mg/day

Infants and Children >3 months: Intrathecal: 1-2 mg/day

Infants and Children <5 years: 2.5 mg/kg/dose every 8 hours

Children >5 years: 1.5-2.5 mg/kg/dose every 8 hours
  Ophthalmic: Solution: 1-2 drops every 2-4 hours, up to 2 drops every hour for severe infections; ointment: 2-3 times/day
  Topical: Apply 3-4 times/day

Adults:
  Intrathecal: 4-8 mg/day
  I.M., I.V.: 3-5 mg/kg/day in divided doses every 8 hours
  Topical: Apply 3-4 times/day
  Ophthalmic: Solution: 1-2 drops every 2-4 hours; ointment: 2-3 times/day

Dosage Forms
Cream, topical (Garamycin®, G-myticin®): 0.1% (15 g)
Infusion, in D_5W, as sulfate: 60 mg, 80 mg, 100 mg
Infusion, in NS, as sulfate: 40 mg, 60 mg, 80 mg, 90 mg, 100 mg, 120 mg
Injection, as sulfate: 40 mg/mL (1 mL, 1.5 mL, 2 mL)
  Pediatric, as sulfate: 10 mg/mL (2 mL)
  Intrathecal, preservative free, as sulfate (Garamycin®): 2 mg/mL (2 mL)
Ointment:
  Ophthalmic:
    Gent-AK®, Gentacidin®, Gentrasul®: 0.3% (3.5 g)
    Sulfate (Garamycin®, Genoptic® S.O.P.): 0.3% (3.5 g)
    Topical (Garamycin®, G-myticin®): 0.1% (15 g)
Solution, ophthalmic (Garamycin®, Genoptic®, Gentacidin®, Gent-AK®, Gentrasul®): 0.3% (1 mL, 5 mL, 15 mL)

gentian violet (jen' shun)

Brand Names Genapax® Vaginal
Synonyms crystal violet; methylrosaniline chloride
Therapeutic Category Antibacterial, Topical; Antifungal Agent, Topical
Use Treatment of cutaneous or mucocutaneous infections caused by *Candida albicans* and other superficial skin infections
Usual Dosage
Infants: 3-4 drops of a 0.5% solution is applied under the tongue or on lesion after feedings

Children and Adults: Apply 0.5% to 2% with cotton to lesion 2-3 times/day for 3 days, do not swallow
(Continued)

gentian violet *(Continued)*
Dosage Forms
Solution, topical: 1% (30 mL); 2% (30 mL)
Tampons: 5 mg (12s)

Gentran® *see* dextran *on page 135*

Gentrasul® Ophthalmic *see* gentamicin sulfate *on previous page*

Gen-XENE® *see* clorazepate dipotassium *on page 109*

Geocillin® *see* carbenicillin *on page 73*

Geref® Injection *see* sermorelin acetate *on page 429*

Geridium® *see* phenazopyridine hydrochloride *on page 368*

german measles vaccine *see* rubella virus vaccine, live *on page 423*

Germinal® *see* ergoloid mesylates *on page 173*

Gesterol® Injection *see* progesterone *on page 397*

Gesterol® L.A. Injection *see* hydroxyprogesterone caproate *on page 240*

Gevrabon® [OTC] *see* vitamin B complex *on page 498*

GG *see* guaifenesin *on page 217*

GG-Cen® [OTC] *see* guaifenesin *on page 217*

Glaucon® Ophthalmic *see* epinephrine *on page 171*

glibenclamide *see* glyburide *on next page*

glipizide (glip' i zide)
Brand Names Glucotrol®
Synonyms glydiazinamide
Therapeutic Category Antidiabetic Agent; Hypoglycemic Agent, Oral; Sulfonylurea Agent
Use Management of noninsulin-dependent diabetes mellitus (type II)
Usual Dosage Adults: Oral: 2.5-40 mg/day; doses larger than 15-20 mg/day should be divided and given twice daily
Dosage Forms Tablet: 5 mg, 10 mg

glucagon (gloo' ka gon)
Therapeutic Category Antihypoglycemic Agent
Use Hypoglycemia; diagnostic aid in the radiologic examination of GI tract when a hypotonic state is needed; used with some success as a cardiac stimulant in management of severe cases of beta-adrenergic blocking agent overdosage
Usual Dosage
Hypoglycemia or insulin shock therapy: I.M., I.V., S.C.:
Neonates: 0.3 mg/kg/dose; maximum: 1 mg/dose
Children: 0.025-0.1 mg/kg/dose, not to exceed 1 mg/dose, repeated in 20 minutes as needed
Adults: 0.5-1 mg, may repeat in 20 minutes as needed
Diagnostic aid: Adults: I.M., I.V.: 0.25-2 mg 10 minutes prior to procedure
Dosage Forms Powder for injection, lyophilized: 1 mg [1 unit]; 10 mg [10 units]

glucocerebrosidase *see* alglucerase *on page 12*

glucose, instant
Brand Names B-D Glucose® [OTC]; Glutose® [OTC]; Insta-Glucose® [OTC]
Therapeutic Category Antihypoglycemic Agent
Use Management of hypoglycemia

Usual Dosage Oral: 10-20 g
Dosage Forms
 Gel, oral (Glutose®, Insta-Glucose®): Dextrose 40% (25 g, 30.8 g, 80 g)
 Tablet, chewable (B-D Glucose®): 5 g

glucose polymers (gloo' kose)
Brand Names Moducal® [OTC]; Polycose® [OTC]; Sumacal® [OTC]
Therapeutic Category Nutritional Supplement
Use Supplies calories for those persons not able to meet the caloric requirement with usual food intake
Usual Dosage Dose is individualized
Dosage Forms
 Liquid (Polycose®): 126 mL
 Powder (Moducal®, Polycose®, Sumacal®): 350 g, 368 g, 400 g

Glucostix® [OTC] see diagnostic aids (in vitro), blood on page 137

Glucotrol® see glipizide on previous page

Glukor® see chorionic gonadotropin on page 101

glutamic acid hydrochloride (gloo tam' ik)
Therapeutic Category Gastrointestinal Agent, Miscellaneous
Use Treatment of hypochlorhydria and achlorhydria
Usual Dosage Adults: Oral: 340 mg to 1.02 g 3 times/day before meals or food
Dosage Forms
 Capsule, as hydrochloride: 340 mg
 Powder: 100 g
 Tablet: 500 mg

glutethimide (gloo teth' i mide)
Brand Names Doriden®
Therapeutic Category Hypnotic; Sedative
Use Short-term treatment of insomnia
Usual Dosage Oral:
 Adults: 250-500 mg at bedtime, dose may be repeated but not less than 4 hours before intended awakening; maximum: 1 g/day

 Elderly/debilitated patients: Total daily dose should not exceed 500 mg
Dosage Forms Tablet: 250 mg, 500 mg

Glutose® [OTC] see glucose, instant on previous page

Glyate® [OTC] see guaifenesin on page 217

glyburide (glye' byoor ide)
Brand Names Diaβeta®; Glynase™ Prestab™; Micronase®
Synonyms glibenclamide
Therapeutic Category Antidiabetic Agent; Hypoglycemic Agent, Oral; Sulfonylurea Agent
Use Management of noninsulin-dependent diabetes mellitus (type II)
Usual Dosage Adults: Oral: 1.25-5 mg to start then 1.25-20 mg maintenance dose/day divided in 1-2 doses
 Prestab™: Initial: 0.75-3 mg/day, increase by 1.5 mg/day in weekly intervals; maximum: 12 mg/day
Dosage Forms
 Tablet (Diaβeta®, Micronase®): 1.25 mg, 2.5 mg, 5 mg
 Tablet, micronized (Glynase™ Prestab™): 1.5 mg, 3 mg

glycerin (glis' er in)
Brand Names Fleet® Babylax® Rectal [OTC]; Ophthalgan® Ophthalmic; Osmoglyn® Ophthalmic; Sani-Supp® Suppository [OTC]
Synonyms glycerol
Therapeutic Category Laxative, Hyperosmolar
Use Constipation; reduction of intraocular pressure; reduction of corneal edema; glycerin has been administered orally to reduce intracranial pressure
Usual Dosage
Constipation: Rectal:
Neonates: 0.5 mL/kg/dose
Children <6 years: 1 infant suppository 1-2 times/day as needed or 2-5 mL as an enema
Children >6 years and Adults: 1 adult suppository 1-2 times/day as needed or 5-15 mL as an enema

Children and Adults:
Reduction of intraocular pressure: Oral: 1-1.8 g/kg 1-1$\frac{1}{2}$ hours preoperatively; additional doses may be administered at 5-hour intervals
Reduction of corneal edema: Instill 1-2 drops in eye(s) every 3-4 hours
Reduction of intracranial pressure: Oral: 1.5 g/kg/day divided every 4 hours; dose of 1 g/kg/dose every 6 hours has also been used
Dosage Forms
Solution:
Ophthalmic, sterile (Ophthalgan®): Glycerin with chlorobutanol 0.55% (7.5 mL)
Oral (lime flavor)(Osmoglyn®): 50% (220 mL)
Rectal (Fleet® Babylax®): 4 mL/applicator (6's)
Suppository, rectal (Sani-Supp®): Glycerin with sodium stearate (infant and adult sizes)

glycerin, lanolin and peanut oil
Brand Names Massé® Breast Cream [OTC]
Therapeutic Category Topical Skin Product
Use Nipple care of pregnant and nursing women
Usual Dosage Topical: Apply as often as needed
Dosage Forms Cream: 2 oz

glycerol see glycerin on this page

glycerol guaiacolate see guaifenesin on page 217

Glycerol-T® see theophylline and guaifenesin on page 461

glycerol triacetate see triacetin on page 474

glyceryl trinitrate see nitroglycerin on page 336

Glycofed® see guaifenesin and pseudoephedrine on page 220

glycopyrrolate (glye koe pye' roe late)
Brand Names Robinul®; Robinul® Forte
Synonyms glycopyrronium bromide
Therapeutic Category Anticholinergic Agent; Antispasmodic Agent, Gastrointestinal
Use Adjunct in treatment of peptic ulcer disease; inhibit salivation and excessive secretions of the respiratory tract preoperatively; reversal of neuromuscular blockade; control of upper airway secretions
Usual Dosage
Children: Control of secretions:
Oral: 40-100 µg/kg/dose 3-4 times/day
I.M., I.V.: 4-10 µg/kg/dose every 3-4 hours; maximum: 0.2 mg/dose or 0.8 mg/24 hours
Children:
Intraoperative: I.V.: 4 µg/kg not to exceed 0.1 mg; repeat at 2- to 3-minute intervals as needed

Preoperative: I.M.:
    <2 years: 4.4-8.8 µg/kg 30-60 minutes before procedure
    >2 years: 4.4 µg/kg 30-60 minutes before procedure
Children and Adults: Reverse neuromuscular blockade: I.V.: 0.2 mg for each 1 mg of neostigmine or 5 mg of pyridostigmine administered
Adults:
    Intraoperative: I.V.: 0.1 mg repeated as needed at 2- to 3-minute intervals
    Peptic ulcer:
        Oral: 1-2 mg 2-3 times/day
        I.M., I.V.: 0.1-0.2 mg 3-4 times/day
    Preoperative: I.M.: 4.4 µg/kg 30-60 minutes before procedure
Dosage Forms
Injection (Robinul®): 0.2 mg/mL (1 mL, 2 mL, 5 mL, 20 mL)
Tablet:
    Robinul®: 1 mg
    Robinul® Forte: 2 mg

glycopyrronium bromide see glycopyrrolate *on previous page*
Glycotuss® [OTC] see guaifenesin *on page 217*
Glycotuss-dM® [OTC] see guaifenesin and dextromethorphan *on page 218*
Glydeine® see guaifenesin and codeine *on page 218*
glydiazinamide see glipizide *on page 212*
Glynase™ Prestab™ see glyburide *on page 213*
Gly-Oxide® Oral [OTC] see carbamide peroxide *on page 73*
Glytuss® [OTC] see guaifenesin *on page 217*
GM-CSF see sargramostim *on page 426*
G-myticin® Topical see gentamicin sulfate *on page 211*
Go-Evac® see polyethylene glycol-electrolyte solution *on page 383*

gold sodium thiomalate
Brand Names Myochrysine® Injection
Therapeutic Category Gold Compound
Use Treatment of progressive rheumatoid arthritis
Usual Dosage I.M.:
    Children: Initial: Test dose of 10 mg I.M. is recommended, followed by 1 mg/kg I.M. weekly for 20 weeks; not to exceed 50 mg in a single injection; maintenance: 1 mg/kg/dose at 2- to 4-week intervals thereafter for as long as therapy is clinically beneficial and toxicity does not develop. Administration for 2-4 months is usually required before clinical improvement is observed
    Adults: 10 mg first week; 25 mg second week; then 25-50 mg/week until 1 g cumulative dose has been given. If improvement occurs without adverse reactions, give 25-50 mg every 2-3 weeks, then every 3-4 weeks.
Dosage Forms Injection: 25 mg/mL (1 mL); 50 mg/mL (1 mL, 10 mL)

GoLYTELY® see polyethylene glycol-electrolyte solution *on page 383*

gonadorelin (goe nad oh rell' in)
Brand Names Factrel® Injection; Lutrepulse® Injection
Synonyms LRH
Therapeutic Category Diagnostic Agent, Gonadotrophic Hormone; Gonadotropin
Use Evaluation of the functional capacity and response of gonadotrophic hormones; used to evaluate abnormal gonadotropin regulation as in precocious puberty and delayed puberty
(Continued)

gonadorelin *(Continued)*

Usual Dosage Female:

Diagnostic test: Children >12 years and Adults: I.V., S.C. hydrochloride salt: 100 μg administered in women during early phase of menstrual cycle (day 1-7)

Primary hypothalamic amenorrhea: Adults: Acetate: I.V.: 5 μg every 90 minutes via Lutrepulse® pump kit at treatment intervals of 21 days (pump will pulsate every 90 minutes for 7 days)

Dosage Forms

Injection, as acetate (Lutrepulse®): 0.8 mg, 3.2 mg

Injection, as hydrochloride (Factrel®): 100 μg, 500 μg

Gonak™ [OTC] *see* hydroxypropyl methylcellulose *on page 241*

Gonic® *see* chorionic gonadotropin *on page 101*

gonioscopic ophthalmic solution *see* hydroxypropyl methylcellulose *on page 241*

Goniosol® [OTC] *see* hydroxypropyl methylcellulose *on page 241*

Gonodecten® *see* diagnostic aids (*in vitro*), other *on page 138*

Gonozyme® *see* diagnostic aids (*in vitro*), other *on page 138*

Gordofilm® Liquid *see* salicylic acid *on page 424*

Gormel® Creme [OTC] *see* urea *on page 487*

goserelin acetate (goe' se rel in)

Brand Names Zoladex® Implant

Therapeutic Category Gonadotropin Releasing Hormone Analog

Use Palliative treatment of advanced prostate cancer

Usual Dosage Adults: S.C.: 3.6 mg as a depot injection every 28 days into upper abdominal wall using sterile technique under the supervision of a physician. At the physician's option, local anesthesia may be used prior to injection. The injection should be repeated every 28 days as long as the patient can tolerate the side effects and there is satisfactory disease regression. While a delay of a few days is permissible, every effort should be made to adhere to the 28-day schedule.

Dosage Forms Injection, implant: 3.6 mg single-dose syringe

granisetron (gra ni' se tron)

Brand Names Kytril® Injection

Therapeutic Category Antiemetic

Use Prophylaxis and treatment of chemotherapy-related emesis

Usual Dosage

Clinicals used 40 μg/kg for 1-3 doses; however the FDA stated patients should use 10 μg/kg/dose, usually single doses are recommended. Doses (regardless of 10 or 40) should be administered as a single IVPB over 5 minutes to 1 hour, given just prior to chemotherapy (15-60 minutes before).

As intervention therapy for breakthrough nausea and vomiting, during the first 24 hours following chemotherapy, 2 or 3 repeat infusions (same dose) have been administered, separated by at least 10 minutes

Dosing interval in renal impairment: Creatinine clearance values have no relationship to granisetron clearance

Dosage Forms Injection

Granulex *see* trypsin, balsam peru, and castor oil *on page 484*

granulocyte colony stimulating factor *see* filgrastim *on page 195*

granulocyte-macrophage colony stimulating factor *see* sargramostim *on page 426*

Grifulvin® V *see griseofulvin on this page*

Grisactin® *see griseofulvin on this page*

Grisactin® Ultra *see griseofulvin on this page*

griseofulvin (gri see oh ful' vin)

Brand Names Fulvicin® P/G; Fulvicin-U/F®; Grifulvin® V; Grisactin®; Grisactin® Ultra; Gris-PEG®

Synonyms griseofulvin microsize; griseofulvin ultramicrosize

Therapeutic Category Antifungal Agent, Systemic

Use Treatment of susceptible tinea infections of the skin, hair, and nails

Usual Dosage Oral:

Children:

Microsize: 10-15 mg/kg/day in single or divided doses;

Ultramicrosize: >2 months: 5.5-7.3 mg/kg/day in single or divided doses

Adults:

Microsize: 500-1000 mg/day in single or divided doses

Ultramicrosize: 330-375 mg/day in single or divided doses; doses up to 750 mg/day have been used for infections more difficult to eradicate such as tinea unguium

Duration of therapy depends on the site of infection:

Tinea corporis: 2-4 weeks

Tinea capitis: 4-6 weeks or longer

Tinea pedis: 4-8 weeks

Tinea unguium: 3-6 months

Dosage Forms

Griseofulvin Microsize:

Capsule (Grisactin®): 125 mg, 250 mg

Suspension, oral (Grifulvin® V): 125 mg/5 mL with alcohol 0.2% (120 mL)

Tablet:

Fulvicin-U/F®, Grifulvin® V: 250 mg

Fulvicin-U/F®, Grifulvin® V, Grisactin®: 500 mg

Griseofulvin Ultramicrosize:

Tablet:

Fulvicin® P/G: 165 mg, 330 mg

Fulvicin® P/G, Grisactin® Ultra, Gris-PEG®: 125 mg, 250 mg

Grisactin® Ultra: 330 mg

griseofulvin microsize *see griseofulvin on this page*

griseofulvin ultramicrosize *see griseofulvin on this page*

Gris-PEG® *see griseofulvin on this page*

guaifenesin (gwye fen' e sin)

Brand Names Amonidrin® [OTC]; Anti-Tuss® Expectorant [OTC]; Breonesin® [OTC]; Fenesin™ [OTC]; Gee Gee® [OTC]; Genatuss® [OTC]; GG-Cen® [OTC]; Glyate® [OTC]; Glycotuss® [OTC]; Glytuss® [OTC]; GuiaCough® Expectorant [OTC]; Guiatuss® [OTC]; Halotussin® [OTC]; Humibid® L.A. [OTC]; Humibid® Sprinkle [OTC]; Hytuss® [OTC]; Hytuss-2X® [OTC]; Liquibid®; Malotuss® [OTC]; Medi-Tuss® [OTC]; Mytussin® [OTC]; Naldecon® Senior EX [OTC]; Pneumomist®; Robitussin® [OTC]; Scot-Tussin® [OTC]; Sinumist®-SR Capsulets® [OTC]; Uni-tussin® [OTC]

Synonyms GG; glycerol guaiacolate

Therapeutic Category Expectorant

Use Temporary control of cough due to minor throat and bronchial irritation

Usual Dosage Oral:

Children:

<2 years: 12 mg/kg/day in 6 divided doses

(Continued)

guaifenesin *(Continued)*
2-5 years: 50-100 mg (2.5-5 mL) every 4 hours, not to exceed 600 mg/day
6-11 years: 100-200 mg (5-10 mL) every 4 hours, not to exceed 1.2 g/day

Children >12 years and Adults: 200-400 mg (10-20 mL) every 4 hours to a maximum of 2.4 g/day (60 mL/day)

Dosage Forms
Capsule (Breonesin®, GG-Cen®, Hytuss-2X®): 200 mg
Capsule, sustained release (Humibid® Sprinkle): 300 mg
Liquid (Naldecon® Senior EX): 200 mg/5 mL (118 mL, 480 mL)
Syrup (Anti-Tuss® Expectorant, Genatuss®, Glyate®, GuiaCough® Expectorant, Guia-tuss®, Halotussin®, Malotuss®, Medi-Tuss®, Mytussin®, Robitussin®, Scot-tussin®, Uni-Tussin®): 100 mg/5 mL (30 mL, 120 mL, 240 mL, 473 mL, 946 mL)
Tablet:
Amonidrin®, Gee Gee®, Glytuss®: 200 mg
Glycotuss®, Hytuss®: 100 mg
Sustained release:
Fenesin™, Humibid® L.A., Pneumomist®, Sinumist®-SR Capsulets®: 600 mg

Guaifenesin AC® *see guaifenesin and codeine on this page*

guaifenesin and codeine
Brand Names Cheracol®; Glydeine®; Guaifenesin AC®; Guaituss AC®; Guiatussin® with Codeine; Halotussin® AC; Medi-Tuss® AC; Mytussin® AC; Robitussin® A-C
Synonyms codeine and guaifenesin
Therapeutic Category Antitussive; Cough Preparation; Expectorant
Use Temporary control of cough due to minor throat and bronchial irritation
Usual Dosage Oral:
Children:
2-6 years: 1-1.5 mg/kg codeine/day divided into 4 doses administered every 4-6 hours
6-12 years: 5 mL every 4 hours, not to exceed 30 mL/24 hours
>12 years: 10 mL every 4 hours, up to 60 mL/24 hours

Adults: 10 mL every 6-8 hours
Dosage Forms Syrup: Guaifenesin 100 mg and codeine phosphate 10 mg per 5 mL (60 mL, 120 mL, 480 mL)

guaifenesin and dextromethorphan
Brand Names Benylin® Expectorant [OTC]; Cheracol® D [OTC]; Contac® Cough Formula Liquid [OTC]; Extra Action Cough Syrup [OTC]; Genatuss DM® [OTC]; Glycotuss-dM® [OTC]; GuiaCough® [OTC]; Guiatuss DM® [OTC]; Halotussin® DM [OTC]; Humibid® DM [OTC]; Kolephrin® GG/DM [OTC]; Mytussin® DM [OTC]; Naldecon® Senior DX [OTC]; Phanatuss® [OTC]; Queltuss® [OTC]; Rhinosyn-DMX® [OTC]; Robitussin®-DM [OTC]; Syracol-CF® [OTC]; Tolu-Sed® DM [OTC]; Tuss-DM® [OTC]; Uni-tussin® DM [OTC]
Synonyms dextromethorphan and guaifenesin
Therapeutic Category Antitussive; Cough Preparation; Expectorant
Use Temporary control of cough due to minor throat and bronchial irritation
Usual Dosage Oral:
Children:
2-5 years: 2.5 mL every 6-8 hours; maximum: 10 mL/day
6-12 years: 5 mL every 6-8 hours; maximum: 20 mL/24 hours
>12 years: 10 mL every 6-8 hours; maximum: 40 mL/24 hours
Alternatively: 0.1-0.15 mL/kg/dose every 6-8 hours as needed

Adults: 10 mL every 6-8 hours
Dosage Forms
Syrup:
Benylin® Expectorant: Guaifenesin 100 mg and dextromethorphan hydrobromide 5 mg per 5 mL (118 mL, 236 mL)

Cheracol® D, Genatuss DM®, Mytussin® DM, Robitussin®-DM, Tolu-Sed® DM: Guaifenesin 100 mg and dextromethorphan hydrobromide 10 mg per 5 mL (5 mL, 10 mL, 120 mL, 240 mL, 360 mL, 480 mL, 3780 mL)

Contac® Cough Formula Liquid: Guaifenesin 67 mg and dextromethorphan hydrobromide 10 mg per 5 mL (120 mL)

Extra Action Cough Syrup, GuiaCough®, Guiatuss DM®, Halotussin® DM, Rhinosyn-DMX®, Uni-Tussin® DM: Guaifenesin 100 mg and dextromethorphan hydrobromide 15 mg per 5 mL (120 mL, 240 mL, 480 mL)

Kolephrin® GG/DM: Guaifenesin 150 mg and dextromethorphan hydrobromide 10 mg per 5 mL (120 mL)

Naldecon® Senior DX: Guaifenesin 200 mg and dextromethorphan hydrobromide 15 mg per 5 mL (118 mL, 480 mL)

Phanatuss®: Guaifenesin 85 mg and dextromethorphan hydrobromide 10 mg per 5 mL

Tablet:

Extended release (Humibid® DM): Guaifenesin 600 mg and dextromethorphan hydrobromide 30 mg

Glycotuss-dM®: Guaifenesin 100 mg and dextromethorphan hydrobromide 10 mg

Queltuss®: Guaifenesin 100 mg and dextromethorphan hydrobromide 15 mg

Syracol-CF®: Guaifenesin 200 mg and dextromethorphan hydrobromide 15 mg

Tuss-DM®: Guaifenesin 200 mg and dextromethorphan hydrobromide 10 mg

guaifenesin and hydrocodone *see* hydrocodone and guaifenesin
on page 235

guaifenesin and phenylpropanolamine

Brand Names Ami-Tex LA®; Codimal® Expectorant [OTC]; Conex® [OTC]; Contuss® XT; Despec® Capsule; Dura-Vent®; Entex® LA; Genamin® Expectorant [OTC]; Gentab-LA®; Guiapax®; Myminic® Expectorant [OTC]; Naldecon-EX® Children's Syrup [OTC]; Nolex® LA; Partuss® LA; Phenylfenesin® I A ; Rymed-TR®; Snaplets-EX® [OTC]; Theramin® Expectorant [OTC]; Triaminic® Expectorant [OTC]; Tri-Clear® Expectorant [OTC]; Triphenyl® Expectorant [OTC]; ULR-LA®; Vanex-LA®

Synonyms phenylpropanolamine and guaifenesin

Therapeutic Category Decongestant; Expectorant

Use Symptomatic relief of those respiratory conditions where tenacious mucous plugs and congestion complicate the problem such as sinusitis, pharyngitis, bronchitis, asthma, and as an adjunctive therapy in serous otitis media

Usual Dosage Oral:

Children:

2-6 years: 2.5 mL every 4 hours

6-12 years: ¹/₂ tablet every 12 hours or 5 mL every 4 hours

Children >12 years and Adults: 1 tablet every 12 hours or 10 mL every 4 hours

Dosage Forms

Caplet (Gentab-LA®, Rymed-TR®): Guaifenesin 400 mg and phenylpropanolamine hydrochloride 75 mg

Capsule (Despec®): Guaifenesin 400 mg and phenylpropanolamine hydrochloride 75 mg

Granules (Snaplets-EX®): Guaifenesin 50 mg and phenylpropanolamine hydrochloride 6.25 mg (pack)

Liquid:

Codimal® Expectorant: Guaifenesin 100 mg and phenylpropanolamine hydrochloride 25 mg per 5 mL (120 mL)

Conex®, Genamin® Expectorant, Myminic® Expectorant, Theramine® Expectorant, Triaminic® Expectorant, Tri-Clear® Expectorant, Triphenyl® Expectorant: Guaifenesin 100 mg and phenylpropanolamine hydrochloride 12.5 mg per 5 mL (120 mL, 240 mL, 480 mL, 3780 mL)

Naldecon-EX® Children's Syrup: Guaifenesin 100 mg and phenylpropanolamine hydrochloride 6.25 mg per 5 mL (120 mL)

(Continued)

guaifenesin and phenylpropanolamine *(Continued)*

Tablet, extended release:

Ami-Tex LA®, Contuss® XT, Entex® LA, Guiapax®, Nolex® LA, Partuss® LA, Phenyl-fenesin® L.A., ULR-LA®, Vanex-LA®: Guaifenesin 400 mg and phenylpropanol-amine hydrochloride 75 mg

Dura-Vent®: Guaifenesin 600 mg and phenylpropanolamine hydrochloride 75 mg

guaifenesin and pseudoephedrine

Brand Names Congess® Jr; Congess® Sr; Congestac®; Deconsal® II; Entex® PSE; Eudal-SR®; Fedahist® Expectorant [OTC]; Fedahist® Expectorant Pediatric [OTC]; Glycofed®; Guiafed® [OTC]; Guiafed-PD®; GuiaMax-D®; Guiatab®; Guiatuss PE® [OTC]; Halotussin® PE [OTC]; Histalet X®; Respaire®-60 SR; Respaire®-120 SR; Robitussin-PE® [OTC]; Ru-Tuss® DE; Rymed®; Sinufed® Timecelles®; Touro LA®; Tuss-LA®; V-Dec-M®; Versacaps®; Zephrex®; Zephrex LA®

Synonyms pseudoephedrine and guaifenesin

Therapeutic Category Decongestant; Expectorant

Use Enhance the output of respiratory tract fluid and reduce mucosal congestion and edema in the nasal passage

Usual Dosage Oral:

Children:

2-6 years: 2.5 mL every 4 hours not to exceed 15 mL/24 hours

6-12 years: 5 mL every 4 hours not to exceed 30 mL/24 hours

Children >12 years and Adults: 10 mL every 4 hours not to exceed 60 mL/24 hours

Dosage Forms

Capsule (Rymed®): Guaifenesin 250 mg and pseudoephedrine hydrochloride 30 mg

Capsule, extended release:

Congess® Jr: Guaifenesin 125 mg and pseudoephedrine hydrochloride 60 mg

Congess® Sr, Guaifed®, Respaire®-120 SR,: Guaifenesin 250 mg and pseudoephe-drine hydrochloride 120 mg

Guiafed-PD®, Sinufed® Timecelles®, Versacaps®: Guaifenesin 300 mg and pseu-doephedrine hydrochloride 60 mg

Respaire®-60 SR: Guaifenesin 200 mg and pseudoephedrine hydrochloride 60 mg

Tuss-LA® Capsule: Guaifenesin 500 mg and pseudoephedrine hydrochloride 120 mg

Drops, oral (Fedahist® Expectorant Pediatric): Guaifenesin 40 mg and pseudoephedrine hydrochloride 7.5 mg per mL (30 mL)

Syrup:

Fedahist® Expectorant, Guiafed®: Guaifenesin 200 mg and pseudoephedrine hydro-chloride 30 mg per 5 mL (120 mL, 240 mL)

Guiatuss® PE, Halotussin® PE, Robitussin-PE®, Rymed®: Guaifenesin 100 mg and pseudoephedrine hydrochloride 30 mg per 5 mL (120 mL, 240 mL, 480 mL)

Histalet X®: Guaifenesin 200 mg and pseudoephedrine hydrochloride 45 mg per 5 mL (473 mL)

Tablet:

Congestac®, Guiatab®, Zephrex®: Guaifenesin 400 mg and pseudoephedrine hydro-chloride 60 mg

Glycofed®: Guaifenesin 100 mg and pseudoephedrine hydrochloride 30 mg

Tablet, extended release:

Deconsal® II: Guaifenesin 600 mg and pseudoephedrine hydrochloride 60 mg

Entex® PSE, GuiaMax-D®, Ru-Tuss® DE, Zephrex LA®: Guaifenesin 600 mg and pseu-doephedrine hydrochloride 120 mg

Eudal-SR®, Histalex® X, Touro LA®: Guaifenesin 400 mg and pseudoephedrine hydro-chloride 120 mg

Tuss-LA® Tablet, V-Dec-M®: Guaifenesin 5mg and pseudoephedrine hydrochloride 120 mg

guaifenesin, phenylpropanolamine, and dextromethorphan

Brand Names Anatuss® [OTC]; Guiatuss CF® [OTC]; Naldecon® DX Adult Liquid [OTC]; Robafen® CF [OTC]; Robitussin-CF® [OTC]

Therapeutic Category Cough Preparation; Decongestant; Expectorant

Use Temporarily relieves nasal congestion and controls cough due to minor throat and bronchial irritation; helps loosen phlegm and thin bronchial secretions to make coughs more productive

Usual Dosage Oral:
Children:
2-6 years: 2.5 mL every 4 hours not to exceed 15 mL/24 hours
6-12 years: 5 mL every 4 hours not to exceed 30 mL/24 hours

Children >12 years and Adults: 10 mL every 4 hours not to exceed 60 mL/24 hours

Dosage Forms
Syrup:
Anatuss®: Guaifenesin 100 mg, phenylpropanolamine hydrochloride 25 mg, and dextromethorphan hydrobromide 15 mg per 5 mL (120 mL, 473 mL)
Guiatuss® CF, Robafen® CF, Robitussin-CF®: Guaifenesin 100 mg, phenylpropanolamine hydrochloride 12.5 mg, and dextromethorphan hydrobromide 10 mg per 5 mL (120 mL, 240 mL, 360 mL, 480 mL)
Naldecon® DX Adult: Guaifenesin 200 mg, phenylpropanolamine hydrochloride 12.5 mg, and dextromethorphan hydrobromide 10 mg per 5 mL (120 mL, 473 mL)
Tablet: (Anatuss®): Guaifenesin 100 mg, phenylpropanolamine hydrochloride 25 mg, and dextromethorphan hydrobromide 15 mg

guaifenesin, phenylpropanolamine, and phenylephrine
Brand Names Contuss®; Despec® Liquid; Dura-Gest®; Enomine®; Entex®; Guiatex®; Respinol-G®; ULR®

Therapeutic Category Decongestant; Expectorant

Use Symptomatic relief of sinusitis, bronchitis, pharyngitis associated with nasal congestion and thick mucous secretions in lower respiratory tract

Usual Dosage Children >12 years and Adults: 1 capsule 4 times/day (every 6 hours) with food or fluid

Dosage Forms
Capsule (Contuss®, Dura-Gest®, Enomine®, Entex®, Guiatex®, ULR®): Guaifenesin 200 mg, phenylpropanolamine hydrochloride 45 mg, and phenylephrine hydrochloride 5 mg
Liquid (Contuss®, Despec®, Entex®): Guaifenesin 100 mg, phenylpropanolamine hydrochloride 20 mg, and phenylephrine hydrochloride 5 mg per 5 mL (118 mL, 480 mL)
Tablet (Respinol-G®): Guaifenesin 200 mg, phenylpropanolamine hydrochloride 45 mg, and phenylephrine hydrochloride 5 mg

guaifenesin, pseudoephedrine, and codeine
Brand Names Codafed® Expectorant; Decohistine® Expectorant; Deproist® Expectorant with Codeine; Dihistine® Expectorant; Guiatuss DAC®; Guiatussin® DAC; Halotussin® DAC; Isoclor® Expectorant; Mytussin® DAC; Novahistine® Expectorant; Nucofed®; Nucofed® Pediatric Expectorant; Nucotuss®; Phenhist® Expectorant; Robitussin®-DAC; Ryna-CX®

Therapeutic Category Cough Preparation; Decongestant; Expectorant

Use Temporarily relieves nasal congestion and controls cough due to minor throat and bronchial irritation; helps loosen phlegm and thin bronchial secretions to make coughs more productive

Usual Dosage Oral:
Children 6-12 years: 5 mL every 4 hours, not to exceed 40 mL/24 hours

Children >12 years and Adults: 10 mL every 4 hours, not to exceed 40 mL/24 hours

Dosage Forms Liquid:
Codafed® Expectorant, Decohistine® Expectorant, Deproist® Expectorant with Codeine, Dihistine® Expectorant, Guiatuss DAC®, Guiatussin® DAC, Halotussin® DAC, Isoclor® Expectorant, Mytussin® DAC, Novahistine® Expectorant, Nucofed® Pediatric Expectorant, Phenhist® Expectorant, Robitussin®-DAC, Ryna-CX®: Guaifenesin 100 mg, pseudoephedrine hydrochloride 30 mg, and codeine phosphate 10 mg per 5 mL (120 mL, 480 mL, 4000 mL)
Nucofed®, Nucotuss®: Guaifenesin 200 mg, pseudoephedrine hydrochloride 60 mg, and codeine phosphate 20 mg per 5 mL (480 mL)

Guaituss AC® *see* guaifenesin and codeine *on page 218*

guanabenz acetate (gwahn' a benz)
Brand Names Wytensin®
Therapeutic Category Alpha-Adrenergic Agonist
Use Management of hypertension
Usual Dosage Adults: Oral: Initial: 4 mg twice daily, increase in increments of 4-8 mg/day every 1-2 weeks to a maximum of 32 mg twice daily
Dosage Forms Tablet: 4 mg, 8 mg

guanadrel sulfate (gwahn' a drel)
Brand Names Hylorel®
Therapeutic Category Alpha-Adrenergic Agonist
Use Considered a second line agent in the treatment of hypertension, usually with a diuretic
Usual Dosage Initial: 10 mg/day (5 mg twice daily); adjust dosage until blood pressure is controlled, usual dosage: 20-75 mg/day, given twice daily
Dosage Forms Tablet: 10 mg, 25 mg

guanethidine monosulfate (gwahn eth' i deen)
Brand Names Ismelin®
Therapeutic Category Alpha-Adrenergic Agonist
Use Treatment of moderate to severe hypertension
Usual Dosage
Children: Initial dose: 0.2 mg/kg/day, given daily; maximum dose: up to 3 mg/kg/24 hours
Adults: Initial dose: 10-12.5 mg/day, then 25-50 mg/day in 3 divided doses
Dosage Forms Tablet: 10 mg, 25 mg

guanfacine hydrochloride (gwahn' fa seen)
Brand Names Tenex®
Therapeutic Category Alpha-Adrenergic Agonist
Use Management of hypertension
Usual Dosage Adults: Oral: 1 mg usually at bedtime, may increase if needed at 3- to 4-week intervals to a maximum of 3 mg/day; 1 mg/day is most common dose
Dosage Forms Tablet: 1 mg

guanidine hydrochloride (gwahn' i deen)
Therapeutic Category Cholinergic Agent
Use Reduction of the symptoms of muscle weakness associated with the myasthenic syndrome of Eaton-Lambert, not for myasthenia gravis
Usual Dosage Adults: Oral: Initial: 10-15 mg/kg/day in 3-4 divided doses, gradually increase to 35 mg/kg/day
Dosage Forms Tablet: 125 mg

GuiaCough® [OTC] *see* guaifenesin and dextromethorphan *on page 218*
GuiaCough® Expectorant [OTC] *see* guaifenesin *on page 217*
Guiafed® [OTC] *see* guaifenesin and pseudoephedrine *on page 220*
Guiafed-PD® *see* guaifenesin and pseudoephedrine *on page 220*
GuiaMax-D® *see* guaifenesin and pseudoephedrine *on page 220*
Guiapax® *see* guaifenesin and phenylpropanolamine *on page 219*
Guiatab® *see* guaifenesin and pseudoephedrine *on page 220*

Guiatex® *see* guaifenesin, phenylpropanolamine, and phenylephrine *on page 221*

Guiatuss® [OTC] *see* guaifenesin *on page 217*

Guiatuss CF® [OTC] *see* guaifenesin, phenylpropanolamine, and dextromethorphan *on page 220*

Guiatuss DAC® *see* guaifenesin, pseudoephedrine, and codeine *on page 221*

Guiatuss DM® [OTC] *see* guaifenesin and dextromethorphan *on page 218*

Guiatussin® DAC *see* guaifenesin, pseudoephedrine, and codeine *on page 221*

Guiatussin® with Codeine *see* guaifenesin and codeine *on page 218*

Guiatuss PE® [OTC] *see* guaifenesin and pseudoephedrine *on page 220*

gum benjamin *see* benzoin *on page 49*

G-well® Lotion *see* lindane *on page 274*

G-well® Shampoo *see* lindane *on page 274*

Gynecort® Topical [OTC] *see* hydrocortisone *on page 236*

Gyne-Lotrimin® Vaginal [OTC] *see* clotrimazole *on page 109*

Gyne-Sulf® Vaginal *see* sulfabenzamide, sulfacetamide, and sulfathiazole *on page 446*

Gynogen L.A.® Injection *see* estradiol *on page 178*

Gynol II® [OTC] *see* nonoxynol 9 *on page 338*

Habitrol™ Patch *see* nicotine *on page 334*

***Haemophilus* b oligosaccharide conjugate vaccine** *see* hemophilus b conjugate vaccine *on page 226*

***Haemophilus* b polysaccharide vaccine** *see* hemophilus b conjugate vaccine *on page 226*

halazepam (hal az' e pam)
Brand Names Paxipam®
Therapeutic Category Antianxiety Agent; Benzodiazepine
Use Management of anxiety disorders; short-term relief of the symptoms of anxiety
Usual Dosage Adults: Oral: 20-40 mg 3 or 4 times daily
Dosage Forms Tablet: 20 mg, 40 mg

halcinonide (hal sin' oh nide)
Brand Names Halog-E® Topical; Halog® Topical
Therapeutic Category Corticosteroid, Topical (High Potency)
Use Inflammation of corticosteroid-responsive dermatoses
Usual Dosage Children and Adults: Topical: Apply sparingly 1-3 times/day, occlusive dressing may be used for severe or resistant dermatoses
Dosage Forms
Cream (Halog®): 0.025% (15 g, 60 g, 240 g); 0.1% (15 g, 30 g, 60 g, 240 g)
Cream, emollient base (Halog®-E) : 0.1% (15 g, 30 g, 60 g)
Ointment, topical (Halog®): 0.1% (15 g, 30 g, 60 g, 240 g)
Solution (Halog®): 0.1% (20 mL, 60 mL)

Halcion® *see* triazolam *on page 476*

Haldol® Decanoate Injection *see* haloperidol *on next page*

Haldol® Injection *see* haloperidol *on next page*

Haldol® Oral *see* haloperidol *on next page*

Halenol® [OTC] *see* acetaminophen *on page 2*

Haley's M-O® [OTC] *see* magnesium hydroxide and mineral oil emulsion *on page 282*

halobetasol propionate (hal oh bay' ta sol)
Brand Names Ultravate™ Topical
Therapeutic Category Corticosteroid, Topical (Very High Potency)
Use Relief of inflammatory and pruritic manifestations of corticosteroid-response dermatoses
Usual Dosage Children and Adults: Topical: Apply sparingly to skin twice daily, rub in gently and completely
Dosage Forms
 Cream: 0.05% (15 g, 45 g)
 Ointment, topical: 0.05% (15 g, 45 g)

Halodrin® *see* ethinyl estradiol and fluoxymesterone *on page 183*
Halog-E® Topical *see* halcinonide *on previous page*
Halog® Topical *see* halcinonide *on previous page*

haloperidol (ha loe per' i dole)
Brand Names Haldol® Decanoate Injection; Haldol® Injection; Haldol® Oral
Therapeutic Category Antipsychotic Agent
Use Treatment of psychoses, Tourette's disorder, and severe behavioral problems in children; may be used for the emergency sedation of severely agitated or delirious patients
Usual Dosage
 Children:
  <3 years: Not recommended
  3-6 years: Dose and indications are not well established
   Control of agitation or hyperkinesia in disturbed children: Oral: 0.01-0.03 mg/kg/day once daily
   Infantile autism: Oral: Daily doses of 0.5-4 mg have been reported to be helpful in this disorder
  6-12 years: Dose not well established
   I.M.: 1-3 mg/dose every 4-8 hours, up to a maximum of 0.1 mg/kg/day
   Acute psychosis: Oral: Begin with 0.5-1.5 mg/day and increase gradually in increments of 0.5 mg/day, to a maintenance dose of 2-4 mg/day (0.05-0.1 mg/kg/day).
   Tourette's syndrome and mental retardation with hyperkinesia: Oral: Begin with 0.5 mg/day and increase by 0.5 mg/day each day until symptoms are controlled or a maximum dose of 15 mg is reached
 Children >12 years and Adults:
  I.M.:
   Acute psychosis: 2-5 mg/dose every 1-8 hours PRN up to a total of 10-30 mg, until control of symptoms is achieved
   Mental retardation with hyperkinesia: Begin with 20 mg/day in divided doses, then increase slowly, up to a maximum of 60 mg/day; change to oral administration as soon as symptoms are controlled
  Oral:
   Acute psychosis: Begin with 1-15 mg/day in divided doses, then gradually increase until symptoms are controlled, up to a maximum of 100 mg/day; after control of symptoms is achieved, reduce dose to the minimal effective dose
   Tourette's syndrome: Begin with 6-15 mg/day in divided doses, increase in increments of 2-10 mg/day until symptoms are controlled or adverse reactions become disabling; when symptoms are controlled, reduce to approximately 9 mg/day for maintenance
Dosage Forms
 Concentrate, oral, as lactate: 2 mg/mL (5 mL, 10 mL, 15 mL, 120 mL, 240 mL)

Injection, as decanoate: 50 mg/mL (1 mL, 5 mL); 100 mg/mL (1 mL, 5 mL)
Injection, as lactate: 5 mg/mL (1 mL, 2 mL, 2.5 mL, 10 mL)
Tablet: 0.5 mg, 1 mg, 2 mg, 5 mg, 10 mg, 20 mg

haloprogin (ha loe proe' jin)
Brand Names Halotex® Topical
Therapeutic Category Antifungal Agent, Topical
Use Topical treatment of tinea pedis, tinea cruris, tinea corporis, tinea manuum caused by *Trichophyton rubrum*, *Trichophyton tonsurans*, *Trichophyton mentagrophytes*, *Microsporum canis*, or *Epidermophyton floccosum*
Usual Dosage Children and Adults: Topical: Twice daily for 2-3 weeks; intertriginous areas may require up to 4 weeks of treatment
Dosage Forms
Cream: 1% (15 g, 30 g)
Solution, topical: 1% with alcohol 75% (10 mL, 30 mL)

Halotestin® *see* fluoxymesterone *on page 203*
Halotex® Topical *see* haloprogin *on this page*

halothane (ha' loe thane)
Brand Names Fluothane®
Therapeutic Category General Anesthetic
Use General induction and maintenance of anesthesia (inhalation)
Usual Dosage Maintenance concentration varies from 0.5% to 1.5%
Dosage Forms Liquid: 125 mL, 250 mL

Halotussin® [OTC] *see* guaifenesin *on page 217*
Halotussin® AC *see* guaifenesin and codeine *on page 218*
Halotussin® DAC *see* guaifenesin, pseudoephedrine, and codeine *on page 221*
Halotussin® DM [OTC] *see* guaifenesin and dextromethorphan *on page 218*
Halotussin® PE [OTC] *see* guaifenesin and pseudoephedrine *on page 220*
Haltran® [OTC] *see* ibuprofen *on page 245*
hamamelis water *see* witch hazel *on page 501*
HBCV *see* hemophilus b conjugate vaccine *on next page*
HBIG *see* hepatitis b immune globulin *on page 227*
H-BIG® *see* hepatitis b immune globulin *on page 227*
HCG *see* chorionic gonadotropin *on page 101*
HCTZ *see* hydrochlorothiazide *on page 233*
HD 85® *see* radiological/contrast media (ionic) *on page 413*
HD 200 Plus® *see* radiological/contrast media (ionic) *on page 413*
HDCV *see* rabies virus vaccine, human diploid *on page 413*
HDRS *see* rabies virus vaccine, human diploid *on page 413*
Head & Shoulders® [OTC] *see* pyrithione zinc *on page 410*
Healon® Injection *see* sodium hyaluronate *on page 436*
Hemabate™ *see* carboprost tromethamine *on page 75*
Hema-Chek® [OTC] *see* diagnostic aids (*in vitro*), feces *on page 138*
Hema-Combistix® [OTC] *see* diagnostic aids (*in vitro*), urine *on page 139*
Hemastix® [OTC] *see* diagnostic aids (*in vitro*), urine *on page 139*
Hematest® [OTC] *see* diagnostic aids (*in vitro*), feces *on page 138*

hemiacidrin *see* citric acid bladder mixture *on page 103*

hemin
Brand Names Panhematin®
Therapeutic Category Blood Modifiers
Use Treatment of recurrent attacks of acute intermittent porphyria (AIP) only after an appropriate period of alternate therapy has been tried
Usual Dosage I.V.: 1-4 mg/kg/day administered over 10-15 minutes for 3-14 days; may be repeated no earlier than every 12 hours; not to exceed 6 mg/kg in any 24-hour period
Dosage Forms Powder for injection, preservative free: 313 mg/vial [hematin 7 mg/mL] (43 mL)

Hemoccult® II [OTC] *see* diagnostic aids (*in vitro*), feces *on page 138*

Hemoccult® Slides *see* diagnostic aids (*in vitro*), feces *on page 138*

Hemocyte® [OTC] *see* ferrous fumarate *on page 193*

Hemofil® M *see* antihemophilic factor *on page 29*

hemophilus b conjugate vaccine (hem off' fil us)
Brand Names HibTITER®; PedvaxHIB™; ProHIBiT®
Synonyms diphtheria crm$_{197}$ protein conjugate; diphtheria toxoid conjugate; *Haemophilus* b oligosaccharide conjugate vaccine; *Haemophilus* b polysaccharide vaccine; HBCV; Hib polysaccharide conjugate; PRP-D
Therapeutic Category Vaccine, Inactivated Bacteria
Use Immunization of children 24 months to 6 years of age against diseases caused by *H. influenzae* type b
Dosage Forms Injection:
HibTITER®: Capsular oligosaccharide 10 μg and diphtheria CRM$_{197}$ protein ~25 μg per 0.5 mL (0.5 mL, 2.5 mL, 5 mL)
PedvaxHIB™: Purified capsular polysaccharide 15 μg and *Neisseria meningitidis* OMPC 250 μg per dose (0.5 mL)
ProHIBiT®: Purified capsular polysaccharide 25 μg and conjugated diphtheria toxoid protein 18 μg per dose (0.5 mL, 2.5 mL, 5 mL)

heparin (hep' a rin)
Brand Names Calciparine® Injection; Hep-Lock® Injection; Liquaemin® Injection
Synonyms heparin calcium; heparin lock flush; heparin sodium
Therapeutic Category Anticoagulant
Use Prophylaxis and treatment of thromboembolic disorders
Usual Dosage Note: For full-dose heparin (ie, nonlow-dose), the dose should be titrated according to PTT results. For anticoagulation, an APTT 1.5-2.5 times normal is usually desired. APTT is usually measured prior to heparin therapy, 6-8 hours after initiation of a continuous infusion (following a loading dose), and 6-8 hours after changes in the infusion rate; increase or decrease infusion by 2-4 units/kg/hour dependent on PTT. Continuous I.V. infusion is preferred vs I.V. intermittent injections. For intermittent I.V. injections, PTT is measured 3.5-4 hours after I.V. injection.

Children:
Intermittent I.V.: Initial: 50-100 units/kg, then 50-100 units/kg every 4 hours
I.V. infusion: Initial: 50 units/kg, then 15-25 units/kg/hour; increase dose by 2-4 units/kg/hour every 6-8 hours as required

Adults:
Prophylaxis (low-dose heparin): S.C.: 5000 units every 8-12 hours
Intermittent I.V.: Initial: 10,000 units, then 50-70 units/kg (5000-10,000 units) every 4-6 hours
I.V. infusion: Initial: 75-100 units/kg, then 15 units/kg/hour with dose adjusted according to PTT results; usual range: 10-30 units/kg/hour

Dosage Forms

Heparin sodium:
  Lock flush injection:
    Beef lung source: 10 units/mL (1 mL, 2 mL, 2.5 mL, 3 mL, 5 mL, 10 mL, 30 mL); 100 units/mL (1 mL, 2 mL, 2.5 mL, 3 mL, 5 mL, 10 mL, 30 mL)
    Porcine intestinal mucosa source: 10 units/mL (1 mL, 2 mL, 10 mL, 30 mL); 100 units/mL (1 mL, 2 mL, 10 mL, 30 mL)
    Porcine intestinal mucosa source, preservative free: 10 units/mL (1 mL); 100 units/mL (1 mL)
  Multiple-dose vial injection:
    Beef lung source, with preservative: 1000 units/mL (5 mL, 10 mL, 30 mL); 5000 units/mL (10 mL); 10,000 units/mL (4 mL, 5 mL, 10 mL); 20,000 units/mL (2 mL, 5 mL, 10 mL); 40,000 units/mL (5 mL)
    Porcine intestinal mucosa source, with preservative: 1000 units/mL (10 mL, 30 mL); 5000 units/mL (10 mL); 10,000 units/mL (4 mL); 20,000 units/mL (2 mL, 5 mL)
  Single-dose vial injection:
    Beef lung source: 1000 units/mL (1 mL); 5000 units/mL (1 mL); 10,000 units/mL (1 mL); 20,000 units/mL (1 mL); 40,000 units/mL (1 mL)
    Porcine intestinal mucosa: 1000 units/mL (1 mL); 5000 units/mL (1 mL); 10,000 units/mL (1 mL); 20,000 units/mL (1 mL); 40,000 units/mL (1 mL)
  Unit dose injection:
    Porcine intestinal mucosa source, with preservative: 1000 units/dose (1 mL, 2 mL); 2500 units/dose (1 mL); 5000 units/dose (0.5 mL, 1 mL); 7500 units/dose (1 mL); 10,000 units/dose (1 mL); 15,000 units/dose (1 mL); 20,000 units/dose (1 mL)

Heparin sodium infusion, porcine intestinal mucosa source:
  D_5W: 40 units/mL (500 mL); 50 units/mL (250 mL, 500 mL); 100 units/mL (100 mL, 250 mL)
  NaCl 0.45%: 2 units/mL (500 mL, 1000 mL); 50 units/mL (250 mL); 100 units/mL (250 mL)
  NaCl 0.9%: 2 units/mL (500 mL, 1000 mL); 5 units/mL (1000 mL); 50 units/mL (250 mL, 500 mL, 1000 mL)

Heparin calcium:
  Unit dose injection, porcine intestinal mucosa, preservative free (Calciparine®): 5000 units/dose (0.2 mL); 12,500 units/dose (0.5 mL); 20,000 units/dose (0.8 mL)

heparin calcium *see* heparin *on previous page*

heparin lock flush *see* heparin *on previous page*

heparin sodium *see* heparin *on previous page*

hepatitis b immune globulin
Brand Names H-BIG®; Hep-B-Gammagee®; HyperHep®
Synonyms HBIG
Therapeutic Category Immune Globulin
Use Provide prophylactic passive immunity to hepatitis B infection to those individuals exposed. Hepatitis B immune globulin is not indicated for treatment of active hepatitis B infections and is ineffective in the treatment of chronic active hepatitis B infection.
Usual Dosage I.M.:
  Newborns: Hepatitis B: 0.5 mL as soon after birth as possible (within 12 hours)
  Adults: Postexposure prophylaxis: 0.06 mL/kg; usual dose: 3-5 mL; maximum dose: 5 mL as soon as possible after exposure (within 7 days); repeat at 28-30 days after exposure
Dosage Forms Injection:
  H-BIG®: 4 mL, 5 mL
  Hep-B-Gammagee®: 5 mL
  HyperHep®: 0.5 mL, 1 mL, 5 mL

hepatitis b inactivated virus vaccine (plasma derived) *see* hepatitis b vaccine *on this page*

hepatitis b inactivated virus vaccine (recombinant dna) *see* hepatitis b vaccine *on this page*

hepatitis b vaccine
Brand Names Engerix-B®; Recombivax HB®
Synonyms hepatitis b inactivated virus vaccine (plasma derived); hepatitis b inactivated virus vaccine (recombinant dna)
Therapeutic Category Vaccine, Inactivated Virus
Use Immunization against infection caused by all known subtypes of hepatitis B virus in individuals considered at high risk of potential exposure to hepatitis B virus or HB_sAg-positive materials
Usual Dosage I.M.:
Neonates born to HB_sAg-positive mothers: 5 μg

Children:
≤11 years: 2.5 μg doses
11-19 years: 5 μg doses

Adults >20 years: 10 μg doses
Dosage Forms Injection:
Recombinant DNA (Engerix-B®): Hepatitis B surface antigen 20 μg/mL (1 mL)
Pediatric, recombinant DNA (Engerix-B®): Hepatitis B surface antigen 10 μg/0.5 mL (0.5 mL)
Recombinant DNA (Recombivax HB®): Hepatitis B surface antigen 10 μg/mL (1 mL, 3 mL)
Dialysis formulation, recombinant DNA (Recombivax HB®): Hepatitis B surface antigen 40 μg/mL (1 mL)

Hep-B-Gammagee® *see* hepatitis b immune globulin *on previous page*
Hep-Lock® Injection *see* heparin *on page 226*
Herplex® Ophthalmic *see* idoxuridine *on page 245*
HES *see* hetastarch *on this page*
Hespan® *see* hetastarch *on this page*

hetastarch (het' a starch)
Brand Names Hespan®
Synonyms HES; hydroxyethyl starch
Therapeutic Category Plasma Volume Expander
Use Blood volume expander used in treatment of shock or impending shock when blood or blood products are not available
Usual Dosage Up to 1500 mL/day
Dosage Forms Infusion, in sodium chloride 0.9%: 6% (500 mL)

Hexabrix™ *see* radiological/contrast media (ionic) *on page 413*
hexachlorocyclohexane *see* lindane *on page 274*

hexachlorophene (hex a klor' oh feen)
Brand Names pHisoHex®; Septisol®
Therapeutic Category Antibacterial, Topical; Soap
Use As surgical scrub and as a bacteriostatic skin cleanser; to control an outbreak of gram-positive infection when other procedures have been unsuccessful
Usual Dosage Children and Adults: Topical: Apply 5 mL cleanser and water to area to be cleansed; lather and rinse thoroughly under running water

Dosage Forms
Foam (Septisol®): 0.23% with alcohol 56% (180 mL, 600 mL)
Liquid, topical (pHisoHex®): 3% (8 mL, 150 mL, 500 mL, 3840 mL)

Hexadrol® Phosphate Injection *see* dexamethasone *on page 132*

Hexadrol® Tablet *see* dexamethasone *on page 132*

Hexalen® *see* altretamine *on page 14*

hexamethylenetetramine *see* methenamine *on page 299*

hexamethylmelamine *see* altretamine *on page 14*

H.H.R.® *see* hydralazine, hydrochlorothiazide, and reserpine *on page 232*

Hibiclens® Topical [OTC] *see* chlorhexidine gluconate *on page 90*

Hibistat® Topical [OTC] *see* chlorhexidine gluconate *on page 90*

Hib polysaccharide conjugate *see* hemophilus b conjugate vaccine *on page 226*

HibTITER® *see* hemophilus b conjugate vaccine *on page 226*

Hi-Cor-1.0® Topical *see* hydrocortisone *on page 236*

Hi-Cor-2.5® Topical *see* hydrocortisone *on page 236*

Hiprex® *see* methenamine *on page 299*

Hismanal® *see* astemizole *on page 36*

Histaject® Injection *see* brompheniramine maleate *on page 59*

Histalet X® *see* guaifenesin and pseudoephedrine *on page 220*

histamine acid phosphate *see* histamine phosphate *on this page*

histamine diphosphate *see* histamine phosphate *on this page*

histamine phosphate
Synonyms histamine acid phosphate; histamine diphosphate
Therapeutic Category Diagnostic Agent, Achlorhydria and Pheochromocytoma
Use Diagnostic test for achlorhydria and pheochromocytoma
Usual Dosage Adults:
Gastric: Function test: S.C.: 0.0275 mg/kg histamine phosphate (10 μg/kg histamine)
Pheochromocytoma: I.V.: 10 μg (histamine), then 50 μg 5 minutes later if no response after first dose
Dosage Forms Injection:
Gastric test: 0.55 mg/mL [0.2 mg base] (5 mL); 2.75 mg/mL [1 mg base] (1 mL)
Pheochromocytoma test: 0.275 mg/mL [0.1 mg base] (1 mL)

Histerone® Injection *see* testosterone *on page 456*

Histolyn-CYL® Injection *see* histoplasmin *on this page*

histoplasmin (hiss toe plaz' min)
Brand Names Histolyn-CYL® Injection
Synonyms histoplasmosis skin test antigen
Therapeutic Category Diagnostic Agent, Skin Test
Use Diagnosing histoplasmosis; to assess cell-mediated immunity
Usual Dosage Adults: Intradermally: 0.1 mL of 1:100 dilution 5-10 cm apart into volar surface of forearm; induration of ≥5 mm in diameter indicates a positive reaction
Dosage Forms Injection: 1:100 (0.1 mL, 1.3 mL)

histoplasmosis skin test antigen *see* histoplasmin *on this page*

Histor-D® Liquid *see* chlorpheniramine and phenylephrine *on page 93*

Histor-D® Timecelles® *see* chlorpheniramine, phenylephrine, and methscopolamine *on page 95*

histrelin (his trel' in)
Brand Names Supprelin™ Injection
Therapeutic Category Gonadotropin Releasing Hormone Analog
Use Central idiopathic precocious puberty, endometriosis, leiomyomata uteri
Usual Dosage
Central idiopathic precocious puberty: S.C.: Usual dose is 10 µg/kg/day given as a single daily dose at the same time each day

Acute intermittent porphyria in women:
S.C.: 5 µg/day
Intranasal: 400-800 µg/day

Endometriosis: S.C.: 100 µg/day

Leiomyomata uteri: S.C.: 20-50 µg/day or 4 µg/kg/day
Dosage Forms Injection: 7-day kits of single use: 120 µg/0.6 mL; 300 µg/0.6 mL; 600 µg/0.6 mL

Histrodrix® [OTC] *see* dexbrompheniramine and pseudoephedrine *on page 134*

Hivid® *see* zalcitabine *on page 502*

HMS Liquifilm® Ophthalmic *see* medrysone *on page 289*

HN₂ *see* mechlorethamine hydrochloride *on page 287*

Hold® DM [OTC] *see* dextromethorphan hydrobromide *on page 136*

homatropine and hydrocodone *see* hydrocodone and homatropine *on page 235*

homatropine hydrobromide (hoe ma' troe peen)
Brand Names AK-Homatropine® Ophthalmic; Isopto® Homatropine Ophthalmic
Therapeutic Category Anticholinergic Agent, Ophthalmic; Ophthalmic Agent, Mydriatic
Use Producing cycloplegia and mydriasis for refraction; treatment of acute inflammatory conditions of the uveal tract
Usual Dosage
Children:
Mydriasis and cycloplegia for refraction: 1 drop of 2% solution immediately before the procedure; repeat at 10-minute intervals as needed
Uveitis: 1 drop of 2% solution 2-3 times/day
Adults:
Mydriasis and cycloplegia for refraction: 1-2 drops of 2% solution or 1 drop of 5% solution before the procedure; repeat at 5- to 10-minute intervals as needed
Uveitis: 1-2 drops 2-3 times/day up to every 3-4 hours as needed
Dosage Forms Solution, ophthalmic:
2% (1 mL, 5 mL); 5% (1 mL, 2 mL, 5 mL)
AK-Homatropine®: 5% (15 mL)
Isopto® Homatropine 2% (5 mL, 15 mL); 5% (5 mL, 15 mL)

horse anti-human thymocyte gamma globulin *see* lymphocyte immune globulin, anti-thymocyte globulin (equine) *on page 280*

H.P. Acthar® Gel *see* corticotropin *on page 116*

human growth hormone
Brand Names Humatrope® Injection; Protropin® Injection
Synonyms somatrem; somatropin
Therapeutic Category Growth Hormone

Use Long-term treatment of growth failure from lack of adequate endogenous growth hormone secretion

Usual Dosage Children: I.M., S.C.:
Somatrem: Up to 0.1 mg (0.26 units)/kg/dose 3 times/week
Somatropin: Up to 0.06 mg (0.16 units)/kg/dose 3 times/week
Therapy should be discontinued when patient has reached satisfactory adult height, when epiphyses have fused, or when the patient ceases to respond

Dosage Forms Injection:
Somatropin: Humatrope®: 5 mg ~13 units (5 mL)
Somatrem: Protropin®: 5 mg ~13 units (10 mL)

Humate-P® *see* antihemophilic factor *on page 29*

Humatin® *see* paromomycin sulfate *on page 357*

Humatrope® Injection *see* human growth hormone *on previous page*

Humibid® DM [OTC] *see* guaifenesin and dextromethorphan *on page 218*

Humibid® L.A. [OTC] *see* guaifenesin *on page 217*

Humibid® Sprinkle [OTC] *see* guaifenesin *on page 217*

Humorsol® Ophthalmic *see* demecarium bromide *on page 129*

Humulin® *see* insulin preparations *on page 250*

Hurricaine® *see* benzocaine *on page 48*

hyaluronic acid *see* sodium hyaluronate *on page 436*

hyaluronidase (hye al yoor on' i dase)
Brand Names Wydase® Injection
Therapeutic Category Antidote, Extravasation
Use Increase the dispersion and absorption of other drugs; increase rate of absorption of parenteral fluids given by hypodermoclysis; enhance diffusion of locally irritating or toxic drugs in the management of I.V. extravasation
Usual Dosage
Infants and Children:
Management of I.V. extravasation: Reconstitute the 150 unit vial of lyophilized powder with 1 mL normal saline; take 0.1 mL of this solution and dilute with 0.9 mL normal saline to yield 15 units/mL; using a 25- or 26-gauge needle, five 0.2 mL injections are made subcutaneously or intradermally into the extravasation site at the leading edge, changing the needle after each injection
Hypodermoclysis: S.C.: 15 units is added to each 100 mL of I.V. fluid to be administered

Adults: Absorption and dispersion of drugs: 150 units is added to the vehicle containing the drug
Dosage Forms
Injection, stabilized solution: 150 units/mL (1 mL, 10 mL)
Powder for injection, lyophilized: 150 units, 1500 units

Hyate®:C *see* factor viii:c (porcine) *on page 189*

Hybalamin® Injection *see* hydroxocobalamin *on page 240*

Hybolin™ Decanoate Injection *see* nandrolone *on page 324*

Hybolin™ Improved Injection *see* nandrolone *on page 324*

Hycodan® *see* hydrocodone and homatropine *on page 235*

Hycomine® *see* hydrocodone and phenylpropanolamine *on page 235*

Hycomine® Pediatric *see* hydrocodone and phenylpropanolamine *on page 235*

Hycort® Topical *see* hydrocortisone *on page 236*

Hycotuss® Expectorant Liquid *see* hydrocodone and guaifenesin *on page 235*

Hydeltrasol® Injection *see* prednisolone *on page 391*

Hydeltra-T.B.A.® Injection *see* prednisolone *on page 391*

Hydergine® *see* ergoloid mesylates *on page 173*

Hydergine® LC *see* ergoloid mesylates *on page 173*

hydralazine and hydrochlorothiazide
Brand Names Apresazide®; Hydrazide®; Hy-Zide®
Synonyms hydrochlorothiazide and hydralazine
Therapeutic Category Antihypertensive, Combination
Use Management of moderate to severe hypertension and treatment of congestive heart failure
Usual Dosage Adults: Oral: 1 capsule twice daily
Dosage Forms Capsule:
25/25: Hydralazine hydrochloride 25 mg and hydrochlorothiazide 25 mg
50/50: Hydralazine hydrochloride 50 mg and hydrochlorothiazide 50 mg
100/50: Hydralazine hydrochloride 100 mg and hydrochlorothiazide 50 mg

hydralazine hydrochloride (hye dral' a zeen)
Brand Names Alazine® Oral; Apresoline® Injection; Apresoline® Oral
Therapeutic Category Vasodilator
Use Management of moderate to severe hypertension, congestive heart failure, hypertension secondary to pre-eclampsia/eclampsia
Usual Dosage
Children:
Oral: Initial: 0.75-1 mg/kg/day in 2-4 divided doses, not to exceed 25 mg/dose; increase over 3-4 weeks to maximum of 7.5 mg/kg/day in 2-4 divided doses; maximum daily dose: 200 mg/day
I.M., I.V.: 0.1-0.5 mg/kg/dose (initial dose not to exceed 20 mg) every 4-6 hours as needed
Adults:
Oral: Initial: 10 mg 4 times/day, increase by 10-25 mg/dose every 2-5 days to maximum of 300 mg/day
I.M., I.V.:
Hypertensive initial: 10-20 mg/dose every 4-6 hours as needed, may increase to 40 mg/dose
Pre-eclampsia/eclampsia: 5 mg/dose then 5-10 mg every 20-30 minutes as needed
Dosage Forms
Injection (Apresoline®): 20 mg/mL (1 mL)
Tablet (Alazine®, Apresoline®): 10 mg, 25 mg, 50 mg, 100 mg

hydralazine, hydrochlorothiazide, and reserpine
Brand Names Cam-ap-es®; H.H.R.®; Hydrap-ES®; Marpres®; Ser-A-Gen®; Ser-Ap-Es®; Serathide®; Tri-Hydroserpine®; Unipres®
Therapeutic Category Antihypertensive, Combination
Use Hypertensive disorders
Usual Dosage Adults: Oral: 1-2 tablets 3 times/day
Dosage Forms Tablet: Hydralazine 25 mg, hydrochlorothiazide 15 mg, and reserpine 0.1 mg

Hydramine® Oral [OTC] *see* diphenhydramine hydrochloride *on page 152*

Hydramyn® Syrup [OTC] *see* diphenhydramine hydrochloride *on page 152*

Hydrap-ES® *see* hydralazine, hydrochlorothiazide, and reserpine *on this page*

hydrated chloral *see* chloral hydrate *on page 87*

Hydrate®️ Injection *see* dimenhydrinate *on page 150*

Hydrazide®️ *see* hydralazine and hydrochlorothiazide *on previous page*

Hydrea®️ *see* hydroxyurea *on page 241*

Hydrex®️ *see* benzthiazide *on page 50*

Hydrisalic™️ Gel *see* salicylic acid *on page 424*

Hydrobexan®️ Injection *see* hydroxocobalamin *on page 240*

Hydrocet®️ *see* hydrocodone and acetaminophen *on next page*

hydrochlorothiazide (hye droe klor oh thye' a zide)
Brand Names Aquazide-H®️; Diaqua®️; Esidrix®️; Ezide®️; HydroDIURIL®️; Hydro-Par®️; Hydro-T®️; Mictrin®️; Oretic®️

Synonyms HCTZ

Therapeutic Category Diuretic, Thiazide

Use Management of mild to moderate hypertension; treatment of edema in congestive heart failure and nephrotic syndrome

Usual Dosage Oral:
Children (daily dosages should be decreased if used with other antihypertensives):
<6 months: 2-3 mg/kg/day in 2 divided doses
>6 months: 2 mg/kg/day in 2 divided doses

Adults: 25-50 mg/day in 1-2 doses; maximum: 200 mg/day

Dosage Forms Tablet: 25 mg, 50 mg, 100 mg

hydrochlorothiazide and amiloride *see* amiloride and hydrochlorothiazide *on page 18*

hydrochlorothiazide and hydralazine *see* hydralazine and hydrochlorothiazide *on previous page*

hydrochlorothiazide and methyldopa *see* methyldopa and hydrochlorothiazide *on page 305*

hydrochlorothiazide and reserpine
Brand Names Hydropres®️; Hydro-Serp®️; Hydroserpine®️

Synonyms reserpine and hydrochlorothiazide

Therapeutic Category Antihypertensive, Combination

Use Management of mild to moderate hypertension; treatment of edema in congestive heart failure and nephrotic syndrome

Usual Dosage Adults: Oral: 1-2 tablets once or twice daily

Dosage Forms Tablet:
25 Hydrochlorothiazide 25 mg and reserpine 0.125 mg
50 Hydrochlorothiazide 50 mg and reserpine 0.125 mg

hydrochlorothiazide and spironolactone
Brand Names Alazide®️; Aldactazide®️; Spironazide®️; Spirozide®️

Synonyms spironolactone and hydrochlorothiazide

Therapeutic Category Antihypertensive, Combination; Diuretic, Combination

Use Management of mild to moderate hypertension; treatment of edema in congestive heart failure and nephrotic syndrome

Usual Dosage Oral:
Children: 1.66-3.3 mg/kg/day (of spironolactone) in 2-4 divided doses
Adults: 1-8 tablets in 1-2 divided doses

Dosage Forms Tablet:
25/25: Hydrochlorothiazide 25 mg and spironolactone 25 mg
50/50: Hydrochlorothiazide 50 mg and spironolactone 50 mg

hydrochlorothiazide and triamterene

Brand Names Dyazide®; Maxzide®

Synonyms triamterene and hydrochlorothiazide

Therapeutic Category Diuretic, Combination

Use Management of mild to moderate hypertension; treatment of edema in congestive heart failure and nephrotic syndrome

Usual Dosage Adults: 1-2 capsules twice daily after meals

Dosage Forms

Capsule (Dyazide®): Hydrochlorothiazide 25 mg and triamterene 50 mg
Tablet:

Maxzide®-25: Hydrochlorothiazide 25 mg and triamterene 37.5 mg
Maxzide®: Hydrochlorothiazide 50 mg and triamterene 75 mg

Hydrocil® [OTC] *see* psyllium *on page 407*

Hydro-Cobex® Injection *see* hydroxocobalamin *on page 240*

hydrocodone and acetaminophen

Brand Names Anexsia®; Anodynos-DHC®; Bancap HC®; Co-Gesic®; Dolacet®; DuoCet™; Duradyne DHC®; Hydrocet®; Hydrogesic®; Hy-Phen®; Lorcet®; Lorcet® 10/650; Lorcet®-HD; Lorcet® Plus; Margesic® H; Norcet®; Panacet® 5/500; Stagesic®; T-Gesic®; Vicodin®; Vicodin® ES; Zydone®

Synonyms acetaminophen and hydrocodone

Therapeutic Category Analgesic, Narcotic

Use Relief of moderate to severe pain; antitussive (hydrocodone)

Usual Dosage Doses should be titrated to appropriate analgesic effect

Adults: 1-2 tablets or capsules every 4-6 hours

Dosage Forms

Capsule:

Bancap HC®, Dolacet®, Hydrocet®, Hydrogesic®, Lorcet®-HD, Margesic® H, Norcet®, Stagesic®, T-Gesic®, Zydone®: Hydrocodone bitartrate 5 mg and acetaminophen 500 mg

Solution, oral (tropical fruit punch flavor) (Lortab®): Hydrocodone bitartrate 2.5 mg and acetaminophen 120 mg per 5 mL with alcohol 7% (480 mL)

Tablet:

Lortab® 2.5/500: Hydrocodone bitartrate 2.5 mg and acetaminophen 500 mg
Anexsia® 5/500, Anodynos-DHC®, Co-Gesic®, DuoCet™, Duradyne DHC®, Hy-Phen®, Lorcet®, Lortab®® 5/500, Panacet® 5/500, Vicodin®: Hydrocodone bitartrate 5 mg and acetaminophen 500 mg
Lorcet® 7.5/500: Hydrocodone bitartrate 7.5 mg and acetaminophen 500 mg
Anexsia® 7.5/650, Lorcet® Plus: Hydrocodone bitartrate 7.5 mg and acetaminophen 650 mg
Vicodin® ES: Hydrocodone bitartrate 7.5 mg and acetaminophen 750 mg
Lorcet® 10/650: Hydrocodone bitartrate 10 mg and acetaminophen 650 mg

hydrocodone and aspirin (hye droe koe' done)

Brand Names Azdone®; Damason-P®; Lortab® ASA; Panasal® 5/500

Therapeutic Category Analgesic, Narcotic

Use Relief of moderate to moderately severe pain

Usual Dosage Adults: Oral: 1-2 tablets every 4-6 hours as needed for pain

Dosage Forms Tablet: Hydrocodone bitartrate 5 mg and aspirin 500 mg

hydrocodone and chlorpheniramine

Formerly Known As Hydrocodone and Phenyltoloxamine

Brand Names Tussionex®

Therapeutic Category Antitussive; Cough Preparation

Use Symptomatic relief of cough
Usual Dosage Oral:
Children 6-12 years: 2.5 mL every 12 hours; do not exceed 5 mL/24 hours
Adults: 5 mL every 12 hours; do not exceed 10 mL/24 hours
Dosage Forms Syrup, alcohol free: Hydrocodone polistirex 10 mg and chlorpheniramine polistirex 8 mg per 5 mL (480 mL, 900 mL)

hydrocodone and guaifenesin
Brand Names Codiclear® DH; Hycotuss® Expectorant Liquid; Kwelcof®
Synonyms guaifenesin and hydrocodone
Therapeutic Category Antitussive; Cough Preparation
Use Symptomatic relief of nonproductive coughs associated with upper and lower respiratory tract congestion
Usual Dosage Oral:
Children:
<2 years: 0.3 mg/kg/day (hydrocodone) in 4 divided doses
2-12 years: 2.5 mL every 4 hours, after meals and at bedtime
>12 years: 5 mL every 4 hours, after meals and at bedtime

Adults: 5 mL every 4 hours, after meals and at bedtime, up to 30 mL/24 hours
Dosage Forms Liquid: Hydrocodone bitartrate 5 mg and guaifenesin 100 mg per 5 mL (120 mL, 480 mL)

hydrocodone and homatropine
Brand Names Hycodan®; Hydromet®; Hydropane®; Hydrotropine®; Tussigon®
Synonyms homatropine and hydrocodone
Therapeutic Category Antitussive; Cough Preparation
Use Symptomatic relief of cough
Usual Dosage Oral (based on hydrocodone component):
Children: 0.6 mg/kg/day in 3-4 divided doses; do not administer more frequently than every 4 hours

A single dose should not exceed 10 mg in children >12 years, 5 mg in children 2-12 years, and 1.25 mg in children <2 years of age

Adults: 5-10 mg every 4-6 hours, a single dose should not exceed 15 mg; do not administer more frequently than every 4 hours
Dosage Forms
Syrup (Hycodan®, Hydromet®, Hydropane®, Hydrotropine®): Hydrocodone bitartrate 5 mg and homatropine methylbromide 1.5 mg per 5 mL (120 mL, 480 mL, 4000 mL)
Tablet (Hycodan®, Tussigon®): Hydrocodone bitartrate 5 mg and homatropine methylbromide 1.5 mg

hydrocodone and phenylpropanolamine
Brand Names Codamine®; Codamine® Pediatric; Hycomine®; Hycomine® Pediatric
Synonyms phenylpropanolamine and hydrocodone
Therapeutic Category Cough Preparation; Decongestant
Use Symptomatic relief of cough and nasal congestion
Usual Dosage Oral:
Children 6-12 years: 2.5 mL every 4 hours, up to 6 doses/24 hours
Adults: 5 mL every 4 hours, up to 6 doses/24 hours
Dosage Forms Syrup:
Codamine®, Hycomine®: Hydrocodone bitartrate 5 mg and phenylpropanolamine hydrochloride 25 mg per 5 mL (480 mL, 3780 mL)
Codamine® Pediatric, Hycomine® Pediatric: Hydrocodone bitartrate 2.5 mg and phenylpropanolamine hydrochloride 12.5 mg per 5 mL (480 mL, 3780 mL)

Hydrocodone and Phenyltoloxamine *see* hydrocodone and chlorpheniramine *on page 234*

hydrocodone, phenylephrine, pyrilamine, phenindamine, chlorpheniramine, and ammonium chloride

Brand Names P-V-Tussin®
Therapeutic Category Antihistamine/Decongestant Combination; Cough Preparation
Use Symptomatic relief of cough and nasal congestion
Usual Dosage Adults: Oral: 10 mL every 4-6 hours, up to 40 mL/day
Dosage Forms Syrup: Hydrocodone bitartrate 2.5 mg, phenylephrine hydrochloride 5 mg, pyrilamine maleate 6 mg, phenindamine tartrate 5 mg, chlorpheniramine maleate 2 mg, and ammonium chloride 50 mg per 5 mL with alcohol 5% (480 mL, 3780 mL)

hydrocodone, pseudoephedrine, and guaifenesin

Brand Names Cophene XP®; Detussin® Expectorant; SRC® Expectorant; Tussafin® Expectorant
Therapeutic Category Cough Preparation; Decongestant; Expectorant
Use Symptomatic relief of irritating, nonproductive cough associated with respiratory conditions such as bronchitis, bronchial asthma, tracheobronchitis, and the common cold
Usual Dosage Adults: Oral: 5 mL every 4-6 hours
Dosage Forms Liquid: Hydrocodone bitartrate 5 mg, pseudoephedrine hydrochloride 60 mg, and guaifenesin 200 mg per 5 mL with alcohol 12.5% (480 mL)

hydrocortisone (hye droe kor' ti sone)

Brand Names Acticort® Topical; Aeroseb-HC® Topical; A-hydroCort® Injection; Ala-Cort® Topical; Ala-Scalp® Topical; Anusol® HC-1 Topical [OTC]; Anusol® HC-2.5% Topical [OTC]; Caldecort® Anti-Itch Topical Spray; Caldecort® Topical [OTC]; Cetacort® Topical; Clocort® Maximum Strength [OTC]; CortaGel® Topical [OTC]; Cortaid® Maximum Strength Topical [OTC]; Cortaid® with Aloe Topical [OTC]; Cort-Dome® Topical; Cortef® Feminine Itch Topical; Cortef® Oral; Cortenema® Rectal; Cortifoam® Rectal; Cortizone®-5 Topical [OTC]; Cortizone®-10 Topical [OTC]; Delcort® Topical; Dermacort® Topical; Dermarest Dricort® Topical; Dermolate® Topical [OTC]; Dermtex® HC with Aloe Topical [OTC]; Eldecort® Topical; Gynecort® Topical [OTC]; Hi-Cor-1.0® Topical; Hi-Cor-2.5® Topical; Hycort® Topical; Hydrocortone® Acetate Injection; Hydrocortone® Oral; Hydrocortone® Phosphate Injection; Hydrocort® Topical; Hydro-Tex® Topical [OTC]; Hytone® Topical; LactiCare-HC® Topical; Lanacort® Topical [OTC]; Locoid® Topical; Nutracort® Topical; Orabase® HCA Topical; Penecort® Topical; Proctocort™ Rectal; Scalpicin® Topical; Solu-Cortef® Injection; S-T Cort® Topical; Synacort® Topical; Tegrin®-HC Topical [OTC]; Texacort® Topical; U-Cort™ Topical; Westcort® Topical
Synonyms compound F; cortisol
Therapeutic Category Adrenal Corticosteroid; Anti-inflammatory Agent; Corticosteroid, Rectal; Corticosteroid, Systemic; Corticosteroid, Topical (Low Potency)
Use Management of adrenocortical insufficiency; relief of inflammation of corticosteroid-responsive dermatoses; adjunctive treatment of ulcerative colitis
Usual Dosage
Acute adrenal insufficiency: I.M., I.V.:
Infants and young Children: 1-2 mg/kg/dose bolus, then 25-150 mg/day in divided doses
Older Children: 1-2 mg/kg bolus then 150-250 mg/day in divided doses
Adults: I.M., I.V., S.C.: 15-240 mg every 12 hours

Physiologic replacement: Children:
Oral: 0.5-0.75 mg/kg/day or 20-25 mg/m²/day every 8 hours
I.M.: 0.25-0.35 mg/kg/day or 12-15 mg/m²/day once daily

Anti-inflammatory or immunosuppressive:
Infants and Children:
Oral: 2.5-10 mg/kg/day or 75-300 mg/m²/day every 6-8 hours
I.M., I.V.: 1-5 mg/kg/day or 30-150 mg/m²/day divided every 6-12 hours

Adults: I.M., I.V., S.C.: 15-240 mg every 12 hours

Congenital adrenal hyperplasia: Oral: Initial: 30-36 mg/m^2/day with $\frac{1}{3}$ of dose every morning and $\frac{2}{3}$ every evening or $\frac{1}{4}$ every morning and midday and $\frac{1}{2}$ every evening; maintenance: 20-25 mg/m^2/day in divided doses

Status asthmaticus: Children: Loading: 1-2 mg/kg/dose every 6 hours for 24 hours then maintenance 0.5-1 mg/kg/dose every 6 hours

Shock: I.M., I.V.:
Children: Initial: 50 mg/kg (succinate) and repeated in 4 hours and/or every 24 hours if needed
Adults: 500 mg to 2 g every 2-6 hours (succinate)

Children and Adults:
Rectal: Apply 1 application 1-2 times/day for 2-3 weeks
Topical: Apply 3-4 times/day

Dosage Forms
Acetate:
Aerosol, rectal (Cortifoam®): 10% [90 mg/applicatorful] 20 g
Cream:
CaldeCORT®, Gynecort®, Cortaid® with Aloe, Cortef® Feminine Itch, Lanacort®: 0.5% (15 g, 22.5 g, 30 g)
Anusol-HC-1®, CaldeCORT®, Clocort® Maximum Strength, Cortaid® Maximum Strength, Dermarest Dricort®, U-cort™: 1% (15 g, 21 g, 30 g, 120 g)
Ointment, topical:
Cortaid® with Aloe, Lanacort® 5: 0.5% (15 g, 30 g)
Cortaid® Maximum Strength, Gynecort® 10, Lanacort® 10: 1% (15 g, 30 g)
Injection, suspension (Hydrocortone® Acetate): 25 mg/mL (5 mL, 10 mL); 50 mg/mL (5 mL, 10 mL)
Paste (Orabase® HCA): 0.5% (5 g)
Solution, topical (Scalpicin®): 1%
Base:
Aerosol, topical:
Aeroseb-HC®, CaldeCORT® Anti-Itch Spray, Cortaid®: 0.5% (45 g, 58 g)
Cortaid® Maximum Strength: 1% (45 mL)
Cream:
Cort-Dome®, Cortizone®-5, DermiCort®, Dermolate®, Dermtex® HC with Aloe, HydroSKIN®, Hydro-Tex®: 0.5% (15 g, 30 g, 120 g, 454 g)
Ala-Cort®, Anusol-HC-2.5%®, Cort-Dome®, Delcort®, Dermacort®, DermiCort®, Eldecort®, Hi-Cor 1.0®, Hycort®, Hytone®, Nutracort®, Penecort®, Synacort®: 1% (15 g, 20 g, 30 g, 60 g, 120 g, 240 g, 454 g)
Eldecort®, Hi-Cor-2.5®, Hydrocort®, Hytone®, Synacort®: 2.5% (15 g, 20 g, 30 g, 60 g, 120 g, 240 g, 454 g)
Rectal (Proctocort™): 1% (30 g)
Gel:
CortaGel®: 0.5% (15 g, 30 g)
CortaGel® Extra Strength: 1% (15 g, 30 g)
Lotion:
Cetacort®, DermiCort®, HydroSKIN®, S-T Cort®: 0.5% (60 mL, 120 mL)
Acticort 100®, Cetacort®, Cortizone-10®, Dermacort®, HydroSKIN® Maximum Strength, Hytone®, LactiCare-HC®, Nutracort®: 1% (60 mL, 120 mL)
Ala-Scalp®: 2% (30 mL)
Hytone®, LactiCare-HC®, Nutracort®: 2.5% (60 mL, 120 mL)
Ointment, topical:
Cortizone®-5, HydroSKIN®: 0.5% (30 g)
Cortizone®-10, Hycort®, HydroSKIN®, Hydro-Tex®, Hytone®, Tegrin®-HC: 1% (15 g, 20 g, 30 g, 60 g, 120 g, 240 g, 454 g)
Hytone®: 2.5% (20 g, 30 g)
Suspension, rectal (Cortenema®): 100 mg/60 mL (7s)
Tablet:
Cortef®: 5 mg, 10 mg, 20 mg
(Continued)

237

hydrocortisone *(Continued)*
  Hydrocortone®: 10 mg, 20 mg
 Butyrate (Locoid®):
  Cream: 0.1%
  Ointment, topical: 0.1%
  Solution, topical: 0.1% (20 mL, 60 mL)
 Cypionate:
  Suspension, oral (Cortef®): 10 mg/5 mL (120 mL)
 Sodium phosphate:
  Injection (Hydrocortone® Phosphate): 50 mg/mL (2 mL, 10 mL)
 Sodium succinate (A-hydroCort®, Solu-Cortef®): 100 mg, 250 mg, 500 mg, 1000 mg
 Valerate (Westcort®):
  Cream: 0.2% (15 g, 45 g, 60 g)
  Ointment, topical: 0.2% (15 g, 45 g, 60 g, 120 g)

hydrocortisone and clioquinol *see* clioquinol and hydrocortisone *on page 106*

hydrocortisone and dibucaine *see* dibucaine and hydrocortisone *on page 143*

hydrocortisone and pramoxine *see* pramoxine and hydrocortisone *on page 389*

hydrocortisone and urea *see* urea and hydrocortisone *on page 488*

Hydrocortone® Acetate Injection *see* hydrocortisone *on page 236*

Hydrocortone® Oral *see* hydrocortisone *on page 236*

Hydrocortone® Phosphate Injection *see* hydrocortisone *on page 236*

Hydrocort® Topical *see* hydrocortisone *on page 236*

Hydro-Crysti-12® Injection *see* hydroxocobalamin *on page 240*

HydroDIURIL® *see* hydrochlorothiazide *on page 233*

Hydro-Ergoloid® *see* ergoloid mesylates *on page 173*

hydroflumethiazide *(hye droe floo meth eye' a zide)*
Brand Names Diucardin®; Saluron®
Therapeutic Category Diuretic, Thiazide
Use Management of mild to moderate hypertension; treatment of edema in congestive heart failure and nephrotic syndrome
Usual Dosage Oral: 1 tablet 1-2 times/day
Dosage Forms Tablet: 50 mg

hydroflumethiazide and reserpine
Brand Names Hydro-Fluserpine®; Salutensin®; Salutensin-Demi®
Therapeutic Category Antihypertensive, Combination
Use Management of hypertension
Usual Dosage Determined by individual titration, usually 1 tablet once or twice daily
Dosage Forms
 Tablet (Salutensin®): Hydroflumethiazide 50 mg and reserpine 0.125 mg
 Tablet (Hydro-Fluserpine®, Salutensin-Demi®): Hydroflumethiazide 25 mg and reserpine 0.125 mg

Hydro-Fluserpine® *see* hydroflumethiazide and reserpine *on this page*

hydrogenated ergot alkaloids *see* ergoloid mesylates *on page 173*

Hydrogesic® *see* hydrocodone and acetaminophen *on page 234*

hydromagnesium aluminate *see* magaldrate *on page 281*

Hydromet® *see* hydrocodone and homatropine *on page 235*

hydromorphone hydrochloride (hye droe mor' fone)

Brand Names Dilaudid-HP® Injection; Dilaudid® Injection; Dilaudid® Oral; Dilaudid® Suppository

Synonyms dihydromorphinone

Therapeutic Category Analgesic, Narcotic; Antitussive

Use Management of moderate to severe pain; antitussive at lower doses

Usual Dosage Doses should be titrated to appropriate analgesic effects; when changing routes of administration, note that oral doses are less than half as effective as parenteral doses (may be only $^1/_5$ as effective)

Pain: Older children and Adults: Oral, I.M., I.V., S.C.: 1-4 mg/dose every 4-6 hours as needed; usual adult dose: 2 mg/dose

Antitussive: Oral:
Children 6-12 years: 0.5 mg every 3-4 hours as needed
Children >12 years and Adults: 1 mg every 3-4 hours as needed

Dosage Forms

Injection:
Dilaudid®: 1 mg/mL (1 mL); 2 mg/mL (1 mL, 20 mL); 3 mg/mL (1 mL); 4 mg/mL (1 mL)
Dilaudid-HP®: 10 mg/mL (1 mL, 2 mL, 5 mL)
Suppository, rectal: 3 mg (6s)
Tablet: 1 mg, 2 mg, 3 mg, 4 mg

Hydromox® *see* quinethazone *on page 411*

Hydropane® *see* hydrocodone and homatropine *on page 235*

Hydro-Par® *see* hydrochlorothiazide *on page 233*

Hydrophen® *see* theophylline, ephedrine, and hydroxyzine *on page 462*

Hydropres® *see* hydrochlorothiazide and reserpine *on page 233*

hydroquinone (hye' droe kwin one)

Brand Names Eldopaque Forte® Topical; Eldopaque® Topical [OTC]; Eldoquin® Forte® Topical; Eldoquin® Topical [OTC]; Esoterica® Facial Topical [OTC]; Esoterica® Regular Topical [OTC]; Esoterica® Sensitive Skin Formula [OTC]; Esoterica® Topical Sunscreen [OTC]; Melanex® Topical; Porcelana® Topical [OTC]; Solaquin Forte® Topical; Solaquin® Topical [OTC]

Therapeutic Category Depigmenting Agent

Use Gradual bleaching of hyperpigmented skin conditions

Usual Dosage Topical: Apply thin layer and rub in twice daily

Dosage Forms

Cream, topical:
Esoterica® Sensitive Skin Formula: 1.5% (85 g)
Eldopaque®, Eldoquin®, Esoterica® Facial, Esoterica® Regular, Porcelana®: 2% (14.2 g, 28.4 g, 60 g, 85 g, 120 g)
Eldopaque Forte®, Eldoquin® Forte®: 4% (14.2 g, 28.4 g)
Cream, topical, with sunscreen:
Esoterica® Sunscreen, Porcelana®, Solaquin®: 2% (28.4 g, 120 g)
Solaquin Forte®: 4% (14.2 g, 28.4 g)
Gel, topical, with sunscreen (Solaquin Forte®): 4% (14.2 g, 28.4 g)
Lotion (Eldoquin®): 2% (15 mL)
Solution, topical (Melanex®): 3% (30 mL)

Hydro-Serp® *see* hydrochlorothiazide and reserpine *on page 233*

Hydroserpine® *see* hydrochlorothiazide and reserpine *on page 233*

Hydro-T® *see* hydrochlorothiazide *on page 233*

Hydro-Tex® Topical [OTC] *see* hydrocortisone *on page 236*

Hydrotropine® *see* hydrocodone and homatropine *on page 235*

Hydroxacen® Injection *see* hydroxyzine *on next page*

hydroxocobalamin (hye drox oh koe bal' a min)
Brand Names Alphamin® Injection; Codroxomin® Injection; Hybalamin® Injection; Hydrobexan® Injection; Hydro-Cobex® Injection; Hydro-Crysti-12® Injection; LA-12® Injection
Synonyms vitamin B_{12a}
Therapeutic Category Vitamin, Water Soluble
Use Pernicious anemia, vitamin B_{12} deficiency, increased B_{12} requirements due to pregnancy, thyrotoxicosis, hemorrhage, malignancy, liver or kidney disease
Usual Dosage
Children:
> Congenital pernicious anemia (if evidence of neurologic involvement): I.M.: 1000 μg/day for at least 2 weeks; maintenance: 50 μg/month
> Vitamin B_{12} deficiency: I.M., S.C.: 1-5 mg given in single or S.C. doses of 100 μg over 2 or more weeks

Adults:
> Pernicious anemia: I.M., S.C.: 100 μg/day for 6-7 days
> Vitamin B_{12} deficiency:
> > Oral: Usually not recommended, maximum absorbed from a single oral dose is 2-3 μg
> > I.M., S.C.: 30 μg/day for 5-10 days, followed by 100-200 μg/month

Dosage Forms Injection: 1000 μg/mL (10 mL, 30 mL)

hydroxychloroquine sulfate (hye drox ee klor' oh kwin)
Brand Names Plaquenil®
Therapeutic Category Antimalarial Agent
Use Suppress and treat acute attacks of malaria; treatment of systemic lupus erythematosus (SLE) and rheumatoid arthritis
Usual Dosage Oral:
Children:
> Chemoprophylaxis of malaria: 5 mg/kg (base) once weekly; should not exceed the recommended adult dose; begin 2 weeks before exposure; continue for 4-6 weeks after leaving endemic area
> Acute attack: 10 mg/kg (base) initial dose; followed by 5 mg/kg in 6 hours on day 1; 5 mg/kg in 1 dose on day 2 and on day 3
> Juvenile rheumatoid arthritis or SLE: 3-5 mg/kg/day divided 1-2 times/day to a maximum of 400 mg/day; not to exceed 7 mg/kg/day

Adults:
> Chemoprophylaxis of malaria: 2 tablets weekly on same day each week; begin 2 weeks before exposure; continue for 4-6 weeks after leaving endemic area
> Acute attack: 4 tablets first dose day 1; 2 tablets in 6 hours day 1; 2 tablets in 1 dose day 2; and 2 tablets in 1 dose on day 3
> Rheumatoid arthritis: 2-3 tablets/day to start taken with food or milk; increase dose until optimum response level is reached; usually after 4-12 weeks dose should be reduced by $\frac{1}{2}$ and a maintenance dose of 1-2 tablets/day given
> Lupus erythematosus: 2 tablets every day or twice daily for several weeks depending on response; 1-2 tablets/day for prolonged maintenance therapy

Dosage Forms Tablet: 200 mg [base 155 mg]

25-hydroxycholecalciferol *see* calcifediol *on page 64*

hydroxydaunomycin hydrochloride *see* doxorubicin hydrochloride *on page 161*

hydroxyethyl starch *see* hetastarch *on page 228*

hydroxyprogesterone caproate (hye drox ee proe jess' te rone)
Brand Names Duralutin® Injection; Gesterol® L.A. Injection; Hy-Gestrone® Injection; Hylutin® Injection; Hyprogest® Injection; Pro-Depo® Injection; Prodrox® Injection
Therapeutic Category Progestin

Use Treatment of amenorrhea, abnormal uterine bleeding, submucous fibroids, endometriosis, uterine carcinoma, and testing of estrogen production
Usual Dosage Adults: I.M.:
Amenorrhea: 375 mg; if no bleeding begin cyclic treatment with estradiol valerate

Endometriosis: Start cyclic therapy with estradiol valerate

Uterine carcinoma: 1 g one or more times/day (1-7 g/week) for up to 12 weeks

Test for endogenous estrogen production: 250 mg anytime; bleeding 7-14 days after injection indicate positive test
Dosage Forms Injection:
Pro-Depo®: 125 mg/mL (10 mL)
Duralutin®, Gesterol® L.A., Hy-Gestrone®, Hylutin®, Hyprogest®, Pro-Depo®, Prodrox®: 250 mg/mL (5 mL)

hydroxypropyl methylcellulose (hye drox ee proe' pil meth e sell' yoo lose)
Brand Names Gonak™ [OTC]; Goniosol® [OTC]; Occucoat™
Synonyms gonioscopic ophthalmic solution
Therapeutic Category Ophthalmic Agent, Miscellaneous
Use Ophthalmic surgical aid in cataract extraction and intraocular implantation; gonioscopic examinations
Usual Dosage Introduced into anterior chamber of eye with 20-gauge or larger cannula
Dosage Forms Solution:
Occucoat™: 2% (1 mL syringe with cannula)
Gonak™, Goniosol®: 2.5% (15 mL)

hydroxyurea (hye drox ee yoor ee' a)
Brand Names Hydrea®
Therapeutic Category Antineoplastic Agent, Miscellaneous
Use Treatment of malignant neoplasms including melanoma, granulocytic leukemia, and ovarian carcinomas; also used with radiation in treatment of squamous cell carcinoma of the head and neck
Usual Dosage Refer to individual protocols
Oral:
Children: No dosage regimens have been established. Dosages of 1500-3000 mg/m^2 as a single dose in combination with other agents every 4-6 weeks have been used in the treatment of pediatric astrocytoma, medulloblastoma and primitive neuroectodermal tumors

Adults:
Solid tumors: Intermittent therapy: 80 mg/kg as a single dose every third day; continuous therapy: 20-30 mg/kg/day given as a single dose/day
Concomitant therapy with irradiation: 80 mg/kg as a single dose every third day starting at least 7 days before initiation of irradiation
Resistant chronic myelocytic leukemia: 20-30 mg/kg/day divided daily
Dosage Forms Capsule: 500 mg

25-hydroxyvitamin d₃ see calcifediol on page 64

hydroxyzine (hye drox' i zeen)
Brand Names Anxanil® Oral; Atarax® Oral; Atozine® Oral; Durrax® Oral; E-Vista® Injection; Hydroxacen® Injection; Hy-Pam® Oral; Hyzine-50® Injection; Quiess® Injection; Vamate® Oral; Vistacon-50® Injection; Vistaject-25® Injection; Vistaject-50® Injection; Vistaquel® Injection; Vistaril® Injection; Vistaril® Oral; Vistazine® Injection
Synonyms hydroxyzine hydrochloride; hydroxyzine pamoate
Therapeutic Category Antianxiety Agent; Antiemetic; Antihistamine; Sedative
Use Treatment of anxiety, as a preoperative sedative, an antipruritic, an antiemetic, and in alcohol withdrawal symptoms
(Continued)

hydroxyzine *(Continued)*

Usual Dosage

Children:

Oral: 2 mg/kg/day divided every 6-8 hours

I.M.: 0.5-1 mg/kg/dose every 4-6 hours as needed

Adults:

Antiemetic: I.M.: 25-100 mg/dose every 4-6 hours as needed

Anxiety: Oral: 25-100 mg 4 times/day; maximum dose: 600 mg/day

Preoperative sedation:

Oral: 50-100 mg

I.M.: 25-100 mg

Management of pruritus: Oral: 25 mg 3-4 times/day

Dosage Forms

Hydrochloride:

Injection:

Vistaject-25®, Vistaril®: 25 mg/mL (1 mL, 2 mL, 10 mL)

E-Vista®, Hydroxacen®, Hyzine-50®, Quiess®, Vistacon-50®, Vistaject-50®, Vista-quel®, Vistaril®, Vistazine®: 50 mg/mL (1 mL, 2 mL, 10 mL)

Syrup (Atarax®): 10 mg/5 mL (120 mL, 480 mL, 4000 mL)

Tablet:

Anxanil®: 25 mg

Atarax®: 10 mg, 25 mg, 50 mg, 100 mg

Atozine®: 10 mg, 25 mg, 50 mg

Durrax®: 10 mg, 25 mg

Pamoate:

Capsule:

Hy-Pam®: 25 mg, 50 mg

Vamate®: 25 mg, 50 mg, 100 mg

Vistaril®: 25 mg, 50 mg, 100 mg

Suspension, oral (Vistaril®:) 25 mg/5 mL (120 mL, 480 mL)

hydroxyzine hydrochloride *see* hydroxyzine *on previous page*

hydroxyzine pamoate *see* hydroxyzine *on previous page*

Hy-Gestrone® Injection *see* hydroxyprogesterone caproate *on page 240*

Hygroton® *see* chlorthalidone *on page 99*

Hylorel® *see* guanadrel sulfate *on page 222*

Hylutin® Injection *see* hydroxyprogesterone caproate *on page 240*

hyoscine *see* scopolamine *on page 426*

hyoscyamine, atropine, scopolamine, and phenobarbital

Brand Names Barbidonna®; Barophen®; Donnapine®; Donna-Sed®; Donnatal®; Donphen®; Hyosophen®; Kinesed®; Malatal®; Relaxadon®; Spaslin®; Spasmolin®; Spasmophen®; Spasquid®; Susano®

Therapeutic Category Anticholinergic Agent; Antispasmodic Agent, Gastrointestinal

Use Adjunct in treatment of peptic ulcer disease, irritable bowel, spastic colitis, spastic bladder, and renal colic

Usual Dosage Oral:

Children 2-12 years:

Kinesed® dose: ½ to 1 tablet 3-4 times/day

Donnatal®: 0.1 mL/kg/dose every 4 hours; maximum dose: 5 mL

Adults: 0.125-0.25 mg (1-2 capsules or tablets) 3-4 times/day; or 0.375-0.75 mg (1 Donnatal® Extentab®) in sustained release form every 12 hours; or 5-10 mL elixir 3-4 times/day or every 8 hours

Dosage Forms

Capsule (Donnatal®, Spasmolin®): Hyoscyamine sulfate 0.1037 mg, atropine sulfate 0.0194 mg, scopolamine hydrobromide 0.0065 mg, and phenobarbital 16.2 mg

Elixir (Barophen®, Donna-Sed®, Donnatal®, Hyosophen®, Spasmophen®, Spasquid®, Susano®): Hyoscyamine sulfate 0.1037 mg, atropine sulfate 0.0194 mg, scopolamine hydrobromide 0.0065 mg, and phenobarbital 16.2 mg per 5 mL (120 mL, 480 mL, 4000 mL)
Tablet:
- Barbidonna®: Hyoscyamine hydrobromide 0.1286 mg, atropine sulfate 0.025 mg, scopolamine hydrobromide 0.0074 mg, and phenobarbital 16 mg
- Barbidonna® No. 2: Hyoscyamine hydrobromide 0.1286 mg, atropine sulfate 0.025 mg, scopolamine hydrobromide 0.0074 mg, and phenobarbital 32 mg
- Chewable (Kinesed®): Hyoscyamine hydrobromide 0.12 mg, atropine sulfate 0.12 mg, scopolamine hydrobromide 0.007 mg, and phenobarbital 16 mg
- Donnapine®, Donnatal®, Hyosophen®, Malatal®, Relaxadon®, Spaslin®, Susano®: Hyoscyamine sulfate 0.1037 mg, atropine sulfate 0.0194 mg, scopolamine hydrobromide 0.0065 mg, and phenobarbital 16.2 mg
- Donnatal® No. 2: Hyoscyamine sulfate 0.1037 mg, atropine sulfate 0.0194 mg, scopolamine hydrobromide 0.0065 mg, and phenobarbital 32.4 mg
- Donphen®: Hyoscyamine sulfate 0.1 mg, atropine sulfate 0.02 mg, scopolamine hydrobromide 0.006 mg, and phenobarbital 15 mg
- Long acting (Donnatal®): Hyoscyamine sulfate 0.3111 mg, atropine sulfate 0.0582 mg, scopolamine hydrobromide 0.0195 mg, and phenobarbital 48.6 mg
- Spasmophen®: Hyoscyamine sulfate 0.1037 mg, atropine sulfate 0.0194 mg, scopolamine hydrobromide 0.0065 mg, and phenobarbital 15 mg

hyoscyamine, atropine, scopolamine, kaolin, and pectin
Therapeutic Category Antidiarrheal
Use Antidiarrheal; also used in gastritis, enteritis, colitis, and acute gastrointestinal upsets, and nausea which may accompany any of these conditions
Usual Dosage Oral:
Children:
10-20 lb: 2.5 mL
20-30 lb: 5 mL
>30 lb: 5-10 mL

Adults:
Diarrhea: 30 mL at once and 15-30 mL with each loose stool
Other conditions: 15 mL every 3 hours as needed
Dosage Forms Suspension, oral: Hyoscyamine sulfate 0.1037 mg, atropine sulfate 0.0194 mg, scopolamine hydrobromide 0.0065 mg, kaolin 6 g, and pectin 142.8 mg per 30 mL

hyoscyamine, atropine, scopolamine, kaolin, pectin, and opium
Brand Names Donnapectolin-PG®; Kapectolin PG®
Therapeutic Category Antidiarrheal
Use Treatment of diarrhea
Usual Dosage
Children 6-12 years: Initial: 10 mL and 5-10 mL every 3 hours thereafter
Dosage recommendations (body weight/dosage): 10 lb/2.5 mL; 20 lb/5 mL; 30 lb and over/5-10 mL. Do not administer more than 4 doses in any 24-hour period

Children >12 years and Adults: Initial: 30 mL (1 fluid oz) followed by 15 mL every 3 hours
Dosage Forms Suspension, oral: Hyoscyamine sulfate 0.1037 mg, atropine sulfate 0.0194 mg, scopolamine hydrobromide 0.0065 mg, kaolin 6 g, pectin 142.8 mg, and powdered opium 24 mg per 30 mL with alcohol 5%

hyoscyamine sulfate (hye oh sye' a meen)
Brand Names Anaspaz® Oral; Cystospaz-M® Oral; Cystospaz® Oral; Donnamor® Oral; Gastrosed™ Oral; Levsinex® Oral; Levsin® Injection; Levsin® Oral; Neoquess® Oral Tablet
Synonyms l-hyoscyamine sulfate
Therapeutic Category Anticholinergic Agent; Antispasmodic Agent, Gastrointestinal
Use GI tract disorders caused by spasm, adjunctive therapy for peptic ulcers
(Continued)
243

hyoscyamine sulfate *(Continued)*
Usual Dosage
Children:
    <2 years: $1/4$ adult dosage
    2-10 years: $1/2$ adult dosage

Adults:
    Oral, S.L.: 0.125-0.25 mg 3-4 times/day before meals or food and at bedtime; 0.375-0.75
        mg (timed release) every 12 hours
    I.M., I.V., S.C.: 0.25-0.5 mg every 6 hours
Dosage Forms
Capsule, timed release (Cystospaz-M®, Levsinex®): 0.375 mg
Elixir (Levsin®): 0.125 mg/5 mL with alcohol 20% (480 mL)
Injection (Levsin®): 0.5 mg/mL (1 mL, 10 mL)
Solution, oral (Gastrosed™, Levsin®): 0.125 mg/mL (15 mL)
Tablet:
    Anaspaz®, Donnamar®, Gastrosed™, Levsin®, Neoquess®: 0.125 mg
    Cystospaz®: 0.15 mg

Hyosophen® *see* hyoscyamine, atropine, scopolamine, and phenobarbital *on page 242*

Hy-Pam® Oral *see* hydroxyzine *on page 241*

Hypaque-Cysto® *see* radiological/contrast media (ionic) *on page 413*

Hypaque® Meglumine *see* radiological/contrast media (ionic) *on page 413*

Hypaque® Sodium *see* radiological/contrast media (ionic) *on page 413*

Hyperab® *see* rabies immune globulin, human *on page 413*

HyperHep® *see* hepatitis b immune globulin *on page 227*

Hyperstat® I.V. *see* diazoxide *on page 142*

Hyper-Tet® *see* tetanus immune globulin, human *on page 457*

Hypertussis® *see* pertussis immune globulin, human *on page 367*

Hy-Phen® *see* hydrocodone and acetaminophen *on page 234*

HypRho®-D *see* Rh$_o$(D) immune globulin *on page 419*

HypRho®-D Mini-Dose *see* Rh$_o$(D) immune globulin *on page 419*

Hyprogest® Injection *see* hydroxyprogesterone caproate *on page 240*

Hysone® Topical *see* clioquinol and hydrocortisone *on page 106*

Hytakerol® *see* dihydrotachysterol *on page 149*

Hytinic® [OTC] *see* polysaccharide-iron complex *on page 384*

Hytone® Topical *see* hydrocortisone *on page 236*

Hytrin® *see* terazosin *on page 454*

Hytuss® [OTC] *see* guaifenesin *on page 217*

Hytuss-2X® [OTC] *see* guaifenesin *on page 217*

Hy-Zide® *see* hydralazine and hydrochlorothiazide *on page 232*

Hyzine-50® Injection *see* hydroxyzine *on page 241*

ibenzmethyzin *see* procarbazine hydrochloride *on page 396*

Iberet-Folic-500® *see* ferrous sulfate, ascorbic acid, vitamin B-complex, and folic acid *on page 195*

Iberet®-Liquid [OTC] *see* ferrous sulfate, ascorbic acid, and vitamin B-complex *on page 195*

ibidomide hydrochloride *see* labetalol hydrochloride *on page 265*

Ibuprin® [OTC] *see* ibuprofen *on next page*

ibuprofen (eye byoo proe' fen)

Brand Names Aches-N-Pain® [OTC]; Advil® [OTC]; Children's Motrin®; Excedrin® IB [OTC]; Genpril® [OTC]; Haltran® [OTC]; Ibuprin® [OTC]; Ibuprohm® [OTC]; Ibu-Tab®; Medipren® [OTC]; Menadol® [OTC]; Midol® IB [OTC]; Motrin®; Motrin® IB [OTC]; Nuprin® [OTC]; Pamprin IB® [OTC]; Rufen®; Saleto-200® [OTC]; Saleto-400®; Trendar® [OTC]; Uni-Pro® [OTC]

Synonyms *p*-isobutylhydratropic acid

Therapeutic Category Analgesic, Non-Narcotic; Anti-inflammatory Agent; Nonsteroidal Anti-Inflammatory Agent (NSAID), Oral

Use Inflammatory diseases and rheumatoid disorders including juvenile rheumatoid arthritis; mild to moderate pain; fever; dysmenorrhea; gout

Usual Dosage Oral:

Children:

- Antipyretic: 6 months to 12 years: Temperature <102.5°F (39°C): 5 mg/kg/dose; temperature >102.5°F: 10 mg/kg/dose given every 6-8 hours; maximum daily dose: 40 mg/kg/day
- Juvenile rheumatoid arthritis: 30-50 mg/kg/day in 4 divided doses; start at lower end of dosing range and titrate upward; maximum: 2.4 g/day
- Analgesic: 4-10 mg/kg/dose every 6-8 hours

Adults:

- Inflammatory disease: 400-800 mg/dose 3-4 times/day; maximum dose: 3.2 g/day
- Pain/fever/dysmenorrhea: 200-400 mg/dose every 4-6 hours; maximum daily dose: 1.2 g

Dosage Forms

Suspension, oral: 100 mg/5 mL (120 mL, 480 mL)

Tablet: 200 mg [OTC], 300 mg, 400 mg, 600 mg, 800 mg

Ibuprohm® [OTC] *see* ibuprofen *on this page*

Ibu-Tab® *see* ibuprofen *on this page*

Ictotest® [OTC] *see* diagnostic aids (*in vitro*), urine *on page 139*

Idamycin® *see* idarubicin hydrochloride *on this page*

idarubicin hydrochloride (eye da rue' bi sin)

Brand Names Idamycin®

Synonyms 4-demothoxydaunorubicin; 4-DMDR

Therapeutic Category Antineoplastic Agent, Antibiotic

Use In combination treatment of acute myeloid leukemia (AML), this includes classifications M1 through M7 of the French-American-British (FAB) classification system

Usual Dosage Refer to individual protocols

Adults: Slow I.V. infusion: 12 mg/m^2/day for 3 days in combination with Ara-C

Dosage Forms Powder for injection, lyophilized: 5 mg, 10 mg

idoxuridine (eye dox yoor' i deen)

Brand Names Herplex® Ophthalmic

Synonyms IDU; IUdR

Therapeutic Category Antiviral Agent, Ophthalmic

Use Treatment of herpes simplex keratitis

Usual Dosage Adults: Ophthalmic:

Ointment: Instill 5 times/day (every 4 hours) in the conjunctival sac with last dose at bedtime; continue therapy for 5-7 days after healing appears complete

Solution: Instill 1 drop in eye(s) every hour during day and every 2 hours at night, continue until definite improvement is noted, then reduce daytime dose to 1 drop every 2 hours and every 4 hours at night; continue for 5-7 days after healing appears complete

Dosage Forms Ophthalmic:

Ointment: 0.5% (4 g)

Solution: 0.1% (15 mL)

IDU *see* idoxuridine *on previous page*

Ifex® Injection *see* ifosfamide *on this page*

IFLrA *see* interferon alfa-2a *on page 252*

IFN *see* interferon alfa-2a *on page 252*

IFN-alpha 2 *see* interferon alfa-2b *on page 252*

ifosfamide (eye foss' fa mide)
Brand Names Ifex® Injection
Therapeutic Category Antineoplastic Agent, Alkylating Agent
Use In combination with certain other antineoplastics in treatment of lung cancer, Hodgkin's and non-Hodgkin's lymphoma, breast cancer, acute and chronic lymphocytic leukemia, ovarian cancer, testicular cancer, and sarcomas
Usual Dosage Refer to individual protocols
  I.V.:
  Children: 1800 mg/m^2/day for 3-5 days every 21-28 days or 5000 mg/m^2 as a single 24-hour infusion or 3 g/m^2/day for 2 days

  Adults: 700-2000 mg/m^2/day for 5 days or 2400 mg/m^2/day for 3 days every 21-28 days; 5000 mg/m^2 as a single dose over 24 hours
Dosage Forms Powder for injection: 1 g, 3 g

IG *see* immune globulin, intramuscular *on next page*

IGIM *see* immune globulin, intramuscular *on next page*

Ilopan-Choline® Oral *see* dexpanthenol *on page 134*

Ilopan® Injection *see* dexpanthenol *on page 134*

Ilosone® Oral *see* erythromycin *on page 175*

Ilotycin® Ophthalmic *see* erythromycin, topical *on page 176*

Ilozyme® *see* pancrelipase *on page 354*

Imdur™ *see* isosorbide mononitrate *on page 260*

imidazole carboxamide *see* dacarbazine *on page 124*

imipemide *see* imipenem/cilastatin *on this page*

imipenem/cilastatin (i mi pen' em/sye la stat' in)
Brand Names Primaxin®
Synonyms imipemide
Therapeutic Category Antibiotic, Miscellaneous
Use Treatment of documented multidrug resistant gram-negative infection due to organisms proven or suspected to be susceptible to imipenem/cilastatin; treatment of multiple organism infection in which other agents have an insufficient spectrum of activity or are contraindicated due to toxic potential
Usual Dosage I.V. infusion (dosage recommendation based on imipenem component):

  Children: 60-100 mg/kg/day in 4 divided doses

  Adults:
    Serious infection: 2-4 g/day in 3-4 divided doses
    Mild to moderate infection: 1-2 g/day in 3-4 divided doses
Dosage Forms Powder for injection:
  I.M.:
    Imipenem 500 mg and cilastatin 500 mg
    Imipenem 750 mg and cilastatin 750 mg
  I.V.:
    Imipenem 250 mg and cilastatin 250 mg
    Imipenem 500 mg and cilastatin 500 mg

imipramine (im ip' ra meen)
Brand Names Janimine® Oral; Tofranil® Injection; Tofranil® Oral; Tofranil-PM® Oral
Synonyms imipramine hydrochloride; imipramine pamoate
Therapeutic Category Antidepressant, Tricyclic
Use Treatment of various forms of depression, often in conjunction with psychotherapy; enuresis in children; analgesic for certain chronic and neuropathic pain
Usual Dosage
Children: Oral (safety and efficacy of imipramine therapy for treatment of depression in children <12 years have not been established):
Enuresis: ≥6 years: Initial: 10-25 mg at bedtime, if inadequate response still seen after 1 week of therapy, increase by 25 mg/day; dose should not exceed 2.5 mg/kg/day or 50 mg at bedtime if 6-12 years of age or 75 mg at bedtime if ≥12 years of age
Adjunct in the treatment of cancer pain: Initial: 0.2-0.4 mg/kg at bedtime; dose may be increased by 50% every 2-3 days up to 1-3 mg/kg/dose at bedtime

Adolescents: Oral: Initial: 25-50 mg/day; increase gradually; maximum: 100 mg/day in single or divided doses

Adults:
Oral: Initial: 25 mg 3-4 times/day, increase dose gradually, total dose may be given at bedtime; maximum: 300 mg/day
I.M.: Initial: Up to 100 mg/day in divided doses; change to oral as soon as possible
Dosage Forms
Capsule, as pamoate (Tofranil-PM®): 75 mg, 100 mg, 125 mg, 150 mg
Injection, as hydrochloride (Tofranil®): 12.5 mg/mL (2 mL)
Tablet, as hydrochloride (Janimine®, Tofranil®): 10 mg, 25 mg, 50 mg

imipramine hydrochloride *see* imipramine *on this page*

imipramine pamoate *see* imipramine *on this page*

Imitrex® Injection *see* sumatriptan succinate *on page 450*

immune globulin, intramuscular
Brand Names Gamastan®; Gammar®
Synonyms gamma globulin; IG; IGIM; immune serum globulin; ISG
Therapeutic Category Immune Globulin
Use Prophylaxis against hepatitis A, measles, varicella, and possibly rubella and immunoglobulin deficiency, idiopathic thrombocytopenia purpura, Kawasaki syndrome, lymphocytic leukemia
Usual Dosage I.M.:
Hepatitis A: 0.02 mL/kg
IgG: 1.3 mL/kg then 0.66 mL/kg in 3-4 weeks
Measles: 0.25 mL/kg
Rubella: 0.55 mL/kg
Varicella: 0.6-1.2 mL/kg
Dosage Forms Injection: I.M.: 165 ± 15 mg (of protein)/mL (2 mL, 10 mL)

immune globulin, intravenous
Brand Names Gamimune® N; Gammagard®; Iveegam®; Polygam®; Sandoglobulin®; Venoglobulin®-I
Synonyms IVIG
Therapeutic Category Immune Globulin
Use Immunodeficiency syndrome, idiopathic thrombocytopenic purpura; used in conjunction with appropriate anti-infective therapy to prevent or modify acute bacterial or viral infections in patients with iatrogenically-induced or disease-associated immunodepression; autoimmune neutropenia, bone marrow transplantation patients, Kawasaki disease, Guillain-Barré syndrome, demyelinating polyneuropathies. Therapy should be guided by clinical observation and serial determination of serum IgG levels.
(Continued)

immune globulin, intravenous *(Continued)*

Usual Dosage Children and Adults: I.V. infusion:

Immunodeficiency syndrome: 100-200 mg/kg/dose every month; may increase to 400 mg/kg/dose as needed

Idiopathic thrombocytopenic purpura: 400-1000 mg/kg/dose for 2-5 consecutive days; maintenance dose: 400-1000 mg/kg/dose every 3-6 weeks based on clinical response and platelet count

Kawasaki disease: 400 mg/kg/day for 4 days or 2 g/kg as a single dose

Congenital and acquired antibody deficiency syndrome: 100-400 mg/kg/dose every 3-4 weeks

Bone marrow transplant: 500 mg/kg/week

Severe systemic viral and bacterial infections:
Neonates: 500 mg/kg/day for 2-6 days then once weekly
Children: 500-1000 mg/kg/week

Dosing comments in renal impairment: Cl_{cr} <10 mL/minute: Avoid use

Dosage Forms

Injection: Gamimune® N: 5% [50 mg/mL] with maltose 10% (10 mL, 50 mL, 100 mL)

Powder for injection, lyophilized:
Gammagard®, Polygam®: 0.5 g, 2.5 g, 5 g, 10 g
Gammar®-IV: 2.5 g
Iveegam®: 0.5 g, 1 g, 2.5 g, 5 g
Polygam®: 5 g, 10 g
Sandoglobulin®: 1 g, 3 g, 6 g
Venoglobulin®-I: 2.5 g, 5 g

immune serum globulin *see* immune globulin, intramuscular *on previous page*

Imodium® *see* loperamide hydrochloride *on page 277*

Imodium® A-D [OTC] *see* loperamide hydrochloride *on page 277*

Imogam® *see* rabies immune globulin, human *on page 413*

Imovax® Rabies I.D. Vaccine *see* rabies virus vaccine, human diploid *on page 413*

Imovax® Rabies Vaccine *see* rabies virus vaccine, human diploid *on page 413*

Imuran® *see* azathioprine *on page 40*

I-Naphline® Ophthalmic *see* naphazoline hydrochloride *on page 325*

Inapsine® *see* droperidol *on page 162*

indapamide (in dap' a mide)

Brand Names Lozol®

Therapeutic Category Diuretic, Miscellaneous

Use Management of mild to moderate hypertension; treatment of edema in congestive heart failure and nephrotic syndrome

Usual Dosage Adults: Oral: 2.5-5 mg/day

Dosage Forms Tablet: 1.25 mg, 2.5 mg

Inderal® *see* propranolol hydrochloride *on page 403*

Inderal® LA *see* propranolol hydrochloride *on page 403*

Inderide® *see* propranolol and hydrochlorothiazide *on page 402*

Indocin® I.V. Injection *see* indomethacin *on next page*

Indocin® Oral *see* indomethacin *on next page*

Indocin® SR Oral *see* indomethacin *on next page*

indocyanine green (in doe sye' a neen)
Brand Names Cardio-Green®
Therapeutic Category Diagnostic Agent, Cardiac Function
Use Determining hepatic function, cardiac output and liver blood flow and for ophthalmic angiography
Usual Dosage Dilute dose in sterile water for injection or 0.9% NaCl to final volume of 1 mL if necessary doses may be repeated periodically; total dose should not exceed 2 mg/kg

Infants: 1.25 mg
Children: 2.5 mg
Adults: 5 mg
Dosage Forms Injection: 25 mg, 50 mg

indometacin *see* indomethacin *on this page*

indomethacin (in doe meth' a sin)
Brand Names Indocin® I.V. Injection; Indocin® Oral; Indocin® SR Oral
Synonyms indometacin
Therapeutic Category Analgesic, Non-Narcotic; Anti-inflammatory Agent; Nonsteroidal Anti-Inflammatory Agent (NSAID), Oral; Nonsteroidal Anti-Inflammatory Agent (NSAID), Parenteral
Use Management of inflammatory diseases and rheumatoid disorders; moderate pain; acute gouty arthritis; I.V. form used as alternative to surgery for closure of patent ductus arteriosus in neonates
Usual Dosage
Patent ductus arteriosus:
  Neonates: I.V.: Initial: 0.2 mg/kg; followed with: 2 doses of 0.1 mg/kg at 12- to 24-hour intervals if age <48 hours at time of first dose; 0.2 mg/kg 2 times if 2-7 days old at time of first dose; or 0.25 mg/kg 2 times if over 7 days at time of first dose; discontinue if significant adverse effects occur. Dose should be withheld if patient has anuria or oliguria.

Analgesia:
  Children: Oral: Initial: 1-2 mg/kg/day in 2-4 divided doses; maximum: 4 mg/kg/day; not to exceed 150-200 mg/day
  Adults: Oral, rectal: 25-50 mg/dose 2-3 times/day; maximum dose: 200 mg/day; extended release capsule should be given on a 1-2 times/day schedule
Dosage Forms
Capsule (Indocin®): 25 mg, 50 mg
Capsule, sustained release (Indocin® SR): 75 mg
Powder for injection, as sodium trihydrate (Indocin® I.V.): 1 mg
Suppository, rectal (Indocin®): 50 mg
Suspension, oral (Indocin®): 25 mg/5 mL (5 mL, 10 mL, 237 mL, 500 mL)

Infectrol® Ophthalmic *see* neomycin, polymyxin b, and dexamethasone *on page 328*
InFed™ Injection *see* iron dextran complex *on page 256*
Inflamase® Mild Ophthalmic *see* prednisolone *on page 391*
Inflamase® Ophthalmic *see* prednisolone *on page 391*

influenza virus vaccine
Brand Names Flu-Imune®; Fluogen®; Fluzone®
Synonyms influenza virus vaccine (inactivated whole-virus); influenza virus vaccine (purified surface antigen); influenza virus vaccine (split-virus)
Therapeutic Category Vaccine, Inactivated Virus
Use Provide active immunity to influenza virus strains contained in the vaccine
(Continued)

influenza virus vaccine *(Continued)*

Usual Dosage Annual vaccination with current vaccine. Either whole- or split-virus vaccine may be used.

Dosage Forms Injection:
Purified surface antigen (Flu-Imune®): 5 mL
Split-virus (Fluogen®, Fluzone®): 0.5 mL, 5 mL
Whole-virus (Fluzone®): 5 mL

influenza virus vaccine (inactivated whole-virus) *see* influenza virus vaccine *on previous page*

influenza virus vaccine (purified surface antigen) *see* influenza virus vaccine *on previous page*

influenza virus vaccine (split-virus) *see* influenza virus vaccine *on previous page*

INH *see* isoniazid *on page 258*

Innovar® *see* droperidol and fentanyl *on page 163*

Inocor® *see* amrinone lactate *on page 27*

insect sting kit

Brand Names Ana-Kit®
Synonyms bee sting kit
Therapeutic Category Antidote, Insect Sting
Use Anaphylaxis emergency treatment of insect bites or stings by the sensitive patient that may occur within minutes of insect sting or exposure to an allergic substance
Usual Dosage Children and Adults:
Epinephrine:
<2 years: 0.05-0.1 mL
2-6 years: 0.15 mL
6-12 years: 0.2 mL
>12 years : 0.3 mL

Chlorpheniramine:
<6 years: 1 tablet
6-12 years: 2 tablets
>12 years: 4 tablets
Dosage Forms Kit: Epinephrine hydrochloride 1:1000 (1 mL syringe), chlorpheniramine maleate chewable tablet 2 mg (4), sterile alcohol pads (2), tourniquet

Insta-Glucose® [OTC] *see* glucose, instant *on page 212*
Insulatard® NPH *see* insulin preparations *on this page*

insulin preparations

Brand Names Beef NPH Iletin® II; Beef Regular Iletin® II; Humulin®; Insulatard® NPH; Lente® Iletin® I; Lente® Iletin® II; Lente® Purified Pork Insulin; Mixtard®; Novolin®; NPH Iletin® I; Pork NPH Iletin® II; Pork Regular Iletin® II; Regular [Concentrated] Iletin® II U-500; Regular Iletin® I; Semilente® Iletin® I; Ultralente® Iletin® I; Velosulin®
Synonyms Lente; NPH; Semilente; Ultralente
Therapeutic Category Antidiabetic Agent
Use Treatment of insulin-dependent diabetes mellitus, also noninsulin-dependent diabetes mellitus unresponsive to treatment with diet and/or oral hypoglycemics
Usual Dosage Dose requires continuous medical supervision; only regular insulin may be given I.V. The daily dose should be divided up depending upon the product used and the patient's response, eg, regular insulin every 4-6 hours; NPH insulin every 8-12 hours.

Children and Adults: S.C.: 0.5-1 unit/kg/day

Adolescents (during growth spurt) S.C.: 0.8-1.2 units/kg/day

Diabetic ketoacidosis: Children: I.V. loading dose: 0.1 unit/kg, then maintenance continuous infusion: 0.1 unit/kg/hour (range: 0.05-0.2 units/kg/hour depending upon the rate of decrease of serum glucose – too rapid decrease of serum glucose may lead to cerebral edema).

Optimum rate of decrease (serum glucose): 80-100 mg/dL/hour

Note: Newly diagnosed patients with JODM presenting in DKA and patients with blood sugars <800 mg/dL may be relatively "sensitive" to insulin and should receive loading and initial maintenance doses approximately $1/2$ of those indicated above.

Note: The term "purified" refers to insulin preparations containing no more than 10 ppm proinsulin (purified and human insulins are less immunogenic)

Dosage Forms All insulins are 100 units/mL (10 mL) except where indicated:

Rapid-acting:
Regular beef and pork: Regular Iletin® I
Regular beef (purified): Beef Regular Iletin® II
Regular human:
rDNA: Humulin® R
rDNA, buffered: Humulin® BR
Semisynthetic: Novolin® R, Novolin® R PenFil® (1.5 mL), Velosulin®
Regular pork:
Purified: Pork Regular Iletin® II, Velosulin®
Purified, concentrated: Regular [Concentrated] Iletin® II U-500, 500 units/mL (20 mL)
Regular Insulin:
Zinc suspension, prompt:
Beef: Semilente® Insulin
Beef and pork: Semilente® Iletin® I

Intermediate-acting:
Isophane suspension:
Beef: NPH Insulin
Beef and pork: NPH Iletin® I
Beef (purified): Beef NPH Iletin® II
Human (rDNA): Humulin® N
Human (semisynthetic): Novolin® N, Novolin® N PenFil® (1.5 mL)
Pork (purified): NPH Purified, Pork NPH Iletin® II, Insulatard® NPH
Zinc suspension:
Beef: Lente® Insulin
Beef and pork: Lente® Iletin® I
Beef (purified): Lente® Iletin® II
Human (rDNA): Humulin® L
Human (semisynthetic): Novolin® L
Pork (purified): Lente® Iletin® II, Lente® Purified Pork Insulin

Long-acting:
Zinc suspension, extended:
Beef: Ultralente® Insulin
Beef and pork: Ultralente® Iletin® I
Human (rDNA): Humulin® U

Combinations:
Isophane insulin suspension (50%) and insulin injection (50%) human (rDNA): Humulin® 50/50
Isophane insulin suspension (70%) and insulin injection (30%) human (rDNA): Humulin® 70/30
Isophane insulin suspension (70%) and insulin injection (30%) human (semisynthetic): Mixtard® Human 70/30, Novolin® 70/30
Isophane insulin suspension (70%) and insulin injection (30%) human (semisynthetic): Novolin® 70/30 PenFil® (1.5 mL)
Isophane insulin suspension (70%) and insulin injection (30%) pork (purified): Mixtard®

Intal® Inhalation Capsule see cromolyn sodium on page 118

Intal® Nebulizer Solution *see* cromolyn sodium *on page 118*

Intal® Oral Inhaler *see* cromolyn sodium *on page 118*

Intercept™ [OTC] *see* nonoxynol 9 *on page 338*

α-2-interferon *see* interferon alfa-2b *on this page*

interferon alfa-2a (in ter feer' on)
Brand Names Roferon-A®
Synonyms IFLrA; IFN; rIFN-A
Therapeutic Category Antineoplastic Agent, Miscellaneous; Interferon
Use Hairy cell leukemia, AIDS related Kaposi's sarcoma in patients >18 years of age, condyloma acuminata, multiple unlabeled uses. Indications and dosage regimens are specific for a particular brand of interferon.
Usual Dosage Refer to individual protocols
Children: S.C.: Pulmonary hemangiomatosis: 1-3 million units/m²/day once daily

Adults >18 years:
Hairy cell leukemia: I.M., S.C.: Induction dose is 3 million units/day for 16-24 weeks; maintenance: 3 million units 3 times/week
AIDS-related Kaposi's sarcoma: I.M., S.C.: Induction dose is 36 million units for 10-12 weeks; maintenance: 36 million units 3 times/week (may begin with dose escalation from 3-9-18 million units each day over 3 consecutive days followed by 36 million units daily for the remainder of the 10-12 weeks of induction)
Dosage Forms
Injection: 3 million units/mL (1 mL); 6 million units/mL (3 mL); 9 million units/mL (3 mL); 36 million units/mL (1 mL)
Powder for injection: 6 million units/mL when reconstituted

interferon alfa-2b
Brand Names Intron® A
Synonyms IFN-alpha 2; α-2-interferon; rLFN-α2
Therapeutic Category Antineoplastic Agent, Miscellaneous; Biological Response Modulator; Interferon
Use Induce hairy-cell leukemia remission; treatment of AIDS related Kaposi's sarcoma; condylomata acuminata; chronic hepatitis C
Usual Dosage Refer to individual protocols
Adults:
Adults:
Hairy cell leukemia: I.M., S.C.: 2 million units/m² 3 times/week
AIDS-related Kaposi's sarcoma: I.M., S.C.: 30 million units/m² 3 times/week or 50 million units/m² I.V. 5 days/week every other week
Condylomata acuminata: Intralesionally: 1 million units/lesion 3 times/week for 3 weeks; not to exceed 5 million units per treatment (maximum: 5 lesions at one time)
Chronic hepatitis C: I.M., S.C.: 3 million units 3 times/week for approximately a 6-month course
Dosage Forms Powder for injection, lyophilized: 3 million units, 5 million units, 10 million units, 18 million units, 25 million units, 50 million units

interferon alfa-n3
Brand Names Alferon® N
Therapeutic Category Antineoplastic Agent, Miscellaneous; Interferon
Use Intralesional treatment of refractory or recurring genital or venereal warts; useful in patients who do not respond or are not candidates for usual treatments; indications and dosage regimens are specific for a particular brand of interferon
Usual Dosage Refer to individual protocols
Adults: Inject 250,000 units (0.05 mL) in each wart twice weekly for a maximum of 8 weeks; therapy should not be repeated for at least 3 months after the initial 8-week course of

therapy
Dosage Forms Injection: 5 million units (1 mL)

interferon beta-1b
Brand Names Betaseron®
Synonyms rIFN-b
Therapeutic Category Interferon
Use Reduce the frequency of clinical exacerbations in ambulatory patients with relapsing-remitting multiple sclerosis
Usual Dosage Adults: S.C.: 0.25 mg every other day
Dosage Forms Powder for injection, lyophilized: 0.3 mg [9.6 μ units]

interferon gamma-1b
Brand Names Actimmune®
Therapeutic Category Biological Response Modulator
Use Reduce the frequency and severity of serious infections associated with chronic granulomatous disease
Usual Dosage Adults: S.C.:
>0.5 m² (body surface area): 50 μg/m² (1.5 million units/m²) three times weekly
≤ >0.5 m² (body surface area): 1.5 μg/kg/dose three times weekly
Dosage Forms Injection: 100 μg [3 million units]

interleukin-2 *see* aldesleukin *on page 11*
Intralipid® *see* fat emulsion *on page 190*

intravascular perfluorochemical emulsion
Brand Names Fluosol®
Therapeutic Category Blood Modifiers
Use To prevent or diminish myocardial ischemia as manifested by decreased ventricular wall motion and global ejection fraction, occurring during percutaneous transluminal angioplasty (PTCA) in patients at high risk of ischemic complications of angioplasty.
Dosage Forms Emulsion, intravascular: 20% [200 mg/mL] (400 mL)

intravenous fat emulsion *see* fat emulsion *on page 190*
Intron® A *see* interferon alfa-2b *on previous page*
Intropin® Injection *see* dopamine hydrochloride *on page 159*
Inversine® *see* mecamylamine hydrochloride *on page 287*
iocetamic acid *see* radiological/contrast media (ionic) *on page 413*
iodamide meglumine *see* radiological/contrast media (ionic) *on page 413*
Iodex® Regular *see* povidone-iodine *on page 389*

iodinated glycerol (eye' oh di nay ted gli' ser ole)
Brand Names Iophen®; Organidin®; Par Glycerol®; R-Gen®
Therapeutic Category Expectorant
Use Mucolytic expectorant in adjunctive treatment of bronchitis, bronchial asthma, pulmonary emphysema, cystic fibrosis, or chronic sinusitis
Usual Dosage Oral:
Children: 30 mg 4 times/day
Adults: 60 mg 4 times/day
Dosage Forms Organically bound iodine in brackets
Elixir (Iophen®, Organidin®, Par Glycerol®, R-Gen®): 60 mg/5 mL [30 mg/5 mL] (120 mL, 480 mL)
(Continued)

iodinated glycerol *(Continued)*
Solution, oral (Iophen®, Organidin®): 50 mg/mL [25 mg/mL] (30 mL)
Tablet (Iophen®, Organidin®): 30 mg [15 mg]

iodinated glycerol and codeine
Brand Names Iophen-C®; IoTuss®; Par Glycerol C®; Tussi-Organidin®; Tussi-R-Gen®
Therapeutic Category Antitussive; Cough Preparation; Expectorant
Use Symptomatic relief of irritating, nonproductive cough associated with respiratory conditions such as bronchitis, bronchial asthma, tracheobronchitis, and the common cold
Usual Dosage Oral:
Children: 2.5-5 mL every 4 hours
Adults: 5-10 mL every 4 hours
Dosage Forms Liquid: Iodinated glycerol 30 mg and codeine phosphate 10 mg per 5 mL

iodinated glycerol and dextromethorphan
Brand Names Iophen® DM; IoTuss-DM®; Par Glycerol DM®; Tussi-Organidin® DM; Tussi-R-Gen DM®; Tusso-DM®
Therapeutic Category Antitussive; Cough Preparation; Expectorant
Use Symptomatic relief of irritating, nonproductive cough associated with respiratory tract conditions
Usual Dosage Oral:
Children: 2.5-5 mL every 4 hours
Adults: 5-10 mL every 4 hours
Dosage Forms Liquid: Iodinated glycerol 30 mg and dextromethorphan hydrobromide 10 mg per 5 mL (120 mL, 480 mL, 4000 mL)

iodine
Therapeutic Category Topical Skin Product
Use Preoperatively to reduce vascularity of the thyroid gland prior to thyroidectomy; management of thyrotoxic crisis or recurrent hyperthyroidism
Usual Dosage Apply topically as necessary to affected areas of skin
Dosage Forms
Solution: 2%
Tincture: 2%

iodine injection *see* trace metals *on page 472*

iodipamide meglumine *see* radiological/contrast media (ionic) *on page 413*

iodochlorhydroxyquin *see* clioquinol *on page 106*

iodochlorhydroxyquin and hydrocortisone *see* clioquinol and hydrocortisone *on page 106*

Iodopen® *see* trace metals *on page 472*

iodoquinol (eye oh doe kwin' ole)
Formerly Known As diiodohydroxyquin
Brand Names Yodoxin®
Therapeutic Category Amebicide
Use Treatment of acute and chronic intestinal amebiasis; asymptomatic cyst passers; *Blastocystis hominis* infections
Usual Dosage Oral:
Children: 30-40 mg/kg/day in 3 divided doses for 20 days; not to exceed 1.95 g/day
Adults: 650 mg 3 times/day after meals for 20 days; not to exceed 2 g/day
Dosage Forms
Powder: 25 g
Tablet: 210 mg, 650 mg

iodoquinol and hydrocortisone
Brand Names Vytone® Topical
Therapeutic Category Antifungal Agent, Topical; Corticosteroid, Topical (Low Potency)
Use Treatment of eczema; infectious dermatitis; chronic eczematoid otitis externa; mycotic dermatoses
Usual Dosage Topical: Apply 3-4 times/day
Dosage Forms Cream: Iodoquinol 1% and hydrocortisone 1% (30 g)

iohexol *see* radiological/contrast media (non-ionic) *on page 415*

Ionamin® *see* phentermine hydrochloride *on page 371*

iopamidol *see* radiological/contrast media (non-ionic) *on page 415*

iopanoic acid *see* radiological/contrast media (ionic) *on page 413*

Iophen® *see* iodinated glycerol *on page 253*

Iophen-C® *see* iodinated glycerol and codeine *on previous page*

Iophen® DM *see* iodinated glycerol and dextromethorphan *on previous page*

Iopidine® *see* apraclonidine hydrochloride *on page 31*

iothalamate meglumine and iothalamate sodium *see* radiological/contrast media (ionic) *on page 413*

iothalamate sodium *see* radiological/contrast media (ionic) *on page 413*

IoTuss® *see* iodinated glycerol and codeine *on previous page*

IoTuss-DM® *see* iodinated glycerol and dextromethorphan *on previous page*

ioversol *see* radiological/contrast media (non-ionic) *on page 415*

I-Paracaine® Ophthalmic *see* proparacaine hydrochloride *on page 401*

ipecac syrup (ip' e kak)
Therapeutic Category Antidote, Emetic
Use Treatment of acute oral drug overdosage and in certain poisonings
Usual Dosage Oral:
Children:
   6-12 months: 5-10 mL followed by 10-20 mL/kg of water; repeat dose one time if vomiting does not occur within 20 minutes
   1-12 years: 15 mL followed by 10-20 mL/kg of water; repeat dose one time if vomiting does not occur within 20 minutes
Adults: 30 mL followed by 200-300 mL of water; repeat dose one time if vomiting does not occur within 20 minutes
Dosage Forms Syrup: 70 mg/mL (15 mL, 30 mL, 473 mL, 4000 mL)

I-Pentolate® Ophthalmic *see* cyclopentolate hydrochloride *on page 121*

I-Phrine® Ophthalmic Solution *see* phenylephrine hydrochloride *on page 372*

I-Picamide® Ophthalmic *see* tropicamide *on page 484*

ipodate calcium *see* radiological/contrast media (ionic) *on page 413*

ipodate sodium *see* radiological/contrast media (ionic) *on page 413*

IPOL™ *see* poliovirus vaccine, inactivated *on page 382*

ipratropium bromide (i pra troe' pee um)
Brand Names Atrovent® Aerosol Inhalation
Therapeutic Category Anticholinergic Agent; Bronchodilator
Use Bronchodilator used in bronchospasm associated with COPD, bronchitis, and emphysema
Usual Dosage Children >12 years and Adults: 2 inhalations 4 times/day up to 12 inhalations/24 hours
Dosage Forms Solution, inhalation: 18 μg/actuation (14 g)

iproveratril hydrochloride *see* verapamil hydrochloride *on page 493*

IPV *see* poliovirus vaccine, inactivated *on page 382*

Ircon® [OTC] *see* ferrous fumarate *on page 193*

iron dextran complex
Brand Names InFed™ Injection
Therapeutic Category Iron Salt
Use Treatment of microcytic hypochromic anemia resulting from iron deficiency in whom oral administration is infeasible or ineffective
Usual Dosage I.M., I.V.:
A 0.5 mL test dose (0.25 mL in infants) should be given prior to starting iron dextran therapy

Total replacement dosage of iron dextran (mL) = 0.0476 x weight (kg) x (Hb_n-Hb_o) + 1 mL/ per 5 kg body weight (up to maximum of 14 mL)
Hb_n = desired hemoglobin (g/dL)
Hb_o = measured hemoglobin (g/dL)

Maximum daily dose:
Infants <5 kg: 25 mg iron
Children:
5-10 kg: 50 mg iron
10-50 kg: 100 mg iron
Adults >50 kg: 100 mg iron
Dosage Forms Injection: 50 mg/mL (2 mL)

ISD *see* isosorbide dinitrate *on page 259*

ISDN *see* isosorbide dinitrate *on page 259*

ISG *see* immune globulin, intramuscular *on page 247*

Ismelin® *see* guanethidine monosulfate *on page 222*

ISMN *see* isosorbide mononitrate *on page 260*

Ismo™ *see* isosorbide mononitrate *on page 260*

Ismotic® *see* isosorbide *on page 259*

isoamyl nitrite *see* amyl nitrite *on page 27*

isobamate *see* carisoprodol *on page 76*

Iso-Bid® *see* isosorbide dinitrate *on page 259*

Isocaine® HCl Injection *see* mepivacaine hydrochloride *on page 293*

isocarboxazid (eye soe kar box' a zid)
Brand Names Marplan®
Therapeutic Category Antidepressant, Monoamine Oxidase Inhibitor
Use Symptomatic treatment of depressed patients refractory to or intolerant to tricyclic antidepressants or electroconvulsive therapy
Usual Dosage Oral: 10 mg 3 times/day; reduce to 10-20 mg/day in divided doses when condition improves
Dosage Forms Tablet: 10 mg

Isocet® *see* butalbital compound *on page 63*

Isoclor® Expectorant *see* guaifenesin, pseudoephedrine, and codeine *on page 221*

Isoclor® Tablet *see* chlorpheniramine and pseudoephedrine *on page 94*

Isoclor® Timesules® *see* chlorpheniramine and pseudoephedrine *on page 94*

ALPHABETICAL LISTING OF DRUGS

Isocult® for Bacteriuria *see* diagnostic aids (*in vitro*), urine *on page 139*

Isocult® for *Neisseria gonorrhoeae* *see* diagnostic aids (*in vitro*), other *on page 138*

Isocult® for *Pseudomonas aeruginosa* *see* diagnostic aids (*in vitro*), urine *on page 139*

Isocult® for *Staphylococcus aureus* *see* diagnostic aids (*in vitro*), other *on page 138*

Isocult® for *Trichomonas vaginalis* *see* diagnostic aids (*in vitro*), other *on page 138*

Isocult® Throat Streptococci *see* diagnostic aids (*in vitro*), other *on page 138*

Isodine® [OTC] *see* povidone-iodine *on page 389*

isoethadione *see* paramethadione *on page 357*

isoetharine (eye soe eth' a reen)
Brand Names Arm-a-Med® Isoetharine Inhalation Solution; Beta-2® Inhalation Solution; Bronkometer® Aerosol; Bronkosol® Inhalation Solution; Dey-Lute® Isoetharine Inhalation Solution
Synonyms isoetharine hydrochloride; isoetharine mesylate
Therapeutic Category Adrenergic Agonist Agent; Bronchodilator
Use Bronchodilator in bronchial asthma and for reversible bronchospasm occurring with bronchitis and emphysema
Usual Dosage Treatments are usually not repeated more often than every 4 hours, except in severe cases, and may be repeated up to 5 times/day if necessary

Nebulizer: Children: 0.1-0.2 mg/kg/dose every 2-6 hours as needed; adult: 0.5 mL diluted in 2-3 mL normal saline or 4 inhalations of undiluted 1% solution
Dosage Forms
Aerosol, oral, as mesylate: 340 µg/metered spray
Solution, inhalation, as hydrochloride: 0.062% (4 mL); 0.08% (3.5 mL); 0.1% (2.5 mL, 5 mL); 0.125% (4 mL); 0.167% (3 mL); 0.17% (3 mL); 0.2% (2.5 mL); 0.25% (2 mL, 3.5 mL); 0.5% (0.5 mL); 1% (0.5 mL, 0.25 mL, 10 mL, 14 mL, 30 mL)

isoetharine hydrochloride *see* isoetharine *on this page*

isoetharine mesylate *see* isoetharine *on this page*

isoflurane (eye soe flure' ane)
Brand Names Forane®
Therapeutic Category General Anesthetic
Use General induction and maintenance of anesthesia (inhalation)
Usual Dosage 1.5% to 3%
Dosage Forms Solution: 100 mL, 125 mL, 250 mL

isoflurophate (eye soe flure' oh fate)
Brand Names Floropryl® Ophthalmic
Synonyms DFP; diisopropyl fluorophosphate; dyflos; fluostigmin
Therapeutic Category Cholinergic Agent, Ophthalmic; Ophthalmic Agent, Miotic
Use Treat primary open-angle glaucoma and conditions that obstruct aqueous outflow and to treat accommodative convergent strabismus
Usual Dosage Adults: Ophthalmic:
Glaucoma: Instill ¹/₄" strip in eye every 8-72 hours
Strabismus: Instill ¹/₄" strip to each eye every night for 2 weeks then reduce to ¹/₄" every other night to once weekly for 2 months
Dosage Forms Ointment, ophthalmic: 0.025% in polyethylene mineral oil gel (3.5 g)

257

Isollyl Improved® see butalbital compound *on page 63*

Isonate® see isosorbide dinitrate *on next page*

isoniazid (eye soe nye' a zid)
Brand Names Laniazid® Oral; Nydrazid® Injection
Synonyms INH; isonicotinic acid hydrazide
Therapeutic Category Antitubercular Agent
Use Treatment of susceptible tuberculosis infections and prophylactically to those individuals exposed to tuberculosis
Usual Dosage Oral, I.M.:
Children: 10-20 mg/kg/day in 1-2 divided doses (maximum: 300 mg total dose)
Prophylaxis: 10 mg/kg/day given daily (up to 300 mg total dose) for 12 months

Adults: 5 mg/kg/day given daily (usual dose is 300 mg)
Disseminated disease: 10 mg/kg/day in 1-2 divided doses
Treatment should be continued for 9 months with rifampin or for 6 months with rifampin and pyrazinamide
Prophylaxis: 300 mg/day given daily for 12 months

American Thoracic Society and CDC currently recommend twice weekly therapy as part of a short-course regimen which follows 1-2 months of daily treatment for uncomplicated pulmonary tuberculosis in compliant patients
Children: 20-40 mg/kg/dose (up to 900 mg) twice weekly
Adults: 15 mg/kg/dose (up to 900 mg) twice weekly
Dosage Forms
Injection: 100 mg/mL (10 mL)
Syrup: 50 mg/5 mL (473 mL)
Tablet: 50 mg, 100 mg, 300 mg

isonicotinic acid hydrazide see isoniazid *on this page*

isonipecaine hydrochloride see meperidine hydrochloride *on page 292*

isoprenaline hydrochloride see isoproterenol *on this page*

isopropamide iodide (eye soe proe' pa mide)
Brand Names Darbid®
Therapeutic Category Anticholinergic Agent; Antispasmodic Agent, Gastrointestinal
Use Adjunctive therapy for peptic ulcer, irritable bowel syndrome
Usual Dosage Children >12 years and Adults: Oral: 5-10 mg every 12 hours
Dosage Forms Tablet: 5 mg

isoproterenol (eye soe proe ter' e nole)
Brand Names Arm-a-Med® Isoproterenol Inhalation Solution; Dey-Dose® Isoproterenol Inhalation Solution; Dispos-a-Med® Isoproterenol Inhalation Solution; Isuprel® Glossets®; Isuprel® Inhalation Solution; Isuprel® Injection; Isuprel® Oral; Medihaler-Iso® Inhalation Aerosol
Synonyms isoprenaline hydrochloride
Therapeutic Category Adrenergic Agonist Agent; Bronchodilator
Use Asthma or COPD (reversible airway obstruction); A-V nodal block; hemodynamically compromised bradyarrhythmias or atropine-resistant bradyarrhythmias, temporary use in 3rd degree A-V block until pacemaker insertion; low cardiac output; vasoconstrictive shock states
Usual Dosage
Children:
Bronchodilation: Inhalation 1-2 metered doses up to 5 times/day
Nebulization: 0.01 mL/kg; minimum dose: 0.1 mL; maximum dose: 0.5 mL diluted in 2-3 mL normal saline
I.V. infusion: 0.05-2 μg/kg/minute; rate (mL/hour) = dose (μg/kg/minute) x weight (kg) x 60 minutes/hour divided by concentration (μg/mL)

Adults:
Bronchodilation: 1-2 inhalations 4-6 times/day
A-V nodal block: I.V. infusion: 2-20 μg/minute
Dosage Forms
Inhalation: Aerosol: 0.2% [2 mg/mL = 1:500] (15 mL, 22.5 mL); 0.25% [2.5 mg/mL = 1:400] (15 mL)
Injection: 0.02% [0.2 mg/mL = 1:5000] (1 mL, 5 mL, 10 mL)
Solution for nebulization: 0.031% (4 mL); 0.062% (4 mL); 0.25% (0.5 mL, 30 mL); 0.5% (0.5 mL, 10 mL, 60 mL); 1% (10 mL)
Tablet, sublingual: 10 mg, 15 mg

isoproterenol and phenylephrine (eye soe proe ter' e nole & fen ill ef' rin)
Brand Names Duo-Medihaler® Aerosol
Therapeutic Category Adrenergic Agonist Agent
Use Treatment of bronchospasm associated with acute and chronic bronchial asthma, bronchitis, pulmonary emphysema, and bronchiectasis
Usual Dosage Daily maintenance: 1-2 inhalations 4-6 times/day, no more than 2 inhalations at any one time or more than 6 in any 1 hour within 24 hours
Dosage Forms Aerosol: Each actuation releases isoproterenol hydrochloride 0.16 mg and phenylephrine bitartrate 0.24 mg (15 mL, 22.5 mL)

Isoptin® see verapamil hydrochloride on page 493

Isopto® Atropine Ophthalmic see atropine sulfate on page 37

Isopto® Carbachol Ophthalmic see carbachol on page 72

Isopto® Carpine Ophthalmic see pilocarpine on page 377

Isopto® Eserine Ophthalmic see physostigmine on page 376

Isopto® Frin Ophthalmic Solution see phenylephrine hydrochloride on page 372

Isopto® Homatropine Ophthalmic see homatropine hydrobromide on page 230

Isopto® Hyoscine Ophthalmic see scopolamine on page 426

Isopto® Plain [OTC] see artificial tears on page 33

Isopto® Tears [OTC] see artificial tears on page 33

Isordil® see isosorbide dinitrate on this page

isosorbide (eye soe sor' bide)
Brand Names Ismotic®
Therapeutic Category Diuretic, Osmotic; Ophthalmic Agent, Osmotic
Use Short-term emergency treatment of acute angle-closure glaucoma
Usual Dosage Adults: Oral: Initial: 1.5 g/kg with a usual range of 1-3 g/kg 2-4 times/day
Dosage Forms Solution: 45% [450 mg/mL] (220 mL)

isosorbide dinitrate (eye soe sor' bide)
Brand Names Dilatrate®-SR; Iso-Bid®; Isonate®; Isordil®; Isotrate®; Sorbitrate®
Synonyms ISD; ISDN
Therapeutic Category Antianginal Agent; Nitrate; Vasodilator, Coronary
Use Prevention and treatment of angina pectoris; for congestive heart failure; to relieve pain, dysphagia, and spasm in esophageal spasm with GE reflux
Usual Dosage Adults:
Chew: 5-10 mg every 2-3 hours
Oral: 5-30 mg 4 times/day or 40 mg every 6-12 hours in sustained-released dosage form
Sublingual: 2.5-10 mg every 4-6 hours
Dosage Forms
Capsule, sustained release: 40 mg

(Continued)

259

isosorbide dinitrate *(Continued)*
Tablet:
Chewable: 5 mg, 10 mg
Oral: 5 mg, 10 mg, 20 mg, 30 mg, 40 mg
Sublingual: 2.5 mg, 5 mg, 10 mg
Sustained release: 40 mg

isosorbide mononitrate
Brand Names Imdur™; Ismo™; Monoket®
Synonyms ISMN
Therapeutic Category Antianginal Agent; Vasodilator, Coronary
Use Long-acting metabolite of the vasodilator isosorbide dinitrate used for the prophylactic treatment of angina pectoris
Usual Dosage Oral: Adults:
Regular tablet: 20 mg twice daily separated by 7 hours; maintenance doses as high as 120 mg have been used
Extended release tablet: 30 mg ($\frac{1}{2}$ of 60 mg tablet) or 60 mg (given as a single tablet) once daily; after several days the dosage may be increased to 120 mg (given as two 60 mg tablets) once daily; the daily dose should be taken in the morning upon arising
Dosage Forms
Tablet (Ismo™, Monoket®): 10 mg, 20 mg
Tablet, extended release (Imdur™): 60 mg

isosulfan blue *see* radiological/contrast media (ionic) *on page 413*
Isotrate® *see* isosorbide dinitrate *on previous page*

isotretinoin (eye soe tret' i noyn)
Brand Names Accutane®
Synonyms 13-*cis*-retinoic acid
Therapeutic Category Acne Product; Retinoic Acid Derivative; Vitamin A Derivative
Use Treatment of severe recalcitrant cystic and/or conglobate acne unresponsive to conventional therapy; used investigationally for the treatment of children with metastatic neuroblastoma or leukemia that does not respond to conventional therapy
Usual Dosage Oral:
Children: Maintenance therapy for neuroblastoma: 100-250 mg/m^2/day in 2 divided doses has been used investigationally

Children and Adults: 0.5-2 mg/kg/day in 2 divided doses for 15-20 weeks
Dosage Forms Capsule: 10 mg, 20 mg, 40 mg

Isovex® *see* ethaverine hydrochloride *on page 181*
Isovue® *see* radiological/contrast media (non-ionic) *on page 415*

isoxsuprine hydrochloride (eye sox' syoo preen)
Brand Names Vasodilan®
Therapeutic Category Vasodilator
Use Treatment of peripheral vascular diseases, such as arteriosclerosis obliterans and Raynaud's disease
Usual Dosage Adults: Oral: 10-20 mg 3-4 times/day
Dosage Forms Tablet: 10 mg, 20 mg

isradipine (is ra' di peen)
Brand Names DynaCirc®
Therapeutic Category Calcium Channel Blocker
Use Management of hypertension, alone or concurrently with thiazide-type diuretics

Usual Dosage Adults: Oral: Initial: 2.5 mg twice daily, if satisfactory response does not occur after 2-4 weeks the dose may be adjusted in increments of 5 mg/day at 2- to 4-week intervals up to a maximum of 20 mg/day
Dosage Forms Capsule: 2.5 mg, 5 mg

I-Sulfacet® Ophthalmic *see* sodium sulfacetamide *on page 439*
Isuprel® Glossets® *see* isoproterenol *on page 258*
Isuprel® Inhalation Solution *see* isoproterenol *on page 258*
Isuprel® Injection *see* isoproterenol *on page 258*
Isuprel® Oral *see* isoproterenol *on page 258*
Itch-X® [OTC] *see* pramoxine hydrochloride *on page 390*

itraconazole (i tra koe' na zole)
Brand Names Sporanox® Oral
Therapeutic Category Antifungal Agent, Systemic
Use Treatment of susceptible fungal infections in immunocompromised and nonimmunocompromised patients including blastomycosis and histoplasmosis
Usual Dosage Adults: Oral: 200 mg once daily, if obvious improvement or there is evidence of progressive fungal disease, increase the dose in 100 mg increments to a maximum of 400 mg/day; doses >200 mg/day are given in 2 divided doses
Life-threatening: Loading dose: 200 mg give 3 times/day (600 mg/day) should be given for the first 3 days
Dosage Forms Capsule: 100 mg

I-Tropine® Ophthalmic *see* atropine sulfate *on page 37*
IUdR *see* idoxuridine *on page 245*
Iveegam® *see* immune globulin, intravenous *on page 247*
IVIG *see* immune globulin, intravenous *on page 247*
Janimine® Oral *see* imipramine *on page 247*

Japanese encephalitis virus vaccine, inactivated
Brand Names JE-VAX®
Synonyms JE vaccine
Therapeutic Category Vaccine, Inactivated Virus
Use Active immunization against Japanese encephalitis for persons spending a month or longer in endemic areas, especially if travel will include rural areas
Usual Dosage S.C. (given on days 0, 7, and 30):
Children 1-3 years: 3 doses of 0.5 mL; booster doses of 0.5 mL may given 2 years after primary immunization series
Children >3 years and Adults: 3 doses of 1 mL; booster doses of 1 mL may be given 2 years after primary immunization series
Dosage Forms Powder for injection, lyophilized: 1 mL, 10 mL

Jenamicin® Injection *see* gentamicin sulfate *on page 211*
JE vaccine *see* Japanese encephalitis virus vaccine, inactivated *on this page*
JE-VAX® *see* Japanese encephalitis virus vaccine, inactivated *on this page*
Kabikinase® *see* streptokinase *on page 443*
Kalcinate® *see* calcium gluconate *on page 68*

kanamycin sulfate (kan a mye' sin)
Brand Names Kantrex® Injection; Kantrex® Oral
Therapeutic Category Antibiotic, Aminoglycoside
Use
Oral: Preoperative bowel preparation in the prophylaxis of infections and adjunctive treatment of hepatic coma (oral kanamycin is not indicated in the treatment of systemic infections)
Parenteral: Initial therapy of severe infections where the strain is thought to be susceptible in patients allergic to other antibiotics, or in mixed staphylococcal or gram-negative infections
Usual Dosage
Children: Infections: I.M., I.V.: 15 mg/kg/day in divided doses every 8-12 hours
Adults:
Infections: I.M., I.V.: 15 mg/kg/day in divided doses every 8-12 hours
Preoperative intestinal antisepsis: Oral: 1 g every 4-6 hours for 36-72 hours
Dosage Forms
Capsule: 500 mg
Injection:
Pediatric: 75 mg (2 mL)
Adults: 500 mg (2 mL); 1 g (3 mL)

Kantrex® Injection see kanamycin sulfate on this page
Kantrex® Oral see kanamycin sulfate on this page
Kaochlor® S-F see potassium chloride on page 386
Kaodene® [OTC] see kaolin and pectin on this page

kaolin and pectin
Brand Names Kaodene® [OTC]; Kao-Spen® [OTC]; Kapectolin® [OTC]
Synonyms pectin and kaolin
Therapeutic Category Antidiarrheal
Use Treatment of uncomplicated diarrhea
Usual Dosage Oral:
Children:
<6 years: Do not use
6-12 years: 30-60 mL after each loose stool
Adults: 60-120 mL after each loose stool
Dosage Forms Suspension, oral: Kaolin 975 mg and pectin 22 mg per 5 mL

kaolin and pectin with opium
Brand Names Parepectolin®
Therapeutic Category Antidiarrheal
Use Symptomatic relief of diarrhea
Usual Dosage Oral:
Children:
3-6 years: 7.5 mL with each loose bowel movement, not to exceed 30 mL in 12 hours
6-12 years: 5-10 mL with each loose bowel movement, not to exceed 40 mL in 12 hours
Children >12 years and Adults: 15-30 mL with each loose bowel movement, not to exceed 120 mL in 12 hours
Dosage Forms Suspension, oral: Kaolin 5.5 g, pectin 162 mg, and opium 15 mg per 30 mL [3.7 mL paregoric] (240 mL)

Kaon® see potassium gluconate on page 387
Kaon-CL® see potassium chloride on page 386

Kaopectate® Advanced Formula [OTC] *see* attapulgite *on page 38*

Kaopectate® II [OTC] *see* loperamide hydrochloride *on page 277*

Kaopectate® Maximum Strength Caplets *see* attapulgite *on page 38*

Kao-Spen® [OTC] *see* kaolin and pectin *on previous page*

Kapectolin® [OTC] *see* kaolin and pectin *on previous page*

Kapectolin PG® *see* hyoscyamine, atropine, scopolamine, kaolin, pectin, and opium *on page 243*

Karidium® *see* fluoride *on page 201*

Karigel® *see* fluoride *on page 201*

Karigel®-N *see* fluoride *on page 201*

Kasof® [OTC] *see* docusate *on page 157*

Kato® *see* potassium chloride *on page 386*

Kaybovite-1000® *see* cyanocobalamin *on page 120*

Kayexalate® *see* sodium polystyrene sulfonate *on page 438*

KCl *see* potassium chloride *on page 386*

K-Dur® *see* potassium chloride *on page 386*

Keflex® *see* cephalexin monohydrate *on page 84*

Keflin® Injection *see* cephalothin sodium *on page 84*

Keftab® *see* cephalexin monohydrate *on page 84*

Kefurox® Injection *see* cefuroxime *on page 83*

Kefzol® *see* cefazolin sodium *on page 79*

Kemadrin® *see* procyclidine hydrochloride *on page 397*

Kenacort® Oral *see* triamcinolone *on page 474*

Kenaject® Injection *see* triamcinolone *on page 474*

Kenalog® Injection *see* triamcinolone *on page 474*

Kenalog® in Orabase® *see* triamcinolone *on page 474*

Kenalog® Topical *see* triamcinolone *on page 474*

Kenonel® Topical *see* triamcinolone *on page 474*

Keralyt® Gel *see* salicylic acid and propylene glycol *on page 425*

Kerlone® Oral *see* betaxolol hydrochloride *on page 53*

Kestrone® Injection *see* estrone *on page 180*

Ketalar® Injection *see* ketamine hydrochloride *on this page*

ketamine hydrochloride (keet' a meen)

Brand Names Ketalar® Injection
Therapeutic Category General Anesthetic
Use Induction of anesthesia; short procedures; supplement nitrous oxide; dressing changes
Usual Dosage
Children:
I.M.: 3-7 mg/kg
I.V.: Range: 0.5-2 mg/kg, use smaller doses (0.5-1 mg/kg) for sedation for minor procedures; usual induction dosage: 1-2 mg/kg

Adults:
I.M.: 3-8 mg/kg
I.V.: Range: 1-4.5 mg/kg; usual induction dosage: 1-2 mg/kg

Children and Adults: Maintenance: Supplemental doses of $\frac{1}{3}$ to $\frac{1}{2}$ of initial dose
Dosage Forms Injection: 10 mg/mL (20 mL, 25 mL, 50 mL); 50 mg/mL (10 mL); 100 mg/mL (5 mL)

ketoconazole (kee toe koe' na zole)
Brand Names Nizoral® Oral; Nizoral® Topical
Therapeutic Category Antifungal Agent, Systemic; Antifungal Agent, Topical
Use Treatment of susceptible fungal infections, including candidiasis, oral thrush, blastomycosis, histoplasmosis, paracoccidioidomycosis, chronic mucocutaneous candidiasis, as well as certain recalcitrant cutaneous dermatophytoses; used topically for treatment of tinea corporis, tinea cruris, tinea versicolor and cutaneous candidiasis
Usual Dosage
Children: Oral: 5-10 mg/kg/day divided every 12-24 hours until lesions clear
Adults:
  Oral: 200-400 mg/day as a single daily dose
  Topical: Rub gently into the affected area once daily to twice daily for two weeks
Dosage Forms
Cream: 2% (15 g, 30 g, 60 g)
Shampoo: 2% (120 mL)
Suspension, oral: 100 mg/5 mL (120 mL)
Tablet: 200 mg

Keto-Diastix® [OTC] *see* diagnostic aids (*in vitro*), urine *on page 139*

ketoprofen (kee toe proe' fen)
Brand Names Orudis®; Oruvail®
Therapeutic Category Analgesic, Non-Narcotic; Anti-inflammatory Agent; Nonsteroidal Anti-Inflammatory Agent (NSAID), Oral
Use Acute or long-term treatment of rheumatoid arthritis and osteoarthritis; primary dysmenorrhea; mild to moderate pain
Usual Dosage Oral:
Children 3 months to 14 years: Fever: 0.5-1 mg/kg every 6-8 hours
Children >12 years and Adults:
  Rheumatoid arthritis or osteoarthritis: 50-75 mg 3-4 times/day up to a maximum of 300 mg/day
  Mild to moderate pain: 25-50 mg every 6-8 hours up to a maximum of 300 mg/day
Dosage Forms
Capsule (Orudis®): 25 mg, 50 mg, 75 mg
Capsule, extended release (Oruvail®): 200 mg

ketorolac tromethamine (kee' toe role ak)
Brand Names Acular® Ophthalmic; Toradol® Injection; Toradol® Oral
Therapeutic Category Analgesic, Non-Narcotic; Anti-inflammatory Agent; Nonsteroidal Anti-Inflammatory Agent (NSAID), Oral; Nonsteroidal Anti-Inflammatory Agent (NSAID), Parenteral
Use Short-term management of pain; first parenteral NSAID for analgesia; 30 mg provides the analgesia comparable to 12 mg of morphine or 100 mg of meperidine
Usual Dosage Adults: Pain relief usually begins within 10 minutes
Oral: 10 mg every 4-6 hours for a maximum of 40 mg/day
I.M.: Initial: 30 mg then 15 mg every 6 hours thereafter, or 60 mg initially, then 30 mg every 6 hours thereafter; maximum dose in the first 24 hours: 150 mg with 120 mg/24 hours thereafter
Dosage Forms
Injection: 15 mg/mL (1 mL); 30 mg/mL (1 mL, 2 mL)
Solution, ophthalmic: 0.5% (5 mL)
Tablet: 10 mg

Ketostix® [OTC] *see* diagnostic aids (*in vitro*), urine *on page 139*
Key-Pred® Injection *see* prednisolone *on page 391*

Key-Pred-SP® Injection *see* prednisolone *on page 391*

KI *see* potassium iodide *on page 387*

K-Ide® *see* potassium bicarbonate and potassium citrate, effervescent *on page 386*

Kinesed® *see* hyoscyamine, atropine, scopolamine, and phenobarbital *on page 242*

Kinevac® *see* sincalide *on page 432*

Klerist-D® *see* chlorpheniramine and pseudoephedrine *on page 94*

Klonopin™ *see* clonazepam *on page 108*

K-Lor™ *see* potassium chloride *on page 386*

Klor-con® *see* potassium chloride *on page 386*

Klor-con®/EF *see* potassium bicarbonate and potassium citrate, effervescent *on page 386*

Klorvess® *see* potassium chloride *on page 386*

Klotrix® *see* potassium chloride *on page 386*

K-Lyte® *see* potassium bicarbonate and potassium citrate, effervescent *on page 386*

K-Lyte/CL® *see* potassium chloride *on page 386*

Koate®-HP *see* antihemophilic factor *on page 29*

Koate®-HS *see* antihemophilic factor *on page 29*

KoGENate® *see* antihemophilic factor *on page 29*

Kolephrin® GG/DM [OTC] *see* guaifenesin and dextromethorphan *on page 218*

Kolyum® *see* potassium gluconate *on page 387*

Konakion® Injection *see* phytonadione *on page 376*

Kondon's Nasal® [OTC] *see* ephedrine sulfate *on page 170*

Konsyl® [OTC] *see* psyllium *on page 407*

Konsyl-D® [OTC] *see* psyllium *on page 407*

Konyne® 80 *see* factor ix complex (human) *on page 189*

Koromex® [OTC] *see* nonoxynol 9 *on page 338*

K-Phos® Neutral *see* potassium phosphate and sodium phosphate *on page 388*

K-Phos® Original *see* potassium acid phosphate *on page 385*

Kronofed-A-Jr® *see* chlorpheniramine and pseudoephedrine *on page 94*

K-Tab® *see* potassium chloride *on page 386*

Ku-Zyme® HP *see* pancrelipase *on page 354*

K-Vescent® *see* potassium bicarbonate and potassium citrate, effervescent *on page 386*

Kwelcof® *see* hydrocodone and guaifenesin *on page 235*

Kwell® Cream *see* lindane *on page 274*

Kwell® Lotion *see* lindane *on page 274*

Kwell® Shampoo *see* lindane *on page 274*

Kytril® Injection *see* granisetron *on page 216*

***L*-3-hydroxytyrosine** *see* levodopa *on page 270*

LA-12® Injection *see* hydroxocobalamin *on page 240*

labetalol hydrochloride (la bet' a lole)

Brand Names Normodyne® Injection; Normodyne® Oral; Trandate® Injection; Trandate® Oral

Synonyms ibidomide hydrochloride

(Continued)

labetalol hydrochloride *(Continued)*

Therapeutic Category Alpha-/Beta- Adrenergic Blocker
Use Treatment of mild to severe hypertension; I.V. for hypertensive emergencies
Usual Dosage

Children: Limited information regarding labetalol use in pediatric patients is currently available in literature. Some centers recommend initial oral doses of 4 mg/kg/day in 2 divided doses. Reported oral doses have started at 3 mg/kg/day and 20 mg/kg/day and have increased up to 40 mg/kg/day.

I.V., intermittent bolus doses of 0.3-1 mg/kg/dose have been reported

For treatment of pediatric hypertensive emergencies, initial continuous infusions of 0.4-1 mg/kg/hour with a maximum of 3 mg/kg/hour have been used.

Due to limited documentation of its use, labetalol should be initiated cautiously in pediatric patients with careful dosage adjustment and blood pressure monitoring

Adults:

Oral: Initial: 100 mg twice daily, may increase as needed every 2-3 days by 100 mg until desired response is obtained; usual dose: 200-400 mg twice daily; not to exceed 2.4 g/day

I.V.: 20 mg or 1-2 mg/kg whichever is lower, IVP over 2 minutes, may give 40-80 mg at 10-minute intervals, up to 300 mg total dose

I.V. infusion: Initial: 2 mg/minute; titrate to response

Dosage Forms

Injection: 5 mg/mL (20 mL, 40 mL, 60 mL)
Tablet: 100 mg, 200 mg, 300 mg

Labstix® [OTC] *see* diagnostic aids *(in vitro)*, urine *on page 139*

Lac-Hydrin® *see* lactic acid with ammonium hydroxide *on next page*

Lactaid® [OTC] *see* lactase enzyme *on this page*

---

lactase enzyme (lak' tase)

Brand Names Dairy Ease® [OTC]; Lactaid® [OTC]; Lactrase® [OTC]
Therapeutic Category Nutritional Supplement
Use Help digest lactose in milk for patients with lactose intolerance
Usual Dosage

Capsule: 1-2 capsules taken with milk or meal; pretreat milk with 1-2 capsules per quart of milk
Liquid: 5-15 drops per quart of milk
Tablet: 1-3 tablets with meals

Dosage Forms

Caplet: 3000 FCC lactase units
Capsule: 250 mg
Liquid: 1250 neutral lactase units/5 drops
Tablet, chewable: 3300 FCC lactase units

---

lactic acid and salicylic acid *see* salicylic acid and lactic acid *on page 424*

---

lactic acid and sodium-PCA

Brand Names LactiCare® [OTC]
Synonyms sodium-PCA and lactic acid
Therapeutic Category Topical Skin Product
Use Lubricate and moisturize the skin counteracting dryness and itching
Usual Dosage Apply as needed
Dosage Forms Lotion, topical: Lactic acid 5% and sodium-PCA 2.5% (240 mL)

lactic acid with ammonium hydroxide
Brand Names Lac-Hydrin®
Synonyms ammonium lactate
Therapeutic Category Topical Skin Product
Use Treatment of moderate to severe xerosis and ichthyosis vulgaris
Usual Dosage Shake well; apply to affected areas, use twice daily, rub in well
Dosage Forms Lotion: Lactic acid 12% with ammonium hydroxide (150 mL)

LactiCare® [OTC] *see* lactic acid and sodium-PCA *on previous page*
LactiCare-HC® Topical *see* hydrocortisone *on page 236*
Lactinex® [OTC] *see* lactobacillus *on this page*
Lactisol® Liquid *see* salicylic acid *on page 424*

lactobacillus (lak toe ba sil' us)
Brand Names Bacid® [OTC]; Lactinex® [OTC]; More-Dophilus® [OTC]
Synonyms *Lactobacillus acidophilus* and *lactobacillus bulgaricus*
Therapeutic Category Antidiarrheal
Use Uncomplicated diarrhea particularly that caused by antibiotic therapy; re-establish normal physiologic and bacterial flora of the intestinal tract
Usual Dosage Children and Adults: Oral:
Capsule: Take 2 capsules 2-4 times daily
Granules: 1 packet added to or taken with cereal, food, milk, fruit juice, or water, 3-4 times/day
Tablet, chewable: 4 tablets 3-4 times/day; may follow each dose with a small amount of milk, fruit juice, or water
Recontamination protocol for BMT unit: 1 packet 3 times/day for 6 doses for those patients who refuse yogurt.
Dosage Forms
Capsule: 50s, 100s
Granules: 1 g/packet (12 packets/box)
Powder: 12 oz
Tablet, chewable: 50's

Lactobacillus acidophilus* and *lactobacillus bulgaricus *see* lactobacillus *on this page*
lactoflavin *see* riboflavin *on page 419*
Lactrase® [OTC] *see* lactase enzyme *on previous page*

lactulose (lak' tyoo lose)
Brand Names Cephulac®; Cholac®; Chronulac®; Constilac®; Constulose®; Duphalac®; Enulose®; Lactulose PSE®
Therapeutic Category Ammonium Detoxicant; Laxative, Miscellaneous
Use Adjunct in the prevention and treatment of portal-systemic encephalopathy; treatment of chronic constipation
Usual Dosage Oral:
Infants: 2.5-10 mL/day divided 3-4 times/day
Children: 40-90 mL/day divided 3-4 times/day
Adults:
Acute episodes of portal systemic encephalopathy: 30-45 mL at 1- to 2-hour intervals until laxative effect observed
Chronic therapy: 30-45 mL/dose 3-4 times/day; titrate dose to produce 2-3 soft stools per day
Rectal: 300 mL diluted with 700 mL of water or normal saline, and given via a rectal balloon catheter and retained for 30-60 minutes; may give every 4-6 hours
Dosage Forms Syrup: 10 g/15 mL (15 mL, 30 mL, 237 mL, 473 mL, 946 mL, 1890 mL)

Lactulose PSE® *see* lactulose *on previous page*

ladakamycin *see* azacitidine *on page 40*

Lamisil® Topical *see* terbinafine hydrochloride *on page 454*

Lamprene® *see* clofazimine palmitate *on page 107*

Lanacort® Topical [OTC] *see* hydrocortisone *on page 236*

Lanaphilic® Topical [OTC] *see* urea *on page 487*

Laniazid® Oral *see* isoniazid *on page 258*

lanolin, cetyl alcohol, glycerin, and petrolatum
Brand Names Lubriderm® [OTC]
Therapeutic Category Topical Skin Product
Use Treatment of dry skin
Usual Dosage Topical: Apply to skin as necessary
Dosage Forms Lotion: 480 mL

Lanophyllin-GG® *see* theophylline and guaifenesin *on page 461*

Lanorinal® *see* butalbital compound *on page 63*

Lanoxicaps® *see* digoxin *on page 147*

Lanoxin® *see* digoxin *on page 147*

Lanvisone® Topical *see* clioquinol and hydrocortisone *on page 106*

Largon® Injection *see* propiomazine hydrochloride *on page 401*

Lariam® *see* mefloquine hydrochloride *on page 290*

Larodopa® *see* levodopa *on page 270*

Lasan™ *see* anthralin *on page 29*

Lasix® Injection *see* furosemide *on page 207*

Lasix® Oral *see* furosemide *on page 207*

Lassar's zinc paste *see* zinc oxide *on page 503*

Lavacol® [OTC] *see* alcohol, ethyl *on page 11*

Lax-Pills® [OTC] *see* phenolphthalein *on page 370*

LazerSporin-C® Otic *see* neomycin, polymyxin b, and hydrocortisone *on page 329*

***l*-bunolol hydrochloride** *see* levobunolol hydrochloride *on page 270*

L-carnitine *see* levocarnitine *on page 270*

L.C.D. *see* coal tar *on page 110*

LCR *see* vincristine sulfate *on page 496*

L-deprenyl *see* selegiline hydrochloride *on page 428*

***l*-dopa** *see* levodopa *on page 270*

Ledercillin® VK Oral *see* penicillin V potassium *on page 362*

Lederplex® [OTC] *see* vitamin B complex *on page 498*

Legatrin® [OTC] *see* quinine sulfate *on page 412*

Lente *see* insulin preparations *on page 250*

Lente® Iletin® I *see* insulin preparations *on page 250*

Lente® Iletin® II *see* insulin preparations *on page 250*

Lente® Purified Pork Insulin *see* insulin preparations *on page 250*

leucovorin calcium (loo koe vor' in)
Brand Names Wellcovorin® Injection; Wellcovorin® Oral
Synonyms calcium leucovorin; citrovorum factor; folinic acid; 5-formyl tetrahydrofolate
Therapeutic Category Antidote, Methotrexate; Folic Acid Derivative

Use Antidote for folic acid antagonists, prevention of hematopoietic effects of folic acid antagonists, treatment of megaloblastic anemias when folate is deficient as in infancy, sprue, pregnancy, and nutritional deficiency when oral folate therapy is not possible and I.V. folic acid cannot be used; in combination with fluorouracil in the treatment of malignancy

Usual Dosage Children and Adults:

Adjunctive therapy with antimicrobial agents (pyrimethamine): Oral: 2-15 mg/day for 3 days or until blood counts are normal or 5 mg every 3 days; doses of 6 mg/day are needed for patients with platelet counts <100,000/mm^3

Folate deficient megaloblastic anemia: I.M.: 1 mg/day

Megaloblastic anemia secondary to congenital deficiency of dihydrofolate reductase: I.M.: 3-6 mg/day

Rescue dose: I.V.: 10 mg/m^2 to start, then 10 mg/m^2 every 6 hours orally for 72 hours; if serum creatinine 24 hours after methotrexate is elevated 50% or more **or** the serum MTX concentration is >5 x 10^{-6}M, increase dose to 100 mg/m^2/dose every 3 hours until serum methotrexate level is less than 1 x 10^{-8}M

Dosage Forms
Injection: 3 mg/mL (1 mL)
Powder for injection: 25 mg, 50 mg, 100 mg, 350 mg
Powder for oral solution: 1 mg/mL (60 mL)
Tablet: 5 mg, 10 mg, 15 mg, 25 mg

Leukeran® *see* chlorambucil *on page 88*

Leukine™ *see* sargramostim *on page 426*

leuprolide acetate (loo proe' lide)

Brand Names Lupron® Injection
Synonyms leuprorelin acetate
Therapeutic Category Antineoplastic Agent, Hormone (Gonadotropin Hormone-Releasing Antigen); Gonadotropin Releasing Hormone Analog
Use Palliative treatment of advanced prostate carcinoma, precocious puberty, endometriosis

Usual Dosage Refer to individual protocols
Children: S.C.: Precocious puberty: 20-45 µg/kg/day

Adults: Advanced prostatic carcinoma:
S.C.: 1 mg/day **or**
I.M. (suspension): 7.5 mg/dose given monthly

Endometriosis: ≥18 years: I.M.: 3.75 mg/month for 6 months

Dosage Forms
Injection: 5 mg/mL (2.8 mL)
Suspension, Depot®: 3.75 mg/mL; 7.5 mg/mL; 11.25 mg/mL; 15 mg/mL

leuprorelin acetate *see* leuprolide acetate *on this page*

leurocristine *see* vincristine sulfate *on page 496*

Leustatin™ *see* cladribine *on page 104*

levamisole hydrochloride (lee vam' i sole)

Brand Names Ergamisol®
Therapeutic Category Immune Modulator
Use Adjuvant treatment with fluorouracil in Dukes stage C colon cancer
Usual Dosage Oral: Initial: 50 mg every 8 hours for 3 days, then 50 mg every 8 hours for 3 days every 2 weeks (fluorouracil is always given concomitantly)
Dosage Forms Tablet, as base: 50 mg

levarterenol bitartrate *see* norepinephrine bitartrate *on page 338*

Levatol® *see* penbutolol sulfate *on page 359*

Levlen® *see* ethinyl estradiol and levonorgestrel *on page 183*

levobunolol hydrochloride (lee voe byoo' noe lole)
Brand Names Betagan® Liquifilm® Ophthalmic
Synonyms *l*-bunolol hydrochloride
Therapeutic Category Beta-Adrenergic Blocker, Ophthalmic
Use Lower intraocular pressure in chronic open-angle glaucoma or ocular hypertension
Usual Dosage Adults: 1-2 drops of 0.5% solution in eye(s) once daily or 1-2 drops of 0.25% solution twice daily
Dosage Forms Solution: 0.25% [2.5 mg/mL] (2 mL, 5 mL, 10 mL, 15 mL); 0.5% [5 mg/mL] (2 mL, 5 mL, 10 mL, 15 mL)

levocarnitine (lee voe kar' ni teen)
Brand Names Carnitor® Injection; Carnitor® Oral; Vitacarn® Oral
Synonyms L-carnitine
Therapeutic Category Dietary Supplement
Use Therapy in patients with primary systemic carnitine deficiency
Usual Dosage Oral:
Children: 50-100 mg/kg/day divided 2-3 times/day, maximum: 3 g/day; dosage must be individualized based upon patient response; higher dosages have been used

Adults: 1-3 g/day for 50 kg subject; start at 1 g/day, increase slowly assessing tolerance and response
Dosage Forms
Capsule: 250 mg
Injection: 1 g/5 mL (5 mL)
Liquid (cherry flavor): 100 mg/mL (10 mL)
Tablet: 330 mg

levodopa (lee voe doe' pa)
Brand Names Dopar®; Larodopa®
Synonyms *L*-3-hydroxytyrosine; *l*-dopa
Therapeutic Category Antiparkinson Agent
Use Treatment of Parkinson's disease; used as a diagnostic agent for growth hormone deficiency
Usual Dosage Children: Oral (given as a single dose to evaluate growth hormone deficiency): 0.5 g/m^2
or
<30 lbs: 125 mg
30-70 lbs: 250 mg
>70 lbs: 500 mg
Dosage Forms
Capsule: 100 mg, 250 mg, 500 mg
Tablet: 100 mg, 250 mg, 500 mg

levodopa and carbidopa (lee voe doe' pa & kar bi doe' pa
Brand Names Sinemet®
Synonyms carbidopa and levodopa
Therapeutic Category Antiparkinson Agent
Use Treatment of Parkinsonian syndrome
Usual Dosage Adults: Oral (carbidopa/levodopa): 75/300 to 150/1500 mg/day in 3-4 divided doses; can increase up to 200/2000 mg/day
Dosage Forms Tablet:
10/100: Carbidopa 10 mg and levodopa 100 mg
25/100: Carbidopa 25 mg and levodopa 100 mg

25/250: Carbidopa 25 mg and levodopa 250 mg
Sustained release: Carbidopa 50 mg and levodopa 200 mg

Levo-Dromoran® Injection *see* levorphanol tartrate *on this page*
Levo-Dromoran® Oral *see* levorphanol tartrate *on this page*
levomepromazine *see* methotrimeprazine hydrochloride *on page 302*

levomethadyl acetate hydrochloride (lee voe meth' a dil)
Brand Names ORLAAM®
Therapeutic Category Analgesic, Narcotic
Use Management of opiate dependence
Usual Dosage Adults: Oral: 20-40 mg 3 times/week; range: 10 mg to as high as 140 mg 3 times/week
Dosage Forms Solution, oral: 10 mg/mL (474 mL)

levonorgestrel (lee' voe nor jess trel)
Brand Names Norplant® Implant
Therapeutic Category Contraceptive, Implant; Contraceptive, Progestin Only; Progestin
Use Prevention of pregnancy
Usual Dosage Each Norplant® silastic capsule releases 80 μg of drug/day for 6-18 months, following which a rate of release of 25-30 μg/day is maintained for ≤5 years.
Dosage Forms Capsule, subdermal implantation: 36 mg (6s)

levonorgestrel and ethinyl estradiol *see* ethinyl estradiol and levonorgestrel *on page 183*
Levophed® Injection *see* norepinephrine bitartrate *on page 338*
Levoprome® *see* methotrimeprazine hydrochloride *on page 302*

levorphanol tartrate (lee vor' fa nole)
Brand Names Levo-Dromoran® Injection; Levo-Dromoran® Oral
Synonyms levorphan tartrate
Therapeutic Category Analgesic, Narcotic
Use Relief of moderate to severe pain; also used parenterally for preoperative sedation and an adjunct to nitrous oxide/oxygen anesthesia
Usual Dosage Adults: Oral, S.C.: 2 mg, up to 3 mg if necessary
Dosage Forms
Injection: 2 mg/mL (1 mL, 10 mL)
Tablet: 2 mg

levorphan tartrate *see* levorphanol tartrate *on this page*
Levothroid® Injection *see* levothyroxine sodium *on this page*
Levothroid® Oral *see* levothyroxine sodium *on this page*

levothyroxine sodium (lee voe thye rox' een)
Brand Names Levothroid® Injection; Levothroid® Oral; Levoxine® Oral; Synthroid® Injection; Synthroid® Oral
Synonyms L-thyroxine sodium; T_4 thyroxine sodium
Therapeutic Category Thyroid Product
Use Replacement or supplemental therapy in hypothyroidism, myxedema, coma or stupor
Usual Dosage
Children:
Oral:
0-6 months: 8-10 μg/kg/day
6-12 months: 6-8 μg/kg/day
(Continued)

271

levothyroxine sodium (Continued)

     1-5 years: 5-6 µg/kg/day
     6-12 years: 4-5 µg/kg/day
     >12 years: 2-3 µg/kg/day
     I.M., I.V.: 75% of the oral dose

Adults:
     Oral: 12.5-50 µg/day to start, then increase by 25-50 µg/day at intervals of 2-4 weeks; average adult dose: 100-200 µg/day
     I.M., I.V.: 50% of the oral dose

Myxedema coma or stupor: I.V.: 200-500 µg one time, then 100-300 µg the next day if necessary

Dosage Forms
Powder for injection, lyophilized: 0.2 mg/vial (6 mL, 10 mL); 0.5 mg/vial (6 mL, 10 mL)
Tablet: 0.0125 mg, 0.025 mg, 0.05 mg, 0.075 mg, 0.088 mg, 0.1 mg, 0.112 mg, 0.125 mg, 0.15 mg, 0.175 mg, 0.2 mg, 0.3 mg

Levoxine® Oral see levothyroxine sodium on previous page

Levsinex® Oral see hyoscyamine sulfate on page 243

Levsin® Injection see hyoscyamine sulfate on page 243

Levsin® Oral see hyoscyamine sulfate on page 243

levulose, dextrose and phosphoric acid see phosphorated carbohydrate solution on page 375

***l*-hyoscyamine sulfate** see hyoscyamine sulfate on page 243

Librax® see clidinium and chlordiazepoxide on page 105

Libritabs® see chlordiazepoxide on page 89

Librium® see chlordiazepoxide on page 89

Lice-Enz® [OTC] see pyrethrins on page 408

Lida-Mantle HC® Topical see lidocaine and hydrocortisone on this page

Lidex-E® Topical see fluocinonide on page 200

Lidex® Topical see fluocinonide on page 200

lidocaine and epinephrine

Brand Names Octocaine® Injection; Xylocaine® With Epinephrine
Therapeutic Category Local Anesthetic, Injectable
Use Local infiltration anesthesia
Usual Dosage Children (dosage varies with the anesthetic procedure): Use lidocaine concentrations of 0.5% or 1% (or even more dilute) to decrease possibility of toxicity; lidocaine dose should not exceed 4.5 mg/kg/dose; do not repeat within 2 hours
Dosage Forms Injection with epinephrine:
     1:200,000: Lidocaine hydrochloride 0.5% [5 mg/mL] (50 mL); 1% [10 mg/mL] (30 mL); 1.5% [15 mg/mL] (5 mL, 10 mL, 30 mL); 2% [20 mg/mL] (20 mL)
     1:100,000: Lidocaine hydrochloride 1% [10 mg/mL] (20 mL, 50 mL); 2% [20 mg/mL] (1.8 mL, 20 mL, 50 mL)
     1:50,000: Lidocaine hydrochloride 2% [20 mg/mL] (1.8 mL)

lidocaine and hydrocortisone

Brand Names Lida-Mantle HC® Topical
Therapeutic Category Corticosteroid, Topical (Low Potency); Local Anesthetic, Topical
Use Topical anti-inflammatory and anesthetic for skin disorders
Usual Dosage Topical: Apply 2-4 times/day
Dosage Forms Cream: Lidocaine 3% and hydrocortisone 0.5% (15 g, 30 g)

lidocaine and prilocaine
Brand Names EMLA® Topical
Therapeutic Category Analgesic, Topical; Antipruritic, Topical; Local Anesthetic, Topical
Use Topical anesthetic for use on normal intact skin to provide local analgesia for minor procedures such as I.V. cannulation or venipuncture; has also been used for painful procedures such as lumbar puncture and skin graft harvesting
Usual Dosage Children and Adults: Topical: Apply a thick layer of cream to intact skin and cover with an occlusive dressing; for minor procedures, apply 2.5 g/site for at least 60 minutes; for painful procedures, apply 2 g/10 cm² of skin and leave on for at least 2 hours
Dosage Forms Cream: Lidocaine 2.5% and prilocaine 2.5% [2 Tegaderm® dressings] (5 g, 30 g)

lidocaine hydrochloride (lye' doe kane)
Brand Names Anestacon® Topical Solution; Dalcaine® Injection; Dilocaine® Injection; Duo-Trach® Injection; LidoPen® I.M. Injection Auto-Injector; Nervocaine® Injection; Solarcaine® Topical; Xylocaine® HCl I.V. Injection for Cardiac Arrhythmias; Xylocaine® Oral; Xylocaine® Topical Ointment; Xylocaine® Topical Solution; Xylocaine® Topical Spray
Synonyms lignocaine hydrochloride
Therapeutic Category Antiarrhythmic Agent, Class Ib; Local Anesthetic, Injectable; Local Anesthetic, Topical
Use Local anesthetic and acute treatment of ventricular arrhythmias from myocardial infarction, cardiac manipulation, digitalis intoxication
Usual Dosage
Topical: Apply to affected area as needed; maximum: 3 mg/kg/dose; do not repeat within 2 hours
Injectable local anesthetic: Varies with procedure, degree of anesthesia needed, vascularity of tissue, duration of anesthesia required, and physical condition of patient; maximum: 4.5 mg/kg/dose; do not repeat within 2 hours

Children: Endotracheal, I.O., I.V.: Loading dose: 1 mg/kg; may repeat in 10-15 minutes to a maximum total dose of 5 mg/kg; after loading dose, start I.V. continuous infusion 20-50 μg/kg/minute. Use 20 μg/kg/minute in patients with shock, hepatic disease, mild congestive heart failure (CHF); moderate to severe CHF may require ½ loading dose and lower infusion rates to avoid toxicity. Endotracheal doses should be diluted to 1-2 mL with normal saline prior to endotracheal administration and may need 2-3 times the I.V. dose.

Adults: Antiarrhythmic:
Endotracheal: Total dose: 5 mg/kg; follow with 0.5 mg/kg in 10 minutes if effective
I.M.: 300 mg may be repeated in 1-1½ hours
I.V.: Loading dose: 1 mg/kg/dose, then 50-100 mg bolus over 2-3 minutes; may repeat in 5-10 minutes up to 200-300 mg in a 1-hour period; continuous infusion of 20-50 μg/kg/minute or 1-4 mg/minute; decrease the dose in patients with CHF, shock, or hepatic disease
Dosage Forms
Injection: 0.5% [5 mg/mL] (50 mL); 1% [10 mg/mL] (2 mL, 5 mL, 10 mL, 20 mL, 30 mL, 50 mL); 1.5% [15 mg/mL] (20 mL); 2% [20 mg/mL] (2 mL, 5 mL, 10 mL, 20 mL, 30 mL, 50 mL); 4% [40 mg/mL] (5 mL); 10% [100 mg/mL] (10 mL); 20% [200 mg/mL] (10 mL, 20 mL)
Injection:
I.M. use: 10% [100 mg/mL] (3 mL, 5 mL)
Direct I.V.: 1% [10 mg/mL] (5 mL, 10 mL); 20 mg/mL (5 mL)
I.V. admixture, preservative free: 4% [40 mg/mL] (25 mL, 30 mL); 10% [100 mg/mL] (10 mL); 20% [200 mg/mL] (5 mL, 10 mL)
I.V. infusion, in D₅W: 0.2% [2 mg/mL] (500 mL); 0.4% [4 mg/mL] (250 mL, 500 mL, 1000 mL); 0.8% [8 mg/mL] (250 mL, 500 mL)
Jelly, topical: 2% (30 mL)
Liquid, viscous: 2% (20 mL, 100 mL)
Ointment, topical: 2.5% [OTC], 5% (35 g)
Solution, topical: 2% [20 mg/mL] (15 mL, 240 mL); 4% [40 mg/mL] (50 mL)

ALPHABETICAL LISTING OF DRUGS

LidoPen® I.M. Injection Auto-Injector *see* lidocaine hydrochloride *on previous page*

Lidox® *see* clidinium and chlordiazepoxide *on page 105*

LIG *see* lymphocyte immune globulin, anti-thymocyte globulin (equine) *on page 280*

lignocaine hydrochloride *see* lidocaine hydrochloride *on previous page*

Limbitrol® *see* amitriptyline and chlordiazepoxide *on page 21*

Lincocin® Injection *see* lincomycin hydrochloride *on this page*

Lincocin® Oral *see* lincomycin hydrochloride *on this page*

lincomycin hydrochloride (lin koe mye' sin)
Brand Names Lincocin® Injection; Lincocin® Oral; Lincorex® Injection
Therapeutic Category Antibiotic, Macrolide
Use Treatment of susceptible bacterial infections, mainly those caused by streptococci and staphylococci
Usual Dosage
Children >1 month:
Oral: 30-60 mg/kg/day in 3-4 divided doses
I.M.: 10 mg/kg every 12-24 hours
I.V.: 10-20 mg/kg/day in divided doses 2-3 times/day

Adults:
Oral: 500 mg every 6-8 hours
I.M.: 600 mg every 12-24 hours
I.V.: 600-1 g every 8-12 hours up to 8 g/day
Dosage Forms
Capsule: 250 mg, 500 mg
Injection: 300 mg/mL (2 mL, 10 mL)

Lincorex® Injection *see* lincomycin hydrochloride *on this page*

lindane (lin' dane)
Brand Names G-well® Lotion; G-well® Shampoo; Kwell® Cream; Kwell® Lotion; Kwell® Shampoo; Scabene® Lotion; Scabene® Shampoo
Synonyms benzene hexachloride; gamma benzene hexachloride; hexachlorocyclohexane
Therapeutic Category Antiparasitic Agent, Topical; Pediculocide; Scabicidal Agent; Shampoos
Use Treatment of scabies (*Sarcoptes scabiei*) and pediculosis (*Pediculus capitis* – head lice, *Pediculus pubis* – crab lice)
Usual Dosage Children and Adults: Topical:
Scabies: Apply a thin layer of lotion and massage it on skin from the neck to the toes. For adults, bathe and remove the drug after 8-12 hours; for children, wash off 6 hours after application.

Pediculosis: 15-30 mL of shampoo is applied and lathered for 4-5 minutes; rinse hair thoroughly and comb with a fine tooth comb to remove nits; repeat treatment in 7 days if lice or nits are still present
Dosage Forms
Cream: 1% (60 g, 454 g)
Lotion: 1% (60 mL, 473 mL, 4000 mL)
Shampoo: 1% (60 mL, 473 mL, 4000 mL)

Lioresal® *see* baclofen *on page 43*

liothyronine sodium (lye oh thye' roe neen)
Brand Names Cytomel® Oral; Triostat™ Injection
Synonyms sodium L-tri-iodothyronine; T_3 thyronine sodium
Therapeutic Category Thyroid Product

Use Replacement or supplemental therapy in hypothyroidism, management of nontoxic goiter, chronic lymphocytic thyroiditis, as an adjunct in thyrotoxicosis and as a diagnostic aid

Usual Dosage

Mild hypothyroidism: 25 μg/day; daily dosage may then be increased by 12.5 or 25 μg/day every 1 or 2 weeks; maintenance: 25-75 μg/day

Myxedema: 5μg/day; may be increased by 5-10 μg/day every 1-2 weeks; when 25 μg is reached, dosage may often be increased by 12.5 or 25 μg every 1 or 2 weeks; maintenance: 50-100 μg/day

Cretinism: 5 μg/day with a 5 μg increment every 3-4 days until the desired response is achieved

Simple (nontoxic) goiter: 5 μg/day; may be increased every week or two by 5 or 10 μg; when 25 μg/day is reached, dosage may be increased every week or two by 12.5 or 25 μg; maintenance: 75 μg/day

T_3 Suppression Test: I^{131} thyroid uptake is in the borderline-high range, administer 75-100 μg/day for 7 days then repeat I^{131} thyroid uptake test

In the elderly or children: Start therapy with 5 μg/day; increase only by 5 μg increments at the recommended intervals

Dosage Forms
Injection: 10 μg/mL (1 mL)
Tablet: 5 μg, 25 μg, 50 μg

liotrix (lye' oh trix)
Brand Names Euthroid®; Thyrolar®
Synonyms T_3/T_4 liotrix
Therapeutic Category Thyroid Hormone
Use Replacement or supplemental therapy in hypothyroidism
Usual Dosage
Congenital hypothyroidism: Oral:
Children (dose/day):
0-6 months: 8-10 μg/kg
6-12 months: 6-8 μg/kg
1-5 years: 5-6 μg/kg
6-12 years: 4-5 μg/kg
>12 years: 2-3 μg/kg
Adults: 30 mg/day, increasing by 15 mg/day at 2- to 3-week intervals to a maximum of 180 mg/day
Dosage Forms Tablet: 30 mg, 60 mg, 120 mg, 180 mg [thyroid equivalent]

lipancreatin see pancrelipase on page 354
Liposyn® see fat emulsion on page 190
Lipovite® [OTC] see vitamin B complex on page 498
Liquaemin® Injection see heparin on page 226
Liquibid® see guaifenesin on page 217
Liqui-Char® [OTC] see charcoal on page 86
liquid antidote see charcoal on page 86
Liquid Barosperse® see radiological/contrast media (ionic) on page 413
Liquid Pred® Oral see prednisone on page 393
Liqui-E® see tocophersolan on page 470
Liquipake® see radiological/contrast media (ionic) on page 413

lisinopril (lyse in' oh pril)
Brand Names Prinivil®; Zestril®
Therapeutic Category Angiotensin Converting Enzyme (ACE) Inhibitors
Use Treatment of hypertension, either alone or in combination with other antihypertensive agents
(Continued)

lisinopril (Continued)
Usual Dosage Adults: Oral: 10-40 mg/day in a single dose
Dosage Forms Tablet: 5 mg, 10 mg, 20 mg, 40 mg

Listermint® with Fluoride [OTC] see fluoride on page 201

Lithane® see lithium on this page

lithium (lith' ee um)
Brand Names Cibalith-S®; Eskalith®; Lithane®; Lithobid®; Lithonate®; Lithotabs®
Synonyms lithium carbonate; lithium citrate
Therapeutic Category Antimanic Agent
Use Management of acute manic episodes, bipolar disorders, and depression
Usual Dosage Oral: Monitor serum concentrations and clinical response (efficacy and toxicity) to determine proper dose

Children: 15-60 mg/kg/day in 3-4 divided doses; dose not to exceed usual adult dosage

Adults: 300 mg 3-4 times/day; usual maximum maintenance dose: 2.4 g/day
Dosage Forms
Capsule, as carbonate: 150 mg, 300 mg, 600 mg
Syrup, as citrate: 300 mg/5 mL (5 mL, 10 mL, 480 mL)
Tablet, as carbonate: 300 mg
Tablet:
    Controlled release, as carbonate: 450 mg
    Slow release, as carbonate: 300 mg

lithium carbonate see lithium on this page

lithium citrate see lithium on this page

Lithobid® see lithium on this page

Lithonate® see lithium on this page

Lithostat® see acetohydroxamic acid on page 5

Lithotabs® see lithium on this page

LKV-Drops® [OTC] see vitamin, multiple (pediatric) on page 499

l-lysine hydrochloride (lye' seen)
Brand Names Enisyl® [OTC]; Lycolan® Elixir [OTC]
Therapeutic Category Dietary Supplement
Use Improves utilization of vegetable proteins
Usual Dosage Adults: Oral: 334-1500 mg/day
Dosage Forms
Capsule: 500 mg
Elixir: 100 mg/15 mL with glycine 1800 mg/15 mL and alcohol 12%
Tablet: 312 mg, 334 mg, 500 mg, 1000 mg

8-L-lysine vasopressin see lypressin on page 280

LMD® see dextran on page 135

Lobac® see chlorzoxazone on page 99

Locoid® Topical see hydrocortisone on page 236

Lodine® see etodolac on page 187

Lodosyn® see carbidopa on page 73

lodoxamide tromethamine (loe dox' a mide)
Brand Names Alomide® Ophthalmic
Therapeutic Category Ophthalmic Agent, Miscellaneous
Use Treatment of vernal keratoconjunctivitis, vernal conjunctivitis, and vernal keratitis

Usual Dosage Children >2 years of age and Adults: 1-2 drops in eye(s) 4 times daily
Dosage Forms Solution, ophthalmic: 0.1% (10 mL)

Loestrin® *see* ethinyl estradiol and norethindrone *on page 183*
Lofene® *see* diphenoxylate and atropine *on page 153*
Logen® *see* diphenoxylate and atropine *on page 153*
Lomanate® *see* diphenoxylate and atropine *on page 153*

lomefloxacin hydrochloride (loe me flox' a sin)
Brand Names Maxaquin® Oral
Therapeutic Category Antibiotic, Quinolone
Use Quinolone antibiotic for skin and skin structure, lower respiratory and urinary tract infections, and sexually transmitted diseases
Usual Dosage Oral: Adults: 400 mg once daily for 10-14 days
Dosage Forms Tablet: 400 mg

Lomodix® *see* diphenoxylate and atropine *on page 153*
Lomotil® *see* diphenoxylate and atropine *on page 153*

lomustine (loe mus' teen)
Brand Names CeeNU® Oral
Synonyms CCNU
Therapeutic Category Antineoplastic Agent, Alkylating Agent (Nitrosourea)
Use Treatment of brain tumors, Hodgkin's and non-Hodgkin's lymphomas
Usual Dosage Refer to individual protocols
Oral:
Children: 75-150 mg/m^2 as a single dose every 6 weeks. Subsequent doses are readjusted after initial treatment according to platelet and leukocyte counts

Adults: 100-130 mg/m^2 as a single dose every 6 weeks; readjust after initial treatment according to platelet and leukocyte counts
Dosage Forms
Capsule: 10 mg, 40 mg, 100 mg
Dose Pack: 10 mg (2s); 100 mg (2s); 40 mg (2s)

Loniten® Oral *see* minoxidil *on page 314*
Lonox® *see* diphenoxylate and atropine *on page 153*
Lo/Ovral® *see* ethinyl estradiol and norgestrel *on page 185*

loperamide hydrochloride (loe per' a mide)
Brand Names Imodium®; Imodium® A-D [OTC]; Kaopectate® II [OTC]; Pepto® Diarrhea Control [OTC
Therapeutic Category Antidiarrheal
Use Treatment of acute diarrhea and chronic diarrhea associated with inflammatory bowel disease; to decrease the volume of ileostomy discharge
Usual Dosage Oral:
Children:
Acute diarrhea: 0.4-0.8 mg/kg/day divided every 6-12 hours, maximum: 2 mg/dose
Chronic diarrhea: 0.08-0.24 mg/kg/day divided 2-3 times/day, maximum: 2 mg/dose

Adults: 4 mg (2 capsules) initially, followed by 2 mg after each loose stool, up to 16 mg/day (8 capsules)
Dosage Forms
Capsule: 2 mg
(Continued)

loperamide hydrochloride *(Continued)*
Liquid, oral: 1 mg/5 mL (60 mL, 90 mL, 120 mL)
Tablet: 2 mg

Lopid® *see gemfibrozil on page 210*
lopremone *see protirelin on page 405*
Lopressor® *see metoprolol on page 309*
Loprox® *see ciclopirox olamine on page 102*
Lorabid™ *see loracarbef on this page*

loracarbef *(loe ra kar' bef)*
Brand Names Lorabid™
Therapeutic Category Antibiotic, Carbacephem
Use Infections caused by susceptible organisms involving the respiratory tract, otitis media, sinusitis, skin and skin structure, bone and joint, and urinary tract and gynecologic as well as septicemia
Usual Dosage Oral:
Acute otitis media: Children: 15 mg/kg twice a day for 10 days
Urinary tract infections: Women: 200 mg once a day for 7 days
Dosage Forms
Capsule: 200 mg
Suspension, oral: 100 mg/5 mL; 200 mg/5 mL

loratadine *(lor at' a deen)*
Brand Names Claritin®
Therapeutic Category Antihistamine
Use Perennial and seasonal allergic rhinitis and other allergic symptoms including urticaria
Usual Dosage Adults: Oral: 10 mg daily on an empty stomach
Dosage Forms Tablet: 10 mg

lorazepam *(lor a' ze pam)*
Brand Names Ativan®
Therapeutic Category Antianxiety Agent; Benzodiazepine; Hypnotic; Sedative
Use Management of anxiety, status epilepticus, preoperative sedation, and amnesia
Usual Dosage
Anxiety and sedation:
Infants and Children: Oral, I.V.: Usual: 0.05 mg/kg/dose (range: 0.02-0.09 mg/kg) every 4-8 hours
Adults: Oral: 1-10 mg/day in 2-3 divided doses; usual dose: 2-6 mg/day in divided doses
Insomnia: Adults: Oral: 2-4 mg at bedtime
Preoperative: Adults:
I.M.: 0.05 mg/kg administered 2 hours before surgery; maximum: 4 mg/dose
I.V.: 0.044 mg/kg 15-20 minutes before surgery; usual maximum: 2 mg/dose
Operative amnesia: Adults: I.V.: up to 0.05 mg/kg; maximum: 4 mg/dose
Status epilepticus: I.V.:
Neonates: 0.05 mg/kg over 2-5 minutes; may repeat in 10-15 minutes (see warning regarding benzyl alcohol)
Infants and Children: 0.1 mg/kg slow I.V. over 2-5 minutes, do not exceed 4 mg/single dose; may repeat second dose of 0.05 mg/kg slow I.V. in 10-15 minutes if needed
Adolescents: 0.07 mg/kg slow I.V. over 2-5 minutes; maximum: 4 mg/dose; may repeat in 10-15 minutes
Adults: 4 mg/dose given slowly over 2-5 minutes; may repeat in 10-15 minutes; usual maximum dose: 8 mg

Dosage Forms
Injection: 2 mg/mL (1 mL, 10 mL); 4 mg/mL (1 mL, 10 mL)
Solution, oral concentrated, alcohol and dye free: 2 mg/mL (30 mL)
Tablet: 0.5 mg, 1 mg, 2 mg

Lorcet® *see* hydrocodone and acetaminophen *on page 234*

Lorcet® 10/650 *see* hydrocodone and acetaminophen *on page 234*

Lorcet®-HD *see* hydrocodone and acetaminophen *on page 234*

Lorcet® Plus *see* hydrocodone and acetaminophen *on page 234*

Lorelco® *see* probucol *on page 395*

Loroxide® [OTC] *see* benzoyl peroxide *on page 49*

Lortab® ASA *see* hydrocodone and aspirin *on page 234*

Losec® *see* omeprazole *on page 343*

Lotensin® *see* benazepril hydrochloride *on page 46*

Lotrimin AF® Topical [OTC] *see* clotrimazole *on page 109*

Lotrimin® Topical *see* clotrimazole *on page 109*

Lotrisone® *see* betamethasone dipropionate and clotrimazole *on page 53*

lovastatin (loe' va sta tin)
Brand Names Mevacor®
Synonyms mevinolin; monacolin K
Therapeutic Category Antilipemic Agent; HMG-COA Reductase Inhibitor
Use Adjunct to dietary therapy to decrease elevated serum total and LDL cholesterol concentrations in primary hypercholesterolemia
Usual Dosage Adults: Oral: Initial: 20 mg with evening meal, then adjust at 4-week intervals; maximum dose: 80 mg/day
Dosage Forms Tablet: 10 mg, 20 mg, 40 mg

Lovenox® Injection *see* enoxaparin sodium *on page 170*

Low-Quel® *see* diphenoxylate and atropine *on page 153*

loxapine (lox' a peen)
Brand Names Loxitane® I.M. Injection; Loxitane® Oral
Synonyms oxilapine succinate
Therapeutic Category Antipsychotic Agent
Use Management of psychotic disorders
Usual Dosage Adults:
Oral: 10 mg twice daily, increase dose until psychotic symptoms are controlled; usual dose range: 60-100 mg/day in divided doses 2-4 times/day; dosages >250 mg/day are not recommended
I.M.: 12.5-50 mg every 4-6 hours or longer as needed and change to oral therapy as soon as possible
Dosage Forms
Capsule: 5 mg, 10 mg, 25 mg, 50 mg
Concentrate, oral: 25 mg/mL (120 mL dropper bottle)
Injection: 50 mg/mL (1 mL)

Loxitane® I.M. Injection *see* loxapine *on this page*

Loxitane® Oral *see* loxapine *on this page*

Lozol® *see* indapamide *on page 248*

L-PAM *see* melphalan *on page 290*

LRH *see* gonadorelin *on page 215*

L-sarcolysin *see* melphalan *on page 290*

L-thyroxine sodium *see* levothyroxine sodium *on page 271*

Lubriderm® [OTC] *see* lanolin, cetyl alcohol, glycerin, and petrolatum *on page 268*

Ludiomil® *see* maprotiline hydrochloride *on page 285*

Lufyllin® *see* dyphylline *on page 165*

Lugol's solution *see* potassium iodide *on page 387*

Luminal® *see* phenobarbital *on page 369*

Lung Check® *see* diagnostic aids (*in vitro*), other *on page 138*

Lupron® Injection *see* leuprolide acetate *on page 269*

Luride® *see* fluoride *on page 201*

Luride® Lozi-Tab® *see* fluoride *on page 201*

Luride®-SF Lozi-Tab® *see* fluoride *on page 201*

Lutrepulse® Injection *see* gonadorelin *on page 215*

Lycolan® Elixir [OTC] *see* l-lysine hydrochloride *on page 276*

Lymphazurin® *see* radiological/contrast media (ionic) *on page 413*

lymphocyte immune globulin, anti-thymocyte globulin (equine)
Brand Names Atgam®
Synonyms ATG; horse anti-human thymocyte gamma globulin; LIG
Therapeutic Category Immunosuppressant Agent
Use Prevention and treatment of acute renal allograft rejection; treatment of moderate to severe aplastic anemia in patients not considered suitable candidates for bone marrow transplantation; prevention of graft-vs-host disease following bone marrow transplantation
Usual Dosage An intradermal skin test is recommended prior to administration of the initial dose of ATG. Use 0.1 mL of a 1:1000 dilution of ATG in normal saline

Aplastic anemia protocol: I.V.: 10-20 mg/kg/day for 8-14 days, then give every other day for 7 more doses

Rejection prevention: Children and Adults: I.V.: 15 mg/kg/day for 14 days, then give every other day for 7 more doses; initial dose should be administered within 24 hours before or after transplantation

Rejection treatment: Children and Adults: I.V. 10-15 mg/kg/day for 14 days, then give every other day for 7 more doses
Dosage Forms Injection: 50 mg/mL (5 mL)

Lyphocin® Injection *see* vancomycin hydrochloride *on page 490*

lypressin (lye press' in)
Brand Names Diapid® Nasal Spray
Synonyms 8-L-lysine vasopressin
Therapeutic Category Antidiuretic Hormone Analog
Use Control or prevent signs and complications of neurogenic diabetes insipidus
Usual Dosage Children and Adults: 1-2 sprays into one or both nostrils 4 times/day; approximately 2 USP posterior pituitary pressor units per spray
Dosage Forms Spray, nasal: 0.185 mg/mL (8 mL)

Lysodren® *see* mitotane *on page 315*

Maalox® [OTC] *see* aluminum hydroxide and magnesium hydroxide *on page 16*

Maalox® Plus [OTC] *see aluminum hydroxide, magnesium hydroxide, and simethicone on page 16*

Maalox® Therapeutic Concentrate [OTC] *see aluminum hydroxide and magnesium hydroxide on page 16*

Macrobid® *see nitrofurantoin on page 335*

Macrodantin® *see nitrofurantoin on page 335*

Macrodex® *see dextran on page 135*

mafenide acetate (ma' fe nide)
Brand Names Sulfamylon® Topical
Therapeutic Category Antibacterial, Topical; Antibiotic, Topical
Use Adjunct in the treatment of second and third degree burns to prevent septicemia caused by susceptible organisms
Usual Dosage Children and Adults: Topical: Apply once or twice daily with a sterile gloved hand; apply to a thickness of approximately 16 mm; the burned area should be covered with cream at all times
Dosage Forms Cream, topical: 85 mg/g (60 g, 120 g, 435 g)

magaldrate (mag' al drate)
Brand Names Riopan® [OTC]
Synonyms hydromagnesium aluminate
Therapeutic Category Antacid
Use Symptomatic relief of hyperacidity associated with peptic ulcer, gastritis, peptic esophagitis and hiatal hernia
Usual Dosage Adults: Oral: 540-1080 mg between meals and at bedtime
Dosage Forms Suspension, oral: 540 mg/5 mL (360 mL)

magaldrate and simethicone
Brand Names Riopan Plus® [OTC]
Synonyms simethicone and magaldrate
Therapeutic Category Antacid; Antiflatulent
Use Relief of hyperacidity associated with peptic ulcer, gastritis, peptic esophagitis and hiatal hernia which are accompanied by symptoms of gas
Usual Dosage Adults: Oral: 5-10 mL between meals and at bedtime
Dosage Forms Suspension, oral: Magaldrate 480 mg and simethicone 20 mg per 5 mL (360 mL)

magnesia magma *see magnesium hydroxide on next page*

magnesium chloride
Brand Names Slow-Mag® [OTC]
Therapeutic Category Magnesium Salt
Use Correct or prevent hypomagnesemia
Usual Dosage I.V. in TPN:
Children: 2-10 mEq/day; the usual recommended pediatric maintenance intake of magnesium ranges from 0.2-0.6 mEq/kg/day. The dose of magnesium may also be based on the caloric intake; on that basis, 3-10 mEq/day of magnesium are needed; maximum maintenance dose: 8-16 mEq/day

Adults: 8-24 mEq/day
Dosage Forms
Injection: 200 mg/mL [1.97 mEq/mL] (30 mL, 50 mL)
Tablet: Elemental magnesium 64 mg

magnesium citrate
Brand Names Citro-Nesia™ [OTC]; Evac-Q-Mag® [OTC]
Synonyms citrate of magnesia
Therapeutic Category Laxative, Saline
Use To evacuate bowel prior to certain surgical and diagnostic procedures
Usual Dosage Cathartic: Oral:
Children:
<6 years: 2-4 mL/kg given as a single daily dose or in divided doses
6-12 years: $\frac{1}{3}$ to $\frac{1}{2}$ bottle

Adults ≥12 years: $\frac{1}{2}$ to 1 full bottle
Dosage Forms Solution, oral: 300 mL

magnesium gluconate
Brand Names Magonate® [OTC]
Therapeutic Category Magnesium Salt
Use Dietary supplement for treatment of magnesium deficiencies
Usual Dosage The recommended dietary allowance (RDA) of magnesium is 4.5 mg/kg which is a total daily allowance of 350-400 mg for adult men and 280-300 mg for adult women. During pregnancy the RDA is 300 mg and during lactation the RDA is 355 mg. Average daily intakes of dietary magnesium have declined in recent years due to processing of food. The latest estimate of the average American dietary intake was 349 mg/day.

Dietary supplement: Oral:
Children: 3-6 mg/kg/day in divided doses 3-4 times/day; maximum: 400 mg/day
Adults: 27-54 mg 2-3 times/day or 100 mg 4 times/day
Dosage Forms Tablet: 500 mg [elemental magnesium 27 mg]

magnesium hydroxide
Brand Names Phillips'® Milk of Magnesia [OTC]
Synonyms magnesia magma; milk of magnesia; MOM
Therapeutic Category Antacid; Laxative, Saline; Magnesium Salt
Use Short-term treatment of occasional constipation and symptoms of hyperacidity
Usual Dosage Oral:
Laxative:
<2 years: 0.5 mL/kg/dose
2-5 years: 5-15 mL/day or in divided doses
6-12 years: 15-30 mL/day or in divided doses
≥12 years: 30-60 mL/day or in divided doses

Antacid:
Children: 2.5-5 mL as needed
Adults: 5-15 mL as needed
Dosage Forms
Liquid: 390 mg/5 mL (10 mL, 15 mL, 20 mL, 30 mL, 100 mL, 120 mL, 180 mL, 360 mL, 720 mL)
Liquid, concentrate: 10 mL equivalent to 30 mL milk of magnesia USP
Suspension, oral: 2.5 g/30 mL (10 mL, 15 mL, 30 mL)
Tablet: 300 mg, 600 mg

magnesium hydroxide and aluminum hydroxide *see* aluminum hydroxide and magnesium hydroxide *on page 16*

magnesium hydroxide and mineral oil emulsion
Brand Names Haley's M-O® [OTC]
Synonyms mom/mineral oil emulsion
Therapeutic Category Laxative, Lubricant; Laxative, Saline
Use Short-term treatment of occasional constipation
Usual Dosage Oral: Adults: 5-45 mL at bedtime with a glass of water

Dosage Forms Suspension, oral: Equivalent to magnesium hydroxide 24 mL/mineral oil emulsion 6 mL (30 mL unit dose)

magnesium oxide
Brand Names Maox®
Therapeutic Category Antacid
Use Short-term treatment of occasional constipation and symptoms of hyperacidity
Usual Dosage Oral:
Antacid: 250 mg to 1.5 g with water or milk 4 times/day after meals and at bedtime

Laxative: 2-4 g at bedtime with full glass of water
Dosage Forms
Capsule: 140 mg
Tablet: 400 mg, 425 mg

magnesium sulfate
Synonyms epsom salts
Therapeutic Category Anticonvulsant, Miscellaneous; Electrolyte Supplement, Parenteral; Laxative, Saline; Magnesium Salt
Use Treatment and prevention of hypomagnesemia and in seizure prevention in severe pre-eclampsia or eclampsia, pediatric acute nephritis; also used as short-term treatment of constipation
Usual Dosage The recommended dietary allowance (RDA) of magnesium is 4.5 mg/kg which is a total daily allowance of 350-400 mg for adult men and 280-300 mg for adult women. During pregnancy the RDA is 300 mg and during lactation the RDA is 355 mg. Average daily intakes of dietary magnesium have declined in recent years due to processing of food. The latest estimate of the average American dietary intake was 349 mg/day. Dose represented as $MgSO_4$ unless stated otherwise.

Note: Serum magnesium is poor reflection of repletional status as the majority of magnesium is intracellular; serum levels may be transiently normal for a few hours after a dose is given, therefore, aim for consistently high normal serum levels in patients with normal renal function for most efficient repletion
Hypomagnesemia:
Neonates: I.V.: 25-50 mg/kg/dose (0.2-0.4 mEq/kg/dose) every 8-12 hours for 2-3 doses
Children: I.M., I.V.: 25-50 mg/kg/dose (0.2-0.4 mEq/kg/dose) every 4-6 hours for 3-4 doses, maximum single dose: 2000 mg (16 mEq), may repeat if hypomagnesemia persists (higher dosage up to 100 mg/kg/dose $MgSO_4$ I.V. has been used); maintenance: I.V.: 30-60 mg/kg/day (0.25-0.5 mEq/kg/day)
Management of seizures and hypertension:
Children:
Oral: 100-200 mg/kg/dose 4 times/day
I.M., I.V.: 20-100 mg/kg/dose every 4-6 hours as needed; in severe cases doses as high as 200 mg/kg/dose have been used
Adults:
Oral: 3 g every 6 hours for 4 doses as needed
I.M., I.V.: 1 g every 6 hours for 4 doses; for severe hypomagnesemia: 8-12 g $MgSO_4$/day in divided doses has been used
Eclampsia, pre-eclampsia: Adults:
I.M.: 1-4 g every 4 hours
I.V.: Initial: 4 g, then switch to I.M. or 1-4 g/hour by continuous infusion
Maximum dose should not exceed 30-40 g/day; maximum rate of infusion: 1-2 g/hour
Maintenance electrolyte requirements:
Daily requirements: 0.2-0.5 mEq/kg/24 hours or 3-10 mEq/1000 kcal/24 hours
Maximum: 8-16 mEq/24 hours

(Continued)

magnesium sulfate (Continued)

Cathartic: Oral:
  Children: 0.25 g/kg every 4-6 hours
  Adults: 10-15 g in a glass of water

Dosing adjustment/comments in renal impairment: Cl_{cr} <25 mL: Do not administer or monitor serum magnesium levels carefully

Dosage Forms
Granules: ~40 mEq magnesium/5 g (240 g)
Injection: 100 mg/mL (20 mL); 125 mg/mL (8 mL); 250 mg/mL (150 mL); 500 mg/mL (2 mL, 5 mL, 10 mL, 30 mL, 50 mL)
Solution, oral: 50% [500 mg/mL] (30 mL)

Magnevist® *see* radiological/contrast media (ionic) *on page 413*

Magonate® [OTC] *see* magnesium gluconate *on page 282*

Maigret-50 *see* phenylpropanolamine hydrochloride *on page 373*

Malatal® *see* hyoscyamine, atropine, scopolamine, and phenobarbital *on page 242*

malathion (mal a thye' on)

Brand Names Ovide™ Topical
Therapeutic Category Pediculocide
Use Treatment of head lice and their ova
Usual Dosage Sprinkle Ovide™ lotion on dry hair and rub gently until the scalp is thoroughly moistened; pay special attention to the back of the head and neck. Allow to dry naturally – use no heat and leave uncovered. After 8-12 hours, the hair should be washed with a nonmedicated shampoo; rinse and use a fine-toothed comb to remove dead lice and eggs. If required, repeat with second application in 7-9 days. Further treatment is generally not necessary. Other family members should be evaluated to determine if infested and if so, receive treatment.
Dosage Forms Lotion: 0.5% (59 mL)

Mallamint® [OTC] *see* calcium carbonate *on page 65*

Mallazine® Eye Drops [OTC] *see* tetrahydrozoline hydrochloride *on page 459*

Mallergan-VC® With Codeine *see* promethazine, phenylephrine, and codeine *on page 399*

Malotuss® [OTC] *see* guaifenesin *on page 217*

malt soup extract

Brand Names Maltsupex® [OTC]
Therapeutic Category Laxative, Bulk-Producing
Use Short-term treatment of constipation
Usual Dosage Oral:
Infants >1 month:
  Breast fed: 1-2 teaspoonfuls in 2-4 oz of water or fruit juice 1-2 times/day
  Bottle fed: $\frac{1}{2}$ to 2 tablespoonfuls/day in formula for 3-4 days, then 1-2 teaspoonfuls/day
Children 2-11 years: 1-2 tablespoonfuls 1-2 times/day
Adults ≥12 years: 2 tablespoonfuls twice daily for 3-4 days, then 1-2 tablespoonfuls every evening
Dosage Forms
Liquid: Nondiastatic barley malt extract 16 g/15 mL
Powder: Nondiastatic barley malt extract 16 g/heaping tablespoonful
Tablet: Nondiastatic barley malt extract 750 mg

Maltsupex® [OTC] *see* malt soup extract *on this page*

Mandelamine® *see* methenamine *on page 299*

Mandol® *see* cefamandole nafate *on page 78*

mandrake *see* podophyllum resin *on page 382*

manganese injection *see* trace metals *on page 472*

mannitol (man' i tole)
Brand Names Osmitrol® Injection; Resectisol® Irrigation Solution
Synonyms D-mannitol
Therapeutic Category Diuretic, Osmotic
Use Reduction of increased intracranial pressure associated with cerebral edema; promotion of diuresis in the prevention and/or treatment of oliguria or anuria due to acute renal failure; reduction of increased intraocular pressure; promoting urinary excretion of toxic substances
Usual Dosage
Children:
Test dose (to assess adequate renal function): 200 mg/kg over 3-5 minutes to produce a urine flow of at least 1 mL/kg/hour for 1-3 hours
Initial: 0.5-1 g/kg
Maintenance: 0.25-0.5 g/kg/hour given every 4-6 hours

Adults:
Test dose: 12.5 g (200 mg/kg) over 3-5 minutes to produce a urine flow of at least 30-50 mL of urine per hour over the next 2-3 hours
Initial: 0.5-1 g/kg
Maintenance: 0.25-0.5 g/kg every 4-6 hours
Dosage Forms
Injection: 5% [50 mg/mL] (1000 mL); 10% [100 mg/mL] (500 mL, 1000 mL); 15% [150 mg/mL] (150 mL, 500 mL); 20% [200 mg/mL] (150 mL, 250 mL, 500 mL); 25% [250 mg/mL] (50 mL, 500 mL)
Solution, urogenital: 0.54% [5.4 mg/mL] (2000 mL)

Manoplax® *see* flosequinan *on page 197*

Mantoux *see* tuberculin tests *on page 484*

Maolate® *see* chlorphenesin carbamate *on page 93*

Maox® *see* magnesium oxide *on page 283*

maprotiline hydrochloride (ma proe' ti leen)
Brand Names Ludiomil®
Therapeutic Category Antidepressant, Tetracyclic
Use Treatment of depression and anxiety associated with depression
Usual Dosage Oral:
Children 6-14 years: 10 mg/day, increase to a maximum daily dose of 75 mg
Adults: 75 mg/day to start, increase by 25 mg every 2 weeks up to 150-225 mg/day; given in 3 divided doses or in a single daily dose
Dosage Forms Tablet: 25 mg, 50 mg, 75 mg

Marax® *see* theophylline, ephedrine, and hydroxyzine *on page 462*

Marazide® *see* benzthiazide *on page 50*

Marbaxin® *see* methocarbamol *on page 300*

Marcaine® *see* bupivacaine hydrochloride *on page 61*

Marcillin® *see* ampicillin *on page 26*

Marezine® [OTC] *see* cyclizine *on page 120*

Margesic® H *see* hydrocodone and acetaminophen *on page 234*

Margesic® No. 3 *see* acetaminophen and codeine *on page 3*
Marinol® *see* dronabinol *on page 162*
Marmine® Injection *see* dimenhydrinate *on page 150*
Marmine® Oral [OTC] *see* dimenhydrinate *on page 150*
Marnal® *see* butalbital compound *on page 63*
Marplan® *see* isocarboxazid *on page 256*
Marpres® *see* hydralazine, hydrochlorothiazide, and reserpine *on page 232*
Marthritic® *see* salsalate *on page 425*

masoprocol (may so pro' kol)
  Brand Names Actinex® Topical
  Therapeutic Category Topical Skin Product; Topical Skin Product, Acne
  Use Treatment of actinic keratosis
  Usual Dosage Apply twice daily
  Dosage Forms Cream: 10% (30 g)

Massé® Breast Cream [OTC] *see* glycerin, lanolin and peanut oil *on page 214*
Matulane® *see* procarbazine hydrochloride *on page 396*
Maxair™ Inhalation Aerosol *see* pirbuterol acetate *on page 379*
Maxaquin® Oral *see* lomefloxacin hydrochloride *on page 277*
Max-Caro® [OTC] *see* beta-carotene *on page 52*
Maxidex® Ophthalmic *see* dexamethasone *on page 132*
Maxiflor® Topical *see* diflorasone diacetate *on page 146*
Maximum Strength Nytol® [OTC] *see* diphenhydramine hydrochloride
  on page 152
Maxitrol® Ophthalmic *see* neomycin, polymyxin b, and dexamethasone
  on page 328
Maxivate® Topical *see* betamethasone *on page 52*
Maxolon® *see* metoclopramide *on page 308*
Maxzide® *see* hydrochlorothiazide and triamterene *on page 234*
may apple *see* podophyllum resin *on page 382*
MCH *see* microfibrillar collagen hemostat *on page 312*

m-cresyl acetate
  Brand Names Cresylate®
  Therapeutic Category Otic Agent, Anti-infective
  Use Provides an acid medium; for external otitis infections caused by susceptible bacteria
  or fungus
  Usual Dosage Otic: Instill 2-4 drops as required
  Dosage Forms Solution: 25% with isopropanol 25%, chlorobutanol 1%, benzyl alcohol 1%,
  and castor oil 5% in propylene glycol (15 mL dropper bottle)

MCT Oil® [OTC] *see* medium chain triglycerides *on page 289*
MD-Gastroview® *see* radiological/contrast media (ionic) *on page 413*

measles and rubella vaccines, combined
  Brand Names M-R-VAX® II
  Synonyms rubella and measles vaccines, combined
  Therapeutic Category Vaccine, Live Virus

Use Simultaneous immunization against measles and rubella
Usual Dosage S.C.: Inject into outer aspect of upper arm
Dosage Forms Injection: 1000 TCID$_{50}$ each of live attenuated measles virus vaccine and live rubella virus vaccine

measles, mumps and rubella vaccines, combined
Brand Names M-M-R® II
Synonyms MMR; mumps, measles and rubella vaccines, combined; rubella, measles and mumps vaccines, combined
Therapeutic Category Vaccine, Live Virus
Use Measles, mumps, and rubella prophylaxis
Usual Dosage S.C.: Inject in outer aspect of the upper arm to children ≥15 months of age; each dose contains 1000 TCID$_{50}$ (tissue culture infectious doses) of 5 attenuated measle virus vaccine, 5000 TCID$_{50}$ of live mumps virus vaccine and 1000 TCID$_{50}$ of live rubella virus vaccine
Dosage Forms Injection: 1000 TCID$_{50}$ each of measles virus vaccine and rubella virus vaccine, 5000 TCID$_{50}$ mumps virus vaccine

measles virus vaccine, live, attenuated
Brand Names Attenuvax®
Synonyms more attenuated enders strain; rubeola vaccine
Therapeutic Category Vaccine, Live Virus
Use Immunization against measles (rubeola) in persons ≥15 months of age
Usual Dosage Children >15 months and Adults: S.C.: 0.5 mL in outer aspect of the upper arm
Dosage Forms Injection: 1000 TCID$_{50}$/dose

Measurin® [OTC] *see* aspirin *on page 34*
Mebaral® *see* mephobarbital *on page 293*

mebendazole (me ben' da zole)
Brand Names Vermox®
Therapeutic Category Anthelmintic
Use Treatment of pinworms, whipworms, roundworms, and hookworms
Usual Dosage Children and Adults: Oral:
Pinworms: Single chewable tablet; may need to repeat after 2 weeks

Whipworms, roundworms, hookworms: 1 tablet twice daily, morning and evening on 3 consecutive days; if patient is not cured within 3-4 weeks, a second course of treatment may be administered
Dosage Forms Tablet, chewable: 100 mg

mecamylamine hydrochloride (mek a mill' a meen)
Brand Names Inversine®
Therapeutic Category Ganglionic Blocking Agent
Use Treatment of moderately severe to severe hypertension and in uncomplicated malignant hypertension
Usual Dosage Adults: Oral: 2.5 mg twice daily after meals for 2 days; increased by increments of 2.5 mg at intervals of ≥2 days until desired blood pressure response is achieved
Dosage Forms Tablet: 2.5 mg

mechlorethamine hydrochloride (me klor eth' a meen)
Brand Names Mustargen® Hydrochloride
Synonyms HN$_2$; mustine; nitrogen mustard
Therapeutic Category Antineoplastic Agent, Alkylating Agent (Nitrogen Mustard)
(Continued)

287

mechlorethamine hydrochloride (Continued)

Use Combination therapy of Hodgkin's disease, brain tumors, non-Hodgkin's lymphoma and malignant lymphomas; palliative treatment of bronchogenic, breast and ovarian carcinoma; may be used by intracavitary injection for treatment of metastatic tumors, pleural and other malignant effusions

Usual Dosage Refer to individual protocols

Children: MOPP: I.V.: 6 mg/m^2 on days 1 and 8 of a 28-day cycle

Adults:

I.V.: 0.4 mg/kg or 12-16 mg/m^2 for one dose or divided into 0.1 mg/kg/day for 4 days
Intracavitary: 10-20 mg or 0.2-0.4 mg/kg

Dosage Forms Powder for injection: 10 mg

Meclan® Topical see meclocycline sulfosalicylate on this page

meclizine hydrochloride (mek' li zeen)

Brand Names Antivert®; Antrizine®; Bonine® [OTC]; Dizmiss® [OTC]; Dramamine® II [OTC]; Meni-D®; Ru-Vert-M®; Vergon® [OTC]

Synonyms meclozine hydrochloride

Therapeutic Category Antiemetic; Antihistamine

Use Prevention and treatment of motion sickness; management of vertigo with diseases affecting the vestibular system

Usual Dosage Children >12 years and Adults: Oral:

Motion sickness: 25-50 mg 1 hour before travel, repeat dose every 24 hours if needed

Vertigo: 25-100 mg/day in divided doses

Dosage Forms

Capsule: 15 mg, 25 mg, 30 mg
Tablet: 12.5 mg, 25 mg, 50 mg
Tablet:
    Chewable: 25 mg
    Film coated: 25 mg

meclocycline sulfosalicylate (me kloe sye' kleen)

Brand Names Meclan® Topical

Therapeutic Category Antibiotic, Topical; Topical Skin Product, Acne

Use Topical treatment of inflammatory acne vulgaris

Usual Dosage Apply to affected areas twice daily

Dosage Forms Cream, topical: 1% (20 g, 45 g)

meclofenamate sodium (me kloe fen am' ate)

Brand Names Meclomen® Oral

Therapeutic Category Analgesic, Non-Narcotic; Anti-inflammatory Agent; Nonsteroidal Anti-Inflammatory Agent (NSAID), Oral

Use Treatment of inflammatory disorders

Usual Dosage Adults: Oral: 200-300 mg 3-4 times/day

Dosage Forms Capsule: 50 mg, 100 mg

Meclomen® Oral see meclofenamate sodium on this page

meclozine hydrochloride see meclizine hydrochloride on this page

medicinal carbon see charcoal on page 86

medicinal charcoal see charcoal on page 86

Medigesic® see butalbital compound on page 63

Medihaler-Epi® Inhalation Aerosol [OTC] see epinephrine on page 171

Medihaler Ergotamine™ see ergotamine derivatives on page 174

Medihaler-Iso® Inhalation Aerosol *see* isoproterenol *on page 258*

Medilax® [OTC] *see* phenolphthalein *on page 370*

Mediplast® Plaster [OTC] *see* salicylic acid *on page 424*

Medipren® [OTC] *see* ibuprofen *on page 245*

Medi-Quick® Topical Ointment [OTC] *see* bacitracin, neomycin, and polymyxin b *on page 43*

Medi-Tuss® [OTC] *see* guaifenesin *on page 217*

Medi-Tuss® AC *see* guaifenesin and codeine *on page 218*

medium chain triglycerides
Brand Names MCT Oil® [OTC]
Synonyms triglycerides, medium chain
Therapeutic Category Nutritional Supplement
Use Dietary supplement for those who cannot digest long chain fats
Usual Dosage Oral: 15 mL 3-4 times/day
Dosage Forms Oil: 14 g/15 mL (960 mL)

Medralone® Injection *see* methylprednisolone *on page 306*

Medrol® Acetate Topical *see* methylprednisolone *on page 306*

Medrol® Oral *see* methylprednisolone *on page 306*

medroxyprogesterone acetate (me drox' ee proe jess' te rone)
Brand Names Amen® Oral; Curretab® Oral; Cycrin® Oral; Depo-Provera® Injection; Provera® Oral
Synonyms acetoxymethylprogesterone; methylacetoxyprogesterone
Therapeutic Category Contraceptive, Progestin Only; Progestin
Use Endometrial carcinoma or renal carcinoma as well as secondary amenorrhea or abnormal uterine bleeding due to hormonal imbalance; prevention of pregnancy
Usual Dosage
Adolescents and Adults: Oral:
Amenorrhea: 5-10 mg/day for 5-10 days or 2.5 mg/day
Abnormal uterine bleeding: 5-10 mg for 5-10 days starting on day 16 or 21 of cycle
Accompanying cyclic estrogen therapy, postmenopausal: 2.5-10 mg the last 10-13 days of estrogen dosing each month

Adults:
Contraception: Deep I.M.: 150 mg every 3 months or 450 mg every 6 months
Endometrial or renal carcinoma: I.M.: 400-1000 mg/week

Dosing adjustment in hepatic impairment: Dose needs to be lowered in patients with alcoholic cirrhosis
Dosage Forms
Injection, suspension: 100 mg/mL (5 mL); 150 mg/mL (1 mL); 400 mg/mL (1 mL, 2.5 mL, 10 mL)
Tablet: 2.5 mg, 5 mg, 10 mg

medrysone (me' dri sone)
Brand Names HMS Liquifilm® Ophthalmic
Therapeutic Category Anti-inflammatory Agent, Ophthalmic; Corticosteroid, Ophthalmic
Use Treatment of allergic conjunctivitis, vernal conjunctivitis, episcleritis, ophthalmic epinephrine sensitivity reaction
Usual Dosage Children and Adults: Ophthalmic: 1 drop in conjunctival sac 2-4 times/day up to every 4 hours; may use every 1-2 hours during first 1-2 days
Dosage Forms Solution, ophthalmic: 1% (5 mL)

mefenamic acid (me fe nam' ik)
Brand Names Ponstel®
Therapeutic Category Analgesic, Non-Narcotic; Nonsteroidal Anti-Inflammatory Agent (NSAID), Oral
Use Short-term relief of mild to moderate pain including primary dysmenorrhea
Usual Dosage Children >14 years and Adults: Oral: 500 mg to start then 250 mg every 4 hours as needed; maximum therapy: 1 week
Dosage Forms Capsule: 250 mg

mefloquine hydrochloride (me' floe kwin)
Brand Names Lariam®
Therapeutic Category Antimalarial Agent
Use Treatment of acute malarial infections and prevention of malaria
Usual Dosage Adults: Oral:
Mild to moderate malaria infection: 5 tablets (1250 mg) as a single dose with at least 8 oz of water

Malaria prophylaxis: 1 tablet (250 mg) once weekly for 4 weeks, then 1 tablet every other week; start treatment 1 week prior to departure to an endemic area; to avoid development of malaria after return from an endemic area, continue prophylaxis for 4 additional weeks; for prolonged stays in an endemic area this prophylaxis be achieved by continuing the recommended dosage schedule, once weekly for 4 weeks, then once every other week, until traveler has taken 3 doses following return to a malaria-free area
Dosage Forms Tablet: 250 mg

Mefoxin® *see* cefoxitin sodium *on page 81*

Mega-B® [OTC] *see* vitamin B complex *on page 498*

Megace® *see* megestrol acetate *on this page*

Megaton™ [OTC] *see* vitamin B complex *on page 498*

megestrol acetate (me jess' trole)
Brand Names Megace®
Therapeutic Category Antineoplastic Agent, Hormone; Progestin
Use Palliative treatment of breast and endometrial carcinomas, appetite stimulation and promotion of weight gain in cachexia
Usual Dosage Refer to individual protocols
Adults: Oral:
Breast carcinoma: 40 mg 4 times/day
Endometrial: 40-320 mg/day in divided doses
Dosage Forms Tablet: 20 mg, 40 mg

Melanex® Topical *see* hydroquinone *on page 239*

Mellaril® *see* thioridazine *on page 465*

Mellaril-S® *see* thioridazine *on page 465*

melphalan (mel' fa lan)
Brand Names Alkeran®
Synonyms L-PAM; L-sarcolysin; phenylalanine mustard
Therapeutic Category Antineoplastic Agent, Alkylating Agent (Nitrogen Mustard)
Use Palliative treatment of multiple myeloma and nonresectable epithelial ovarian carcinoma; neuroblastoma, rhabdomyosarcoma
Usual Dosage Refer to individual protocols
Children: I.V. (Investigational, distributed under the auspices of the NCI for authorized studies):

Pediatric rhabdomyosarcoma: 10-35 mg/m^2 bolus every 21-28 days
Chemoradiotherapy supported by marrow infusions for neuroblastoma: 70-140 mg/m^2 on day 7 and 6 before BMT

Adults: Oral:
Multiple myeloma: 6 mg/day or 10 mg/day for 7-10 days, or 0.15 mg/kg/day for 7 days
Ovarian carcinoma: 0.2 mg/kg/day for 5 days, repeat in 4-5 weeks
Dosage Forms
Powder for injection: 50 mg
Tablet: 2 mg

menadiol sodium diphosphate (men a dye' ole)
Brand Names Synkayvite®
Synonyms vitamin K$_4$
Therapeutic Category Vitamin, Water Soluble
Use Prevention and treatment of hypoprothrombinemia caused by vitamin K deficiency secondary to oral anti-infective therapy and salicylates, inadequate absorption and synthesis of vitamin K due to lack of bile salts, eg, cystic fibrosis, obstructive jaundice, biliary fistula
Usual Dosage
Hypoprothrombinemia (vitamin K deficiency, liver disease or malabsorption): Oral, I.M., I.V., S.C.:
Term infants >1 month: 2.5-5 mg/dose; repeat every 12-24 hours as needed
Children: 5-10 mg/dose; repeat every 12-24 hours as needed
Adults: 5-15 mg/dose 1-2 times/day

Minimum daily requirement not well established
Infants: 1-5 μg/kg/day
Adults: 0.03 μg/kg/day
Dosage Forms
Injection: 5 mg/mL (1 mL); 10 mg/mL (1 mL); 37.5 mg/mL (2 mL)
Tablet: 5 mg

Menadol® [OTC] see ibuprofen on page 245

Menest® see estrogens, esterified on page 179

Meni-D® see meclizine hydrochloride on page 288

meningococcal polysaccharide vaccine, groups A, C, Y and W-135
Brand Names Menomune®-A/C/Y/W-135
Therapeutic Category Vaccine, Live Bacteria
Use Immunization against infection caused by Neisseria meningitidis groups A,C,Y, and W-135 in persons ≥2 years
Usual Dosage Do not inject intradermally or I.V.; inject S.C. only. The immunizing dose is one S.C. injection of 0.5 mL.
Dosage Forms Injection: 10 dose, 50 dose

Menomune®-A/C/Y/W-135 see meningococcal polysaccharide vaccine, groups A, C, Y and W-135 on this page

menotropins (men oh troe' pins)
Brand Names Pergonal®
Therapeutic Category Gonadotropin; Ovulation Stimulator
Use Used sequentially with hCG to induce ovulation and pregnancy in the infertile woman with functional anovulation; used with hCG in men to stimulate spermatogenesis in those with primary hypogonadotropic hypogonadism
(Continued)

menotropins *(Continued)*

Usual Dosage I.M.:

Male: Following pretreatment with hCG, 1 ampul 3 times/week and hCG 2000 units twice weekly until sperm is detected in the ejaculate (4-6 months) then may be increased to 2 ampuls of menotropins 3 times/week

Female: 1 ampul/day (75 units of FSH and LH) for 9-12 days followed by 10,000 units hCG 1 day after the last dose; repeated at least twice at same level before increasing dosage to 2 ampuls

Dosage Forms Injection: Follicle stimulating hormone activity 75 units and luteinizing hormone activity 75 units per 2 mL ampul; follicle stimulating hormone activity 150 units and luteinizing hormone activity 150 units per 2 mL ampul

mepacrine hydrochloride *see* quinacrine hydrochloride *on page 410*

mepenzolate bromide (me pen' zoe late)

Brand Names Cantil®
Therapeutic Category Anticholinergic Agent; Antispasmodic Agent, Gastrointestinal
Use Management of peptic ulcer disease; inhibit salivation and excessive secretions in respiratory tract preoperatively
Usual Dosage Adults: Oral: 25-50 mg 4 times/day with meal and at bedtime
Dosage Forms Tablet, with tartrazine: 25 mg

meperidine hydrochloride (me per' i deen)

Brand Names Demerol® Injection; Demerol® Oral
Synonyms isonipecaine hydrochloride; pethidine hydrochloride
Therapeutic Category Analgesic, Narcotic
Use Management of moderate to severe pain; adjunct to anesthesia and preoperative sedation
Usual Dosage Doses should be titrated to appropriate analgesic effect; when changing route of administration, note that oral doses are about half as effective as parenteral dose

Children: Oral, I.M., I.V., S.C.: 1-1.5 mg/kg/dose every 3-4 hours as needed; 1-2 mg/kg as a single dose preoperative medication may be used; maximum 100 mg/dose

Adults: Oral, I.M., I.V.: S.C.: 50-150 mg/dose every 3-4 hours as needed
Dosage Forms
Injection:
Single-dose: 10 mg/mL (5 mL, 10 mL, 30 mL); 25 mg/dose (0.5 mL, 1 mL); 50 mg/dose (1 mL); 75 mg/dose (1 mL, 1.5 mL); 100 mg/dose (1 mL)
Multiple-dose vials: 50 mg/mL (30 mL); 100 mg/mL (20 mL)
Syrup: 50 mg/5 mL (500 mL)
Tablet: 50 mg, 100 mg

mephentermine sulfate (me fen' ter meen)

Brand Names Wyamine® Sulfate Injection
Therapeutic Category Adrenergic Agonist Agent; Sympathomimetic
Use Treatment of hypotension secondary to ganglionic blockade or spinal anesthesia; may be used as an emergency measure to maintain blood pressure until whole blood replacement becomes available
Usual Dosage
Hypotension: I.M., I.V.:
Children: 0.4 mg/kg
Adults: 0.5 mg/kg

Hypotensive emergency: I.V. infusion: 20-60 mg
Dosage Forms Injection: 15 mg/mL (2 mL, 10 mL); 30 mg/mL (10 mL)

mephenytoin (me fen' i toyn)
Brand Names Mesantoin®
Synonyms methoin; methylphenylethylhydantoin; phenantoin
Therapeutic Category Anticonvulsant, Hydantoin
Use Used for the management of tonic-clonic seizures, partial seizures, partial seizures with motor symptoms, and partial seizures with complex symptomatology in patients refractory to less toxic anticonvulsants
Usual Dosage Oral:
Children: 3-15 mg/kg/day in 3 divided doses; usual maintenance dose: 100-400 mg/day in 3 divided doses

Adults: Initial dose: 50-100 mg/day given daily; increase by 50-100 mg at weekly intervals; usual maintenance dose: 200-600 mg/day in 3 divided doses; maximum: 800 mg/day
Dosage Forms Tablet: 100 mg

mephobarbital (me foe bar' bi tal)
Brand Names Mebaral®
Synonyms methylphenobarbital
Therapeutic Category Anticonvulsant, Barbiturate
Use Prophylactic management of tonic-clonic (grand mal) seizures and absence (petit mal) seizures
Usual Dosage Epilepsy: Oral:
Children: 4-10 mg/kg/day in 2-4 divided doses
Adults: 200-600 mg/day in 2-4 divided doses
Dosage Forms Tablet: 32 mg, 50 mg, 100 mg

Mephyton® Oral see phytonadione *on page 376*

mepivacaine hydrochloride (me piv' a kane)
Brand Names Carbocaine® Injection; Isocaine® HCl Injection; Polocaine® Injection
Therapeutic Category Local Anesthetic, Injectable
Use Local anesthesia by nerve block; infiltration in dental procedures
Usual Dosage
Injectable local anesthetic: Varies with procedure, degree of anesthesia needed, vascularity of tissue, duration of anesthesia required, and physical condition of patient
Topical: Apply to affected area as needed
Dosage Forms Injection: 1% [10 mg/mL] (30 mL, 50 mL); 1.5% [15 mg/mL] (30 mL); 2% [20 mg/mL] (20 mL, 50 mL); 3% [30 mg/mL] (1.8 mL)

meprobamate (me proe ba' mate)
Brand Names Equanil®; Meprospan®; Miltown®; Neuramate®
Therapeutic Category Antianxiety Agent
Use Management of anxiety disorders
Usual Dosage Oral:
Children 6-12 years:
100-200 mg 2-3 times/day
Sustained release: 200 mg twice daily

Adults:
400 mg 3-4 times/day, up to 2400 mg/day
Sustained release; 400-800 mg twice daily
Dosage Forms
Capsule, sustained release: 200 mg, 400 mg
Tablet: 200 mg, 400 mg, 600 mg

meprobamate and aspirin see aspirin and meprobamate *on page 35*

Mepron® *see* atovaquone *on page 37*

Meprospan® *see* meprobamate *on previous page*

merbromin (meer bro' min)
Brand Names Mercurochrome®
Therapeutic Category Topical Skin Product
Use Topical antiseptic
Usual Dosage Topical: Apply freely, until injury has healed
Dosage Forms Solution, topical: 2%

mercaptopurine (mer kap toe pyoor' een)
Brand Names Purinethol®
Synonyms 6-mercaptopurine; 6-MP
Therapeutic Category Antineoplastic Agent, Antimetabolite; Antineoplastic Agent, Purine
Use Treatment of leukemias
Usual Dosage Refer to individual protocols
Oral:
Induction: 2.5 mg/kg/day for several weeks or more; if, after 4 weeks there is no improvement and no myelosuppression, increase dosage up to 5 mg/kg/day
Maintenance: 1.5-2.5 mg/kg/day
Dosage Forms Tablet: 50 mg

6-mercaptopurine *see* mercaptopurine *on this page*

mercuric oxide
Synonyms yellow mercuric oxide
Therapeutic Category Antibiotic, Ophthalmic
Use Treatment of irritation and minor infections of the eyelids
Usual Dosage Ophthalmic: Apply small amount to inner surface of lower eyelid once or twice daily
Dosage Forms Ointment, ophthalmic: 1%, 2% [OTC]

Mercurochrome® *see* merbromin *on this page*

Merlenate® Topical [OTC] *see* undecylenic acid and derivatives *on page 486*

Mersol® [OTC] *see* thimerosal *on page 464*

Meruvax® II *see* rubella virus vaccine, live *on page 423*

mesalamine (me sal' a meen)
Brand Names Asacol® Oral; Pentasa® Oral; Rowasa® Rectal
Synonyms 5-aminosalicylic acid; 5-ASA; fisalamine; mesalazine
Therapeutic Category 5-Aminosalicylic Acid Derivative; Anti-inflammatory Agent, Rectal
Use Treatment of ulcerative colitis, proctosigmoiditis, and proctitis
Usual Dosage Adults (usual course of therapy is 3-6 weeks): Oral: 800 mg 3 times/day
Retention enema: 60 mL (4 g) at bedtime, retained over night, approximately 8 hours
Rectal suppository: Insert 1 suppository in rectum twice daily
Dosage Forms
Capsule, controlled release (Pentasa®): 250 mg
Suppository, rectal (Rowasa®): 500 mg
Suspension, rectal (Rowasa®): 4 g/60 mL (7s)
Tablet, enteric coated (Asacol®): 400 mg

mesalazine *see* mesalamine *on previous page*

Mesantoin® *see* mephenytoin *on page 293*

mesna (mes' na)
Brand Names Mesnex™ Injection
Synonyms sodium 2-mercaptoethane sulfonate
Therapeutic Category Antidote, Cyclophosphamide-induced Hemorrhagic Cystitis; Antidote, Ifosfamide-induced Hemorrhagic Cystitis
Use Detoxifying agent used as a protectant against hemorrhagic cystitis induced by ifosfamide and cyclophosphamide
Usual Dosage Children and Adults (refer to individual protocols):
Ifosfamide: I.V.: 20% W/W of ifosfamide dose at time of administration and 4 and 8 hours after each dose of ifosfamide
Cyclophosphamide: I.V.: 20% W/W of cyclophosphamide dose prior to administration and 3, 6, 9, 12 hours after cyclophosphamide dose (total daily dose = 120% to 180% of cyclophosphamide dose)
Oral dose: 40% W/W of the antineoplastic agent dose in 3 doses at 4-hour intervals
Dosage Forms Injection: 100 mg/mL (2 mL, 4 mL, 10 mL)

Mesnex™ Injection *see* mesna *on this page*

mesoridazine besylate (mez oh rid' a zeen)
Brand Names Serentil®
Therapeutic Category Antipsychotic Agent; Phenothiazine Derivative
Use Symptomatic management of psychotic disorders, including schizophrenia, behavioral problems, alcoholism as well as reducing anxiety and tension occurring in neurosis
Usual Dosage Initial: 25 mg for most patients; may repeat dose in 30-60 minutes, if necessary; the usual optimum dosage range is 25-200 mg/day. Concentrate may be diluted just prior to administration with distilled water, acidified tap water, orange or grape juice; do not prepare and store bulk dilutions.
Dosage Forms
Injection: 25 mg/mL (1 mL)
Liquid, oral: 25 mg/mL (118 mL)
Tablet: 10 mg, 25 mg, 50 mg, 100 mg

Mestinon® Injection *see* pyridostigmine bromide *on page 408*

Mestinon® Oral *see* pyridostigmine bromide *on page 408*

mestranol and norethindrone (mes' tra nole & nor eth in' drone)
Brand Names Norinyl® 1+50; Ortho-Novum™ 1/50
Synonyms norethindrone and mestranol
Therapeutic Category Contraceptive, Low Estrogen/Progestin; Contraceptive, Monophasic; Contraceptive, Oral; Progestin
Use Prevention of pregnancy; treatment of hypermenorrhea, endometriosis, female hypogonadism
Usual Dosage Contraception: Oral: 1 tablet daily, beginning on day 5 of menstrual cycle (first day of menstrual flow is day 1). With 20-tablet and 21-tablet packages, new dosing cycle begins 7 days after last tablet taken; with 28-tablet packages, dosage is 1 tablet daily without interruption; extra tablets are placebos or contain iron. If next menstrual period does not begin on schedule, rule out pregnancy before starting new dosing cycle; if menstrual period begins, start new dosing cycle 7 days after last tablet was taken. If all doses have been taken on schedule and 1 menstrual period is missed, continue dosing cycle; if 2 consecutive menstrual periods are missed, pregnancy test is required before new dosing cycle is started.
Dosage Forms Tablet: Mestranol 0.05 mg and norethindrone 1 mg (21s and 28s)

mestranol and norethynodrel (mes' tra nole & nor e thye' noe drel)
Brand Names Enovid®
Synonyms norethynodrel and mestranol
Therapeutic Category Contraceptive, Oral
Use Prevention of pregnancy; treatment of hypermenorrhea, endometriosis, female hypogonadism
Usual Dosage Adults: Female: Oral:
Endometriosis: 5-10 mg/day for 2 weeks beginning on day 5 of menstrual cycle; increase by 5-10 mg increments at 2-week intervals up to 20 mg/day for 6-9 months

Hypermenorrhea: 20-30 mg/day until bleeding is controlled, then reduce to 10 mg/day and continue through day 24 of cycle; administer 5-10 mg/day from day 5 through day 24 of next 2-3 cycles
Dosage Forms Tablet:
5: Mestranol 0.075 mg and norethynodrel 5 mg
10: Mestranol 0.150 mg and norethynodrel 9.85 mg

metacortandralone *see* prednisolone *on page 391*
Metahydrin® *see* trichlormethiazide *on page 476*
Metamucil® [OTC] *see* psyllium *on page 407*
Metamucil® Instant Mix [OTC] *see* psyllium *on page 407*
Metandren® *see* methyltestosterone *on page 307*
Metaprel® Inhalation Aerosol *see* metaproterenol sulfate *on this page*
Metaprel® Inhalation Solution *see* metaproterenol sulfate *on this page*
Metaprel® Oral *see* metaproterenol sulfate *on this page*

metaproterenol sulfate (met a proe ter' e nol)
Brand Names Alupent® Inhalation Aerosol; Alupent® Inhalation Solution; Alupent® Oral; Arm-a-Med® Metaproterenol Inhalation Solution; Dey-Dose® Metaproterenol Inhalation Solution; Metaprel® Inhalation Aerosol; Metaprel® Inhalation Solution; Metaprel® Oral; Prometa® Oral
Synonyms orciprenaline sulfate
Therapeutic Category Adrenergic Agonist Agent; Beta-2-Adrenergic Agonist Agent; Bronchodilator
Use Bronchodilator in reversible airway obstruction due to asthma or COPD; because of its delayed onset of action (one hour) and prolonged effect (4 or more hours), this may not be the drug of choice for assessing response to a bronchodilator
Usual Dosage
Oral:
Children:
<2 years: 0.4 mg/kg/dose given 3-4 times/day; in infants, the dose can be given every 8-12 hours
2-6 years: 1-2.6 mg/kg/day divided every 6-8 hours
6-9 years: 10 mg/dose given 3-4 times/day
Children >9 years and Adults: 20 mg/dose given 3-4 times/day

Inhalation: Children >12 years and Adults: 2-3 inhalations every 3-4 hours, up to 12 inhalations in 24 hours

Nebulizer:
Infants: 6 mg/dose administered over 5 minutes
Children <12 years: 0.01-0.02 mL/kg of 5% solution; diluted in 2-3 mL normal saline every 4-6 hours (may be given more frequently according to need), maximum dose: 15 mg/dose every 4-6 hours

Adolescents and Adults: 5-20 breaths of full strength 5% metaproterenol **or** 0.2 to 0.3 mL 5% metaproterenol in 2.5-3 mL normal saline nebulized every 4-6 hours (can be given more frequently according to need)

Dosage Forms
Aerosol, oral: 0.65 mg/dose (5 mL, 10 mL)
Solution for inhalation, preservative free: 0.4% [4 mg/mL] (2.5 mL); 0.6% [6 mg/mL] (2.5 mL); 5% [50 mg/mL] (10 mL, 30 mL)
Syrup: 10 mg/5 mL (480 mL)
Tablet: 10 mg, 20 mg

metaraminol bitartrate (met a ram' i nole)
Brand Names Aramine®
Therapeutic Category Adrenergic Agonist Agent
Use Acute hypotensive crisis in the treatment of shock
Usual Dosage Adults:
Prevention of hypotension: I.M., S.C.: 2-10 mg

Adjunctive treatment of hypotension: I.V.: 15-100 mg in 250-500 mL NS or 5% dextrose in water

Severe shock: I.V.: 0.5-5 mg direct I.V. injection then use I.M. dose
Dosage Forms Injection: 10 mg/mL (10 mL)

Metasep® [OTC] *see* parachlorometaxylenol *on page 356*
Metastron® Injection *see* strontium-89 chloride *on page 444*

metaxalone (me tax' a lone)
Brand Names Skelaxin®
Therapeutic Category Skeletal Muscle Relaxant
Use Relief of discomfort associated with acute, painful musculoskeletal conditions
Usual Dosage Children >12 years and Adults: Oral: 800 mg 3-4 times/day
Dosage Forms Tablet: 400 mg

methacholine chloride (meth a kol' leen)
Brand Names Provocholine®
Therapeutic Category Diagnostic Agent, Bronchial Airway Hyperactivity
Use Diagnosis of bronchial airway hyperactivity in subjects who do not have clinically apparent asthma
Usual Dosage Before inhalation challenge, perform baseline pulmonary function tests; the patient must have an FEV_1 of at least 70% of the predicted value. The following is a suggested schedule for administration of methacholine challenge. Calculate cumulative units by multiplying number of breaths by concentration given. Total cumulative units is the sum of cumulative units for each concentration given. See table.

Vial	Serial Concentration (mg/mL)	No. of Breaths	Cumulative Units per Concentration	Total Cumulative Units
E	0.025	5	0.125	0.125
D	0.25	5	1.25	1.375
C	2.5	5	12.5	13.88
B	10	5	50	63.88
A	25	5	125	188.88

(Continued)

methacholine chloride (Continued)

Determine FEV$_1$ within 5 minutes of challenge, a postive challenge is a 20% reduction in FEV$_1$

Dosage Forms Powder for reconstitution, inhalation: 100 mg/5 mL

methadone hydrochloride (meth' a done)

Brand Names Dolophine® Oral
Therapeutic Category Analgesic, Narcotic
Use Management of severe pain, used in narcotic detoxification maintenance programs
Usual Dosage Doses should be titrated to appropriate effects:
Children: Analgesia:
Oral, I.M., S.C.: 0.7 mg/kg/24 hours divided every 4-6 hours as needed or 0.1-0.2 mg/kg every 4-12 hours as needed; maximum: 10 mg/dose
I.V.: 0.1 mg/kg every 4 hours initially for 2-3 doses, then every 6-12 hours as needed; maximum: 10 mg/dose

Adults:
Analgesia: Oral, I.M., I.V., S.C.: 2.5-10 mg every 3-8 hours as needed, up to 5-20 mg every 6-8 hours
Detoxification: Oral: 15-40 mg/day
Maintenance of opiate dependence: Oral: 20-120 mg/day
Dosage Forms
Injection: 10 mg/mL (1 mL, 10 mL, 20 mL)
Solution:
Oral: 5 mg/5 mL (5 mL, 500 mL); 10 mg/5 mL (500 mL)
Oral, concentrate: 10 mg/mL (30 mL)
Tablet: 5 mg, 10 mg
Tablet, dispersible: 40 mg

methaminodiazepoxide hydrochloride see chlordiazepoxide on page 89

methamphetamine hydrochloride (meth am fet' a meen)

Brand Names Desoxyn®
Synonyms desoxyephedrine hydrochloride
Therapeutic Category Amphetamine; Central Nervous System Stimulant, Amphetamine
Use Narcolepsy; exogenous obesity; abnormal behavioral syndrome in children (minimal brain dysfunction)
Usual Dosage
Attention deficit disorder: Children >6 years: 2.5-5 mg 1-2 times/day, may increase by 5 mg increments weekly until optimum response is achieved, usually 20-25 mg/day

Exogenous obesity: Children >12 years and Adults: 5 mg, 30 minutes before each meal, 10-15 mg in morning; treatment duration should not exceed a few weeks
Dosage Forms
Tablet: 5 mg
Tablet, extended release (Gradumet®): 5 mg, 10 mg, 15 mg

methantheline bromide (meth an' tha leen)

Brand Names Banthine®
Synonyms methanthelinium bromide
Therapeutic Category Anticholinergic Agent; Antispasmodic Agent, Gastrointestinal
Use Adjunctive treatment of peptic ulcer, irritable bowel syndrome, pancreatitis, ureteral and urinary bladder spasm; to reduce duodenal motility during diagnostic radiologic procedures and treatment of an uninhibited neurogenic bladder
Usual Dosage Oral:
Neonates: 12.5 mg twice daily then 3 times/day

Children:
<1 year: 12.5-25 mg 4 times/day
>1 year: 12.5-50 mg 4 times/day
Adults: 50-100 mg every 6 hours
Dosage Forms Tablet: 50 mg

methanthelinium bromide *see* methantheline bromide *on previous page*

methazolamide (meth a zoe' la mide)
Brand Names Neptazane®
Therapeutic Category Carbonic Anhydrase Inhibitor; Diuretic, Carbonic Anhydrase Inhibitor
Use Adjunctive treatment of open-angle or secondary glaucoma; short-term therapy of narrow-angle glaucoma when delay of surgery is desired
Usual Dosage Adults: Oral: 50-100 mg 2-3 times/day
Dosage Forms Tablet: 50 mg

methdilazine hydrochloride (meth dill' a zeen)
Brand Names Tacaryl®
Therapeutic Category Antihistamine; Phenothiazine Derivative
Use Symptomatic relief of pruritus associated with urticaria; neuroallergic, atopic, contact, poison ivy or eczematous dermatitis; pruritus ani or drug rash
Usual Dosage Oral:
Children >3 years: 4 mg 2-4 times/day
Adults: 8 mg 2-4 times/day
Dosage Forms
Syrup: 4 mg/5 mL (473 mL)
Tablet: 8 mg
Tablet, chewable: 3.6 mg [methdilazine hydrochloride 4 mg]

methenamine (meth en' a meen)
Brand Names Hiprex®; Mandelamine®; Urex®
Synonyms hexamethylenetetramine
Therapeutic Category Antibiotic, Miscellaneous
Use Prophylaxis or suppression of recurrent urinary tract infections; urinary tract discomfort secondary to hypermotility
Usual Dosage Oral:
Children:
Hippurate: 6-12 years: 25-50 mg/kg/day divided every 12 hours
Mandelate: 50-75 mg/kg/day divided every 6 hours

Adults:
Hippurate: 1 g twice daily
Mandelate: 1 g 4 times/day after meals and at bedtime
Dosage Forms
Granules (orange flavor): 1 g (56s)
Suspension, oral, as mandelate (Mandelamine®): 250 mg/5 mL (coconut flavor), 500 mg/5 mL (cherry flavor)
Tablet, as hippurate (Hiprex®, Urex®): 1 g (Hiprex® contains tartrazine dye)
Tablet, as mandelate, enteric coated (Mandelamine®): 250 mg, 500 mg, 1 g

Methergine® *see* methylergonovine maleate *on page 305*

methicillin sodium (meth i sill' in)
Brand Names Staphcillin®
Synonyms dimethoxyphenyl penicillin sodium; sodium methicillin
Therapeutic Category Antibiotic, Penicillin
(Continued)

methicillin sodium *(Continued)*

Use Treatment of susceptible bacterial infections such as osteomyelitis, septicemia, endocarditis, and CNS infections due to penicillinase-producing strains of *Staphylococcus*

Usual Dosage I.M., I.V.:

Neonates:

0-4 weeks, <1200 g: 50 mg/kg/day divided every 12 hours; meningitis: 100 mg/kg/day divided every 12 hours

Postnatal age <7 days:

1200-2000 g: 50 mg/kg/day divided every 12 hours; meningitis: 100 mg/kg/day divided every 12 hours

>2000 g: 75 mg/kg/day divided every 8 hours; meningitis: 150 mg/kg/day divided every 8 hours

Postnatal age >7 days

1200-2000 g: 75 mg/kg/day divided every 8 hours; meningitis: 150 mg/kg/day divided every 8 hours

>2000 g: 100 mg/kg/day divided every 6 hours; meningitis: 200 mg/kg/day divided every 6 hours

Children: 150-200 mg/kg/day divided every 6 hours; 200-400 mg/kg/day divided every 4-6 hours has been used for treatment of severe infections; maximum dose: 12 g/day

Adults: 4-12 g/day in divided doses every 4-6 hours

Dosage Forms Powder for injection: 1 g, 4 g, 6 g, 10 g

methimazole *(meth im' a zole)*

Brand Names Tapazole®

Synonyms thiamazole

Therapeutic Category Antithyroid Agent

Use Palliative treatment of hyperthyroidism, to return the hyperthyroid patient to a normal metabolic state prior to thyroidectomy, and to control thyrotoxic crisis that may accompany thyroidectomy

Usual Dosage Oral:

Children: Initial: 0.4 mg/kg/day in 3 divided doses; maintenance: 0.2 mg/kg/day in 3 divided doses

Adults: Initial: 10 mg every 8 hours; maintenance dose ranges from 5-30 mg/day

Dosage Forms Tablet: 5 mg, 10 mg

methionine *(me thye' oh neen)*

Brand Names Pedameth®

Therapeutic Category Dietary Supplement

Use Treatment of diaper rash and control of odor, dermatitis and ulceration caused by ammoniacal urine

Usual Dosage Oral:

Children: Control of diaper rash: 75 mg in formula or other liquid 3-4 times/day for 3-5 days

Adults:

Control of odor in incontinent adults: 200-400 mg 3-4 times/day

Dietary supplement: 500 mg/day

Dosage Forms

Capsule: 200 mg, 300 mg, 500 mg

Liquid: 75 mg/5 mL (473 mL)

Tablet: 500 mg

methocarbamol *(meth oh kar' ba mole)*

Brand Names Delaxin®; Marbaxin®; Robaxin®; Robomol®

Therapeutic Category Skeletal Muscle Relaxant

Use Treatment of muscle spasm associated with acute painful musculoskeletal conditions; supportive therapy in tetanus

Usual Dosage
Children: Recommended **only** for use in tetanus I.V.: 15 mg/kg/dose or 500 mg/m^2/dose, may repeat every 6 hours if needed; maximum dose: 1.8 g/m^2/day for 3 days only

Adults: Muscle spasm:
Oral: 1.5 g 4 times/day for 2-3 days, then decrease to 4-4.5 g/day in 3-6 divided doses
I.M., I.V.: 1 g every 8 hours if oral not possible
Dosage Forms
Injection: 100 mg/mL in polyethylene glycol 50% (10 mL)
Tablet: 500 mg, 750 mg

methocarbamol and aspirin
Brand Names Robaxisal®
Therapeutic Category Skeletal Muscle Relaxant
Use Adjunct to rest, physical therapy, and other measures for the relief of discomfort associated with acute, painful musculoskeletal disorders
Usual Dosage Children >12 years and Adults: Oral: 2 tablets 4 times/day
Dosage Forms Tablet: Methocarbamol 400 mg and aspirin 325 mg

methohexital sodium (meth oh hex' i tal)
Brand Names Brevital® Sodium
Therapeutic Category Barbiturate; General Anesthetic; Sedative
Use Induction and maintenance of general anesthesia for short procedures
Usual Dosage Doses must be titrated to effect
Children:
I.M.: Preop: 5-10 mg/kg/dose
I.V.: Induction: 1-2 mg/kg/dose
Rectal: Preop/induction: 20-35 mg/kg/dose; usual: 25 mg/kg/dose; give as 10% aqueous solution

Adults: I.V.: Induction: 50-120 mg to start; 20-40 mg every 4-7 minutes
Dosage Forms Injection: 500 mg, 2.5 g, 5 g

methoin see mephenytoin on page 293

methotrexate (meth oh trex' ate)
Brand Names Folex® Injection; Rheumatrex® Oral
Synonyms amethopterin; MTX
Therapeutic Category Antineoplastic Agent, Antimetabolite
Use Treatment of trophoblastic neoplasms, leukemias, psoriasis, rheumatoid arthritis, osteosarcoma, non-Hodgkin's lymphoma
Usual Dosage Refer to individual protocols
Children:
High-dose MTX for acute lymphocytic leukemia: I.V.: Loading dose of 200 mg/m^2 and a 24-hour infusion of 1200 mg/m^2/day
Induction of remission in acute lymphoblastic leukemias: Oral, I.M., I.V.: 3.3 mg/m^2/day for 4-6 weeks
Leukemia: Remission maintenance: Oral, I.M.: 20-30 mg/m^2 2 times/week
Juvenile rheumatoid arthritis: Oral: 5-15 mg/m^2/week as a single dose or as 3 divided doses given 12 hours apart
Osteosarcoma:
I.T.: 10-15 mg/m^2 (maximum dose: 15 mg) by protocol
I.V.: <12 years: 12 g/m^2 (12-18 g); >12 years: 8 g/m^2 (maximum dose: 18 g)
Non-Hodgkin's lymphoma: I.V.: 200-300 mg/m^2

Adults:
Trophoblastic neoplasms: Oral, I.M.: 15-30 mg/day for 5 days, repeat in 7 days for 3-5 courses
(Continued)
301

methotrexate *(Continued)*
Rheumatoid arthritis: Oral: 7.5 mg once weekly or 2.5 mg every 12 hours for 3 doses/week; not to exceed 20 mg/week
Dosage Forms
Dose Pack: 2.5 mg (4 cards with 3 tablets each)
Injection, as sodium: 2.5 mg/mL (2 mL); 25 mg/mL (2 mL, 4 mL, 8 mL, 10 mL)
Injection, as sodium, preservative free: 25 mg/mL (2 mL, 4 mL, 8 mL, 10 mL)
Powder for injection, as sodium: 20 mg, 25 mg, 50 mg, 100 mg, 250 mg
Tablet, as sodium: 2.5 mg

methotrimeprazine hydrochloride (meth oh trye mep' ra zeen)
Brand Names Levoprome®
Synonyms levomepromazine
Therapeutic Category Analgesic, Non-Narcotic; Phenothiazine Derivative; Sedative
Use Relief of moderate to severe pain in nonambulatory patients; for analgesia and sedation when respiratory depression is to be avoided, as in obstetrics; preanesthetic for producing sedation, somnolence and relief of apprehension and anxiety
Usual Dosage Adults: I.M.:
Sedation analgesia: 10-20 mg every 4-6 hours as needed

Preoperative medication: 2-20 mg, 45 minutes to 3 hours before surgery

Postoperative analgesia: 2.5-7.5 mg every 4-6 hours is suggested as necessary since residual effects of anesthetic may be present

Pre- and postoperative hypotension: I.M.: 5-10 mg
Dosage Forms Injection: 20 mg/mL (10 mL)

methoxamine hydrochloride (meth ox' a meen)
Brand Names Vasoxyl®
Therapeutic Category Adrenergic Agonist Agent
Use Treatment of hypotension occurring during general anesthesia; to terminate episodes of supraventricular tachycardia; treatment of shock
Usual Dosage Adults:
Emergencies: I.V.: 3-5 mg
Supraventricular tachycardia: I.V.: 10 mg
During spinal anesthesia: I.M.: 10-20 mg
Dosage Forms Injection: 20 mg/mL (1 mL)

methoxsalen (meth ox' a len)
Brand Names Oxsoralen®; Oxsoralen-Ultra®
Synonyms methoxypsoralen; 8-MOP
Therapeutic Category Psoralen
Use Symptomatic control of severe, recalcitrant, disabling psoriasis in conjunction with long wave ultraviolet radiation; induce repigmentation in vitiligo topical repigmenting agent in conjunction with controlled doses of ultraviolet A (UVA) or sunlight
Usual Dosage
Psoriasis: Adults: Oral: 10-70 mg 1½-2 hours before exposure to ultraviolet light, 2-3 times at least 48 hours apart; dosage is based upon patient's body weight and skin type

Vitiligo: Children >12 years and Adults:
Oral: 20 mg 2-4 hours before exposure to UVA light or sunlight
Topical: Apply lotion 1-2 hours before exposure to UVA light, no more than once weekly
Dosage Forms
Capsule: 10 mg
Lotion: 1% (30 mL)

methoxyflurane (meth ox ee floo' rane)
Brand Names Penthrane®
Therapeutic Category General Anesthetic
Use Adjunct to provide anesthesia procedures under 4 hours in duration

Usual Dosage 0.3% to 0.8% for analgesia and anesthesia, with 0.1% to 2% for maintenance when used with nitrous oxide
Dosage Forms Liquid: 15 mL, 125 mL

methoxypsoralen *see* methoxsalen *on previous page*

methscopolamine bromide (meth skoe pol' a meen)
Brand Names Pamine®
Therapeutic Category Anticholinergic Agent; Antispasmodic Agent, Gastrointestinal
Use Adjunctive therapy in the treatment of peptic ulcer
Usual Dosage Oral: 2.5 mg 30 minutes before meals or food and 2.5-5 mg at bedtime
Dosage Forms Tablet: 2.5 mg

methsuximide (meth sux' i mide)
Brand Names Celontin®
Therapeutic Category Anticonvulsant, Succinimide
Use Control of absence (petit mal) seizures; useful adjunct in refractory, partial complex (psychomotor) seizures
Usual Dosage Oral:
Children: Initial: 10-15 mg/kg/day in 3-4 divided doses; increase weekly up to maximum of 30 mg/kg/day

Adults: 300 mg/day for the first week; may increase by 300 mg/day at weekly intervals up to 1.2 g in 2-4 divided doses/day
Dosage Forms Capsule: 150 mg, 300 mg

methyclothiazide (meth i kloe thye' a zide)
Brand Names Aquatensen®; Enduron®
Therapeutic Category Diuretic, Thiazide
Use Management of mild to moderate hypertension; treatment of edema in congestive heart failure and nephrotic syndrome
Usual Dosage Adults: Oral:
Edema: 2.5-10 mg/day
Hypertension: 2.5-5 mg/day
Dosage Forms Tablet: 2.5 mg, 5 mg

methyclothiazide and cryptenamine tannates
Brand Names Diutensin®
Synonyms cryptenamine tannates and methyclothiazide
Therapeutic Category Antihypertensive, Combination
Use Management of hypertension
Usual Dosage Oral: 1-4 tablets/day
Dosage Forms Tablet: Methyclothiazide 2.5 mg and cryptenamine tannates 2 mg

methyclothiazide and deserpidine
Brand Names Enduronyl®; Enduronyl® Forte
Therapeutic Category Antihypertensive, Combination
Use Management of mild to moderately severe hypertension
Usual Dosage Oral: Individualized, normally 1-4 tablets/day
Dosage Forms Tablet: Methyclothiazide 5 mg and deserpidine 0.25 mg; methyclothiazide 5 mg and deserpidine 0.5 mg

methyclothiazide and pargyline
Brand Names Eutron®
Synonyms pargyline and methyclothiazide
Therapeutic Category Antihypertensive, Combination
(Continued)
303

methyclothiazide and pargyline *(Continued)*
Use Management of hypertension
Usual Dosage Oral: Individualized, normally 1-4 tablets/day
Dosage Forms Tablet: Methyclothiazide 5 mg and pargyline hydrochloride 25 mg

methylacetoxyprogesterone *see medroxyprogesterone acetate on page 289*

methylbenzethonium chloride (meth ill ben ze thoe' nee um)
Brand Names Diaparene® [OTC]; Puri-Clens™ [OTC]; Sween Cream® [OTC]
Therapeutic Category Topical Skin Product
Use Diaper rash and ammonia dermatitis
Usual Dosage Topical: Apply to area as needed
Dosage Forms
Cream: 0.1% (30 g, 60 g, 120 g)
Ointment, topical: 0.1% (30 g, 60 g, 120 g)
Powder: 0.055% (120 g, 270 g, 420 g)

methylcellulose (meth ill sell' yoo lose)
Brand Names Citrucel® [OTC]
Therapeutic Category Ophthalmic Agent, Miscellaneous
Use
Oral: Adjunct in treatment of constipation
Ophthalmic: Relief of dry eyes and ocular lubricant for artificial eyes and contact lenses
Usual Dosage
Children:
Oral: 5-10 mL 1-2 times/day
Ophthalmic: Instill 1-2 drops of 0.25% to 1% in eye(s) 3-4 times/day

Adults: Oral: 5-20 mL 3 times/day
Dosage Forms
Liquid: 450 mg/5 mL
Powder: 105 mg/g

methyldopa (meth ill doe' pa)
Brand Names Aldomet®
Synonyms methyldopate hydrochloride
Therapeutic Category Alpha-Adrenergic Inhibitors, Central
Use Management of moderate to severe hypertension
Usual Dosage
Children:
Oral: Initial: 10 mg/kg/day in 2-4 divided doses; increase every 2 days as needed to maximum dose of 65 mg/kg/day; do not exceed 3 g/day
I.V.: 5-10 mg/kg/dose every 6-8 hours

Adults:
Oral: Initial: 250 mg 2-3 times/day; increase every 2 days as needed; usual dose 1-1.5 g/day in 2-4 divided doses; maximum dose: 3 g/day
I.V.: 250-1000 mg every 6-8 hours
Dosage Forms
Injection, as methyldopate HCl: 50 mg/mL (5 mL, 10 mL)
Suspension, oral: 250 mg/5 mL (5 mL, 473 mL)
Tablet: 125 mg, 250 mg, 500 mg

methyldopa and chlorothiazide *see chlorothiazide and methyldopa on page 92*

methyldopa and hydrochlorothiazide
Brand Names Aldoril®
Synonyms hydrochlorothiazide and methyldopa
Therapeutic Category Antihypertensive, Combination
Use Management of moderate to severe hypertension
Usual Dosage Oral: 1 tablet 2-3 times/day for first 48 hours, then decrease or increase at intervals of not less than 2 days until an adequate response is achieved
Dosage Forms Tablet:
15: Methyldopa 250 mg and hydrochlorothiazide 15 mg
25: Methyldopa 250 mg and hydrochlorothiazide 25 mg
D50: Methyldopa 500 mg and hydrochlorothiazide 50 mg

methyldopate hydrochloride *see* methyldopa *on previous page*

methylene blue (meth' i leen)
Brand Names Urolene Blue® Oral
Therapeutic Category Antidote, Cyanide; Antidote, Drug Induced Methemoglobinemia
Use Antidote for cyanide poisoning and drug-induced methemoglobinemia, indicator dye, chronic urolithiasis
Usual Dosage
Children:
NADH-methemoglobin reductase deficiency: Oral: 1.5-5 mg/kg/day (maximum: 300 mg/day) given with 5-8 mg/kg/day of ascorbic acid
Methemoglobinemia: I.V.: 1-2 mg/kg over several minutes
Adults:
Genitourinary antiseptic: Oral: 55-130 mg 3 times/day (maximum: 390 mg/day)
Methemoglobinemia: I.V.: 1-2 mg/kg over several minutes; may be repeated in 1 hour if necessary
Dosage Forms
Injection: 10 mg/mL (1 mL, 10 mL)
Tablet: 65 mg

methylergometrine maleate *see* methylergonovine maleate *on this page*

methylergonovine maleate (meth ill er goe noe' veen)
Brand Names Methergine®
Synonyms methylergometrine maleate
Therapeutic Category Ergot Alkaloid
Use Prevention and treatment of postpartum and postabortion hemorrhage caused by uterine atony or subinvolution
Usual Dosage Adults:
Oral: 0.2-0.4 mg every 6-12 hours for 2-7 days
I.M., I.V.: 0.2 mg every 2-4 hours for 5 doses then change to oral dosage
Dosage Forms
Injection: 0.2 mg/mL (1 mL)
Tablet: 0.2 mg

methylmorphine *see* codeine *on page 112*

methylphenidate hydrochloride (meth ill fen' i date)
Brand Names Ritalin®; Ritalin-SR®
Therapeutic Category Central Nervous System Stimulant, Nonamphetamine
Use Treatment of attention deficit disorder and symptomatic management of narcolepsy
(Continued)

methylphenidate hydrochloride *(Continued)*
Usual Dosage Oral:

Children ≥6 years: Attention deficit disorder: Initial: 0.3 mg/kg/dose or 2.5-5 mg/dose given before breakfast and lunch; increase by 0.1 mg/kg/dose or by 5-10 mg/day at weekly intervals; usual dose: 0.5-1 mg/kg/day; maximum dose: 2 mg/kg/day or 60 mg/day

Adults: Narcolepsy: 10 mg 2-3 times/day, up to 60 mg/day
Dosage Forms
Tablet: 5 mg, 10 mg, 20 mg
Tablet, sustained release: 20 mg

methylphenobarbital *see* mephobarbital *on page 293*

methylphenylethylhydantoin *see* mephenytoin *on page 293*

methylphenyl isoxazolyl penicillin *see* oxacillin sodium *on page 347*

methylphytyl napthoquinone *see* phytonadione *on page 376*

methylprednisolone (meth ill pred niss' oh lone)
Brand Names Adlone® Injection; A-methaPred® Injection; depMedalone® Injection; Depoject® Injection; Depo-Medrol® Injection; Depopred® Injection; D-Med® Injection; Duralone® Injection; Medralone® Injection; Medrol® Acetate Topical; Medrol® Oral; M-Prednisol® Injection; Rep-Pred® Injection; Solu-Medrol® Injection
Synonyms 6-α-methylprednisolone
Therapeutic Category Adrenal Corticosteroid; Anti-inflammatory Agent; Corticosteroid, Systemic; Corticosteroid, Topical (Low Potency)
Use Primarily as an anti-inflammatory or immunosuppressant agent in the treatment of a variety of diseases including those of hematologic, allergic, inflammatory, neoplastic, and autoimmune origin
Usual Dosage Methylprednisolone sodium succinate is highly soluble and has a rapid effect by I.M. and I.V. routes. Methylprednisolone acetate has a low solubility and has a sustained I.M. effect.

Children:
Anti-inflammatory or immunosuppressive: Oral, I.M., I.V. (sodium succinate): 0.16-0.8 mg/kg/day or 5-25 mg/m^2/day in divided doses every 6-12 hours
Status asthmaticus: I.V. (sodium succinate): Loading dose: 2 mg/kg/dose, then 0.5-1 mg/kg/dose every 6 hours for up to 5 days
Lupus nephritis:
I.V. (sodium succinate): 30 mg/kg every other day for 6 doses
Topical: Apply sparingly 2-4 times/day

Adults:
Anti-inflammatory or immunosuppressive: Oral: 4-48 mg/day to start, followed by gradual reduction in dosage to the lowest possible level consistent with maintaining an adequate clinical response
I.M. (sodium succinate): 10-80 mg/day once daily
I.M. (acetate): 40-120 mg every 1-2 weeks
I.V. (sodium succinate): 10-40 mg over a period of several minutes and repeated I.V. or I.M. at intervals depending on clinical response; when high dosages are needed, give 30 mg/kg over a period of 10-20 minutes and may be repeated every 4-6 hours for 48 hours
Status asthmaticus: I.V. (sodium succinate): Loading dose: 2 mg/kg/dose, then 0.5-1 mg/kg/dose every hours for up to 5 days
Lupus nephritis:
I.V. (sodium succinate): 1 g/day for 3 days
Topical: Apply sparingly 2-4 times/day
Intra-articular (acetate):
Large joints: 20-80 mg
Small joints: 4-10 mg

Intralesional (acetate): 20-60 mg
Dosage Forms
Injection, as sodium succinate: 40 mg (1 mL, 3 mL); 125 mg (2 mL, 5 mL); 500 mg (1 mL, 4 mL, 8 mL, 20 mL); 1000 mg (1 mL, 8 mL, 50 mL); 2000 mg (30.6 mL)
Injection, as acetate: 20 mg/mL (5 mL, 10 mL); 40 mg/mL (1 mL, 5 mL, 10 mL); 80 mg/mL (1 mL, 5 mL)
Ointment, topical, as acetate: 0.25% (30 g); 1% (30 g)
Tablet: 2 mg, 4 mg, 8 mg, 16 mg, 24 mg, 32 mg
Tablet, dose pack: 4 mg (21s)

6-α-methylprednisolone *see* methylprednisolone *on previous page*

methylrosaniline chloride *see* gentian violet *on page 211*

methyltestosterone (meth ill tess toss' te rone)
Brand Names Android®; Metandren®; Oreton® Methyl; Testred®; Virilon®
Therapeutic Category Androgen
Use
Male: Hypogonadism; delayed puberty; impotence and climacteric symptoms
Female: Palliative treatment of metastatic breast cancer; postpartum breast pain and/or engorgement
Usual Dosage Adults:
Male:
Oral: 10-40 mg/day
Buccal: 5-20 mg/day

Female:
Breast pain/engorgement:
Oral: 80 mg/day for 3-5 days
Buccal: 40 mg/day for 3-5 days
Breast cancer:
Oral: 200 mg/day
Buccal: 100 mg/day
Dosage Forms
Capsule: 10 mg
Tablet: 10 mg, 25 mg
Tablet, buccal: 5 mg, 10 mg

methysergide maleate (meth i ser' jide)
Brand Names Sansert®
Therapeutic Category Ergot Alkaloid
Use Prophylaxis of vascular headache
Usual Dosage Oral: 4-8 mg/day with meals; if no improvement is noted after 3 weeks, drug is unlikely to be beneficial; must not be given continuously for longer than 6 months, and a drug-free interval of 3-4 weeks must follow each 6-month course; dosage should be tapered over the 2-3 week period before drug discontinuation to avoid rebound headaches
Dosage Forms Tablet: 2 mg

Meticorten® Oral *see* prednisone *on page 393*

Metimyd® Ophthalmic *see* sodium sulfacetamide and prednisolone *on page 439*

metipranolol hydrochloride (met i pran' oh lol)
Brand Names OptiPranolol® Ophthalmic
Therapeutic Category Beta-Adrenergic Blocker, Ophthalmic
Use Agent for lowering intraocular pressure
(Continued)
307

metipranolol hydrochloride *(Continued)*
Usual Dosage Ophthalmic: Adults: 1 drop in the affected eye(s) twice daily
Dosage Forms Solution, ophthalmic: 0.3% (5 mL, 10 mL)

Metizol® Oral *see* metronidazole *on next page*

metoclopramide (met oh kloe pra' mide)
Brand Names Clopra®; Maxolon®; Octamide®; Reglan®
Therapeutic Category Antiemetic
Use Symptomatic treatment of diabetic gastric stasis, gastroesophageal reflux; prevention of nausea associated with chemotherapy or postsurgery and facilitates intubation of the small intestine
Usual Dosage
Children:
> Gastroesophageal reflux: Oral: 0.1 mg/kg/dose up to 4 times/day; efficacy of continuing metoclopramide beyond 12 weeks in reflux has not been determined; total daily dose should not exceed 0.5 mg/kg/day
> Gastrointestinal hypomotility: Oral, I.M., I.V.: 0.1 mg/kg/dose up to 4 times/day, not to exceed 0.5 mg/kg/day
> Antiemetic: I.V.: 1-2 mg/kg 30 minutes before chemotherapy and every 2-4 hours
> Facilitate intubation: I.V.: <6 years: 0.1 mg/kg; 6-14 years: 2.5-5 mg

Adults:
> Stasis/reflux: Oral: 10-15 mg/dose up to 4 times/day 30 minutes before meals or food and at bedtime; efficacy of continuing metoclopramide beyond 12 weeks in reflux has not been determined
> Gastrointestinal hypomotility: Oral, I.M., I.V.: 10 mg 30 minutes before each meal and at bedtime
> Antiemetic: I.V.: 1-2 mg/kg 30 minutes before chemotherapy and every 2-4 hours
> Facilitate intubation: I.V.: 10 mg

Dosage Forms
Injection: 5 mg/mL (2 mL, 10 mL, 30 mL, 50 mL, 100 mL)
Solution, oral, concentrated: 10 mg/mL (10 mL, 30 mL)
Syrup, sugar free: 5 mg/5 mL (10 mL, 480 mL)
Tablet: 5 mg, 10 mg

metocurine iodide (met oh kyoor' een)
Brand Names Metubine® Iodide
Synonyms dimethyl tubocurarine iodide
Therapeutic Category Neuromuscular Blocker Agent, Nondepolarizing
Use Adjunct to anesthesia to induce skeletal muscle relaxation
Usual Dosage
Children:
> Chronic respiratory paralysis in neonates: Start 0.25-0.5 mg/kg/dose (repeat once if paralysis is not achieved in 3 minutes); maintenance: repeat previous dose as soon as movement is observed. The dose should be titrated to achieve a dosage interval of 3-4 hours, then plateau at 10-20 mg/kg/24 hours
> Neuromuscular blockade for surgery: Initial: 0.2-0.4 mg/kg/dose; maintenance: 0.1-0.25 mg/kg/dose every 25-90 minutes

Adults:
> Surgery: 0.2-0.4 mg/kg (initial); supplement dose: 0.5-1 mg; use of anesthetics that potentiate effect of neuromuscular blocking drug requires less metocurine
> Electric shock therapy: 1.75-5.5 mg
Dosage Forms Injection: 2 mg/mL (20 mL)

metolazone (me tole' a zone)
Brand Names Diulo®; Mykrox®; Zaroxolyn®
Therapeutic Category Diuretic, Miscellaneous
Use Management of mild to moderate hypertension; treatment of edema in congestive heart failure and nephrotic syndrome; impaired renal function
Usual Dosage Oral:
Children: 0.2-0.4 mg/kg/day divided every 12-24 hours
Adults:
Edema: 5-20 mg/dose every 24 hours
Hypertension: 2.5-5 mg/dose every 24 hours
Dosage Forms Tablet:
Diulo®, Zaroxolyn®: 2.5 mg, 5 mg, 10 mg
Mykrox®: 0.5 mg

Metopirone® *see* metyrapone tartrate *on next page*

metoprolol (me toe' proe lole)
Brand Names Lopressor®; Toprol XL®
Therapeutic Category Beta-Adrenergic Blocker
Use Treatment of hypertension and angina pectoris; prevention of myocardial infarction; selective inhibitor of beta$_1$-adrenergic receptors
Usual Dosage Safety and efficacy in children have not been established.
Children: Oral: 1-5 mg/kg/24 hours divided twice daily; allow 3 days between dose adjustments
Adults:
Oral: 100-450 mg/day in 2-3 divided doses, begin with 50 mg twice daily and increase doses at weekly intervals to desired effect
I.V.: 5 mg every 2 minutes for 3 doses in early treatment of myocardial infarction; thereafter give 50 mg orally every 6 hours 15 minutes after last I.V. dose and continue for 48 hours; then administer a maintenance dose of 100 mg twice daily
Dosage Forms
Injection: 1 mg/mL (5 mL)
Tablet: 50 mg, 100 mg
Tablet, sustained release: 50 mg, 100 mg, 200 mg

Metreton® Ophthalmic *see* prednisolone *on page 391*

metrizamide *see* radiological/contrast media (non-ionic) *on page 415*

Metrodin® Injection *see* urofollitropin *on page 488*

MetroGel® Topical *see* metronidazole *on this page*

MetroGel®-Vaginal *see* metronidazole *on this page*

Metro I.V.® Injection *see* metronidazole *on this page*

metronidazole (me troe ni' da zole)
Brand Names Flagyl® Oral; Metizol® Oral; MetroGel® Topical; MetroGel®-Vaginal; Metro I.V.® Injection; Protostat® Oral
Therapeutic Category Amebicide; Antibiotic, Anaerobic; Antibiotic, Topical; Antiprotozoal
Use Treatment of susceptible anaerobic bacterial and protozoal infections in the following conditions: amebiasis, symptomatic and asymptomatic trichomoniasis; skin and skin structure infections; CNS infections; intra-abdominal infections; systemic anaerobic infections; topically for the treatment of acne rosacea; treatment of antibiotic-associated pseudomembranous colitis (AAPC); bacterial vaginosis
Usual Dosage
Neonates: Anaerobic infections: Oral, I.V.:
0-4 weeks: <1200 g: 7 5 mg/kg every 48 hours
(Continued)

metronidazole *(Continued)*
Postnatal age <7 days:
  1200-2000 g: 7.5 mg/kg/day given every 24 hours
  >2000 g: 15 mg/kg/day in divided doses every 12 hours
Postnatal age >7 days:
  1200-2000 g: 15 mg/kg/day in divided doses every 12 hours
  >2000 g: 30 mg/kg/day in divided doses every 12 hours

Infants and Children:
  Amebiasis: Oral: 35-50 mg/kg/day in divided doses every 8 hours
  Other parasitic infections: Oral: 15-30 mg/kg/day in divided doses every 8 hours
  Anaerobic infections: Oral, I.V.: 30 mg/kg/day in divided doses every 6 hours
  Clostridium difficile (antibiotic-associated colitis): Oral: 20 mg/kg/day divided every 6 hours
  Maximum dose: 2 g/day

Adults:
  Amebiasis: Oral: 500-750 mg every 8 hours
  Other parasitic infections: Oral: 250 mg every 8 hours or 2 g as a single dose
  Anaerobic infections: Oral, I.V.: 30 mg/kg/day in divided doses every 6 hours; not to exceed 4 g/day
  AAPC: Oral: 250-500 mg 3-4 times/day for 10-14 days
  Topical: Apply a thin film twice daily to affected areas
  Vaginal: One applicatorful in vagina each morning and evening, as needed
Dosage Forms
Gel, topical: 0.75% [7.5 mg/mL] (30 g)
Gel, vaginal: 0.75% [7.5 mg/mL] (70 g)
Injection, ready to use, in normal saline: 5 mg/mL (100 mL)
Powder for injection, as hydrochloride: 500 mg
Tablet: 250 mg, 500 mg

Metubine® Iodide *see metocurine iodide on page 308*

metyrapone tartrate (me teer' a pone)
Brand Names Metopirone®
Therapeutic Category Diagnostic Agent, Hypothalmic-Pituitary ACTH Function
Use Diagnostic test for hypothalamic-pituitary ACTH function

Unlabeled use: Controlling cortisol secretion in Cushing syndrome
Usual Dosage Discontinue all corticosteroid therapy prior to and during testing
  Day 1: Control period: Collect 24-hour urine to measure 17-hydroxycorticosteroids (17-OHCS) or 17-ketogenic steroids (17-KGS)
  Day 2: ACTH test: Standard ACTH test (ie, administer 50 units ACTH by infusion over 8 hours and measure 24-hour urinary steroids); if results indicate adequate response, proceed with test
  Day 3 to 4: Rest period
  Day 5: Administer metyrapone, preferably with milk or a snack
    Adults: 750 mg every 4 hours for 6 doses; single dose is approximately equivalent to 15 mg/kg
    Children: 15 mg/kg every 4 hours for 6 doses; use a minimal 250 mg single dose
  Day 6: Determine 24-hour urinary steroids for effect
Dosage Forms Tablet: 250 mg

metyrosine (me tye' roe seen)
Brand Names Demser®
Synonyms AMPT; OGMT
Therapeutic Category Tyrosine Hydroxylase Inhibitor
Use Short-term management of pheochromocytoma before surgery, long-term management when surgery is contraindicated or when malignant

Usual Dosage Children >12 years and Adults: Initial: 250 mg 4 times/day, increased by 250-500 mg/day up to 4 g/day; maintenance: 2-3 g/day in 4 divided doses; for preoperative preparation, give optimum effective dosage for 5-7 days
Dosage Forms Capsule: 250 mg

Mevacor® *see* lovastatin *on page 279*
mevinolin *see* lovastatin *on page 279*

mexiletine hydrochloride (mex' i le teen)
Brand Names Mexitil®
Therapeutic Category Antiarrhythmic Agent, Class Ib
Use Management of serious ventricular arrhythmias; suppression of PVCs
Usual Dosage Oral:
Children: Range: 1.4-5 mg/kg/dose (mean: 3.3 mg/kg/dose) given every 8 hours; start with lower initial dose and increase according to effects and serum concentrations

Adults: Initial: 200 mg every 8 hours (may load with 400 mg if necessary); adjust dose every 2-3 days; usual dose: 200-300 mg every 8 hours; maximum dose: 1.2 g/day (some patients respond to every 12-hour dosing)
Dosage Forms Capsule: 150 mg, 200 mg, 250 mg

Mexitil® *see* mexiletine hydrochloride *on this page*
Mezlin® *see* mezlocillin sodium *on this page*

mezlocillin sodium (mez loe sill' in)
Brand Names Mezlin®
Therapeutic Category Antibiotic, Penicillin
Use Treatment of infections caused by susceptible gram-negative aerobic bacilli (*Klebsiella*, *Proteus*, *Escherichia coli*, *Enterobacter*, *Pseudomonas aeruginosa*, *Serratia*) involving the skin and skin structure, bone and joint, respiratory tract, urinary tract, gastrointestinal tract, as well as septicemia
Usual Dosage I.M., I.V.:
Neonates:
Postnatal age <7 days: 150 mg/kg/day divided every 12 hours
Postnatal age >7 days: 225 mg/kg/day divided every 8 hours

Children: 200-300 mg/kg/day divided every 4-6 hours; maximum: 24 g/day

Adults:
Uncomplicated urinary tract infection: 1.5-2 g every 6 hours
Serious infections: 3-4 g every 4-6 hours
Dosage Forms Powder for injection: 1 g, 2 g, 3 g, 4 g, 20 g

Miacalcin® *see* calcitonin (salmon) *on page 65*
Micatin® Topical [OTC] *see* miconazole *on this page*

miconazole (mi kon' a zole)
Brand Names Micatin® Topical [OTC]; Monistat-Derm™ Topical; Monistat i.v.™ Injection; Monistat™ Vaginal
Synonyms miconazole nitrate
Therapeutic Category Antifungal Agent, Topical; Antifungal Agent, Vaginal
Use
I.V.: Treatment of severe systemic fungal infections and fungal meningitis that are refractory to standard treatment
Topical: Treatment of vulvovaginal candidiasis and a variety of skin and mucous membrane fungal infections
(Continued)

miconazole *(Continued)*

Usual Dosage
Children:
    I.V.: 20-40 mg/kg/day divided every 8 hours
    Topical: Apply twice daily for 2-4 weeks
    Vaginal: Insert contents of one applicator of vaginal cream or 100 mg suppository at
        bedtime for 7 days, or 200 mg suppository at bedtime for 3 days

Adults:
    I.T.: 20 mg every 3-7 days
    I.V.: Candidiasis: 600-1800 mg/day divided every 8 hours
    Topical: Apply twice daily for 2-4 weeks
    Vaginal: Insert contents of one applicator of vaginal cream or 100 mg suppository at
        bedtime for 7 days, or 200 mg suppository at bedtime for 3 days
    Coccidioidomycosis: 1800-3600 mg/day divided every 8 hours
    Cryptococcosis: 1200-2400 mg/day divided every 8 hours
    Paracoccidioidomycosis: 200-1200 mg/day divided every 8 hours

Dosage Forms
Cream:
    Topical, as nitrate: 2% [20 mg/g] (15 g, 30 g, 85 g)
    Vaginal, as nitrate: 2% [20 mg/g] (45 g is equivalent to 7 doses)
Injection: 1% [10 mg/mL] (20 mL)
Lotion, as nitrate: 2% [20 mg/g] (30 mL, 60 mL)
Powder, topical: 2% [20 mg/g] (45 g, 90 g)
Spray, topical: 2% [20 mg/g] (105 mL)
Suppository, vaginal, as nitrate: 100 mg (7s); 200 mg (3s)

miconazole nitrate *see* miconazole *on previous page*

MICRhoGAM™ *see* Rh$_o$(D) immune globulin *on page 419*

microfibrillar collagen hemostat

Brand Names Avitene®
Synonyms MCH
Therapeutic Category Hemostatic Agent
Use Adjunct to hemostasis when control of bleeding by ligature in ineffective or impractical
Usual Dosage Apply dry directly to source of bleeding
Dosage Forms
Fibrous: 1 g, 5 g
Nonwoven web: 70 mm x 70 mm x 1 mm; 70 mm x 35 mm x 1 mm

Micro-K® *see* potassium chloride *on page 386*

Micronase® *see* glyburide *on page 213*

microNefrin® Inhalation Solution [OTC] *see* epinephrine *on page 171*

Micronor® *see* norethindrone *on page 338*

Microstix-3® *see* diagnostic aids *(in vitro),* urine *on page 139*

Microsulfon® *see* sulfadiazine *on page 447*

MicroTrak® HSV 1/HSV 2 Culture Identification/Typing Test *see* diagnostic
aids *(in vitro),* blood *on page 137*

Mictrin® *see* hydrochlorothiazide *on page 233*

Midamor® *see* amiloride hydrochloride *on page 19*

midazolam hydrochloride (mid' ay zoe lam)

Brand Names Versed®
Therapeutic Category Benzodiazepine; Hypnotic; Sedative
Use Preoperative sedation and provide conscious sedation prior to diagnostic or radio-
graphic procedures

Usual Dosage The dose of midazolam needs to be individualized based on the patient's age, underlying diseases, and concurrent medications. Personnel and equipment needed for standard respiratory resuscitation should be immediately available during midazolam administration.

Children:
Preoperative sedation:
I.M.: 0.07-0.08 mg/kg 30-60 minutes presurgery
I.V.: 0.035 mg/kg/dose, repeat over several minutes as required to achieve the desired sedative effect up to a total dose of 0.1-0.2 mg/kg
Conscious sedation during mechanical ventilation: I.V.: Loading dose: 0.05-0.2 mg/kg then follow with initial continuous infusion: 1-2 μg/kg/minute; titrate to the desired effect; usual range: 0.4-6 μg/kg/minute
Conscious sedation for procedures:
Oral, Intranasal: 0.2-0.4 mg/kg (maximum: 15 mg) 30-45 minutes before the procedure
I.V.: 0.05 mg/kg 3 minutes before procedure
Adolescents >12 years: I.V.: 0.5 mg every 3-4 minutes until effect achieved

Adults:
Preoperative sedation: I.M.: 0.07-0.08 mg/kg 30-60 minutes presurgery; usual dose: 5 mg
Conscious sedation: I.V.: Initial: 0.5-2 mg slow I.V. over at least 2 minutes; slowly titrate to effect by repeating doses every 2-3 minutes if needed; usual total dose: 2.5-5 mg; use decreased doses in elderly

Adults, healthy <60 years: Some patients respond to doses as low as 1 mg; no more than 2.5 mg should be administered over a period of 2 minutes. Additional doses of midazolam may be administered after a 2-minute waiting period and evaluation of sedation after each dose increment. A total dose >5 mg is generally not needed. If narcotics or other CNS depressants are administered concomitantly, the midazolam dose should be reduced by 30%.
Dosage Forms Injection: 1 mg/mL (2 mL, 5 mL, 10 mL); 5 mg/mL (1 mL, 2 mL, 5 mL, 10 mL)

Midol® IB [OTC] *see* ibuprofen *on page 245*

Midrin® *see* acetaminophen and isometheptene mucate *on page 3*

Miflex® *see* chlorzoxazone *on page 99*

MIH *see* procarbazine hydrochloride *on page 396*

milk of magnesia *see* magnesium hydroxide *on page 282*

Milontin® *see* phensuximide *on page 371*

Milophene® *see* clomiphene citrate *on page 108*

milrinone lactate (mil' ri none)
Brand Names Primacor®
Therapeutic Category Cardiovascular Agent, Other
Use Short-term I.V. therapy of congestive heart failure
Usual Dosage Adults: I.V.: Loading dose: 50 μg/kg administered over 10 minutes, then 0.375-0.75 μg/kg/min as a continuous infusion for a total daily dose of 0.59-1.13 mg/kg
Dosage Forms Injection: 1 mg/mL (5 mL, 10 mL, 20 mL)

Miltown® *see* meprobamate *on page 293*

Mini-Gamulin® Rh *see* Rh₀(D) immune globulin *on page 419*

Minipress® *see* prazosin hydrochloride *on page 391*

Minitran® Patch *see* nitroglycerin *on page 336*

Minizide® *see* prazosin and polythiazide *on page 391*

Minocin® IV Injection *see minocycline hydrochloride on this page*

Minocin® Oral *see minocycline hydrochloride on this page*

minocycline hydrochloride (mi noe sye' kleen)
Brand Names Dynacin® Oral; Minocin® IV Injection; Minocin® Oral
Therapeutic Category Antibiotic, Tetracycline Derivative
Use Treatment of susceptible bacterial infections of both gram-negative and gram-positive organisms; acne
Usual Dosage
Children 8-12 years: 4 mg/kg stat, then 4 mg/kg/day (maximum: 200 mg/day) in divided doses every 12 hours

Adults:
Infection: Oral, I.V.: 200 mg stat, 100 mg every 12 hours
Acne: Oral: 50 mg 1-3 times/day
Dosage Forms
Capsule: 50 mg, 100 mg
Capsule, pellet-filled: 50 mg, 100 mg
Injection: 100 mg
Suspension, oral: 50 mg/5 mL (60 mL)

minoxidil (mi nox' i dill)
Brand Names Loniten® Oral; Rogaine® Topical
Therapeutic Category Vasodilator
Use Management of severe hypertension; treatment of male pattern baldness (alopecia androgenetica)
Usual Dosage
Children <12 years: Hypertension: Oral: Initial: 0.1-0.2 mg/kg once daily; maximum: 5 mg/day; increase gradually every 3 days; usual dosage: 0.25-1 mg/kg/day in 1-2 divided doses; maximum: 50 mg/day

Adults:
Hypertension: Oral: Initial: 5 mg once daily, increase gradually every 3 days; usual dose: 10-40 mg/day in 1-2 divided doses; maximum: 100 mg/day
Alopecia: Topical: Apply twice daily
Dosage Forms
Solution, topical: 2% = 20 mg/metered dose (60 mL)
Tablet: 2.5 mg, 10 mg

Mintezol® *see thiabendazole on page 462*

Minute-Gel® *see fluoride on page 201*

Miochol® *see acetylcholine chloride on page 6*

Miostat® Intraocular *see carbachol on page 72*

misoprostol (mye soe prost' ole)
Brand Names Cytotec®
Therapeutic Category Prostaglandin
Use Prevention of NSAID induced gastric ulcers
Usual Dosage Oral: 200 μg 4 times/day with food
Dosage Forms Tablet: 100 μg, 200 μg

Mithracin® *see plicamycin on page 381*

mithramycin *see plicamycin on page 381*

mitomycin (mye toe mye' sin)
Brand Names Mutamycin®
Synonyms mitomycin-C; MTC
Therapeutic Category Antineoplastic Agent, Antibiotic
Use Therapy of disseminated adenocarcinoma of stomach or pancreas in combination with other approved chemotherapeutic agents; bladder cancer
Usual Dosage Refer to individual protocols
Children and Adults (refer to individual protocols): I.V.: 10-20 mg/m^2/dose every 6-8 weeks, or 2 mg/m^2/day for 5 days, stop for 2 days then repeat; subsequent doses should be adjusted to platelet and leukocyte response.
Dosage Forms Powder for injection: 5 mg, 20 mg, 40 mg

mitomycin-C *see* mitomycin *on this page*

mitotane (mye' toe tane)
Brand Names Lysodren®
Synonyms o,p'-DDD
Therapeutic Category Antiadrenal Agent; Antineoplastic Agent, Miscellaneous
Use Treatment of inoperable adrenal cortical carcinoma
Usual Dosage Refer to individual protocols
Oral:
Children: 1-2 g/day in divided doses increasing gradually to a maximum of 5-7 g/day

Adults: Start at 1-6 g/day in divided doses, then increase incrementally to 8-10 g/day in 3-4 divided doses; dose is changed on basis of side effect with aim of giving as high a dose as tolerated; maximum daily dose: 18 g
Dosage Forms Tablet: 500 mg

mitoxantrone hydrochloride (mye toe zan' trone)
Brand Names Novantrone®
Synonyms DHAD
Therapeutic Category Antineoplastic Agent, Antibiotic; Antineoplastic Agent, Anthracycline
Use FDA approved for the treatment of acute nonlymphocytic leukemia (ANLL) in adults; mitoxantrone is also found to be very active against various leukemias, lymphoma, and breast cancer, and moderately active against pediatric sarcoma
Usual Dosage Refer to individual protocols
I.V.:
Leukemias:
Children ≤2 years: 0.4 mg/kg/day once daily for 3-5 days
Children >2 years and Adults: 8-12 mg/m^2/day once daily for 5 days or 12 mg/m^2/day once daily for 3 days

Solid tumors:
Children: 18-20 mg/m^2 every 3-4 weeks
Adults: 12-14 mg/m^2 every 3-4 weeks
Dosage Forms Injection, as base: 2 mg/mL (10 mL, 12.5 mL, 15 mL)

Mitran® Oral *see* chlordiazepoxide *on page 89*
Mitrolan® Chewable Tablet [OTC] *see* calcium polycarbophil *on page 69*
Mivacron® *see* mivacurium chloride *on this page*

mivacurium chloride (mye va kyoo' ree um)
Brand Names Mivacron®
Therapeutic Category Neuromuscular Blocker Agent, Nondepolarizing
Use Produces skeletal muscle relaxation during surgery after induction of general anesthesia, increases pulmonary compliance during assisted respiration, facilitates endotracheal intubation
(Continued)

mivacurium chloride *(Continued)*
Usual Dosage I.V.:
Children 2-12 years: 0.2 mg/kg over 5-15 seconds; continuous infusion: 14 µg/kg

Adults: Initial: 0.15 mg/kg administered over 5-15 seconds
Dosage Forms
Infusion, in D$_5$W: 0.5 mg/mL (50 mL)
Injection: 2 mg/mL (5 mL, 10 mL)

Mixtard® *see* insulin preparations *on page 250*
MMR *see* measles, mumps and rubella vaccines, combined *on page 287*
M-M-R® II *see* measles, mumps and rubella vaccines, combined *on page 287*
Moban® *see* molindone hydrochloride *on this page*
Moctanin® *see* monoctanoin *on next page*
Modane® [OTC] *see* phenolphthalein *on page 370*
Modane® Bulk [OTC] *see* psyllium *on page 407*
Modane® Plus [OTC] *see* docusate and phenolphthalein *on page 158*
Modane® Soft [OTC] *see* docusate *on page 157*
Modicon™ *see* ethinyl estradiol and norethindrone *on page 183*
modified Dakin's solution *see* sodium hypochlorite solution *on page 436*
modified Shohl's solution *see* sodium citrate and citric acid *on page 435*
Moducal® [OTC] *see* glucose polymers *on page 213*
Moduretic® *see* amiloride and hydrochlorothiazide *on page 18*
Moi-Stir® [OTC] *see* saliva substitute *on page 425*
1/6 molar sodium lactate *see* sodium lactate *on page 436*

molindone hydrochloride *(moe lin' done)*
Brand Names Moban®
Therapeutic Category Antipsychotic Agent
Use Management of psychotic disorder
Usual Dosage Oral: 50-75 mg/day; up to 225 mg/day
Dosage Forms
Concentrate, oral: 20 mg/mL (120 mL)
Tablet: 5 mg, 10 mg, 25 mg, 50 mg, 100 mg

Mol-Iron® [OTC] *see* ferrous sulfate *on page 194*
molybdenum injection *see* trace metals *on page 472*
Molypen® *see* trace metals *on page 472*
MOM *see* magnesium hydroxide *on page 282*

mometasone furoate *(moe met' a sone)*
Brand Names Elocon® Topical
Therapeutic Category Corticosteroid, Topical (Medium Potency)
Use Relief of inflammatory and pruritic manifestations of corticosteroid-responsive dermatoses
Usual Dosage Apply to area once daily, do not use occlusive dressings
Dosage Forms
Cream: 0.1% (15 g, 45 g)
Lotion: 0.1% (30 mL, 60 mL)
Ointment, topical: 0.1% (15 g, 45 g)

mom/mineral oil emulsion *see* magnesium hydroxide and mineral oil emulsion *on page 282*

monacolin K *see* lovastatin *on page 279*

Monilia **skin test** *see* Candida albicans (*Monilia*) *on page 70*

Monistat-Derm™ Topical *see* miconazole *on page 311*

Monistat i.v.™ Injection *see* miconazole *on page 311*

Monistat™ Vaginal *see* miconazole *on page 311*

Monocid® *see* cefonicid sodium *on page 80*

Monoclate-P® *see* antihemophilic factor *on page 29*

monoclonal antibody *see* muromonab-CD3 *on page 320*

monoctanoin (mon oh ock' ta noyn)
Brand Names Moctanin®
Synonyms monooctanoin
Therapeutic Category Gallstone Dissolution Agent
Use Solubilize cholesterol gallstones that are retained in the biliary tract after cholecystectomy
Usual Dosage Administer via T-tube into common bile duct at rate of 3-5 mL/hour at pressure of 10 mL water for 7-21 days
Dosage Forms Solution: 120 mL

Mono-Diff® *see* diagnostic aids (*in vitro*), blood *on page 137*

Monodox® Oral *see* doxycycline *on page 161*

Mono-Gesic® *see* salsalate *on page 425*

Monoket® *see* isosorbide mononitrate *on page 260*

Mono-Lisa® *see* diagnostic aids (*in vitro*), blood *on page 137*

Mononine® *see* factor ix complex (human) *on page 189*

monooctanoin *see* monoctanoin *on this page*

Monopril® *see* fosinopril *on page 206*

Monospot® *see* diagnostic aids (*in vitro*), blood *on page 137*

Monosticon® *see* diagnostic aids (*in vitro*), blood *on page 137*

Monosticon® Dri-Dot® *see* diagnostic aids (*in vitro*), blood *on page 137*

Mono-Sure® *see* diagnostic aids (*in vitro*), blood *on page 137*

Mono-Test® *see* diagnostic aids (*in vitro*), blood *on page 137*

8-MOP *see* methoxsalen *on page 302*

more attenuated enders strain *see* measles virus vaccine, live, attenuated *on page 287*

More-Dophilus® [OTC] *see* lactobacillus *on page 267*

moricizine hydrochloride (mor i' siz een)
Brand Names Ethmozine®
Therapeutic Category Antiarrhythmic Agent, Class I
Use Treatment of ventricular tachycardia and life-threatening ventricular arrhythmias; a Class I antiarrhythmic agent
Usual Dosage Adults: Oral: 200-300 mg every 8 hours, adjust dosage at 150 mg/day at 3-day intervals
Dosage Forms Tablet: 200 mg, 250 mg, 300 mg

morphine sulfate
Brand Names Astramorph™ PF Injection; Duramorph® Injection; MS Contin® Oral; MSIR® Oral; OMS® Oral; Oramorph SR™ Oral; RMS® Rectal; Roxanol™ Oral; Roxanol SR™ Oral
Synonyms MS
Therapeutic Category Analgesic, Narcotic
Use Relief of moderate to severe acute and chronic pain; pain of myocardial infarction; relieves dyspnea of acute left ventricular failure and pulmonary edema; preanesthetic medication
Usual Dosage Doses should be titrated to appropriate effect; when changing routes of administration in chronically treated patients, please note that oral doses are approximately $\frac{1}{6}$ as effective as parenteral dose

Infants and Children:
    Oral: Tablet and solution (prompt release): 0.2-0.5 mg/kg/dose every 4-6 hours as needed; tablet (controlled release): 0.3-0.6 mg/kg/dose every 12 hours
    I.M., I.V., S.C.: 0.1-0.2 mg/kg/dose every 2-4 hours as needed; usual maximum: 15 mg/dose; may initiate at 0.05 mg/kg/dose
    I.V., S.C. continuous infusion: Sickle cell or cancer pain: 0.025-2 mg/kg/hour; postoperative pain: 0.01-0.04 mg/kg/hour
    Sedation/analgesia for procedures: I.V.: 0.05-0.1 mg/kg 5 minutes before the procedure

Adolescents >12 years: Sedation/analgesia for procedures: I.V.: 3-4 mg and repeat in 5 minutes if necessary

Adults:
    Oral: Prompt release: 10-30 mg every 4 hours as needed; controlled release: 15-30 mg every 8-12 hours
    I.M., I.V., S.C.: 2.5-20 mg/dose every 2-6 hours as needed; usual: 10 mg/dose every 4 hours as needed
    I.V., S.C. continuous infusion: 0.8-10 mg/hour; may increase depending on pain relief/adverse effects; usual range up to 80 mg/hour
    Epidural: Initial: 5 mg in lumbar region; if inadequate pain relief within 1 hour, give 1-2 mg, maximum dose: 10 mg/24 hours
    Intrathecal ($\frac{1}{10}$ of epidural dose): 0.2-1 mg/dose; repeat doses **not** recommended
Dosage Forms
Injection: 0.5 mg/mL (10 mL); 1 mg/mL (10 mL, 30 mL, 60 mL); 2 mg/mL (1 mL, 2 mL, 60 mL); 3 mg/mL (50 mL); 4 mg/mL (1 mL, 2 mL); 5 mg/mL (1 mL, 30 mL); 8 mg/mL (1 mL, 2 mL); 10 mg/mL (1 mL, 2 mL, 10 mL); 15 mg/mL (1 mL, 2 mL, 20 mL)
Injection:
    Preservative free: 0.5 mg/mL (2 mL, 10 mL); 1 mg/mL (2 mL, 10 mL); 10 mg/mL (20 mL); 25 mg/mL (20 mL)
    I.V. via PCA pump: 1 mg/mL (10 mL, 30 mL, 60 mL); 5 mg/mL (30 mL)
    I.V. infusion preparation: 25 mg/mL (4 mL, 10 mL, 20 mL)
Solution, oral: 10 mg/5 mL (5 mL, 10 mL, 100 mL, 120 mL, 500 mL); 20 mg/5 mL (2.5 mL, 5 mL, 100 mL, 120 mL, 500 mL); 20 mg/mL (30 mL)
Suppository, rectal: 5 mg, 10 mg, 20 mg, 30 mg
Tablet: 15 mg, 30 mg
Tablet:
    Controlled release: 15 mg, 30 mg, 60 mg, 100 mg
    Soluble: 10 mg, 15 mg, 30 mg
    Sustained release: 30 mg, 60 mg, 100 mg

morrhuate sodium (mor' yoo ate)
Brand Names Scleromate®
Therapeutic Category Sclerosing Agent
Use Treatment of small, uncomplicated varicose veins of the lower extremities
Usual Dosage I.V.:
Children 1-18 years: Esophageal hemorrhage: 2, 3, or 4 mL of 5% solution repeated every 3-4 days until bleeding is controlled, then every 6 weeks until varices obliterated

Adults: 50-250 mg, repeated at 5- to 7-day intervals (50-100 mg for small veins, 150-250 mg for large veins)
Dosage Forms Injection: 50 mg/mL (5 mL)

Motofen® *see* difenoxin and atropine *on page 146*

Motrin® *see* ibuprofen *on page 245*

Motrin® IB [OTC] *see* ibuprofen *on page 245*

6-MP *see* mercaptopurine *on page 294*

M-Prednisol® Injection *see* methylprednisolone *on page 306*

M-R-VAX® II *see* measles and rubella vaccines, combined *on page 286*

MS *see* morphine sulfate *on previous page*

MS Contin® Oral *see* morphine sulfate *on previous page*

MSIR® Oral *see* morphine sulfate *on previous page*

MSTA *see* mumps skin test antigen *on this page*

MTC *see* mitomycin *on page 315*

M.T.E.-4® *see* trace metals *on page 472*

M.T.E.-5® *see* trace metals *on page 472*

M.T.E.-6® *see* trace metals *on page 472*

MTX *see* methotrexate *on page 301*

Mucomyst® *see* acetylcysteine *on page 6*

Mucoplex® [OTC] *see* vitamin B complex *on page 498*

Mucosol® *see* acetylcysteine *on page 6*

Multe-Pak-4® *see* trace metals *on page 472*

Multistix® [OTC] *see* diagnostic aids (*in vitro*), urine *on page 139*

Multitest CMI® *see* skin test antigens, multiple *on page 432*

multivitamins/fluoride *see* vitamin, multiple (pediatric) *on page 499*

Multi Vit® Drops [OTC] *see* vitamin, multiple (pediatric) *on page 499*

mumps, measles and rubella vaccines, combined *see* measles, mumps and rubella vaccines, combined *on page 287*

mumps skin test antigen

Synonyms MSTA

Therapeutic Category Diagnostic Agent, Skin Test

Use Assess the status of cell-mediated immunity

Usual Dosage Children and Adults: 0.1 mL intradermally into flexor surface of the forearm; examine reaction site in 24-48 hours; a positive reaction is ≥1.5 mm diameter induration

Dosage Forms Injection: 1 mL (10 tests)

Mumpsvax® *see* mumps virus vaccine, live, attenuated *on this page*

mumps virus vaccine, live, attenuated

Brand Names Mumpsvax®

Therapeutic Category Vaccine, Live Virus

Use Immunization against mumps in children ≥12 months and adults

Usual Dosage 1 vial (5000 units) S.C. in outer aspect of the upper arm

Dosage Forms Injection: Single dose

mupirocin (myoo peer' oh sin)

Brand Names Bactroban® Topical

Synonyms pseudomonic acid A

Therapeutic Category Antibiotic, Topical

Use Topical treatment of impetigo

Usual Dosage Children and Adults: Topical: Apply small amount 3 times/day for 5 days

Dosage Forms Ointment, topical: 2% (15 g)

Murine® Ear Drops [OTC] *see* carbamide peroxide *on page 73*

Murine® Plus Ophthalmic [OTC] *see* tetrahydrozoline hydrochloride *on page 459*

Muro 128® Ophthalmic [OTC] *see* sodium chloride *on page 434*

Murocoll-2® Ophthalmic *see* phenylephrine and scopolamine *on page 372*

muromonab-CD3 (myoo roe moe' nab)
Brand Names Orthoclone® OKT3
Synonyms monoclonal antibody; OKT3
Therapeutic Category Immunosuppressant Agent
Use Treatment of acute allograft rejection in renal transplant patients; effective in reversing acute hepatic, cardiac, and bone marrow transplant rejection episodes resistant to conventional treatment
Usual Dosage I.V. (refer to individual protocols):
Children <30 kg: 2.5 mg/day once daily for 10-14 days

Adults: 5 mg/day once daily for 10-14 days

Children and Adults: Methylprednisolone sodium succinate 1 mg/kg I.V. given prior to first muromonab-CD3 administration and I.V. hydrocortisone sodium succinate 50-100 mg given 30 minutes after administration are strongly recommended to decrease the incidence of reactions to the first dose; patient temperature should not exceed 37.8°C (100°F) at time of administration
Dosage Forms Injection: 5 mg/5 mL

Mus-Lac® *see* chlorzoxazone *on page 99*

Mustargen® Hydrochloride *see* mechlorethamine hydrochloride *on page 287*

mustine *see* mechlorethamine hydrochloride *on page 287*

Mutamycin® *see* mitomycin *on page 315*

M.V.C.® 9 + 3 *see* vitamin, multiple (injectable) *on page 499*

M.V.I.®-12 *see* vitamin, multiple (injectable) *on page 499*

M.V.I.® Concentrate *see* vitamin, multiple (injectable) *on page 499*

M.V.I.® Pediatric *see* vitamin, multiple (injectable) *on page 499*

Myambutol® *see* ethambutol hydrochloride *on page 181*

Myapap® Drops [OTC] *see* acetaminophen *on page 2*

Mycelex®-G Topical *see* clotrimazole *on page 109*

Mycelex®-G Vaginal [OTC] *see* clotrimazole *on page 109*

Mycelex® Troche *see* clotrimazole *on page 109*

Mycifradin® Sulfate Oral *see* neomycin sulfate *on page 330*

Mycifradin® Sulfate Topical *see* neomycin sulfate *on page 330*

Mycitracin® Topical [OTC] *see* bacitracin, neomycin, and polymyxin b *on page 43*

Mycobutin® Oral *see* rifabutin *on page 420*

Mycogen II Topical *see* nystatin and triamcinolone *on page 342*

Mycolog®-II Topical *see* nystatin and triamcinolone *on page 342*

Myconel® Topical *see* nystatin and triamcinolone *on page 342*

Mycostatin® Oral *see* nystatin *on page 341*

Mycostatin® Topical *see* nystatin *on page 341*

Mycostatin® Vaginal *see* nystatin *on page 341*

Mydfrin® Ophthalmic Solution *see* phenylephrine hydrochloride *on page 372*

Mydriacyl®️ Ophthalmic *see* tropicamide *on page 484*

Mykrox®️ *see* metolazone *on page 309*

Mylanta®️ [OTC] *see* aluminum hydroxide, magnesium hydroxide, and simethicone *on page 16*

Mylanta Gas®️ [OTC] *see* simethicone *on page 431*

Mylanta®️-II [OTC] *see* aluminum hydroxide, magnesium hydroxide, and simethicone *on page 16*

Myleran®️ *see* busulfan *on page 62*

Mylicon®️ [OTC] *see* simethicone *on page 431*

Mylosar®️ *see* azacitidine *on page 40*

Myminic®️ Expectorant [OTC] *see* guaifenesin and phenylpropanolamine *on page 219*

Myminic®️ Syrup [OTC] *see* chlorpheniramine and phenylpropanolamine *on page 93*

Myochrysine®️ Injection *see* gold sodium thiomalate *on page 215*

Myoflex®️ [OTC] *see* triethanolamine salicylate *on page 477*

Myotonachol™️ *see* bethanechol chloride *on page 53*

Myphetane DC®️ *see* brompheniramine, phenylpropanolamine, and codeine *on page 60*

Myphetapp®️ [OTC] *see* brompheniramine and phenylpropanolamine *on page 59*

Myprozine®️ Ophthalmic *see* natamycin *on page 326*

Mysoline®️ *see* primidone *on page 394*

Mytelase®️ Caplets®️ *see* ambenonium chloride *on page 17*

Mytrex®️ F Topical *see* nystatin and triamcinolone *on page 342*

Mytussin®️ [OTC] *see* guaifenesin *on page 217*

Mytussin®️ AC *see* guaifenesin and codeine *on page 218*

Mytussin®️ DAC *see* guaifenesin, pseudoephedrine, and codeine *on page 221*

Mytussin®️ DM [OTC] *see* guaifenesin and dextromethorphan *on page 218*

nabilone (na' bi lone)
Brand Names Cesamet®️
Therapeutic Category Antiemetic
Use Treat nausea and vomiting associated with cancer chemotherapy
Usual Dosage Oral:
Children >4 years:
<18 kg: 0.5 mg twice daily
18-30 kg: 1 mg twice daily
>30 kg: 1 mg 3 times/day

Adults: 1-2 mg twice daily beginning 1-3 hours before chemotherapy is administered and continuing around the clock until 1 dose after chemotherapy is completed; maximum daily dose: 6 mg divided in 3 doses
Dosage Forms Capsule: 1 mg

nabumetone (na byoo' me tone)
Brand Names Relafen®️
Therapeutic Category Nonsteroidal Anti-Inflammatory Agent (NSAID), Oral
Use Management of osteoarthritis and rheumatoid arthritis
Usual Dosage Adults: Oral: 1000 mg/day; an additional 500-1000 mg may be needed in some patients to obtain more symptomatic relief; may be administered once or twice daily
Dosage Forms Tablet: 500 mg, 750 mg

N-acetylcysteine *see* acetylcysteine *on page 6*
N-acetyl-L-cysteine *see* acetylcysteine *on page 6*
N-acetyl-P-aminophenol *see* acetaminophen *on page 2*
NaCl *see* sodium chloride *on page 434*

nadolol (nay doe' lole)
Brand Names Corgard®
Therapeutic Category Antianginal Agent; Beta-Adrenergic Blocker
Use Treatment of hypertension and angina pectoris; prevention of myocardial infarction; prophylaxis of migraine headaches
Usual Dosage Adults: Initial: 40 mg once daily; increase gradually; usual dosage: 40-80 mg/day; may need up to 240-320 mg/day; doses as high as 640 mg/day have been used
Dosage Forms Tablet: 20 mg, 40 mg, 80 mg, 120 mg, 160 mg

nafarelin acetate (naf' a re lin)
Brand Names Synarel®
Therapeutic Category Hormone, Posterior Pituitary; Luteinizing Hormone-Releasing Hormone Analog
Use Treatment of endometriosis, including pain and reduction of lesions
Usual Dosage Adults: 1 spray in 1 nostril each morning and evening for 6 months
Dosage Forms Solution, nasal: 2 mg/mL (10 mL)

Nafazair® Ophthalmic *see* naphazoline hydrochloride *on page 325*
Nafcil™ Injection *see* nafcillin sodium *on this page*

nafcillin sodium (naf sill' in)
Brand Names Nafcil™ Injection; Nallpen® Injection; Unipen® Injection; Unipen® Oral
Synonyms ethoxynaphthamido penicillin sodium; sodium nafcillin
Therapeutic Category Antibiotic, Penicillin
Use Treatment of susceptible bacterial infections such as osteomyelitis, septicemia, endocarditis, and CNS infections due to penicillinase-producing strains of *Staphylococcus*
Usual Dosage
Neonates: I.M., I.V.:
  0-4 weeks: <1200 g: 50 mg/kg/day in divided doses every 12 hours
  <7 days:
    1200-2000 g: 50 mg/kg/day in divided doses every 12 hours
    >2000 g: 60 mg/kg/day in divided doses every 8 hours
  >7 days:
    1200-2000 g: 75 mg/kg/day in divided doses every 8 hours
    >2000 g: 100 mg/kg/day in divided doses every 6 hours
Children: I.M., I.V.:
  Mild to moderate infections: 50-100 mg/kg/day in divided doses every 6 hours
  Severe infections: 100-200 mg/kg/day in divided doses every 4-6 hours
  Maximum dose: 12 g/day
  Oral: 50-100 mg/kg/day divided every 6 hours
Adults:
  Oral: 250-500 mg every 4-6 hours, up to 1 g every 4-6 hours for more severe infections
  I.M.: 500 mg every 4-6 hours
  I.V.: 500-2000 mg every 4-6 hours
Dosage Forms
Capsule: 250 mg
Powder for injection: 500 mg, 1 g, 2 g, 4 g, 10 g
Tablet: 500 mg

naftifine hydrochloride (naf' ti feen)
Brand Names Naftin® Topical
Therapeutic Category Antifungal Agent, Topical
Use Topical treatment of tinea cruris and tinea corporis
Usual Dosage Adults: Topical: Apply twice daily
Dosage Forms
Cream: 1% (15 g, 30 g, 60 g)
Gel, topical: 1% (20 g, 40 g, 60 g)

Naftin® Topical *see* naftifine hydrochloride *on this page*

NaHCO₃ *see* sodium bicarbonate *on page 434*

nalbuphine hydrochloride (nal' byoo feen)
Brand Names Nubain®
Therapeutic Category Analgesic, Narcotic
Use Relief of moderate to severe pain
Usual Dosage I.M., I.V., S.C.: 10 mg/70 kg every 3-6 hours
Dosage Forms Injection: 10 mg/mL (1 mL, 10 mL); 20 mg/mL (1 mL, 10 mL)

Naldecon® *see* chlorpheniramine, phenyltoloxamine, phenylpropanolamine, and phenylephrine *on page 96*

Naldecon® DX Adult Liquid [OTC] *see* guaifenesin, phenylpropanolamine, and dextromethorphan *on page 220*

Naldecon-EX® Children's Syrup [OTC] *see* guaifenesin and phenylpropanolamine *on page 219*

Naldecon® Senior DX [OTC] *see* guaifenesin and dextromethorphan *on page 218*

Naldecon® Senior EX [OTC] *see* guaifenesin *on page 217*

Naldelate® *see* chlorpheniramine, phenyltoloxamine, phenylpropanolamine, and phenylephrine *on page 96*

Nalfon® *see* fenoprofen calcium *on page 192*

Nalgest® *see* chlorpheniramine, phenyltoloxamine, phenylpropanolamine, and phenylephrine *on page 96*

nalidixic acid (nal i dix' ik)
Brand Names NegGram®
Synonyms nalidixinic acid
Therapeutic Category Antibiotic, Quinolone
Use Urinary tract infections
Usual Dosage Oral:
Children: 55 mg/kg/day divided every 6 hours; suppressive therapy is 33 mg/kg/day divided every 6 hours

Adults: 1 g 4 times/day for 2 weeks; then suppressive therapy of 500 mg 4 times/day
Dosage Forms
Suspension, oral (raspberry flavor): 250 mg/5 mL (473 mL)
Tablet: 250 mg, 500 mg, 1 g

nalidixinic acid *see* nalidixic acid *on this page*

Nallpen® Injection *see* nafcillin sodium *on previous page*

N-allylnoroxymorphone hydrochloride *see* naloxone hydrochloride *on next page*

naloxone hydrochloride (nal ox' one)
Brand Names Narcan® Injection
Synonyms N-allylnoroxymorphone hydrochloride
Therapeutic Category Antidote, Narcotic Agonist
Use Reverses CNS and respiratory depression in suspected narcotic overdose; neonatal opiate depression; coma of unknown etiology; used investigationally for shock, PCP and alcohol ingestion, and Alzheimer's disease
Usual Dosage I.M., I.V. (preferred), intratracheal, S.C. (give undiluted injection):
Neonates: Narcotic-induced asphyxia: 0.01-0.1 mg/kg every 2-3 minutes as needed; may need to repeat every 1-2 hours

Infants and Children: Postanesthesia narcotic reversal: 0.01 mg/kg; may repeat every 2-3 minutes as needed based on response

Opiate intoxication: Birth (including premature infants) to 5 years or <20 kg: 0.1 mg/kg; re-peat every 2-3 minutes if needed; may need to repeat doses every 20-60 minutes
>5 years or ≥20 kg: 2 mg/dose; if no response, repeat every 2-3 minutes; may need to repeat doses every 20-60 minutes

Children and Adults: Continuous infusion: I.V.: If continuous infusion is required, calculate dosage/hour based on effective intermittent dose used and duration of adequate re-sponse seen, titrate dose

Adults: 0.4-2 mg every 2-3 minutes as needed; may need to repeat doses every 20-60 min-utes; if no response is observed for a total of 10 mg, re-evaluate patient for possibility of a drug or disease process unresponsive to naloxone. **Note:** Use 0.1-0.2 mg increments in patients who are opioid dependent and in postoperative patients to avoid large cardio-vascular changes
Dosage Forms
Injection: 0.4 mg/mL (1 mL, 2 mL, 10 mL); 1 mg/mL (2 mL, 10 mL)
Injection, neonatal: 0.02 mg/mL (2 mL)

Nalspan® *see* chlorpheniramine, phenyltoloxamine, phenylpropanolamine, and phenylephrine *on page 96*

naltrexone hydrochloride (nal trex' one)
Brand Names Trexan™ Oral
Therapeutic Category Antidote, Narcotic Agonist
Use Adjunct to the maintenance of an opioid-free state in detoxified individual
Usual Dosage Do not give until patient is opioid-free for 7-10 days as required by urine analysis

Adults: Oral: 25 mg; if no withdrawal signs within 1 hour give another 25 mg; maintenance regimen is flexible, variable and individualized (50 mg/day to 100-150 mg 3 times/week)
Dosage Forms Tablet: 50 mg

Nandrobolic® Injection *see* nandrolone *on this page*

nandrolone (nan' droe lone)
Brand Names Anabolin® Injection; Androlone®-D Injection; Androlone® Injection; Deca-Durabolin® Injection; Durabolin® Injection; Hybolin™ Decanoate Injection; Hybolin™ Im-proved Injection; Nandrobolic® Injection; Neo-Durabolic Injection
Synonyms nandrolone decanoate; nandrolone phenpropionate
Therapeutic Category Androgen
Use Control of metastatic breast cancer; management of anemia of renal insufficiency
Usual Dosage
Children 2-13 years: 25-50 mg every 3-4 weeks

Adults:
Female: 50-100 mg/week

Male: 100-200 mg/week
Dosage Forms
Injection, as phenpropionate, in oil: 25 mg/mL (5 mL); 50 mg/mL (2 mL)
Injection, as decanoate, in oil: 50 mg/mL (1 mL, 2 mL); 100 mg/mL (1 mL, 2 mL); 200 mg/mL (1 mL)
Injection, repository, as decanoate: 50 mg/mL (2 mL); 100 mg/mL (2 mL); 200 mg/mL (2 mL)

nandrolone decanoate *see* nandrolone *on previous page*
nandrolone phenpropionate *see* nandrolone *on previous page*

naphazoline and antazoline
Brand Names Albalon-A® Ophthalmic; Antazoline-V® Ophthalmic; Vasocon-A® Ophthalmic
Therapeutic Category Ophthalmic Agent, Vasoconstrictor
Use Topical ocular congestion, irritation and itching
Usual Dosage Ophthalmic: 1-2 drops every 3-4 hours
Dosage Forms Solution: Naphazoline hydrochloride 0.05% and antazoline phosphate 0.5% (15 mL)

naphazoline and pheniramine
Brand Names Naphcon-A® Ophthalmic
Synonyms pheniramine and naphazoline
Therapeutic Category Ophthalmic Agent, Vasoconstrictor
Use Topical ocular vasoconstrictor
Usual Dosage Ophthalmic: 1-2 drops every 3-4 hours
Dosage Forms Solution, ophthalmic: Naphazoline hydrochloride 0.025% and pheniramine 0.3% (15 mL)

naphazoline hydrochloride (naf az' oh leen)
Brand Names AK-Con® Ophthalmic; Albalon® Liquifilm® Ophthalmic; Allerest® Eye Drops [OTC]; Clear Eyes® [OTC]; Comfort® Ophthalmic [OTC]; Degest® 2 Ophthalmic [OTC]; Estivin® II Ophthalmic [OTC]; I-Naphline® Ophthalmic; Nafazair® Ophthalmic; Naphcon Forte® Ophthalmic; Naphcon® Ophthalmic [OTC]; Opcon® Ophthalmic; Privine® Nasal [OTC]; VasoClear® Ophthalmic [OTC]; Vasocon Regular® Ophthalmic
Therapeutic Category Adrenergic Agonist Agent, Ophthalmic; Decongestant, Nasal; Nasal Agent, Vasoconstrictor; Ophthalmic Agent, Vasoconstrictor
Use Topical ocular vasoconstrictor; will temporarily relieve congestion, itching, and minor irritation, and to control hyperemia in patients with superficial corneal vascularity
Usual Dosage
Nasal:
Children:
<6 years: Not recommended (especially infants) due to CNS depression
6-12 years: 1 spray of 0.05% into each nostril, repeat in 3 hours if necessary
Children >12 years and Adults: 0.05%, instill 2 drops or sprays every 3-6 hours if needed; therapy should not exceed 3-5 days or more frequently than every 3 hours
Ophthalmic:
Children <6 years: Not recommended for use due to CNS depression (especially in infants)
Children >6 years and Adults: Instill 1-2 drops into conjunctival sac of affected eye(s) every 3-4 hours; therapy generally should not exceed 3-4 days
Dosage Forms Solution:
Nasal:
Drops: 0.05% (20 mL)
Spray: 0.05% (15 mL)
Ophthalmic: 0.012% (7.5 mL, 30 mL); 0.02% (15 mL); 0.03% (15 mL); 0.1% (15 mL)

Naphcon-A® Ophthalmic *see* naphazoline and pheniramine *on previous page*

Naphcon Forte® Ophthalmic *see* naphazoline hydrochloride *on previous page*

Naphcon® Ophthalmic [OTC] *see* naphazoline hydrochloride *on previous page*

Napril® [OTC] *see* chlorpheniramine and pseudoephedrine *on page 94*

Naprosyn® *see* naproxen *on this page*

naproxen (na prox' en)
Brand Names Aleve® [OTC]; Anaprox®; Naprosyn®
Synonyms naproxen sodium
Therapeutic Category Analgesic, Non-Narcotic; Anti-inflammatory Agent; Nonsteroidal Anti-Inflammatory Agent (NSAID), Oral
Use Management of inflammatory disease and rheumatoid disorders (including juvenile rheumatoid arthritis); acute gout; mild to moderate pain; dysmenorrhea; fever
Usual Dosage Oral (as naproxen):
  Children >2 years:
    Antipyretic or analgesic: 5-7 mg/kg/dose every 8-12 hours
    Juvenile rheumatoid arthritis: 10 mg/kg/day, up to a maximum of 1000 mg/day divided twice daily
  Adults:
    Rheumatoid arthritis, osteoarthritis, and ankylosing spondylitis: 500-1000 mg/day in 2 divided doses
    Mild to moderate pain or dysmenorrhea: Initial: 500 mg, then 250 mg every 6-8 hours; maximum: 1250 mg/day
Dosage Forms
  Suspension, oral (Naprosyn®): 125 mg/5 mL (480 mL)
  Tablet, as sodium (Anaprox®): 275 mg (250 mg base); 550 mg (500 mg base)
  Tablet:
    Aleve®: 200 mg
    Naprosyn®: 250 mg, 375 mg, 500 mg

naproxen sodium *see* naproxen *on this page*

Naqua® *see* trichlormethiazide *on page 476*

Narcan® Injection *see* naloxone hydrochloride *on page 324*

Nardil® *see* phenelzine sulfate *on page 368*

Nasacort® *see* triamcinolone *on page 474*

Nasahist B® Injection *see* brompheniramine maleate *on page 59*

Nasalcrom® Nasal Solution *see* cromolyn sodium *on page 118*

Nasalide® Nasal Aerosol *see* flunisolide *on page 199*

Natabec® [OTC] *see* vitamin, multiple (prenatal) *on page 499*

Natabec® FA [OTC] *see* vitamin, multiple (prenatal) *on page 499*

Natabec® Rx *see* vitamin, multiple (prenatal) *on page 499*

Natacyn® Ophthalmic *see* natamycin *on this page*

Natalins® [OTC] *see* vitamin, multiple (prenatal) *on page 499*

Natalins® Rx *see* vitamin, multiple (prenatal) *on page 499*

natamycin (na ta mye' sin)
Brand Names Myprozine® Ophthalmic; Natacyn® Ophthalmic
Synonyms pimaricin
Therapeutic Category Antifungal Agent, Ophthalmic
Use Treatment of blepharitis, conjunctivitis, and keratitis caused by susceptible fungi (*Aspergillus*, *Candida*), *Cephalosporium*, *Curvularia*, *Fusarium*, *Penicillium*, *Microsporum*,

Epidermophyton, Blastomyces dermatitidis, Coccidioides immitis, Cryptococcus neoformans, Histoplasma capsulatum, Sporothrix schenckii, Trichomonas vaginalis
Usual Dosage Adults: 1 drop in conjunctival sac every 1-2 hours, after 3-4 days dose may be reduced to one drop 6-8 times/day; usual course of therapy: 2-3 weeks
Dosage Forms Suspension, ophthalmic: 5% (15 mL)

natural lung surfactant *see beractant on page 51*
Naturetin® *see bendroflumethiazide on page 47*
Naus-A-Way® [OTC] *see phosphorated carbohydrate solution on page 375*
Nausetrol® [OTC] *see phosphorated carbohydrate solution on page 375*
Navane® *see thiothixene on page 466*
N D Clear® *see chlorpheniramine and pseudoephedrine on page 94*
ND-Stat® Injection *see brompheniramine maleate on page 59*
Nebcin® Injection *see tobramycin on page 469*
NebuPent™ Inhalation *see pentamidine isethionate on page 363*

nedocromil sodium (ne doe kroe' mil)
Brand Names Tilade® Inhalation Aerosol
Therapeutic Category Antiasthmatic; Antihistamine, Inhalation
Use Maintenance therapy in patients with mild to moderate bronchial asthma
Usual Dosage Adults: Inhalation: 2 inhalations 4 times daily
Dosage Forms Aerosol: 1.75 mg/activation (16.2 g)

N.E.E.® 1/35 *see ethinyl estradiol and norethindrone on page 183*
NegGram® *see nalidixic acid on page 323*
Neisseria gonorrhoeae *see diagnostic aids (in vitro), other on page 138*
Nelova™ *see ethinyl estradiol and norethindrone on page 183*
Nembutal® *see pentobarbital on page 364*
Neo-Calglucon® [OTC] *see calcium glubionate on page 67*
Neocidin® Ophthalmic Solution *see neomycin, polymyxin b, and gramicidin on page 329*
Neo-Cortef® Ophthalmic *see neomycin and hydrocortisone on next page*
Neo-Cortef® Topical *see neomycin and hydrocortisone on next page*
NeoDecadron® Ophthalmic *see neomycin and dexamethasone on this page*
NeoDecadron® Topical *see neomycin and dexamethasone on this page*
Neo-Durabolic Injection *see nandrolone on page 324*
Neofed® [OTC] *see pseudoephedrine on page 406*
Neo-fradin® Oral *see neomycin sulfate on page 330*
Neoloid® [OTC] *see castor oil on page 77*
Neomixin® Topical *see bacitracin, neomycin, and polymyxin b on page 43*

neomycin and dexamethasone
Brand Names NeoDecadron® Ophthalmic; NeoDecadron® Topical
Synonyms dexamethasone and neomycin
Therapeutic Category Antibiotic, Ophthalmic; Corticosteroid, Ophthalmic
Use Treatment of steroid responsive inflammatory conditions of the palpebral and bulbar conjunctiva, lid, cornea, and anterior segment of the globe
(Continued)

neomycin and dexamethasone *(Continued)*

Usual Dosage Apply thin coat 3-4 times/day until favorable response is observed, then reduce dose to one application/day

Dosage Forms

Cream: Neomycin sulfate 0.5% [5 mg/g] and dexamethasone 0.1% [1 mg/g] (15 g, 30 g)

Ointment, ophthalmic: Neomycin sulfate 0.35% [3.5 mg/g] and dexamethasone 0.05% [0.5 mg/g] (3.5 g)

Solution, ophthalmic: Neomycin sulfate 0.35% [3.5 mg/mL] and dexamethasone 0.1% [1 mg/mL] (15 mL)

neomycin and fluocinolone

Brand Names Neo-Synalar® Topical

Therapeutic Category Antibiotic, Topical; Corticosteroid, Topical (Medium Potency)

Use Treatment of corticosteroid-responsive dermatoses with secondary infection

Usual Dosage Topical: Apply to area in a thin film 2-4 times/day

Dosage Forms Cream: Neomycin sulfate 0.5% and fluocinolone acetonide 0.025% (15 g, 30 g, 60 g)

neomycin and hydrocortisone

Brand Names Neo-Cortef® Ophthalmic; Neo-Cortef® Topical

Therapeutic Category Antibiotic, Topical; Corticosteroid, Topical (Low Potency)

Use Treatment of susceptible topical bacterial infections with associated inflammation

Usual Dosage Topical: Apply to area in a thin film 2-4 times/day

Dosage Forms

Cream: Neomycin sulfate 0.5% and hydrocortisone 1% (20 g)

Ointment, topical: Neomycin sulfate 0.5% and hydrocortisone 0.5% (20 g); neomycin sulfate 0.5% and hydrocortisone 1% (20 g)

Solution, ophthalmic: Neomycin sulfate 0.5% and hydrocortisone 0.5% (5 mL)

neomycin and polymyxin b

Brand Names Neosporin® Cream [OTC]; Neosporin® G.U. Irrigant

Synonyms polymyxin b and neomycin

Therapeutic Category Antibiotic, Urinary Irrigation; Antibiotic, Topical

Use Short-term use as a continuous irrigant or rinse in the urinary bladder to prevent bacteriuria and gram-negative rod septicemia associated with the use of indwelling catheters; to help prevent infection in minor cuts, scrapes, and burns

Usual Dosage Children and Adults:

Topical: Apply cream 2-4 times/day

Bladder irrigation: Continuous irrigant or rinse in the urinary bladder for up to 10 days where 1 mL is added to 1 L of normal saline with administration rate adjusted to patient's urine output; usually no more than 1 L of irrigant is used per day

Dosage Forms

Cream: Neomycin sulfate 3.5 mg and polymyxin b sulfate 10,000 units per g (0.94 g, 15 g)

Solution, irrigant: Neomycin sulfate 40 mg and polymyxin b sulfate 200,000 units per mL (1 mL, 20 mL)

neomycin, polymyxin b, and dexamethasone

Brand Names AK-Trol® Ophthalmic; Dexacidin® Ophthalmic; Dexasporin® Ophthalmic; Infectrol® Ophthalmic; Maxitrol® Ophthalmic; Ocu-Trol® Ophthalmic

Therapeutic Category Antibiotic, Ophthalmic

Use Steroid-responsive inflammatory ocular conditions in which a corticosteroid is indicated and where bacterial infection or a risk of bacterial infection exists

Usual Dosage Children and Adults: Ophthalmic:

Ointment: Place a small amount ($\sim\frac{1}{2}$") in the affected eye 3-4 times/day or apply at bedtime as an adjunct with drops

Solution: Instill 1-2 drops into affected eye(s) every 4-6 hours; in severe disease drops may be used hourly and tapered to discontinuation

Dosage Forms
Ointment, ophthalmic: Neomycin sulfate 3.5 mg, polymyxin b sulfate 10,000 units, and dexamethasone 0.1% per g (3.5 g)
Suspension, ophthalmic: Neomycin sulfate 3.5 mg, polymyxin b sulfate 10,000 units, and dexamethasone 0.1% per mL (5 mL)

neomycin, polymyxin b, and gramicidin
Brand Names AK-Spore® Ophthalmic Solution; Neocidin® Ophthalmic Solution; Neosporin® Ophthalmic Solution; Neotricin® Ophthalmic Solution; Ocu-Spor-G® Ophthalmic Solution; Ocutricin® Ophthalmic Solution; Tri-Thalmic® Ophthalmic Solution
Therapeutic Category Antibiotic, Ophthalmic
Use Treatment of superficial ocular infection, infection prophylaxis in minor skin abrasions
Usual Dosage Ophthalmic: Drops: 1-2 drops 4-6 times/day or more frequently as required for severe infections
Dosage Forms Solution, ophthalmic: Polymyxin b sulfate 10,000 units, neomycin sulfate 1.75 mg, and gramicidin 0.025 mg per mL (1 mL, 2 mL, 10 mL)

neomycin, polymyxin b, and hydrocortisone
Brand Names AK-Spore H.C.® Otic; AntibiOtic® Otic; Bacticort® Otic; Cortatrigen® Otic; Cortisporin® Ophthalmic Suspension; Cortisporin® Otic; Cortisporin® Topical Cream; Drotic® Otic; LazerSporin-C® Otic; Octicair® Otic; Ocutricin® HC Otic; Otocort® Otic; Otomycin-HPN® Otic; Otosporin® Otic; PediOtic® Otic
Therapeutic Category Antibiotic, Ophthalmic; Antibiotic, Otic; Antibiotic, Topical; Corticosteroid, Ophthalmic; Corticosteroid, Otic; Corticosteroid, Topical (Low Potency)
Use Treatment of topical bacterial infections caused by susceptible bacteria and when the use of an anti-inflammatory is indicated
Usual Dosage Duration of use should be limited to 10 days unless otherwise directed by the physician

Adults and Children: Ophthalmic:
Ointment: Apply to the affected eye every 3-4 hours
Suspension: 1 drop every 3-4 hours

Children: Otic: Solution and suspension: 3 drops into affected ear 3-4 times/day

Adults: Otic: Solution and suspension: 4 drops into affected ear 3-4 times/day

Dosage Forms
Cream, topical: Neomycin sulfate 5 mg, polymyxin b sulfate 10,000 units, and hydrocortisone 10 mg per mL (7.5 g)
Solution, otic: Neomycin sulfate 5 mg, polymyxin b sulfate 10,000 units, and hydrocortisone 10 mg per mL (10 mL)
Suspension:
Ophthalmic: Neomycin sulfate 5 mg, polymyxin b sulfate 10,000 units, and hydrocortisone 10 mg per mL (7.5 mL)
Otic: Neomycin sulfate 5 mg, polymyxin b sulfate 10,000 units, and hydrocortisone 10 mg per mL (10 mL)

neomycin, polymyxin b, and prednisolone
Brand Names Poly-Pred® Liquifilm® Ophthalmic
Therapeutic Category Antibiotic, Ophthalmic; Corticosteroid, Ophthalmic
Use Steroid-responsive inflammatory ocular condition in which bacterial infection or a risk of bacterial ocular infection exists
Usual Dosage Children and Adults: Ophthalmic: Instill 1-2 drops every 3-4 hours; acute infections may require every 30-minute instillation initially with frequency of administration reduced as the infection is brought under control. To treat the lids: Instill 1-2 drops every 3-4 hours, close the eye and rub the excess on the lids and lid margins.
(Continued)

neomycin, polymyxin b, and prednisolone *(Continued)*
Dosage Forms Suspension: Neomycin sulfate 0.35%, polymyxin b sulfate 10,000 units, and prednisolone acetate 0.5% per mL (5 mL, 10 mL)

neomycin sulfate *(nee oh mye' sin)*
Brand Names Mycifradin® Sulfate Oral; Mycifradin® Sulfate Topical; Neo-fradin® Oral; Neo-Tabs® Oral
Therapeutic Category Ammonium Detoxicant; Antibiotic, Aminoglycoside; Antibiotic, Topical
Use Given orally to prepare GI tract for surgery; treat minor skin infections; treat diarrhea caused by *E. coli*; adjunct in the treatment of hepatic encephalopathy
Usual Dosage
Neonates: Oral: Necrotizing enterocolitis: 50-100 mg/kg/day divided every 6 hours

Children: Oral:
Preoperative intestinal antisepsis: 90 mg/kg/day divided every 4 hours for 2 days; or 25 mg/kg at 1 PM, 2 PM, and 11 PM on the day preceding surgery as an adjunct to mechanical cleansing of the intestine and in combination with erythromycin base
Hepatic coma: 50-100 mg/kg/day in divided doses every 6-8 hours or 2.5-7 g/m^2/day divided every 4-6 hours for 5-6 days not to exceed 12 g/day

Children and Adults: Topical: Apply ointment 1-4 times/day; topical solutions containing 0.1% to 1% neomycin have been used for irrigation

Adults: Oral:
Preoperative intestinal antisepsis: 1 g each hour for 4 doses then 1 g every 4 hours for 5 doses; or 1 g at 1 PM, 2 PM, and 11 PM on day preceding surgery as an adjunct to mechanical cleansing of the bowel and oral erythromycin; or 6 g/day divided every 4 hours for 2-3 days
Hepatic coma: 500-2000 mg every 6-8 hours or 4-12 g/day divided every 4-6 hours for 5-6 days
Chronic hepatic insufficiency: Oral: 4 g/day for an indefinite period
Dosage Forms
Cream: 0.5% (15 g)
Injection: 500 mg
Ointment, topical: 0.5% (15 g, 30 g, 120 g)
Solution, oral: 125 mg/5 mL (480 mL)
Tablet: 500 mg

neonatal trace metals *see* trace metals *on page 472*
Neopap® [OTC] *see* acetaminophen *on page 2*
Neoquess® Injection *see* dicyclomine hydrochloride *on page 145*
Neoquess® Oral Tablet *see* hyoscyamine sulfate *on page 243*
Neosar® Injection *see* cyclophosphamide *on page 121*
Neosporin® Cream [OTC] *see* neomycin and polymyxin b *on page 328*
Neosporin® G.U. Irrigant *see* neomycin and polymyxin b *on page 328*
Neosporin® Ophthalmic Ointment *see* bacitracin, neomycin, and polymyxin b *on page 43*
Neosporin® Ophthalmic Solution *see* neomycin, polymyxin b, and gramicidin *on previous page*
Neosporin® Topical Ointment [OTC] *see* bacitracin, neomycin, and polymyxin b *on page 43*

neostigmine *(nee oh stig' meen)*
Brand Names Prostigmin® Injection; Prostigmin® Oral
Synonyms neostigmine bromide; neostigmine methylsulfate
Therapeutic Category Antidote, Neuromuscular Blocking Agent; Cholinergic Agent; Diagnostic Agent, Myasthenia Gravis

Use Treatment of myasthenia gravis and to prevent and treat postoperative bladder distention and urinary retention; reversal of the effects of nondepolarizing neuromuscular blocking agents after surgery

Usual Dosage

Myasthenia gravis: Diagnosis: I.M.:
  Children: 0.04 mg/kg as a single dose
  Adults: 0.02 mg/kg as a single dose

Myasthenia gravis: Treatment:
  Children:
    I.M., I.V., S.C.: 0.01-.04 mg/kg every 2-4 hours
    Oral: 2 mg/kg/day divided every 3-4 hours
  Adults:
    I.M., I.V., S.C.: 0.5-2.5 mg every 1-3 hours
    Oral: 15 mg/dose every 3-4 hours

Reversal of nondepolarizing neuromuscular blockade after surgery in conjunction with atropine or glycopyrrolate: I.V.:
  Infants: 0.025-0.1 mg/kg/dose
  Children: 0.025-0.08 mg/kg/dose
  Adults: 0.5-2.5 mg; total dose not to exceed 5 mg

Bladder atony: Adults: I.M., S.C.:
  Prevention: 0.25 mg every 4-6 hours for 2-3 days
  Treatment: 0.5-1 mg every 3 hours for 5 doses after bladder has emptied

Dosage Forms
Injection, as methylsulfate: 0.25 mg/mL (1 mL); 0.5 mg/mL (1 mL, 10 mL); 1 mg/mL (10 mL)
Tablet, as bromide: 15 mg

neostigmine bromide *see* neostigmine *on previous page*

neostigmine methylsulfate *see* neostigmine *on previous page*

Neo-Synalar® Topical *see* neomycin and fluocinolone *on page 328*

Neo-Synephrine® 12 Hour Nasal Solution [OTC] *see* oxymetazoline hydrochloride *on page 350*

Neo-Synephrine® Nasal Solution [OTC] *see* phenylephrine hydrochloride *on page 372*

Neo-Synephrine® Ophthalmic Solution *see* phenylephrine hydrochloride *on page 372*

Neo-Tabs® Oral *see* neomycin sulfate *on previous page*

Neothylline® *see* dyphylline *on page 165*

Neotrace-4® *see* trace metals *on page 472*

Neotricin® Ophthalmic Solution *see* neomycin, polymyxin b, and gramicidin *on page 329*

NeoVadrin® [OTC] *see* vitamin, multiple (prenatal) *on page 499*

NeoVadrin® B Complex [OTC] *see* vitamin B complex *on page 498*

Nephro-Calci® [OTC] *see* calcium carbonate *on page 65*

Nephrocaps® [OTC] *see* vitamin B complex with vitamin C and folic acid *on page 498*

Nephro-Fer™ [OTC] *see* ferrous fumarate *on page 193*

Nephron® Inhalation Solution [OTC] *see* epinephrine *on page 171*

Nephrox Suspension [OTC] *see* aluminum hydroxide *on page 15*

Neptazane® *see* methazolamide *on page 299*

Nervocaine® Injection *see* lidocaine hydrochloride *on page 273*

Nesacaine® *see* chloroprocaine hydrochloride *on page 91*

Nesacaine®-MPF *see* chloroprocaine hydrochloride *on page 91*

Nestrex® *see* pyridoxine hydrochloride *on page 409*

1-*N*-ethyl sisomicin *see* netilmicin sulfate *on this page*

netilmicin sulfate (ne til mye' sin)
Brand Names Netromycin® Injection
Synonyms 1-*N*-ethyl sisomicin
Therapeutic Category Antibiotic, Aminoglycoside
Use Short-term treatment of serious or life-threatening infections including septicemia, peritonitis, intra-abdominal abscess, lower respiratory tract infections, urinary tract infections, skin, bone and joint infections caused by sensitive *Pseudomonas aeruginosa*, *Escherichia coli*, *Proteus*, *Klebsiella*, *Serratia*, *Enterobacter*, *Citrobacter*, and *Staphylococcus*
Usual Dosage I.M., I.V.:

Neonates <6 weeks: 2-3.25 mg/kg/dose every 12 hours

Children 6 weeks to 12 years: 1-2.5 mg/kg/dose every 8 hours

Children >12 years and Adults: 1.5-2 mg/kg/dose every 8-12 hours
Dosage Forms
Injection: 100 mg/mL (1.5 mL)
Injection:
   Neonatal: 10 mg/mL (2 mL)
   Pediatric: 25 mg/mL (2 mL)

Netromycin® Injection *see* netilmicin sulfate *on this page*

Neupogen® Injection *see* filgrastim *on page 195*

Neuramate® *see* meprobamate *on page 293*

Neut® Injection *see* sodium bicarbonate *on page 434*

Neutra-Phos® *see* potassium phosphate and sodium phosphate *on page 388*

Neutra-Phos®-K *see* potassium phosphate *on page 388*

Neutrexin™ Injection *see* trimetrexate glucuronate *on page 480*

Neutrogena® T/Derm *see* coal tar *on page 110*

New Decongestant® *see* chlorpheniramine, phenyltoloxamine, phenylpropanolamine, and phenylephrine *on page 96*

NGT® Topical *see* nystatin and triamcinolone *on page 342*

Niac® [OTC] *see* niacin *on this page*

Niacels™ [OTC] *see* niacin *on this page*

niacin (nye' a sin)
Brand Names Niac® [OTC]; Niacels™ [OTC]; Nicobid® [OTC]; Nicolar® [OTC]; Nicotinex [OTC]; Slo-Niacin® [OTC]
Synonyms nicotinic acid; vitamin B_3
Therapeutic Category Antilipemic Agent; Vitamin, Water Soluble
Use Adjunctive treatment of hyperlipidemias; peripheral vascular disease and circulatory disorders; treatment of pellagra; dietary supplement
Usual Dosage
Children: Pellagra: Oral, I.M., I.V.: 50-100 mg/dose 3 times/day
   Oral: Recommended daily allowances:
      0-1 year: 6-8 mg/day
      2-6 years: 9-11 mg/day
      7-10 years: 16 mg/day
      >10 years: 15-18 mg/day

Adults: Oral:
Hyperlipidemia: 1.5-6 g/day in 3 divided doses with or after meals
Pellagra: 50 mg 3-10 times/day, maximum: 500 mg/day
Niacin deficiency: 10-20 mg/day, maximum: 100 mg/day
Dosage Forms
Capsule, timed release: 125 mg, 250 mg, 300 mg, 400 mg, 500 mg
Elixir: 50 mg/5 mL (473 mL, 4000 mL)
Injection: 100 mg/mL (30 mL)
Tablet: 25 mg, 50 mg, 100 mg, 250 mg, 500 mg
Tablet, timed release: 150 mg, 250 mg, 500 mg, 750 mg

niacinamide (nye a sin' a mide)
Synonyms nicotinamide
Therapeutic Category Vitamin, Water Soluble
Use Prophylaxis and treatment of pellagra
Usual Dosage Oral:
Children: Pellagra: 100-300 mg/day

Adults: 50 mg 3-10 times/day
Pellagra: 300-500 mg/day
Hyperlipidemias: 1-2 g 3 times/day
Dosage Forms Tablet: 50 mg, 100 mg, 125 mg, 250 mg, 500 mg

nicardipine hydrochloride (nye kar' de peen)
Brand Names Cardene®; Cardene® SR
Therapeutic Category Antianginal Agent; Calcium Channel Blocker
Use Chronic stable angina; management of essential hypertension
Usual Dosage Adults:
Oral: 40 mg 3 times/day (allow 3 days between dose increases)
Oral, sustained release: Initial: 30 mg twice daily, titrate up to 60 mg twice daily
I.V.: (Dilute to 0.1 mg/mL) Initial: 5 mg/hour increased by 2.5 mg/hour every 15 minutes to
a maximum of 15 mg/hour
Oral to I.V. dose:
20 mg every 8 hours = I.V. 0.5 mg/hour
30 mg every 8 hours = I.V. 1.2 mg/hour
40 mg every 8 hours = I.V. 2.2 mg/hour
Dosage Forms
Capsule: 20 mg, 30 mg
Capsule, sustained release: 30 mg, 45 mg, 60 mg
Injection: 2.5 mg/mL (10 mL)

Niclocide® see niclosamide *on this page*

niclosamide (ni kloe' sa mide)
Brand Names Niclocide®
Therapeutic Category Anthelmintic
Use Treatment of intestinal beef, fish, and dwarf tapeworm infections
Usual Dosage Oral:
Beef and fish tapeworm:
Children:
11-34 kg: 1 g as a single dose
>34 kg: 1.5 g as a single dose
Adults: 2 g (4 tablets) in a single dose

Dwarf tapeworm:
Children:
11-34 kg: 1 g chewed thoroughly in a single dose the first day, then 0.5 g/day for next
6 days
(Continued)

niclosamide *(Continued)*

>34 kg: 1.5 g in a single dose the first day, then 1 g/day for 6 days
Adults: 2 g in a single daily dose for 7 days
Dosage Forms Tablet, chewable (vanilla flavor): 500 mg

Nicobid® [OTC] *see niacin on page 332*
Nicoderm® Patch *see nicotine on this page*
Nicolar® [OTC] *see niacin on page 332*
Nicorette® DS Gum *see nicotine on this page*
Nicorette® Gum *see nicotine on this page*
nicotinamide *see niacinamide on previous page*

nicotine *(nik oh teen')*
Brand Names Habitrol™ Patch; Nicoderm® Patch; Nicorette® DS Gum; Nicorette® Gum; Nicotrol® Patch; ProStep® Patch
Therapeutic Category Smoking Deterrent
Use Treatment aid to giving up smoking while participating in a behavioral modification program, under medical supervision
Usual Dosage
Gum: Chew 1 piece of gum when urge to smoke, up to 30 pieces/day; most patients require 10-12 pieces of gum/day
Transdermal patches: Apply new patch every 24 hours to nonhairy, clean, dry skin on the upper body or upper outer arm; each patch should be applied to a different site; start with the 21 mg/day or 22 mg/day patch, except those patients with stable coronary artery disease should start with 14 mg/day; most patients the dosage can be reduced after 6-8 weeks; progressively lower doses are used every 2 weeks, with complete nicotine elimination achieved after 10 weeks
Dosage Forms
Patch, transdermal:
Habitrol™: 21 mg/day; 14 mg/day; 7 mg/day (30 systems/box)
Nicoderm®: 21 mg/day; 14 mg/day; 7 mg/day (14 systems/box)
ProStep®: 22 mg/day; 11 mg/day (7 systems/box)
Pieces, chewing gum, as polacrilex: 2 mg/square (96 pieces/box); 4 mg/square (96 pieces/box)

Nicotinex [OTC] *see niacin on page 332*
nicotinic acid *see niacin on page 332*
Nicotrol® Patch *see nicotine on this page*
Nico-Vert® Oral *see dimenhydrinate on page 150*
Nidryl® Oral [OTC] *see diphenhydramine hydrochloride on page 152*

nifedipine *(nye fed' i peen)*
Brand Names Adalat®; Adalat® CC; Procardia®; Procardia XL®
Therapeutic Category Antianginal Agent; Calcium Channel Blocker
Use Angina, hypertrophic cardiomyopathy, hypertension (sustained release only)
Usual Dosage
Children: Oral, S.L.:
Hypertensive emergencies: 0.25-0.5 mg/kg/dose
Hypertrophic cardiomyopathy: 0.6-0.9 mg/kg/24 hours in 3-4 divided doses
Adults: Initial: 10 mg 3 times/day as capsules or 30-60 mg once daily as sustained release tablet; maintenance: 10-30 mg 3-4 times/day (capsules); maximum: 180 mg/24 hours (capsules) or 120 mg/day (sustained release)

Dosage Forms
Capsule, liquid-filled (Adalat®, Procardia®): 10 mg, 20 mg
Tablet, extended release (Adalat® CC): 30 mg, 60 mg, 90 mg
Tablet, sustained release (Procardia XL®): 30 mg, 60 mg, 90 mg

Niferex® [OTC] *see polysaccharide-iron complex on page 384*
Niferex®-PN *see vitamin, multiple (prenatal) on page 499*
Niloric® *see ergoloid mesylates on page 173*
Nilstat® Oral *see nystatin on page 341*
Nilstat® Topical *see nystatin on page 341*
Nilstat® Vaginal *see nystatin on page 341*
Nimbus® *see diagnostic aids (in vitro), urine on page 139*
Nimbus® II *see diagnostic aids (in vitro), urine on page 139*

nimodipine (nye moe' di peen)
Brand Names Nimotop®
Therapeutic Category Calcium Channel Blocker
Use Improvement of neurological deficits due to spasm following subarachnoid hemorrhage from ruptured congenital intracranial aneurysms who are in good neurological condition postictus
Usual Dosage Adults: Oral: 60 mg every 4 hours for 21 days, start therapy within 96 hours after subarachnoid hemorrhage
Dosage Forms Capsule, liquid-filled: 30 mg

Nimotop® *see nimodipine on this page*
Nipent™ Injection *see pentostatin on page 365*
Nipride® *see nitroprusside sodium on page 337*
Nitro-Bid® I.V. Injection *see nitroglycerin on next page*
Nitro-Bid® Ointment *see nitroglycerin on next page*
Nitro-Bid® Oral *see nitroglycerin on next page*
Nitrocine® Oral *see nitroglycerin on next page*
Nitrodisc® Patch *see nitroglycerin on next page*
Nitro-Dur® Patch *see nitroglycerin on next page*
nitrofural *see nitrofurazone on next page*

nitrofurantoin (nye troe fyoor an' toyn)
Brand Names Furadantin®; Furalan®; Furan®; Furanite®; Macrobid®; Macrodantin®
Therapeutic Category Antibiotic, Miscellaneous
Use Prevention and treatment of urinary tract infections caused by susceptible gram-negative and some gram-positive organisms; *Pseudomonas*, *Serratia*, and most species of *Proteus* are generally resistant to nitrofurantoin
Usual Dosage Oral:
Children >1 month: 5-7 mg/kg/day divided every 6 hours; maximum: 400 mg/day
Chronic therapy: 1-2 mg/kg/day in divided doses every 12-24 hours; maximum dose: 400 mg/day
Adults: 50-100 mg/dose every 6 hours (not to exceed 400 mg/24 hours)
Prophylaxis: 50-100 mg/dose at bedtime
Dosage Forms
Capsule: 50 mg, 100 mg
Capsule:
Macrocrystal: 25 mg, 50 mg, 100 mg
(Continued)
335

nitrofurantoin *(Continued)*
Macrocrystal/monohydrate: 100 mg
Suspension, oral: 25 mg/5 mL (470 mL)
Tablet: 50 mg, 100 mg

nitrofurazone (nye troe fyoor' a zone)
Brand Names Furacin® Topical
Synonyms nitrofural
Therapeutic Category Antibacterial, Topical
Use Antibacterial agent used in second and third degree burns and skin grafting
Usual Dosage Children and Adults: Topical: Apply once daily or every few days to lesion or place on gauze
Dosage Forms
Cream: 0.2% (4 g, 28 g)
Powder, topical: 0.2% (14 g)
Soluble dressing, topical: 0.2% (28 g, 56 g, 454 g, 480 g)

Nitrogard® Buccal *see* nitroglycerin *on this page*

nitrogen mustard *see* mechlorethamine hydrochloride *on page 287*

nitroglycerin (nye troe gli' ser in)
Brand Names Deponit® Patch; Minitran® Patch; Nitro-Bid® I.V. Injection; Nitro-Bid® Ointment; Nitro-Bid® Oral; Nitrocine® Oral; Nitrodisc® Patch; Nitro-Dur® Patch; Nitrogard® Buccal; Nitroglyn® Oral; Nitrolingual® Translingual Spray; Nitrol® Ointment; Nitrong® Oral Tablet; Nitrostat® Sublingual; Transdermal-NTG® Patch; Transderm-Nitro® Patch; Tridil® Injection
Synonyms glyceryl trinitrate; nitroglycerol; NTG
Therapeutic Category Antianginal Agent; Nitrate; Vasodilator, Coronary
Use Angina pectoris; I.V. for congestive heart failure (especially when associated with acute myocardial infarction); pulmonary hypertension; hypertensive emergencies occurring perioperatively (especially during cardiovascular surgery)
Usual Dosage Note: Hemodynamic and antianginal tolerance often develops within 24-48 hours of continuous nitrate administration

Children: Pulmonary hypertension: Continuous infusion: Start 0.25-0.5 μg/kg/minute and titrate by 1 μg/kg/minute at 20- to 60-minute intervals to desired effect; usual dose: 1-3 μg/kg/minute; maximum: 5 μg/kg/minute

Adults:
Oral: 2.5-9 mg 2-4 times/day (up to 26 mg 4 times/day)
I.V.: 5 μg/minute, increase by 5 μg/minute every 3-5 minutes to 20 μg/minute; if no response at 20 μg/minute increase by 10 μg/minute every 3-5 minutes, up to 200 μg/minute
Sublingual: 0.2-0.6 mg every 5 minutes for maximum of 3 doses in 15 minutes; may also use prophylactically 5-10 minutes prior to activities which may provoke an attack
Ointment: 1" to 2" every 8 hours up to 4" to 5" every 4 hours
Patch, transdermal: 0.2-0.4 mg/hour initially and titrate to doses of 0.4-0.8 mg/hour; tolerance is minimized by using a patch on period of 12-14 hours and patch off period of 10-12 hours
Translingual: 1-2 sprays into mouth under tongue every 3-5 minutes for maximum of 3 doses in 15 minutes, may also be used 5-10 minutes prior to activities which may provoke an attack prophylactically
Buccal: Initial: 1 mg every 3-5 hours while awake (3 times/day); titrate dosage upward if angina occurs with tablet in place

May need to use nitrate-free interval (10-12 hours/day) to avoid tolerance development; tolerance may possibly be reversed with acetylcysteine; gradually decrease dose in patients receiving NTG for prolonged period to avoid withdrawal reaction

Dosage Forms
Capsule, sustained release: 2.5 mg, 6.5 mg, 9 mg
Injection: 0.5 mg/mL (10 mL); 0.8 mg/mL (10 mL); 5 mg/mL (1 mL, 5 mL, 10 mL, 20 mL); 10 mg/mL (5 mL, 10 mL)
Ointment, topical (Nitrol®): 2% [20 mg/g] (30 g, 60 g)
Patch, transdermal, topical: Systems designed to deliver 2.5, 5, 7.5, 10, or 15 mg NTG over 24 hours
Spray, translingual: 0.4 mg/metered spray (13.8 g)
Tablet:
    Buccal, controlled release: 1 mg, 2 mg, 3 mg
    Sublingual (Nitrostat®): 0.15 mg, 0.3 mg, 0.4 mg, 0.6 mg
    Sustained release: 2.6 mg, 6.5 mg, 9 mg

nitroglycerol *see* nitroglycerin *on previous page*
Nitroglyn® Oral *see* nitroglycerin *on previous page*
Nitrolingual® Translingual Spray *see* nitroglycerin *on previous page*
Nitrol® Ointment *see* nitroglycerin *on previous page*
Nitrong® Oral Tablet *see* nitroglycerin *on previous page*
Nitropress® *see* nitroprusside sodium *on this page*

nitroprusside sodium (nye troe pruss' ide)
Brand Names Nipride®; Nitropress®
Synonyms sodium nitroferricyanide; sodium nitroprusside
Therapeutic Category Vasodilator
Use Management of hypertensive crises; congestive heart failure; used for controlled hypotension to reduce bleeding during surgery
Usual Dosage I.V.:
Children: Continuous infusion:
    Initial: 1 μg/kg/minute by continuous I.V. infusion; increase in increments of 1 μg/kg/minute at intervals of 20-60 minutes; titrating to the desired response
    Usual dose: 3 μg/kg/minute; rarely need >4 μg/kg/minute
    Maximum: 10 μg/kg/minute. Dilute 15 mg x weight (kg) to 250 mL D_5W, then dose in μg/kg/minute = infusion rate in mL/hour

Adults: Begin at 5 μg/kg/minute; increase in increments of 5 μg/kg/minute (up to 20 μg/kg/minute), then in increments of 10-20 μg/kg/minute; titrating to the desired hemodynamic effect or the appearance of headache or nausea. When >500 μg/kg is administered by prolonged infusion of faster than 2 μg/kg/minute, cyanide is generated faster than an unaided patient can handle.
Dosage Forms Injection: 10 mg/mL (5 mL); 25 mg/mL (2 mL)

Nitrostat® Sublingual *see* nitroglycerin *on previous page*
Nix™ Creme Rinse *see* permethrin *on page 366*

nizatidine (ni za' ti deen)
Brand Names Axid®
Therapeutic Category Histamine-2 Antagonist
Use Treatment and maintenance of duodenal ulcer
Usual Dosage Adults: Active duodenal ulcer: Oral:
Treatment: 300 mg at bedtime or 150 mg twice daily
Maintenance: 150 mg/day
Dosage Forms Capsule: 150 mg, 300 mg

Nizoral® Oral *see* ketoconazole *on page 264*

Nizoral® Topical *see* ketoconazole *on page 264*

n-methylhydrazine *see* procarbazine hydrochloride *on page 396*

Noctec® Oral *see* chloral hydrate *on page 87*

Nolamine® *see* chlorpheniramine, phenindamine, and phenylpropanolamine *on page 95*

Nolex® LA *see* guaifenesin and phenylpropanolamine *on page 219*

Nolvadex® Oral *see* tamoxifen citrate *on page 452*

nonoxynol 9 (noe nox' ee nole)
Brand Names Because® [OTC]; Conceptrol® [OTC]; Delfen® [OTC]; Emko® [OTC]; Encare® [OTC]; Gynol II® [OTC]; Intercept™ [OTC]; Koromex® [OTC]; Ramses® [OTC]; Semicid® [OTC]; Shur-Seal® [OTC]
Therapeutic Category Spermicide
Use Spermatocide in contraception
Usual Dosage Insert into vagina at least 15 minutes before intercourse
Dosage Forms Vaginal:
  Cream: 2% (103.5 g)
  Foam: 12.5% (60 g)
  Jelly: 2% (81 g, 126 g)

noradrenaline acid tartrate *see* norepinephrine bitartrate *on this page*

Norcept-E® 1/35 *see* ethinyl estradiol and norethindrone *on page 183*

Norcet® *see* hydrocodone and acetaminophen *on page 234*

Norcuron® *see* vecuronium *on page 493*

nordeoxyguanosine *see* ganciclovir *on page 208*

Nordette® *see* ethinyl estradiol and levonorgestrel *on page 183*

Nordryl® Injection *see* diphenhydramine hydrochloride *on page 152*

Nordryl® Oral *see* diphenhydramine hydrochloride *on page 152*

norepinephrine bitartrate (nor ep i nef' rin)
Brand Names Levophed® Injection
Synonyms levarterenol bitartrate; noradrenaline acid tartrate
Therapeutic Category Adrenergic Agonist Agent; Alpha-Adrenergic Agonist
Use Treatment of shock which persists after adequate fluid volume replacement
Usual Dosage I.V.:
  Children: Initial: 0.05-0.1 μg/kg/minute, titrate to desired effect; rate (mL/hour) = dose (μg/kg/minute) x weight (kg) x 60 minutes/hour divided by concentration (μg/mL)

  Adults: 8-12 μg/minute as an infusion; initiate at 4 μg/minute and titrate to desired response

  Note: Dose stated in terms of norepinephrine base
Dosage Forms Injection: 1 mg/mL (4 mL)

Norethin™ 1/35E *see* ethinyl estradiol and norethindrone *on page 183*

norethindrone (nor eth in' drone)
Brand Names Aygestin®; Micronor®; Norlutate®; Norlutin®; NOR-Q.D.®
Synonyms norethisterone
Therapeutic Category Contraceptive, Oral; Contraceptive, Progestin Only; Progestin
Use Treatment of amenorrhea; abnormal uterine bleeding; endometriosis, oral contraceptive in combination with estrogens

Usual Dosage Adolescents and Adults: Oral:
Amenorrhea and abnormal uterine bleeding: 2.5-10 mg on days 5-25 of menstrual cycle

Endometriosis: 5 mg/day for 14 days; increase at increments of 2.5 mg/day every 2 weeks up to 15 mg/day

Dosage Forms
Tablet: 0.35 mg, 5 mg
Tablet, as acetate: 5 mg

norethindrone acetate and ethinyl estradiol *see* ethinyl estradiol and norethindrone *on page 183*

norethindrone and mestranol *see* mestranol and norethindrone *on page 295*

norethisterone *see* norethindrone *on previous page*

norethynodrel and mestranol *see* mestranol and norethynodrel *on page 296*

Norflex® *see* orphenadrine citrate *on page 346*

norfloxacin (nor flox' a sin)
Brand Names Chibroxin™ Ophthalmic; Noroxin® Oral
Therapeutic Category Antibiotic, Quinolone
Use Complicated and uncomplicated urinary tract infections caused by susceptible gram-negative and gram-positive bacteria
Usual Dosage
Oral: Adults: 400 mg twice daily for 7-21 days depending on infection
Ophthalmic: Children >1 year and Adults: Instill 1-2 drops in affected eye(s) 4 times/day for up to 7 days
Dosage Forms
Solution, ophthalmic: 0.3% [3 mg/mL] (5 mL)
Tablet: 400 mg

Norgesic® *see* orphenadrine, aspirin and caffeine *on page 346*

Norgesic® Forte *see* orphenadrine, aspirin and caffeine *on page 346*

norgestimate and ethinyl estradiol *see* ethinyl estradiol and norgestimate *on page 184*

norgestrel (nor jess' trel)
Brand Names Ovrette®
Therapeutic Category Contraceptive, Oral; Progestin
Use Prevention of pregnancy; treatment of hypermenorrhea, endometriosis, female hypogonadism
Usual Dosage Administer daily, starting the first day of menstruation, take one tablet at the same time each day, every day of the year. If one dose is missed, take as soon as remembered, then next tablet at regular time; if two doses are missed, take one tablet and discard the other, then take daily at usual time; if three doses are missed, use an additional form of birth control until menses or pregnancy is ruled out
Dosage Forms Tablet: 0.075 mg

norgestrel and ethinyl estradiol *see* ethinyl estradiol and norgestrel *on page 185*

Norinyl® 1+35 *see* ethinyl estradiol and norethindrone *on page 183*

Norinyl® 1+50 *see* mestranol and norethindrone *on page 295*

Norlestrin® *see* ethinyl estradiol and norethindrone *on page 183*

Norlutate® *see* norethindrone *on previous page*

Norlutin® *see* norethindrone *on previous page*

ALPHABETICAL LISTING OF DRUGS

normal human serum albumin *see* albumin human *on page 10*

normal saline *see* sodium chloride *on page 434*

normal serum albumin (human) *see* albumin human *on page 10*

Normodyne® Injection *see* labetalol hydrochloride *on page 265*

Normodyne® Oral *see* labetalol hydrochloride *on page 265*

Noroxin® Oral *see* norfloxacin *on previous page*

Norpace® *see* disopyramide phosphate *on page 155*

Norplant® Implant *see* levonorgestrel *on page 271*

Norpramin® *see* desipramine hydrochloride *on page 131*

NOR-Q.D.® *see* norethindrone *on page 338*

Nor-tet® Oral *see* tetracycline *on page 458*

north american coral snake antivenin *see* antivenin (*Micrurus fulvius*) *on page 31*

north and south american antisnake-bite serum *see* antivenin (crotalidae) polyvalent *on page 31*

nortriptyline hydrochloride (nor trip' ti leen)
Brand Names Aventyl® Hydrochloride; Pamelor®
Therapeutic Category Antidepressant, Tricyclic
Use Used in the treatment of various forms of depression, often in conjunction with psychotherapy
Usual Dosage Oral:
Adults: 25 mg 3-4 times/day up to 150 mg/day
Elderly and Adolescents: 30-50 mg/day in divided doses
Dosage Forms
Capsule: 10 mg, 25 mg, 50 mg, 75 mg
Solution: 10 mg/5 mL (473 mL)

Norvasc® *see* amlodipine *on page 22*

Nostrilla® [OTC] *see* oxymetazoline hydrochloride *on page 350*

Nostril® Nasal Solution [OTC] *see* phenylephrine hydrochloride *on page 372*

Novafed® *see* pseudoephedrine *on page 406*

Novafed® A *see* chlorpheniramine and pseudoephedrine *on page 94*

Novahistine® DH *see* chlorpheniramine, pseudoephedrine, and codeine *on page 97*

Novahistine® Elixir [OTC] *see* chlorpheniramine and phenylephrine *on page 93*

Novahistine® Expectorant *see* guaifenesin, pseudoephedrine, and codeine *on page 221*

Novantrone® *see* mitoxantrone hydrochloride *on page 315*

Novocain® Injection *see* procaine hydrochloride *on page 396*

Novolin® *see* insulin preparations *on page 250*

NP-27® [OTC] *see* tolnaftate *on page 471*

NPH *see* insulin preparations *on page 250*

NPH Iletin® I *see* insulin preparations *on page 250*

NSC-102816 *see* azacitidine *on page 40*

NTG *see* nitroglycerin *on page 336*

NTZ® Long Acting Nasal Solution [OTC] *see* oxymetazoline hydrochloride *on page 350*

Nubain® *see* nalbuphine hydrochloride *on page 323*

Nucofed® *see* guaifenesin, pseudoephedrine, and codeine *on page 221*

Nucofed® Pediatric Expectorant *see* guaifenesin, pseudoephedrine, and codeine *on page 221*

Nucotuss® *see* guaifenesin, pseudoephedrine, and codeine *on page 221*

Nu-Iron® [OTC] *see* polysaccharide-iron complex *on page 384*

NuLYTELY® *see* polyethylene glycol-electrolyte solution *on page 383*

Numorphan® Injection *see* oxymorphone hydrochloride *on page 351*

Numorphan® Oral *see* oxymorphone hydrochloride *on page 351*

Nupercainal® Topical [OTC] *see* dibucaine *on page 143*

Nuprin® [OTC] *see* ibuprofen *on page 245*

Nuromax® Injection *see* doxacurium chloride *on page 160*

Nutracort® Topical *see* hydrocortisone *on page 236*

Nutraplus® Topical [OTC] *see* urea *on page 487*

Nydrazid® Injection *see* isoniazid *on page 258*

nylidrin hydrochloride (nye' li drin)

Brand Names Arlidin®
Therapeutic Category Vasodilator, Peripheral
Use Increases blood supply as to treat peripheral disease and circulatory disturbances of the inner ear
Usual Dosage Oral: 3-12 mg 3-4 times/day
Dosage Forms Tablet: 6 mg, 12 mg

nystatin (nye stat' in)

Brand Names Mycostatin® Oral; Mycostatin® Topical; Mycostatin® Vaginal; Nilstat® Oral; Nilstat® Topical; Nilstat® Vaginal; Nystat-Rx®; Nystex® Oral; Nystex® Topical; O-V Staticin® Oral/Vaginal

Therapeutic Category Antifungal Agent, Oral Nonabsorbed; Antifungal Agent, Topical; Antifungal Agent, Vaginal

Use Treatment of susceptible cutaneous, mucocutaneous, and oral cavity fungal infections normally caused by the *Candida* species

Usual Dosage

Oral candidiasis:
Neonates: 100,000 units 4 times/day or 50,000 units to each side of mouth 4 times/day
Infants: 200,000 units 4 times/day or 100,000 units to each side of mouth 4 times/day
Children and Adults: 400,000-600,000 units 4 times/day; troche: 200,000-400,000 units 4-5 times/day

Cutaneous candidal infections: Children and Adults: Topical: Apply 3-4 times/day

Intestinal infections: Adults: Oral: 500,000-1,000,000 units every 8 hours
Vaginal infections: Adults: Vaginal tablets: Insert 1-2 tablets/day at bedtime for 2 weeks

Dosage Forms
Cream: 100,000 units/g (15 g, 30 g)
Ointment, topical: 100,000 units/g (15 g, 30 g)
Powder, for preparation of oral suspension: 50 million units, 1 billion units, 2 billion units, 5 billion units
Powder, topical: 100,000 units/g (15 g)
Suspension, oral: 100,000 units/mL (5 mL, 60 mL, 480 mL)
(Continued)

nystatin *(Continued)*
Tablet:
  Oral: 500,000 units
  Vaginal: 100,000 units (15 and 30/box with applicator)
  Troche: 200,000 units

nystatin and triamcinolone
Brand Names Dermacomb® Topical; Mycogen II Topical; Mycolog®-II Topical; Myconel® Topical; Mytrex® F Topical; NGT® Topical; Nyst-Olone® II Topical; Tri-Statin® II Topical
Synonyms triamcinolone and nystatin
Therapeutic Category Antifungal Agent, Topical; Corticosteroid, Topical (Medium Potency)
Use Treatment of cutaneous candidiasis
Usual Dosage Topical: Apply twice daily
Dosage Forms
  Cream: Nystatin 100,000 units and triamcinolone acetonide 0.1% (15 g, 30 g, 45 g, 60 g, 240 g)
  Ointment, topical: Nystatin 100,000 units and triamcinolone acetonide 0.1% (15 g, 30 g, 60 g, 120 g)

Nystat-Rx® *see* nystatin *on previous page*
Nystex® Oral *see* nystatin *on previous page*
Nystex® Topical *see* nystatin *on previous page*
Nyst-Olone® II Topical *see* nystatin and triamcinolone *on this page*
Nytol® Oral [OTC] *see* diphenhydramine hydrochloride *on page 152*
Occlusal-HP Liquid *see* salicylic acid *on page 424*
Occucoat™ *see* hydroxypropyl methylcellulose *on page 241*
Ocean Nasal Mist [OTC] *see* sodium chloride *on page 434*
OCL® *see* polyethylene glycol-electrolyte solution *on page 383*
Octamide® *see* metoclopramide *on page 308*
Octicair® Otic *see* neomycin, polymyxin b, and hydrocortisone *on page 329*
Octocaine® Injection *see* lidocaine and epinephrine *on page 272*

octreotide acetate (ok tree' oh tide)
Brand Names Sandostatin®
Therapeutic Category Antisecretory Agent; Somatostatin Analog
Use Control of symptoms in patients with metastatic carcinoid and vasoactive intestinal peptide-secreting tumors (VIPomas)
Usual Dosage Adults: S.C.: Initial: 50 µg 1-2 times/day and titrate dose based on patient tolerance and response
  Carcinoid: 100-600 µg/day in 2-4 divided doses
  VIPomas: 200-300 µg/day in 2-4 divided doses
  Diarrhea: Initial: I.V.: 50-100 µg every 8 hours; increase by 100 µg/dose at 48-hour intervals; maximum dose: 500 µg every 8 hours
Dosage Forms Injection: 0.05 mg (1 mL); 0.1 mg (1 mL); 0.5 mg (1 mL)

Ocu-Carpine® Ophthalmic *see* pilocarpine *on page 377*
OcuClear® Ophthalmic [OTC] *see* oxymetazoline hydrochloride *on page 350*
Ocufen® Ophthalmic *see* flurbiprofen sodium *on page 204*
Ocuflox™ Ophthalmic *see* ofloxacin *on next page*
Oculinum® *see* botulinum toxin type A *on page 57*

Ocupress® Ophthalmic *see* carteolol hydrochloride *on page 76*

Ocusert Pilo-20® Ophthalmic *see* pilocarpine *on page 377*

Ocusert Pilo-40® Ophthalmic *see* pilocarpine *on page 377*

Ocu-Spor-G® Ophthalmic Solution *see* neomycin, polymyxin b, and gramicidin *on page 329*

Ocutricin® HC Otic *see* neomycin, polymyxin b, and hydrocortisone *on page 329*

Ocutricin® Ophthalmic Solution *see* neomycin, polymyxin b, and gramicidin *on page 329*

Ocutricin® Topical Ointment *see* bacitracin, neomycin, and polymyxin b *on page 43*

Ocu-Trol® Ophthalmic *see* neomycin, polymyxin b, and dexamethasone *on page 328*

ofloxacin (oh floks' a sin)
Brand Names Floxin® Injection; Floxin® Oral; Ocuflox™ Ophthalmic
Therapeutic Category Antibiotic, Quinolone
Use Quinolone antibiotic for skin and skin structure, lower respiratory and urinary tract infections and sexually transmitted diseases
Usual Dosage Adults:
Oral, I.V.: 200-400 mg every 12 hours for 7-10 days for most infections or for 6 weeks for prostatitis
Ophthalmic: Instill 1-2 drops in affected eye(s) every 2-4 hours for the first 2 days, then use 4 times daily for an additional 5 days
Dosing adjustment/interval in renal impairment:
Cl_{cr} 10-50 mL/minute: Administer 50% of normal dose or administer every 24 hours
Cl_{cr} <10 mL/minute: Administer 25% of normal dose or administer 50% of normal dose every 24 hours
Dosage Forms
Injection: 200 mg (50 mL); 400 mg (10 mL, 20 mL, 100 mL)
Solution, ophthalmic: 0.3% (5 mL)
Tablet: 200 mg, 300 mg, 400 mg

Ogen® Oral *see* estropipate *on page 180*

Ogen® Vaginal *see* estropipate *on page 180*

OGMT *see* metyrosine *on page 310*

OKT3 *see* muromonab-CD3 *on page 320*

old tuberculin *see* tuberculin tests *on page 484*

oleovitamin A *see* vitamin A *on page 496*

oleum ricini *see* castor oil *on page 77*

olsalazine sodium (ole sal' a zeen)
Brand Names Dipentum®
Therapeutic Category 5-Aminosalicylic Acid Derivative; Anti-inflammatory Agent
Use Maintenance of remission of ulcerative colitis in patients intolerant to sulfasalazine
Usual Dosage Adults: Oral: 1 g daily in 2 divided doses
Dosage Forms Capsule: 250 mg

omeprazole (oh me' pray zol)
Formerly Known As Losec®
Brand Names Prilosec™
Therapeutic Category Gastric Acid Secretion Inhibitor
(Continued)

omeprazole *(Continued)*

Use Short-term (4-8 weeks) treatment of severe erosive esophagitis (grade 2 or above), diagnosed by endoscopy and short-term treatment of symptomatic gastroesophageal reflux disease (GERD) poorly responsible to customary medical treatment; pathological hypersecretory conditions

Usual Dosage Adults: Oral:

Active duodenal ulcer: 20 mg/day for 4-8 weeks

GERD or severe erosive esophagitis: 20 mg/day for 4-8 weeks

Pathological hypersecretory conditions: 60 mg once daily to start; doses up to 120 mg 3 times/day have been administered; administer daily doses >80 mg in divided doses

Dosage Forms Capsule: 20 mg

Omnipaque® *see* radiological/contrast media (non-ionic) *on page 415*

Omnipen® *see* ampicillin *on page 26*

Omnipen®-N *see* ampicillin *on page 26*

OMS® Oral *see* morphine sulfate *on page 318*

Oncovin® Injection *see* vincristine sulfate *on page 496*

ondansetron hydrochloride (on dan' se tron)

Brand Names Zofran® Injection; Zofran® Oral

Therapeutic Category Antiemetic

Use May be prescribed for patients who are refractory to or have severe adverse reactions to standard antiemetic therapy; also for young patients (ie, <45 years of age who are more likely to develop extrapyramidal reactions to high-dose metoclopramide) who are to receive highly emetogenic chemotherapeutic agents

Usual Dosage

Oral:

Children 4-11 years: 4 mg 30 minutes before chemotherapy; repeat 4 and 8 hours after initial dose

Children >11 years and Adults: 8 mg 30 minutes before chemotherapy; repeat 4 and 8 hours after initial dose or every 8 hours for a maximum of 48 hours

I.V.: Administer either three 0.15 mg/kg doses or a single 32 mg dose; with the 3-dose regimen, the initial dose is given 30 minutes prior to chemotherapy with subsequent doses administered 4 and 8 hours after the first dose. With the single-dose regimen 32 mg is infused over 15 minutes beginning 30 minutes before the start of emetogenic chemotherapy. Dosage should be calculated based on weight: I.V.:

Children: Pediatric dosing should follow the manufacturer's guidelines for 0.15 mg/kg/dose administered 30 minutes prior to chemotherapy, 4 and 8 hours after the first dose. While not as yet FDA-approved, literature supports the day's total dose administered as a single dose 30 minutes prior to chemotherapy.

Adults:

>80 kg: 12 mg IVPB

45-80 kg: 8 mg IVPB

<45 kg: 0.15 mg/kg/dose IVPB

Dosing in hepatic impairment: Maximum daily dose: 8 mg in cirrhotic patients with severe liver disease

Dosage Forms

Injection: 2 mg/mL (20 mL); 32 mg (single-dose vials)

Tablet: 4 mg, 8 mg

Ony-Clear® Nail Topical *see* triacetin *on page 474*

OP-CCK *see* sincalide *on page 432*

Opcon® Ophthalmic *see* naphazoline hydrochloride *on page 325*

o,p'-DDD *see* mitotane *on page 315*

Ophthacet® Ophthalmic *see* sodium sulfacetamide *on page 439*

Ophthaine® Ophthalmic *see* proparacaine hydrochloride *on page 401*

Ophthalgan® Ophthalmic *see* glycerin *on page 214*

Ophthetic® Ophthalmic *see* proparacaine hydrochloride *on page 401*

Ophthochlor® Ophthalmic *see* chloramphenicol *on page 88*

Ophthocort® Ophthalmic *see* chloramphenicol, polymyxin b, and hydrocortisone *on page 89*

opium alkaloids
Brand Names Pantopon®
Therapeutic Category Analgesic, Narcotic
Use For relief of severe pain
Usual Dosage Adults: I.M., S.C.: 5-20 mg every 4-5 hours
Dosage Forms Injection: 20 mg/mL (1 mL)

opium and belladonna *see* belladonna and opium *on page 46*

opium tincture
Synonyms deodorized opium tincture; DTO
Therapeutic Category Analgesic, Narcotic; Antidiarrheal
Use Treatment of diarrhea or relief of pain
Usual Dosage Oral:
Children:
Diarrhea: 0.005-0.01 mL/kg/dose every 3-4 hours
Analgesia: 0.01-0.02 mL/kg/dose every 3-4 hours

Adults: 0.6 mL 4 times/day
Dosage Forms Liquid: 10% [0.6 mL equivalent to morphine 6 mg]

Optigene® Ophthalmic [OTC] *see* tetrahydrozoline hydrochloride *on page 459*

Optimine® *see* azatadine maleate *on page 40*

OptiPranolol® Ophthalmic *see* metipranolol hydrochloride *on page 307*

Optiray® *see* radiological/contrast media (non-ionic) *on page 415*

Optised® Ophthalmic [OTC] *see* phenylephrine and zinc sulfate *on page 372*

OPV *see* poliovirus vaccine, live, trivalent, oral *on page 382*

Orabase®-B [OTC] *see* benzocaine *on page 48*

Orabase® HCA Topical *see* hydrocortisone *on page 236*

Orabase®-O [OTC] *see* benzocaine *on page 48*

Orabase® Plain [OTC] *see* gelatin, pectin, and methylcellulose *on page 209*

Orabase® With Benzocaine [OTC] *see* benzocaine, gelatin, pectin, and sodium carboxymethylcellulose *on page 48*

Oracit® *see* sodium citrate and citric acid *on page 435*

Oragest SR® *see* chlorpheniramine and phenylpropanolamine *on page 93*

Oragrafin® Calcium *see* radiological/contrast media (ionic) *on page 413*

Oragrafin® Sodium *see* radiological/contrast media (ionic) *on page 413*

Orajel® Brace-Aid Oral Anesthetic [OTC] *see* benzocaine *on page 48*

Orajel® Brace-Aid Rinse [OTC] *see* carbamide peroxide *on page 73*

Orajel® Maximum Strength [OTC] *see* benzocaine *on page 48*

Orajel® Mouth-Aid [OTC] *see* benzocaine *on page 48*

Oraminic® II Injection *see* brompheniramine maleate *on page 59*

Oramorph SR™ Oral *see* morphine sulfate *on page 318*

Orap™ *see* pimozide *on page 378*

Orasone® Oral *see* prednisone *on page 393*

Orazinc® Oral [OTC] *see* zinc sulfate *on page 504*

orciprenaline sulfate *see* metaproterenol sulfate *on page 296*

Ordine AT® Extended Release Capsule *see* caramiphen and phenylpropanolamine *on page 72*

Oretic® *see* hydrochlorothiazide *on page 233*

Oreton® Methyl *see* methyltestosterone *on page 307*

Orex® [OTC] *see* saliva substitute *on page 425*

Orexin® [OTC] *see* vitamin B complex *on page 498*

Organidin® *see* iodinated glycerol *on page 253*

ORG NC 45 *see* vecuronium *on page 493*

Orimune® *see* poliovirus vaccine, live, trivalent, oral *on page 382*

Orinase® Diagnostic Injection *see* tolbutamide *on page 471*

Orinase® Oral *see* tolbutamide *on page 471*

ORLAAM® *see* levomethadyl acetate hydrochloride *on page 271*

Ormazine *see* chlorpromazine hydrochloride *on page 97*

Ornade® Spansule® *see* chlorpheniramine and phenylpropanolamine *on page 93*

Ornidyl® Injection *see* eflornithine hydrochloride *on page 168*

orphenadrine, aspirin and caffeine
Brand Names Norgesic® Forte; Norgesic®
Therapeutic Category Analgesic, Non-Narcotic; Skeletal Muscle Relaxant
Use Relief of discomfort associated with skeletal muscular conditions
Usual Dosage Oral: 1-2 tablets 3-4 times/day
Dosage Forms
  Tablet: Orphenadrine citrate 25 mg, aspirin 385 mg, and caffeine 30 mg
  Tablet (Norgesic® Forte): Orphenadrine citrate 50 mg, aspirin 770 mg, and caffeine 60 mg

orphenadrine citrate (or fen' a dreen)
Brand Names Norflex®
Therapeutic Category Skeletal Muscle Relaxant
Use Treatment of muscle spasm associated with acute painful musculoskeletal conditions; supportive therapy in tetanus
Usual Dosage Adults:
  Oral: 100 mg twice daily
  I.M., I.V.: 60 mg every 12 hours
Dosage Forms
  Injection: 30 mg/mL (2 mL, 10 mL)
  Tablet: 100 mg
  Tablet, sustained release: 100 mg

Ortho-Cept™ *see* ethinyl estradiol and desogestrel *on page 182*

Orthoclone® OKT3 *see* muromonab-CD3 *on page 320*

Ortho® Dienestrol Vaginal *see* dienestrol *on page 145*

Ortho-Est® Oral *see* estropipate *on page 180*

Ortho-Novum™ 1/35 *see* ethinyl estradiol and norethindrone *on page 183*

Ortho-Novum™ 1/50 *see* mestranol and norethindrone *on page 295*

Ortho-Novum™ 7/7/7 *see* ethinyl estradiol and norethindrone *on page 183*

Ortho-Novum™ 10/11 *see* ethinyl estradiol and norethindrone *on page 183*

Ortho™ Tri-Cyclen® *see* ethinyl estradiol and norgestimate *on page 184*

Or-Tyl® Injection *see* dicyclomine hydrochloride *on page 145*

Orudis® *see* ketoprofen *on page 264*

Oruvail® *see* ketoprofen *on page 264*

Os-Cal® 500 [OTC] *see* calcium carbonate *on page 65*

Osmitrol® Injection *see* mannitol *on page 285*

Osmoglyn® Ophthalmic *see* glycerin *on page 214*

OT *see* tuberculin tests *on page 484*

Otic Domeboro® *see* aluminum acetate and acetic acid *on page 15*

Otobiotic® Otic *see* polymyxin b and hydrocortisone *on page 384*

Otocalm® Ear *see* antipyrine and benzocaine *on page 30*

Otocort® Otic *see* neomycin, polymyxin b, and hydrocortisone *on page 329*

Otomycin-HPN® Otic *see* neomycin, polymyxin b, and hydrocortisone *on page 329*

Otosporin® Otic *see* neomycin, polymyxin b, and hydrocortisone *on page 329*

Otrivin® Nasal [OTC] *see* xylometazoline hydrochloride *on page 501*

Ovcon® *see* ethinyl estradiol and norethindrone *on page 183*

Ovide™ Topical *see* malathion *on page 284*

Ovral® *see* ethinyl estradiol and norgestrel *on page 185*

Ovrette® *see* norgestrel *on page 339*

O-V Staticin® Oral/Vaginal *see* nystatin *on page 341*

OvuKIT® Acetest® [OTC] *see* diagnostic aids (*in vitro*), urine *on page 139*

ovulation tests *see* diagnostic aids (*in vitro*), urine *on page 139*

OvuQUICK® *see* diagnostic aids (*in vitro*), urine *on page 139*

oxacillin sodium (ox a sill' in)

Brand Names Bactocill® Injection; Bactocill® Oral; Prostaphlin® Injection; Prostaphlin® Oral
Synonyms methylphenyl isoxazolyl penicillin; sodium oxacillin
Therapeutic Category Antibiotic, Penicillin
Use Treatment of susceptible bacterial infections such as osteomyelitis, septicemia, endocarditis, and CNS infections due to penicillinase-producing strains of *Staphylococcus*
Usual Dosage
Neonates: I.M., I.V.:
Postnatal age <7 days:
<2000 g: 25 mg/kg/dose every 12 hours
>2000 g: 25 mg/kg/dose every 8 hours
Postnatal age >7 days:
<1200 g: 25 mg/kg/dose every 12 hours
1200-2000 g: 30 mg/kg/dose every 8 hours
>2000 g: 37.5 mg/kg/dose every 6 hours

Infants and Children: I.M., I.V.: 150-200 mg/kg/day in divided doses every 6 hours; maximum dose: 12 g/day

Infants and Children: Oral: 50-100 mg/kg/day divided every 6 hours

Adults:
Oral: 500-1000 mg every 4-6 hours for at least 5 days
(Continued)

oxacillin sodium *(Continued)*
I.M., I.V.: 250 mg to 2 g/dose every 4-6 hours
Dosage Forms
Capsule: 250 mg, 500 mg
Powder for injection: 250 mg, 500 mg, 1 g, 2 g, 4 g, 10 g
Powder for oral solution: 250 mg/5 mL (100 mL)

oxamniquine (ox am' ni kwin)
Brand Names Vansil™
Therapeutic Category Anthelmintic
Use Treat all stages of *Schistosoma mansoni* infection
Usual Dosage Oral:
Children <30 kg: 20 mg/kg in 2 divided doses of 10 mg/kg at 2- to 8-hour intervals
Adults: 12-15 mg/kg as a single dose
Dosage Forms Capsule: 250 mg

Oxandrine® *see oxandrolone on this page*

oxandrolone (ox an' droe lone)
Brand Names Oxandrine®
Therapeutic Category Androgen
Use Treatment of catabolic or tissue-depleting processes
Usual Dosage Adults: Oral: 2.5 mg 2-4 times daily
Dosage Forms Tablet: 2.5 mg

oxaprozin (ox a proe' zin)
Brand Names Daypro®
Therapeutic Category Nonsteroidal Anti-Inflammatory Agent (NSAID), Oral
Use Acute and long-term use in the management of signs and symptoms of osteoarthritis and rheumatoid arthritis
Usual Dosage Adults: Oral (individualize the dosage to the lowest effective dose to minimize adverse effects):
Osteoarthritis: 600-1200 mg once daily
Rheumatoid arthritis: 1200 mg once daily
Maximum dose: 1800 mg/day or 26 mg/kg (whichever is lower) in divided doses
Dosage Forms Tablet: 600 mg

oxazepam (ox a' ze pam)
Brand Names Serax®
Therapeutic Category Benzodiazepine
Use Treatment of anxiety and management of alcohol withdrawal; may also be used as an anticonvulsant in management of simple partial seizures
Usual Dosage Oral:
Children: 1 mg/kg/day has been administered
Adults:
Anxiety: 10-30 mg 3-4 times/day
Alcohol withdrawal: 15-30 mg 3-4 times/day
Hypnotic: 15-30 mg
Dosage Forms
Capsule: 10 mg, 15 mg, 30 mg
Tablet: 15 mg

oxiconazole nitrate (ox i kon' a zole)
Brand Names Oxistat® Topical
Therapeutic Category Antifungal Agent, Topical
Use Treatment of tinea pedis, tinea cruris, and tinea corporis
Usual Dosage Topical: Apply once daily to affected areas for 2 weeks to 1 month
Dosage Forms Cream: 1% (15 g, 30 g)

oxilapine succinate *see* loxapine *on page 279*

Oxistat® Topical *see* oxiconazole nitrate *on this page*

oxpentifylline *see* pentoxifylline *on page 365*

Oxsoralen® *see* methoxsalen *on page 302*

Oxsoralen-Ultra® *see* methoxsalen *on page 302*

oxtriphylline (ox trye' fi lin)
Brand Names Choledyl®
Synonyms choline theophyllinate
Therapeutic Category Antiasthmatic; Bronchodilator; Theophylline Derivative
Use Bronchodilator in symptomatic treatment of asthma and reversible bronchospasm
Usual Dosage Oral:
Children:
1-9 years: 6.2 mg/kg/dose every 6 hours
9-16 years: 4.7 mg/kg/dose every 6 hours

Adults: 4.7 mg/kg every 8 hours; sustained release: administer every 12 hours
Dosage Forms
Elixir: 100 mg/5 mL (5 mL, 10 mL, 473 mL)
Syrup: 50 mg/5 mL (473 mL)
Tablet: 100 mg, 200 mg
Tablet, sustained release: 400 mg, 600 mg

Oxy-5® [OTC] *see* benzoyl peroxide *on page 49*

oxybutynin chloride (ox i byoo' ti nin)
Brand Names Ditropan®
Therapeutic Category Antispasmodic Agent, Urinary
Use Antispasmodic for neurogenic bladder
Usual Dosage Oral:
Children:
1-5 years: 0.2 mg/kg/dose 2-4 times/day
>5 years: 5 mg twice daily, up to 5 mg 3 times/day

Adults: 5 mg 2-3 times/day up to 5 mg 4 times/day maximum
Dosage Forms
Syrup: 5 mg/5 mL (473 mL)
Tablet: 5 mg

Oxycel® *see* cellulose, oxidized *on page 83*

oxycodone and acetaminophen
Brand Names Percocet®; Roxicet® 5/500; Roxilox®; Tylox®
Synonyms acetaminophen and oxycodone
Therapeutic Category Analgesic, Narcotic
Use Management of moderate to severe pain
Usual Dosage Oral (doses should be titrated to appropriate analgesic effects):

Children: Oxycodone: 0.05-0.15 mg/kg/dose to 5 mg/dose (maximum) every 4-6 hours as needed
(Continued)

oxycodone and acetaminophen *(Continued)*
Adults: 1-2 tablets every 4-6 hours as needed for pain
  Maximum daily dose of acetaminophen: 8 g/day, in alcoholics: 4 g/day
Dosage Forms
Caplet: Oxycodone hydrochloride 5 mg and acetaminophen 500 mg
Capsule: Oxycodone hydrochloride 5 mg and acetaminophen 500 mg
Solution, oral: Oxycodone hydrochloride 5 mg and acetaminophen 325 mg per 5 mL (5 mL, 500 mL)
Tablet: Oxycodone hydrochloride 5 mg and acetaminophen 325 mg

oxycodone and aspirin
Brand Names Codoxy®; Percodan®; Percodan®-Demi; Roxiprin®
Therapeutic Category Analgesic, Narcotic
Use Relief of moderate to moderately severe pain
Usual Dosage Oral (based on oxycodone combined salts):
Children: 0.05-0.15 mg/kg/dose every 4-6 hours as needed; maximum: 5 mg/dose (1 tablet Percodan® or 2 tablets Percodan®-Demi/dose) **or**
  Alternatively:
  6-12 years: Percodan®-Demi: ¼ tablet every 6 hours as needed for pain
  > 12 years: ½ tablet every 6 hours as needed for pain

Adults: Percodan®: 1 tablet every 6 hours as needed for pain or Percodan®-Demi: 1-2 tablets every 6 hours as needed for pain
Dosage Forms Tablet:
Percodan®: Oxycodone hydrochloride 4.5 mg, oxycodone terephthalate 0.38 mg, and aspirin 325 mg
Percodan®-Demi: Oxycodone hydrochloride 2.25 mg, oxycodone terephthalate 0.19 mg, and aspirin 325 mg

oxycodone hydrochloride (ox i koe' done)
Brand Names Roxicodone™
Synonyms dihydrohydroxycodeinone
Therapeutic Category Analgesic, Narcotic
Use Management of moderate to severe pain, normally used in combination with non-narcotic analgesics
Usual Dosage
Children:
  6-12 years: 1.25 mg every 6 hours as needed
  > 12 years: 2.5 mg every 6 hours as needed

Adults: 5 mg every 6 hours as needed
Dosage Forms
Liquid, oral: 5 mg/5 mL (50 mL)
Solution, oral concentrate: 20 mg/mL (30 mL)
Tablet: 5 mg

oxymetazoline hydrochloride (ox i met az' oh leen)
Brand Names Afrin® Nasal Solution [OTC]; Allerest® 12 Hours Nasal Solution [OTC]; Chlorphed®-LA Nasal Solution [OTC]; Dristan® Long Lasting Nasal Solution [OTC]; Duration® Nasal Solution [OTC]; Neo-Synephrine® 12 Hour Nasal Solution [OTC]; Nōstrilla® [OTC]; NTZ® Long Acting Nasal Solution [OTC]; OcuClear® Ophthalmic [OTC]; Sinarest® 12 Hour Nasal Solution; Vicks Sinex® Long-Acting Nasal Solution [OTC]; Visine® L.R. Ophthalmic [OTC]; 4-Way® Long Acting Nasal Solution [OTC]
Therapeutic Category Adrenergic Agonist Agent; Decongestant, Nasal; Vasoconstrictor, Nasal; Vasoconstrictor, Ophthalmic
Use Symptomatic relief of nasal mucosal congestion and adjunctive therapy of middle ear infections, associated with acute or chronic rhinitis, the common cold, sinusitis, hay fever or other allergies

Usual Dosage
Intranasal:
Children 2-5 years: 0.025% solution: Instill 2-3 drops in each nostril twice daily
Children ≥6 years and Adults: 0.05% solution: Instill 2-3 drops or 2-3 sprays into each nostril twice daily
Ophthalmic: Adults: Instill 1-2 drops into affected eye(s) every 6 hours
Dosage Forms
Solution, nasal:
Drops: 0.05% (20 mL)
Drops, pediatric: 0.025% (20 mL)
Spray: 0.05% (15 mL, 20 mL, 30 mL)
Solution, ophthalmic: 0.025% (15 mL, 30 mL)

oxymetholone (ox i meth' oh lone)
Brand Names Anadrol®
Therapeutic Category Anabolic Steroid
Use Anemias caused by the administration of myelotoxic drugs
Usual Dosage Erythropoietic effects: 1-5 mg/kg/day in 1 daily dose; maximum: 100 mg/day
Dosage Forms Tablet: 50 mg

oxymorphone hydrochloride (ox i mor' fone)
Brand Names Numorphan® Injection; Numorphan® Oral
Therapeutic Category Analgesic, Narcotic
Use Management of moderate to severe pain and preoperatively as a sedative and a supplement to anesthesia
Usual Dosage Adults:
I.M., S.C.: Initial: 0.5 mg, then 1-1.5 mg every 4-6 hours as needed
I.V.: Initial: 0.5 mg
Rectal: 5 mg every 4-6 hours
Dosage Forms
Injection: 1 mg (1 mL); 1.5 mg/mL (1 mL, 10 mL)
Suppository, rectal: 5 mg

oxyphenbutazone (ox i fen byoo' ta zone)
Therapeutic Category Analgesic, Non-Narcotic; Nonsteroidal Anti-Inflammatory Agent (NSAID), Oral
Use Management of inflammatory disorders, as an analgesic in the treatment of mild to moderate pain and as an antipyretic; I.V. form used as an alternate to surgery in management of patent ductus arteriosus in premature neonates; acute gouty arthritis
Usual Dosage Adults: Oral:
Rheumatoid arthritis: 100-200 mg 3-4 times/day until desired effect, then reduce dose to not exceeding 400 mg/day
Acute gouty arthritis: Initial: 400 mg then 100 mg every 4 hours until acute attack subsides
Dosage Forms Tablet: 100 mg

oxyphencyclimine hydrochloride (ox i fen sye' kli meen)
Brand Names Daricon®
Therapeutic Category Anticholinergic Agent; Antispasmodic Agent, Gastrointestinal
Use Adjunctive treatment of peptic ulcer
Usual Dosage Adults: Oral: 10 mg twice daily or 5 mg 3 times/day
Dosage Forms Tablet: 10 mg

oxytetracycline and polymyxin b
Brand Names Terramycin® Ophthalmic Ointment; Terramycin® w/ Polymyxin B Sulfate Vaginal
Synonyms polymyxin b and oxytetracycline
(Continued)
351

oxytetracycline and polymyxin b *(Continued)*
Therapeutic Category Antibiotic, Ophthalmic
Use Treatment of superficial ocular infections involving the conjunctiva and/or cornea
Usual Dosage
    Topical: Apply $\frac{1}{2}$" of ointment onto the lower lid of affected eye 2-4 times/day
    Vaginal: Insert one in vagina twice daily for 2-4 days
Dosage Forms
    Ointment, ophthalmic/otic: Oxytetracycline hydrochloride 5 mg and polymyxin b 10,000 units per g (3.75 g)
    Tablet, vaginal: Oxytetracycline hydrochloride 100 mg and polymyxin b 100,000 units (10s)

oxytetracycline hydrochloride (ox i tet ra sye' kleen)
Brand Names E.P. Mycin® Oral; Terramycin® I.M. Injection; Terramycin® Oral; Uri-Tet® Oral
Therapeutic Category Antibiotic, Tetracycline Derivative
Use Treatment of susceptible bacterial infections; both gram-positive and gram-negative, as well as *Rickettsia* and *Mycoplasma* organisms
Usual Dosage
    Oral:
        Children: 40-50 mg/kg/day in divided doses every 6 hours (maximum: 2 g/24 hours)
        Adults: 250-500 mg/dose every 6 hours
    I.M.:
        Children >8 years: 15-25 mg/kg/day (maximum: 250 mg/dose) in divided doses every 8-12 hours
        Adults: 250-500 mg every 24 hours or 300 mg/day divided every 8-12 hours
Dosage Forms
    Capsule: 250 mg
    Injection, with lidocaine 2%: 5% [50 mg/mL] (2 mL, 10 mL); 12.5% [125 mg/mL] (2 mL)

oxytocin (ox i toe' sin)
Brand Names Pitocin® Injection; Syntocinon® Injection; Syntocinon® Nasal Spray
Synonyms PIT
Therapeutic Category Oxytocic Agent
Use Induce labor at term; control postpartum bleeding; nasal preparation used to promote milk letdown in lactating females
Usual Dosage Adults:
    Induction of labor: I.V.: 0.001-0.002 unit/minute; increase by 0.001-0.002 every 15-30 minutes until contraction pattern has been established
    Postpartum bleeding: I.V.: 0.001-0.002 units/minute as needed
    Promotion of milk letdown: Intranasal: 1 spray or 3 drops in one or both nostrils 2-3 minutes before breast feeding
Dosage Forms
    Injection: 10 units/mL (1 mL, 10 mL)
    Solution, nasal: 40 units/mL (2 mL, 5 mL)

Oyst-Cal 500 [OTC] *see* calcium carbonate *on page 65*
Oystercal® 500 *see* calcium carbonate *on page 65*

paclitaxel (pack li tax' el)
Brand Names Taxol®
Therapeutic Category Antineoplastic Agent, Antimicrotubular
Use Treatment of metastatic carcinoma of the ovary after failure of first-line or subsequent chemotherapy
Usual Dosage Refer to individual protocols
    Adults: I.V.: 135 mg/m^2 over 24 hours every 3 weeks
Dosage Forms Injection: 6 mg/mL (5 mL)

2-PAM *see* pralidoxime chloride *on page 389*

Pamelor® *see* nortriptyline hydrochloride *on page 340*

pamidronate disodium (pa mi droe' nate)
Brand Names Aredia™
Therapeutic Category Antidote, Hypercalcemia; Biphosphonate Derivative
Use Symptomatic treatment of Paget's disease and heterotopic ossification due to spinal cord injury or after total hip replacement, hypercalcemia associated with malignancy
Usual Dosage Drug must be diluted properly before administration and infused slowly (at least over 2 hours)

Adults: I.V.:
    Moderate cancer related hypercalcemia (12-13 mg/dL): 60-90 mg given as a slow infusion over 2-24 hours;
    Severe cancer-related hypercalcemia (>13.5 mg/dL): 90 mg as a slow infusion over 2-24 hours
        A period of 7 days should elapse before the use of second course; repeat infusions every 2-3 weeks have been suggested, however, could be administered every 2-3 months according to the degree and of severity of hypercalcemia and/or the type of malignancy
    Paget's disease: 60 mg as a single 2-24 hour infusion
Dosage Forms Powder for injection, lyophilized: 30 mg

Pamine® *see* methscopolamine bromide *on page 303*

Pamprin IB® [OTC] *see* ibuprofen *on page 245*

Panacet® 5/500 *see* hydrocodone and acetaminophen *on page 234*

Panadol® [OTC] *see* acetaminophen *on page 2*

Panasal® 5/500 *see* hydrocodone and aspirin *on page 234*

Pancrease® *see* pancrelipase *on next page*

Pancrease® MT *see* pancrelipase *on next page*

pancreatin (pan' kree a tin)
Brand Names Creon®; Pancreatin Enseals® [OTC]
Therapeutic Category Pancreatic Enzyme
Use Replacement therapy in symptomatic treatment of malabsorption syndrome caused by pancreatic insufficiency

Pancreatin

Product	Dosage Form	Lipase USP Units	Amylase USP Units	Protease USP Units
Creon®	Capsule delayed release	8000	30,000	13,000
Pancreatin single strength	Tablet	650	8125	8125
Pancreatin 5X	Tablet	12,000	60,000	60,000
Pancreatin 8X	Tablet	22,500	180,000	180,000
Pancreatin Enseals®	Tablet enteric coated	2000	25,000	25,000

Usual Dosage Enteric coated microspheres: The following dosage recommendations are only an approximation for initial dosages. The actual dosage will depend on the digestive requirements of the individual patient.

Children:
    <1 year: 2000 units of lipase with meals/feedings
(Continued)

pancreatin *(Continued)*

1-6 years: 4000-8000 units of lipase with meals and 4,000 units with snacks

7-12 years: 4000-12,000 units of lipase with meals and snacks

Adults: 4000-16,000 units of lipase with meals and with snacks

Dosage Forms See table. *on previous page*

Pancreatin Enseals® [OTC] *see* pancreatin *on previous page*

pancrelipase (pan kre li' pase)

Brand Names Cotazym®; Cotazym-S®; Entolase®; Festal® II; Ilozyme®; Ku-Zyme® HP; Pancrease®; Pancrease® MT; Protilase®; Viokase®; Zymase®

Synonyms lipancreatin

Therapeutic Category Pancreatic Enzyme

Use Replacement therapy in symptomatic treatment of malabsorption syndrome caused by pancreatic insufficiency

Usual Dosage Oral:

Powder: Actual dose depends on the digestive requirements of the patient

Children <1 year: Start with ⅛ teaspoonful with feedings

Enteric coated microspheres and microtablets: The following dosage recommendations are only an approximation for initial dosages. The actual dosage will depend on the digestive requirements of the individual patient.

Children <1 year: 2000 units of lipase with meals/feedings

Children 1-6 years: 4000-8000 units of lipase with meals and 4000 units with snacks

Children 7-12 years: 4000-12,000 units of lipase with meals and snacks

Adults: 4000-16,000 units of lipase with meals and with snacks

Dosage Forms See table.

Pancrelipase

Product	Dosage Form	Lipase USP Units	Amylase USP Units	Protease USP Units
Cotazym® Ku-Zyme® HP	Capsule	8000	30,000	30,000
Cotazym®-S	Capsule, enteric coated spheres	5000	20,000	20,000
Entolase® Pancrease® Protilase®	Capsule, delayed release	4000	20,000	25,000
Festal® II	Tablet, delayed release	6000	30,000	20,000
Ilozyme®	Tablet	11,000	30,000	30,000
Pancrease® MT 4	Capsule, enteric coated microtablets	4000	12,000	12,000
10		10,000	30,000	30,000
16		16,000	48,000	48,000
Viokase®	Powder	16,800 per 0.7 g	70,000 per 0.7 g	70,000 per 0.7 g
	Tablet	8000	30,000	30,000
Zymase®	Capsule, enteric coated spheres	12,000	24,000	24,000

pancuronium bromide (pan kyoo roe' nee um)
Brand Names Pavulon®
Therapeutic Category Neuromuscular Blocker Agent, Nondepolarizing; Skeletal Muscle Relaxant
Use Produces skeletal muscle relaxation during surgery after induction of general anesthesia, increases pulmonary compliance during assisted respiration, facilitates endotracheal intubation
Usual Dosage I.V.:
Neonates: ≤1 month: Initial: 0.03 mg/kg/dose repeated twice at 5- to 10-minute intervals as needed; maintenance: 0.03-0.09 mg/kg/dose every 30 minutes to 4 hours as needed

Infants >1 month, Children, and Adults: 0.04-0.1 mg/kg; maintenance dose: 0.02-0.1 mg/kg/dose every 30-60 minutes as needed
Dosage Forms Injection: 1 mg/mL (10 mL); 2 mg/mL (2 mL, 5 mL)

Panhematin® *see* hemin *on page 226*
Panmycin® Oral *see* tetracycline *on page 458*
PanOxyl® [OTC] *see* benzoyl peroxide *on page 49*
PanOxyl®-AQ *see* benzoyl peroxide *on page 49*
Panscol® Lotion [OTC] *see* salicylic acid *on page 424*
Panscol® Ointment [OTC] *see* salicylic acid *on page 424*
Panthoderm® Cream [OTC] *see* dexpanthenol *on page 134*
Pantopon® *see* opium alkaloids *on page 345*

pantothenic acid
Synonyms calcium pantothenate; vitamin B₅
Therapeutic Category Vitamin, Water Soluble
Use Pantothenic acid deficiency
Usual Dosage Adults: Oral: Recommended daily dose 4-7 mg/day
Dosage Forms Tablet: 25 mg, 50 mg, 100 mg, 218 mg, 250 mg, 500 mg, 545 mg, 1000 mg

pantothenyl alcohol *see* dexpanthenol *on page 134*
Panwarfin® *see* warfarin sodium *on page 500*

papaverine hydrochloride (pa pav' er een)
Brand Names Cerespan® Oral; Genabid® Oral; Pavabid® Oral; Pavased® Oral; Pavatine® Oral; Paverolan® Oral
Therapeutic Category Vasodilator
Use Relief of peripheral and cerebral ischemia associated with arterial spasm
Usual Dosage
Children: I.M., I.V.: 1.5 mg/kg 4 times/day

Adults:
Oral: 100-300 mg 3-5 times/day
Oral, sustained release: 150-300 mg every 12 hours
I.M., I.V.: 30-120 mg every 3 hours as needed
Dosage Forms
Capsule, sustained release: 150 mg
Injection: 30 mg/mL (2 mL, 10 mL)
Tablet: 30 mg, 60 mg, 100 mg, 150 mg, 200 mg, 300 mg
Tablet, timed release: 200 mg

Paplex® Solution *see* salicylic acid *on page 424*
Paplex® Ultra Solution *see* salicylic acid *on page 424*

para-aminosalicylate sodium
Synonyms aminosalicylate sodium; PAS
Therapeutic Category Analgesic, Non-Narcotic; Salicylate
Use Adjunctive treatment of tuberculosis
Usual Dosage Oral:
Children: 240-360 mg/kg/day in 3-4 divided doses
Adults: 12-15 g/day in 3-4 divided doses
Dosage Forms Tablet: 500 mg

parabromdylamine see brompheniramine maleate on page 59

paracetaldehyde see paraldehyde on this page

paracetamol see acetaminophen on page 2

parachlorometaxylenol
Brand Names Metasep® [OTC]
Synonyms PCMX
Therapeutic Category Antiseborrheic Agent, Topical
Use Aid in relief of dandruff and associated conditions
Usual Dosage Massage to a foamy lather, allow to remain on hair for 5 minutes, rinse thoroughly and repeat
Dosage Forms Shampoo: 2% with isopropyl alcohol 9%

Paradione® see paramethadione on next page

Paraflex® see chlorzoxazone on page 99

Parafon Forte™ DSC see chlorzoxazone on page 99

Paral® see paraldehyde on this page

paraldehyde (par al' de hyde)
Brand Names Paral®
Synonyms paracetaldehyde
Therapeutic Category Anticonvulsant, Miscellaneous; Hypnotic; Sedative
Use Treatment of status epilepticus and tetanus induced seizures; has been used as a sedative/hypnotic and in the treatment of alcohol withdrawal symptoms (delirium tremens)
Usual Dosage
Oral: Dilute in milk or iced fruit juice to mask taste and odor; see table.

Paraldehyde

	Sedative	Hypnotic	Seizures
Adult Oral, rectal	5–10 mL	10–30 mL	
I.M.		5 mL	5–10 mL
I.V.		3–5 mL	0.2–0.4 mL/kg
Children Oral, rectal	0.15 mL/kg	0.3 mL/kg	
I.M.			0.15 mL/kg every 4–6 h
I.V.			5 mL in 95 mL normal saline solution

Rectal: Mix paraldehyde 2:1 with oil (cottonseed or olive)
Dosing adjustment in hepatic impairment: Dosage may need to be reduced
Dosage Forms Liquid, oral or rectal: 1 g/mL (30 mL)

paramethad *see* paramethadione *on this page*

paramethadione (par a meth a dye' one)
Brand Names Paradione®
Synonyms isoethadione; paramethad
Therapeutic Category Anticonvulsant, Oxazolidinedione
Use To control absence (petit mal) seizures refractory to other drugs
Usual Dosage Oral:
Children: 300-900 mg/day in 3-4 equally divided doses
Adults: 900 mg to 2.4 g/day in 3-4 equally divided doses
Dosage Forms Capsule: 150 mg, 300 mg

Paraplatin® *see* carboplatin *on page 75*

Parathar™ Injection *see* teriparatide *on page 455*

Par Decon® *see* chlorpheniramine, phenyltoloxamine, phenylpropanolamine, and phenylephrine *on page 96*

Par-Drix® [OTC] *see* dexbrompheniramine and pseudoephedrine *on page 134*

paregoric (par e gor' ik)
Synonyms camphorated tincture of opium
Therapeutic Category Analgesic, Narcotic; Antidiarrheal
Use Treatment of diarrhea or relief of pain; neonatal opiate withdrawal
Usual Dosage
Neonatal opiate withdrawal: Oral: 3-6 drops every 3-6 hours as needed, or initially 0.2 mL every 3 hours; increase dosage by approximately 0.05 mL every 3 hours until withdrawal symptoms are controlled; it is rare to exceed 0.7 mL/dose. Stabilize withdrawal symptoms for 3-5 days, then gradually decrease dosage over a 2- to 4-week period.

Children: 0.25-0.5 mL/kg 1-4 times/day

Adults: 5-10 mL 1-4 times/day
Dosage Forms Liquid: 2 mg morphine equivalent/5 mL [equivalent to 20 mg opium powder] (5 mL, 60 mL, 473 mL, 4000 mL)

Parepectolin® *see* kaolin and pectin with opium *on page 262*

Pargen Fortified® *see* chlorzoxazone *on page 99*

Par Glycerol® *see* iodinated glycerol *on page 253*

Par Glycerol C® *see* iodinated glycerol and codeine *on page 254*

Par Glycerol DM® *see* iodinated glycerol and dextromethorphan *on page 254*

pargyline and methyclothiazide *see* methyclothiazide and pargyline *on page 303*

Parhist SR® *see* chlorpheniramine and phenylpropanolamine *on page 93*

Parlodel® *see* bromocriptine mesylate *on page 58*

Parnate® *see* tranylcypromine sulfate *on page 473*

paromomycin sulfate (par oh moe mye' sin)
Brand Names Humatin®
Therapeutic Category Amebicide
Use Treatment of acute and chronic intestinal amebiasis; preoperatively to suppress intestinal flora; tapeworm infestations; rid bowel of nitrogen forming bacteria in hepatic coma
Usual Dosage Oral:
Intestinal amebiasis: Children and Adults: 25-35 mg/kg/day in 3 divided doses for 5-10 days
(Continued)

paromomycin sulfate *(Continued)*
Tapeworm (fish, dog, bovine, porcine):
    Children: 11 mg/kg every 15 minutes for 4 doses
    Adults: 1 g every 15 minutes for 4 doses
Hepatic coma: Adults: 4 g/day in 2-4 divided doses for 5-6 days
Dwarf tapeworm: Children and Adults: 45 mg/kg/dose every day for 5-7 days
Dosage Forms Capsule: 250 mg

paroxetine (pa rox' e teen)
Brand Names Paxil®
Therapeutic Category Antidepressant; Serotonin Antagonist
Use Treatment of depression
Usual Dosage Adults: Oral: 20 mg once daily, preferably in the morning
Dosage Forms Tablet: 20 mg, 30 mg

Parsidol® *see* ethopropazine hydrochloride *on page 185*

Partuss® LA *see* guaifenesin and phenylpropanolamine *on page 219*

PAS *see* aminosalicylate sodium *on page 20*

PAS *see* para-aminosalicylate sodium *on page 356*

Pathilon® *see* tridihexethyl chloride *on page 477*

Pathocil® *see* dicloxacillin sodium *on page 144*

Pavabid® Oral *see* papaverine hydrochloride *on page 355*

Pavased® Oral *see* papaverine hydrochloride *on page 355*

Pavatine® Oral *see* papaverine hydrochloride *on page 355*

Paverolan® Oral *see* papaverine hydrochloride *on page 355*

Pavulon® *see* pancuronium bromide *on page 355*

Paxil® *see* paroxetine *on this page*

Paxipam® *see* halazepam *on page 223*

PBZ® *see* tripelennamine *on page 481*

PBZ-SR® *see* tripelennamine *on page 481*

PCE® Oral *see* erythromycin *on page 175*

PCMX *see* parachlorometaxylenol *on page 356*

pectin and kaolin *see* kaolin and pectin *on page 262*

Pedameth® *see* methionine *on page 300*

PediaCare® Oral *see* pseudoephedrine *on page 406*

Pediacof® *see* chlorpheniramine, phenylephrine, and codeine *on page 95*

Pediaflor® *see* fluoride *on page 201*

PediaPatch Transdermal Patch [OTC] *see* salicylic acid *on page 424*

Pediapred® Oral *see* prednisolone *on page 391*

Pediazole® Oral *see* erythromycin and sulfisoxazole *on page 176*

Pedi-Boro® [OTC] *see* aluminum acetate *on page 14*

Pedi-Cort V® Topical *see* clioquinol and hydrocortisone *on page 106*

Pedi-Dri Topical *see* undecylenic acid and derivatives *on page 486*

PediOtic® Otic *see* neomycin, polymyxin b, and hydrocortisone *on page 329*

Pedi-Pro Topical [OTC] *see* undecylenic acid and derivatives *on page 486*

Pedituss® *see* chlorpheniramine, phenylephrine, and codeine *on page 95*

Pedte-Pak-5® *see* trace metals *on page 472*

Pedtrace-4® *see* trace metals *on page 472*

PedvaxHIB™ *see* hemophilus b conjugate vaccine *on page 226*

pegademase bovine (peg a' de mase)
Brand Names Adagen™
Therapeutic Category Enzyme, Replacement Therapy
Use Enzyme replacement therapy for adenosine deaminase (ADA) deficiency in patients with severe combined immunodeficiency disease (SCID) who can not benefit from bone marrow transplant
Usual Dosage Children: I.M.: Dose given every 7 days, 10 units/kg the first dose, 15 units/kg the second dose, and 20 units/kg the third; maintenance dose: 20 units/kg/week is recommended depending on patient's ADA level
Dosage Forms Injection: 250 units/mL

Peganone® *see* ethotoin *on page 186*

PEG-ES *see* polyethylene glycol-electrolyte solution *on page 383*

pemoline (pem' oh leen)
Brand Names Cylert®
Synonyms phenylisohydantoin; PIO
Therapeutic Category Central Nervous System Stimulant, Nonamphetamine
Use Treatment of attention deficit disorder with hyperactivity (ADDH); narcolepsy
Usual Dosage
Children: <6 years: Not recommended.
Children ≥6 years and Adults: Initial: 37.5 mg given once daily in the morning, increase by 18.75 mg/day at weekly intervals; effective dose range: 56.25-75 mg/day; maximum: 112.5 mg/day; dosage range: 0.5-3 mg/kg/24 hours
Dosage Forms
Tablet: 18.75 mg, 37.5 mg, 75 mg
Tablet, chewable: 37.5 mg

penbutolol sulfate (pen byoo' toe lole)
Brand Names Levatol®
Therapeutic Category Beta-Adrenergic Blocker
Use Treatment of mild to moderate arterial hypertension
Usual Dosage Adults: Oral: Initial: 20 mg once daily, full effect of a 20 or 40 mg dose is seen by the end of a 2-week period, doses of 40-80 mg have been tolerated but have shown little additional antihypertensive effects
Dosage Forms Tablet: 20 mg

Penecort® Topical *see* hydrocortisone *on page 236*

Penetrex™ Oral *see* enoxacin *on page 170*

pen G *see* penicillin g, oral *on page 361*

penicillamine (pen i sill' a meen)
Brand Names Cuprimine®; Depen®
Synonyms D-3-mercaptovaline; β,β-dimethylcysteine; d-penicillamine
Therapeutic Category Antidote, Copper Toxicity; Antidote, Lead Toxicity; Chelating Agent, Oral
Use Treatment of Wilson's disease, cystinuria, adjunct in the treatment of rheumatoid arthritis; lead poisoning, arsenic poisoning; primary biliary cirrhosis
Usual Dosage Oral:
Rheumatoid arthritis:
Children: Initial: 3 mg/kg/day (≤250 mg/day) for 3 months, then 6 mg/kg/day (≤500 mg/day) in divided doses twice daily for 3 months to a maximum of 10 mg/kg/day in 3-4

(Continued)

penicillamine *(Continued)*

divided doses
Adults: 125-250 mg/day, may increase dose at 1- to 3-month intervals up to 1-1.5 g/day

Wilson's disease (doses titrated to maintain urinary copper excretion >1 mg/day):
Infants <6 months: 250 mg/dose once daily
Children <12 years: 250 mg/dose 2-3 times/day
Adults: 250 mg 4 times/day

Cystinuria:
Children: 30 mg/kg/day in 4 divided doses
Adults: 1-4 g/day in divided doses every 6 hours

Lead poisoning (continue until blood lead level is <60 μg/dL):
Children: 25-40 mg/kg/day in 3 divided doses
Adults: 250 mg/dose every 8-12 hours

Primary biliary cirrhosis: 250 mg/day to start, increase by 250 mg every 2 weeks up to a maintenance dose of 1 g/day, usually given 250 mg 4 times/day

Arsenic poisoning: Children: 100 mg/kg/day in divided doses every 6 hours for 5 days; maximum: 1 g/day

Dosage Forms
Capsule: 125 mg, 250 mg
Tablet: 250 mg

penicillin g benzathine

Brand Names Bicillin® L-A Injection; Permapen® Injection
Synonyms benzathine benzylpenicillin; benzathine penicillin g; benzylpenicillin benzathine
Therapeutic Category Antibiotic, Penicillin
Use Active against most gram-positive organisms; some gram-negative organisms such as *Neisseria gonorrhoeae* and some anaerobes and spirochetes; used only for the treatment of mild to moderately severe infections caused by organisms susceptible to low concentrations of penicillin g, or for prophylaxis of infections caused by these organisms
Usual Dosage I.M.: Give undiluted injection, very slowly released from site of injection, providing uniform levels over 2-4 weeks; higher doses result in more sustained rather than higher levels. Use a penicillin g benzathine-penicillin g procaine combination to achieve early peak levels in acute infections

Neonates >1200 g: 50,000 units as a single dose

Infants and Children:
Group A streptococcal upper respiratory infection: 25,000 units/kg as a single dose; maximum: 1.2 million units
Prophylaxis of recurrent rheumatic fever: 25,000 units/kg every 3-4 weeks; maximum: 1.2 million units/dose
Early syphilis: 50,000 units/kg as a single injection; maximum: 2.4 million units
Syphilis of more than 1-year duration: 50,000 units/kg every week for 3 doses; maximum: 2.4 million units/dose

Adults:
Group A streptococcal upper respiratory infection: 1.2 million units as a single dose
Prophylaxis of recurrent rheumatic fever: 1.2 million units every 3-4 weeks or 600,000 units twice monthly; a single dose of 600,000 to 1,2000,000 units is effective in the prevention of rheumatic fever secondary to streptococcal pharyngitis
Early syphilis: 2.4 million units as a single dose
Syphilis of more than 1-year duration: 2.4 million units once weekly for 3 doses
Dosage Forms Injection: 300,000 units/mL (10 mL); 600,000 units/mL (1 mL, 2 mL, 4 mL)

penicillin g benzathine and procaine combined

Brand Names Bicillin® C-R 900/300 Injection; Bicillin® C-R Injection
Synonyms penicillin g procaine and benzathine combined
Therapeutic Category Antibiotic, Penicillin

Use Active against most gram-positive organisms, mostly streptococcal and pneumococcal
Usual Dosage I.M.:
Children:
<30 lb: 600,000 units in a single dose
30-60 lb: 900,000 units to 1.2 million units in a single dose
Children >60 lb and Adults: 2.4 million units in a single dose
Dosage Forms
Injection:
300,000 units [150,000 units each of penicillin g benzathine and penicillin g procaine] (10 mL)
600,000 units [300,000 units each penicillin g benzathine and penicillin g procaine] (1 mL)
1,200,000 units [600,000 units each penicillin g benzathine and penicillin g procaine] (2 mL)
2,400,000 units [1,200,000 units each penicillin g benzathine and penicillin g procaine] (4 mL)
Injection: Penicillin g benzathine 900,000 units and penicillin g procaine 300,000 units per dose (2 mL)

penicillin g, oral
Brand Names Pentids® Oral
Synonyms pen G
Therapeutic Category Antibiotic, Penicillin
Use Treatment of susceptible bacterial infections including most gram-positive organisms (except *Staphylococcus aureus*), some gram-negative organisms such as *Neisseria gonorrhoeae*, and some anaerobes and spirochetes
Usual Dosage Oral (penicillin V potassium is preferred for oral therapy):
Infants and Children: 25-50 mg/kg/day or 40,000-80,000 units/kg/day divided every 6-8 hours hours
Adults: 125-500 mg every 6-8 hours
Dosage Forms
Powder for oral solution: 400,000 units/5 mL (100 mL, 200 mL)
Tablet: 200,000 units, 250,000 units, 400,000 units, 500,000 units, 800,000 units

penicillin g, parenteral
Brand Names Pfizerpen® Injection
Synonyms benzylpenicillin potassium; benzylpenicillin sodium; crystalline penicillin; penicillin g potassium; penicillin g sodium
Therapeutic Category Antibiotic, Penicillin
Use Active against most gram-positive organisms except *Staphylococcus aureus*; some gram-negative such as *Neisseria gonorrhoeae* and some anaerobes and spirochetes; although ceftriaxone is now the drug of choice for lyme disease and gonorrhea
Usual Dosage I.M., I.V.:
Neonates:
Postnatal age <7 days:
<2000 g: 25,000 units/kg/dose every 12 hours; meningitis: 50,000 units/kg/dose every 12 hours
>2000 g: 20,000 units/kg/dose every 8 hours; meningitis: 50,000 units/kg/dose every 8 hours
Postnatal age >7 days:
<1200 g: 25,000 units/kg/dose every 12 hours; meningitis: 50,000 units/kg/dose every 12 hours
1200-2000 g: 25,000 units/kg/dose every 8 hours; meningitis: 75,000 units/kg/dose every 8 hours
>2000 g: 25,000 units/kg/dose every 6 hours; meningitis: 50,000 units/kg/dose every 6 hours
(Continued)
361

penicillin g, parenteral (Continued)

Infants and Children (sodium salt is preferred in children): 100,000-250,000 units/kg/day in divided doses every 4 hours; maximum: 4.8 million units/24 hours

Severe infections: Up to 400,000 units/kg/day in divided doses every 4 hours; maximum dose: 24 million units/day

Adults: 2-24 million units/day in divided doses every 4 hours

Dosage Forms

Injection, as sodium: 5 million units

Injection:

Frozen premixed, as potassium: 1 million units, 2 million units, 3 million units

Powder, as potassium: 1 million units, 5 million units, 10 million units, 20 million units

penicillin g potassium see penicillin g, parenteral on previous page

penicillin g procaine and benzathine combined see penicillin g benzathine and procaine combined on page 360

penicillin g procaine, aqueous

Brand Names Crysticillin® A.S. Injection; Pfizerpen®-AS Injection; Wycillin® Injection

Synonyms APPG; aqueous procaine penicillin g; procaine benzylpenicillin; procaine penicillin g

Therapeutic Category Antibiotic, Penicillin

Use Moderately severe infections due to *Neisseria gonorrhoeae*, *Treponema pallidum* and other penicillin g-sensitive microorganisms that are susceptible to low but prolonged serum penicillin concentrations

Usual Dosage I.M.:

Newborns: 50,000 units/kg/day given every day (avoid using in this age group since sterile abscesses and procaine toxicity occur more frequently with neonates than older patients)

Children: 25,000-50,000 units/kg/day in divided doses 1-2 times/day; not to exceed 4.8 million units/24 hours

Gonorrhea: 100,000 units/kg one time (in 2 injection sites) along with probenecid 25 mg/kg (maximum: 1 g) orally 30 minutes prior to procaine penicillin

Adults: 0.6-4.8 million units/day in divided doses 1-2 times/day

Uncomplicated gonorrhea: 1 g probenecid orally, then 4.8 million units procaine penicillin divided into 2 injection sites 30 minutes later. When used in conjunction with an aminoglycoside for the treatment of endocarditis caused by susceptible *S. viridans*: 1.2 million units every 6 hours for 2-4 weeks

Dosage Forms Injection, suspension: 300,000 units/mL (10 mL); 500,000 units/mL (1.2 mL); 600,000 units/mL (1 mL, 2 mL, 4 mL)

penicillin g sodium see penicillin g, parenteral on previous page

penicillin V potassium

Brand Names Beepen-VK® Oral; Betapen®-VK Oral; Ledercillin® VK Oral; Pen.Vee® K Oral; Robicillin® VK Oral; V-Cillin K® Oral; Veetids® Oral

Synonyms pen vk; phenoxymethyl penicillin

Therapeutic Category Antibiotic, Penicillin

Use Treatment of moderate to severe susceptible bacterial infections involving the respiratory tract, skin and urinary tract; prophylaxis of pneumococcal infections and rheumatic fever; otitis media and sinusitis

Usual Dosage Oral:

Systemic infections:

Children <12 years: 25-50 mg/kg/day in divided doses every 6-8 hours; maximum dose: 3 g/day

Children >12 years and Adults: 125-500 mg every 6-8 hours

Prophylaxis of pneumococcal infections:
Children <5 years: 125 mg twice daily
Children ≥5 years: 250 mg twice daily

Prophylaxis of recurrent rheumatic fever:
Children <5 years: 125 mg
Children ≥5 years and Adults: 250 mg twice daily

Dosage Forms
Powder for oral solution: 125 mg/5 mL (3 mL, 100 mL, 150 mL, 200 mL); 250 mg/5 mL (100 mL, 150 mL, 200 mL)
Tablet: 125 mg, 250 mg, 500 mg

penicilloyl-polylysine *see* benzylpenicilloyl-polylysine *on page 51*

Pentacef™ *see* ceftazidime *on page 81*

pentaerythritol tetranitrate (pen ta er ith' ri tole te tra nye' trate)
Brand Names Duotrate®; Peritrate®; Peritrate® SA
Synonyms PETN
Therapeutic Category Antianginal Agent; Nitrate; Vasodilator, Coronary
Use Prophylactic long-term management of angina pectoris
Usual Dosage Adults: Oral: 10-20 mg 4 times/day (160 mg/day) up to 40 mg 4 times/day before or after meals and at bedtime; administer sustained release preparation every 12 hours; maximum daily dose: 240 mg
Dosage Forms
Capsule: sustained release: 15 mg, 30 mg
Tablet: 10 mg, 20 mg, 40 mg
Tablet, sustained release: 80 mg

pentagastrin (pen ta gas' trin)
Brand Names Peptavlon®
Therapeutic Category Diagnostic Agent, Gastric Acid Secretory Function
Use Evaluate gastric acid secretory function in pernicious anemia, gastric carcinoma; in suspected duodenal ulcer or Zollinger-Ellison tumor
Usual Dosage Adults: S.C.: 6 µg/kg
Dosage Forms Injection: 0.25 mg/mL (2 mL)

Pentam-300® Injection *see* pentamidine isethionate *on this page*

pentamidine isethionate (pen tam' i deen eye se thi' o nate)
Brand Names NebuPent™ Inhalation; Pentam-300® Injection
Therapeutic Category Antibiotic, Miscellaneous
Use Treatment and prevention of pneumonia caused by *Pneumocystis carinii* (PCP); treatment of trypanosomiasis
Usual Dosage
Children:
Treatment: I.M., I.V. (I.V. preferred): 4 mg/kg/day once daily for 14-21 days
Prevention:
I.M., I.V.: 4 mg/kg monthly or biweekly
Inhalation (aerosolized pentamidine in children ≥5 years): 300 mg/dose given every 3 weeks or monthly via Respirgard® II inhaler (8 mg/kg dose has also been used in children <5 years)
Treatment of trypanosomiasis: I.V.: 4 mg/kg/day once daily for 10 days

(Continued)

pentamidine isethionate (Continued)

Adults:
Treatment: I.M., I.V. (I.V. preferred): 4 mg/kg/day once daily for 14 days
Prevention: Inhalation: 300 mg every 4 weeks via Respirgard® II nebulizer
Dosage Forms
Inhalation: 300 mg
Powder for injection, lyophilized: 300 mg

Pentasa® Oral see mesalamine on page 294

pentazocine (pen taz' oh seen)

Brand Names Talwin®; Talwin® NX
Synonyms pentazocine hydrochloride; pentazocine lactate
Therapeutic Category Analgesic, Narcotic
Use Relief of moderate to severe pain; has also been used as a sedative prior to surgery and as a supplement to surgical anesthesia
Usual Dosage
Children: I.M., S.C.:
5-8 years: 15 mg
8-14 years: 30 mg

Children >12 years and Adults: Oral: 50 mg every 3-4 hours; may increase to 100 mg/dose if needed, but should not exceed 600 mg/day
Adults:
I.M., S.C.: 30-60 mg every 3-4 hours, not to exceed total daily dose of 360 mg
I.V.: 30 mg every 3-4 hours
Dosage Forms
Injection, as lactate: 30 mg/mL (1 mL, 1.5 mL, 2 mL, 10 mL)
Tablet, scored: Pentazocine hydrochloride 50 mg and naloxone hydrochloride 0.5 mg

pentazocine and acetaminophen see pentazocine compound on this page

pentazocine and aspirin see pentazocine compound on this page

pentazocine compound

Brand Names Talacen®; Talwin® Compound
Synonyms acetaminophen and pentazocine; aspirin and pentazocine; pentazocine and acetaminophen; pentazocine and aspirin
Therapeutic Category Analgesic, Narcotic
Use Relief of moderate to severe pain; has also been used as a sedative prior to surgery and as a supplement to surgical anesthesia
Usual Dosage Adults: Oral: 2 tablets 3-4 times/day
Dosage Forms Tablet:
Talacen®: Pentazocine hydrochloride 25 mg and acetaminophen 650 mg
Talwin® Compound: Pentazocine hydrochloride 12.5 mg and aspirin 325 mg

pentazocine hydrochloride see pentazocine on this page
pentazocine lactate see pentazocine on this page
Penthrane® see methoxyflurane on page 302
Pentids® Oral see penicillin g, oral on page 361

pentobarbital (pen toe bar' bi tal)

Brand Names Nembutal®
Synonyms pentobarbital sodium
Therapeutic Category Barbiturate; Sedative

Use Short-term treatment of insomnia; preoperative sedation; high-dose barbiturate coma for treatment of increased intracranial pressure or status epilepticus unresponsive to other therapy

Usual Dosage

Children:

Sedative: Oral: 2-6 mg/kg/day divided in 3 doses; maximum: 100 mg/day

Hypnotic: I.M.: 2-6 mg/kg; maximum: 100 mg/dose

Rectal:

2 months to 1 year (10-20 lb): 30 mg

1-4 years (20-40 lb): 30-60 mg

5-12 years (40-80 lb): 60 mg

12-14 years (80-110 lb): 60-120 mg **or**

<4 years: 3-6 mg/kg/dose

>4 years: 1.5-3 mg/kg/dose

Preoperative/preprocedure sedation: ≥6 months:

Oral, I.M., rectal: 2-6 mg/kg; maximum: 100 mg/dose

I.V.: 1-3 mg/kg to a maximum of 100 mg until asleep

Children 5-12 years: Conscious sedation prior to a procedure: I.V.: 2 mg/kg 5-10 minutes before procedures, may repeat one time

Adolescents: Conscious sedation: Oral, I.V.: 100 mg prior to a procedure

Children and Adults: Barbiturate coma in head injury patients: I.V.: Loading dose: 5-10 mg/kg given slowly over 1-2 hours; monitor blood pressure and respiratory rate; Maintenance infusion: Initial: 1 mg/kg/hour; may increase to 2-3 mg/kg/hour; maintain burst suppression on EEG

Adults:

Hypnotic:

Oral: 100-200 mg at bedtime or 20 mg 3-4 times/day for daytime sedation

I.M.: 150-200 mg

I.V.: Initial: 100 mg, may repeat every 1-3 minutes up to 200-500 mg total dose

Rectal: 120-200 mg at bedtime

Preoperative sedation: I.M.: 150-200 mg

Dosage Forms

Capsule, as sodium: 50 mg, 100 mg

Elixir: 18.2 mg/5 mL (473 mL, 4000 mL)

Injection, as sodium: 50 mg/mL (1 mL, 2 mL, 20 mL, 50 mL)

Suppository, rectal (C-III): 30 mg, 60 mg, 120 mg, 200 mg

pentobarbital sodium see pentobarbital on previous page

pentostatin (pen' toe stat in)

Brand Names Nipent™ Injection

Synonyms DCF; 2'-deoxycoformycin

Therapeutic Category Antineoplastic Agent, Antimetabolite; Antineoplastic Agent, Nonirritant

Use Treatment of adult patients with alpha-interferon-refractory hairy cell leukemia; significant antitumor activity in various lymphoid neoplasms has been demonstrated

Usual Dosage Refer to individual protocols

Refractory hairy cell leukemia: Adults: I.V.: 4 mg/m^2 every other week

Dosage Forms Powder for injection: 10 mg

Pentothal® Sodium see thiopental sodium on page 464

pentoxifylline (pen tox i' fi leen)

Brand Names Trental®

Synonyms oxpentifylline

Therapeutic Category Blood Viscosity Reducer Agent

(Continued)

pentoxifylline *(Continued)*
Use Symptomatic management of peripheral vascular disease, mainly intermittent claudication

Usual Dosage Adults: Oral: 400 mg 3 times/day with meals; may reduce to 400 mg twice daily if GI or CNS side effects occur

Dosage Forms Tablet, controlled release: 400 mg

Pentrax® [OTC] *see coal tar on page 110*

Pen.Vee® K Oral *see penicillin V potassium on page 362*

pen vk *see penicillin V potassium on page 362*

Pepcid® I.V. *see famotidine on page 190*

Pepcid® Oral *see famotidine on page 190*

Peptavlon® *see pentagastrin on page 363*

Pepto-Bismol® [OTC] *see bismuth on page 55*

Pepto® Diarrhea Control [OTC *see loperamide hydrochloride on page 277*

Perchloracap® *see radiological/contrast media (ionic) on page 413*

Percocet® *see oxycodone and acetaminophen on page 349*

Percodan® *see oxycodone and aspirin on page 350*

Percodan®-Demi *see oxycodone and aspirin on page 350*

Percogesic® [OTC] *see acetaminophen and phenyltoloxamine on page 4*

Perdiem® Plain [OTC] *see psyllium on page 407*

pergolide mesylate *(per' go lide)*
Brand Names Permax®

Therapeutic Category Antiparkinson Agent; Ergot Alkaloid

Use Adjunctive treatment to levodopa/carbidopa in the management of Parkinson's Disease

Usual Dosage Adults: Oral: Start with 0.05 mg/day for 2 days, then increase dosage by 0.1 or 0.15 mg/day every 3 days over next 12 days, increase dose by 0.25 mg/day every 3 days until optimal therapeutic dose is achieved

Dosage Forms Tablet: 0.05 mg, 0.25 mg, 1 mg

Pergonal® *see menotropins on page 291*

Periactin® *see cyproheptadine hydrochloride on page 123*

Peri-Colace® [OTC] *see docusate and casanthranol on page 158*

Peridex® Oral Rinse *see chlorhexidine gluconate on page 90*

Peritrate® *see pentaerythritol tetranitrate on page 363*

Peritrate® SA *see pentaerythritol tetranitrate on page 363*

Permapen® Injection *see penicillin g benzathine on page 360*

Permax® *see pergolide mesylate on this page*

permethrin *(per meth' rin)*
Brand Names Elimite™ Cream; Nix™ Creme Rinse

Therapeutic Category Antiparasitic Agent, Topical; Scabicidal Agent

Use Single application treatment of infestation with *Pediculus humanus capitis* (head louse) and its nits, or *Sarcoptes scabiei* (scabies)

Usual Dosage
Head lice: Children >2 months and Adults: Topical: After hair has been washed with shampoo, rinsed with water and towel dried, apply a sufficient volume to saturate the hair and scalp. Leave on hair for 10 minutes before rinsing off with water; remove remaining nits.

Scabies: Apply cream from head to toe; leave on for 8-14 hours before washing off with water
Dosage Forms
Cream: 5% (60 g)
Creme rinse: 1% (60 mL with comb)

Permitil® Oral *see* fluphenazine *on page 203*

Pernox® [OTC] *see* sulfur and salicylic acid *on page 450*

perphenazine (per fen' a zeen)
Brand Names Trilafon®
Therapeutic Category Antiemetic; Antipsychotic Agent; Phenothiazine Derivative
Use Symptomatic management of psychotic disorders, as well as severe nausea and vomiting
Usual Dosage
Children:
Psychoses: Oral:
1-6 years: 4-6 mg/day in divided doses
6-12 years: 6 mg/day in divided doses
>12 years: 4-16 mg 2-4 times/day
I.M.: 5 mg every 6 hours
Nausea/vomiting: I.M.: 5 mg every 6 hours

Adults:
Psychoses:
Oral: 4-16 mg 2-4 times/day not to exceed 64 mg/day
I.M.: 5 mg every 6 hours up to 15 mg/day in ambulatory patients and 30 mg/day in hospitalized patients
Nausea/vomiting:
Oral: 8-16 mg/day in divided doses up to 24 mg/day
I.M.: 5-10 mg every 6 hours as necessary up to 15 mg/day in ambulatory patients and 30 mg/day in hospitalized patients
I.V. (severe): 1 mg at 1- to 2-minute intervals up to a total of 5 mg
Dosage Forms
Concentrate, oral: 16 mg/5 mL (118 mL)
Injection: 5 mg/mL (1 mL)
Tablet: 2 mg, 4 mg, 8 mg, 16 mg

perphenazine and amitriptyline *see* amitriptyline and perphenazine *on page 21*

Persa-Gel® *see* benzoyl peroxide *on page 49*

Persantine® *see* dipyridamole *on page 155*

Pertofrane® *see* desipramine hydrochloride *on page 131*

Pertussin® CS [OTC] *see* dextromethorphan hydrobromide *on page 136*

Pertussin® ES [OTC] *see* dextromethorphan hydrobromide *on page 136*

pertussis immune globulin, human
Brand Names Hypertussis®
Therapeutic Category Immune Globulin
Dosage Forms Injection: 1.25 mL

pethidine hydrochloride *see* meperidine hydrochloride *on page 292*

PETN *see* pentaerythritol tetranitrate *on page 363*

pfa *see* foscarnet *on page 206*

Pfizerpen®-AS Injection *see* penicillin g procaine, aqueous *on page 362*

Pfizerpen® Injection *see* penicillin g, parenteral *on page 361*

PGE₁ *see* alprostadil *on page 13*

PGE₂ *see* dinoprostone *on page 151*

Phanatuss® [OTC] *see* guaifenesin and dextromethorphan *on page 218*

Pharmaflur® *see* fluoride *on page 201*

Phazyme® [OTC] *see* simethicone *on page 431*

Phenameth® DM *see* promethazine with dextromethorphan *on page 399*

Phenameth® Oral *see* promethazine hydrochloride *on page 399*

phenantoin *see* mephenytoin *on page 293*

Phenaphen® With Codeine *see* acetaminophen and codeine *on page 3*

Phenazine® Injection *see* promethazine hydrochloride *on page 399*

phenazopyridine hydrochloride (fen az oh peer' i deen)
Brand Names Azo-Standard®; Geridium®; Pyridiate®; Pyridium®; Urodine®
Synonyms phenylazo diamino pyridine hydrochloride
Therapeutic Category Analgesic, Urinary; Local Anesthetic, Urinary
Use Symptomatic relief of urinary burning, itching, frequency and urgency in association with urinary tract infection or following urologic procedures
Usual Dosage Oral:
Children 6-12 years: 12 mg/kg/day in 3 divided doses administered after meals for 2 days
Adults: 100-200 mg 3-4 times/day for 2 days
Dosage Forms Tablet: 100 mg, 200 mg

Phen DH® w/Codeine *see* chlorpheniramine, pseudoephedrine, and codeine *on page 97*

Phendry® Oral [OTC] *see* diphenhydramine hydrochloride *on page 152*

phenelzine sulfate (fen' el zeen)
Brand Names Nardil®
Therapeutic Category Antidepressant, Monoamine Oxidase Inhibitor
Use Symptomatic treatment of atypical, nonendogenous or neurotic depression
Usual Dosage Adults: Oral: 15 mg 3 times/day; may increase to 60-90 mg/day during early phase of treatment, then reduce to dose for maintenance therapy slowly after maximum benefit is obtained; takes 2-4 weeks for a significant response to occur
Dosage Forms Tablet: 15 mg

Phenergan® Injection *see* promethazine hydrochloride *on page 399*

Phenergan® Oral *see* promethazine hydrochloride *on page 399*

Phenergan® Rectal *see* promethazine hydrochloride *on page 399*

Phenergan® VC *see* promethazine and phenylephrine *on page 398*

Phenergan® VC With Codeine *see* promethazine, phenylephrine, and codeine *on page 399*

Phenergan® with Codeine *see* promethazine and codeine *on page 398*

Phenergan® with Dextromethorphan *see* promethazine with dextromethorphan *on page 399*

Phenetron® Oral *see* chlorpheniramine maleate *on page 94*

Phenhist® Expectorant *see* guaifenesin, pseudoephedrine, and codeine *on page 221*

pheniramine and naphazoline *see* naphazoline and pheniramine *on page 325*

pheniramine, phenylpropanolamine, and pyrilamine
Brand Names Triaminic® Oral Infant Drops
Therapeutic Category Antihistamine/Decongestant Combination
Use Symptomatic relief of nasal congestion and postnasal drip as well as allergic rhinitis
Usual Dosage Infants <1 year: Drops: 0.05 mL/kg/dose 4 times/day
Dosage Forms Drops: Pheniramine maleate 10 mg, phenylpropanolamine hydrochloride 20 mg, and pyrilamine maleate 10 mg per mL (15 mL)

phenobarbital (fee noe bar' bi tal)
Brand Names Barbita®; Luminal®; Solfoton®
Synonyms phenobarbitone; phenylethylmalonylurea
Therapeutic Category Anticonvulsant, Barbiturate; Barbiturate; Hypnotic; Sedative
Use Management of generalized tonic-clonic (grand mal) and partial seizures; prevention of febrile seizures in infants and young children; sedation; may also be used for prevention and treatment of neonatal hyperbilirubinemia and lowering of bilirubin in chronic cholestasis
Usual Dosage
Children:
    Sedation: Oral: 2 mg/kg 3 times/day
    Hypnotic: I.M., I.V., S.C.: 3-5 mg/kg at bedtime
    Hyperbilirubinemia: <12 years: Oral: 3-8 mg/kg/day in 2-3 divided doses; doses up to 12 mg/kg/day have been used
    Preoperative sedation: Oral, I.M., I.V.: 1-3 mg/kg 1-1.5 hours before procedure
Anticonvulsant: Status epilepticus: **Loading dose:** I.V.:
    Neonates: 15-20 mg/kg in a single or divided dose
    Infants, Children and Adults: 15-18 mg/kg in a single or divided dose; usual maximum loading dose: 20 mg/kg; in select patients may give additional 5 mg/kg/dose every 15-30 minutes until seizure is controlled or a total dose of 30 mg/kg is reached
Anticonvulsant maintenance dose: Oral, I.V.:
    Neonates: 3-4 mg/kg/day in 1-2 divided doses; assess serum concentrations; increase to 5 mg/kg/day if needed (usually by second week of therapy)
    Infants: 5-6 mg/kg/day in 1-2 divided doses
    Children:
        1-5 years: 6-8 mg/kg/day in 1-2 divided doses
        5-12 years: 4-6 mg/kg/day in 1-2 divided doses
    Children >12 years and Adults: 1-3 mg/kg/day in divided doses
Adults:
    Sedation: Oral, I.M.: 30-120 mg/day in 2-3 divided doses
    Hypnotic: Oral, I.M., I.V., S.C.: 100-320 mg at bedtime
    Hyperbilirubinemia: Oral: 90-180 mg/day in 2-3 divided doses
    Preoperative sedation: I.M.: 100-200 mg 1-1½ hours before procedure
Dosage Forms
Capsule: 16 mg
Elixir: 15 mg/5 mL (5 mL, 10 mL, 20 mL); 20 mg/5 mL (3.75 mL, 5 mL, 7.5 mL, 120 mL, 473 mL, 946 mL, 4000 mL)
Injection, as sodium: 30 mg/mL (1 mL); 60 mg/mL (1 mL); 65 mg/mL (1 mL); 130 mg/mL (1 mL)
Powder for injection: 120 mg
Tablet: 8 mg, 15 mg, 16 mg, 30 mg, 32 mg, 60 mg, 65 mg, 100 mg

phenobarbitone *see* phenobarbital *on this page*

phenol
Brand Names Baker's P&S Topical [OTC]; Chloraseptic® Oral [OTC]
Synonyms carbolic acid
Therapeutic Category Pharmaceutical Aid
(Continued)

phenol *(Continued)*

Use Relief of sore throat pain, mouth, gum, and throat irritations
Usual Dosage Allow to dissolve slowly in mouth; may be repeated every 2 hours as needed
Dosage Forms
Liquid, topical (Baker's P&S): 1% [10 mg/mL] with sodium chloride, liquid paraffin oil and water (120 mL, 240 mL)
Lozenge (Chloraseptic®): 32.5 mg total phenol, sugar, corn syrup
Mouthwash (Chloraseptic®): 1.4% [14 mg/mL] with thymol, sodium borate, menthol and glycerin (180 mL)
Solution (Liquified Phenol): 88% [880 mg/mL]

Phenolax® [OTC] *see* phenolphthalein *on this page*

phenolphthalein (fee nole thay' leen)

Brand Names Alophen Pills® [OTC]; Espotabs® [OTC]; Evac-U-Gen® [OTC]; Evac-U-Lax® [OTC]; Ex-Lax® [OTC]; Feen-a-Mint® [OTC]; Lax-Pills® [OTC]; Medilax® [OTC]; Modane® [OTC]; Phenolax® [OTC]; Prulet® [OTC]
Therapeutic Category Laxative, Stimulant
Use Stimulant laxative
Usual Dosage Oral:
Children: 15-60 mg
Adults: 60-200 mg preferably at bedtime
Dosage Forms
Gum: 97.2 mg
Tablet: 60 mg, 90 mg, 97.2 mg, 130 mg
Tablet, chewable: 65 mg, 90 mg, 97.2 mg, 120 mg
Wafer: 64.8 mg
Wafer, chewable: 80 mg

phenol red *see* phenolsulfonphthalein *on this page*

phenolsulfonphthalein (fee nole sul fon thay' leen)

Synonyms phenol red; psp
Therapeutic Category Diagnostic Agent, Kidney Function
Use Evaluation of renal blood flow to aid in the determination of renal function
Usual Dosage I.M., I.V.: 6 mg
Dosage Forms Injection: 6 mg/mL (1 mL)

phenoxybenzamine hydrochloride (fen ox ee ben' za meen)

Brand Names Dibenzyline®
Therapeutic Category Alpha-Adrenergic Blocking Agent, Oral; Antihypertensive; Vasodilator, Coronary
Use Symptomatic management of pheochromocytoma; treatment of hypertensive crisis caused by sympathomimetic amines
Usual Dosage Oral:
Children: Initial: 0.2 mg/kg (maximum: 10 mg) once daily, increase by 0.2 mg/kg increments; usual maintenance dose: 1-2 mg/kg/day divided every 6-8 hours, maximum single dose: 10 mg
Adults: 10-40 mg every 8-12 hours
Dosage Forms Capsule: 10 mg

phenoxymethyl penicillin *see* penicillin V potassium *on page 362*

phensuximide (fen sux' i mide)
Brand Names Milontin®
Therapeutic Category Anticonvulsant, Succinimide
Use Control of absence (petit mal) seizures
Usual Dosage Children and Adults: Oral: 0.5-1 g 2-3 times/day
Dosage Forms Capsule: 500 mg

phentermine hydrochloride (fen' ter meen)
Brand Names Adipex-P®; Fastin®; Ionamin®; Zantryl®
Therapeutic Category Anorexiant
Use Short-term adjunct in exogenous obesity
Usual Dosage Children and Adults: Oral: 8 mg 3 times/day 30 minutes before meals or food or 15-37.5 mg/day before breakfast
Dosage Forms
Capsule: 15 mg, 18.75 mg, 30 mg, 37.5 mg
Capsule, resin complex: 15 mg, 30 mg
Tablet: 8 mg, 37.5 mg

phentolamine mesylate (fen tole' a meen)
Brand Names Regitine®
Therapeutic Category Alpha-Adrenergic Blocking Agent, Parenteral; Alpha-Adrenergic Inhibitors, Central; Antidote, Extravasation; Antihypertensive; Diagnostic Agent, Pheochromocytoma; Vasodilator, Coronary
Use Diagnosis of pheochromocytoma and to control or prevent paroxysmal hypertension prior to and during pheochromocytomectomy; as treatment of dermal necrosis after extravasation of drugs with alpha-adrenergic effects (norepinephrine, dopamine, epinephrine)
Usual Dosage
Treatment of extravasation: Infiltrate area S.C. with small amount of solution made by diluting 5-10 mg in 10 mL 0.9% NaCl within 12 hours of extravasation; for children use 0.1-0.2 mg/kg up to a maximum of 10 mg

Children: I.M., I.V.:
Diagnosis of pheochromocytoma: 0.05-0.1 mg/kg/dose, maximum single dose: 5 mg
Hypertension: 0.05-0.1 mg/kg/dose given 1-2 hours before procedure; repeat as needed until hypertension is controlled; maximum single dose: 5 mg

Adults: I.M., I.V.:
Diagnosis of pheochromocytoma: 5 mg
Hypertension: 5 mg given 1-2 hours before procedure
Dosage Forms Injection: 5 mg/mL (1 mL)

phenylalanine mustard *see* melphalan *on page 290*
phenylazo diamino pyridine hydrochloride *see* phenazopyridine hydrochloride *on page 368*

phenylbutazone (fen ill byoo' ta zone)
Brand Names Azolid®; Butazolidin®
Therapeutic Category Analgesic, Non-Narcotic; Anti-inflammatory Agent
Use Management of inflammatory disorders, as an analgesic in the treatment of mild to moderate pain and as an antipyretic; I.V. form used as an alternate to surgery in management of patent ductus arteriosus in premature neonates; acute gouty arthritis
Usual Dosage Adults: Oral:
Rheumatoid arthritis: 100-200 mg 3-4 times/day until desired effect, then reduce dose to not exceeding 400 mg/day
(Continued)

371

phenylbutazone *(Continued)*

Acute gouty arthritis: Initial: 400 mg, 100 mg every 4 hours until acute attack subsides
Dosage Forms
Capsule: 100 mg
Tablet: 100 mg

phenylephrine and chlorpheniramine *see* chlorpheniramine and phenylephrine
on page 93

phenylephrine and cyclopentolate *see* cyclopentolate and phenylephrine
on page 121

phenylephrine and scopolamine

Brand Names Murocoll-2® Ophthalmic
Synonyms scopolamine and phenylephrine
Therapeutic Category Ophthalmic Agent, Mydriatic
Use Mydriasis, cycloplegia and to break posterior synechiae in iritis
Usual Dosage Ophthalmic: Instill 1-2 drops into eye(s); repeat in 5 minutes
Dosage Forms Solution, ophthalmic: Phenylephrine hydrochloride 10% and scopolamine
hydrobromide 0.3% (7.5 mL)

phenylephrine and zinc sulfate

Brand Names Optised® Ophthalmic [OTC]; Phenylzin® Ophthalmic [OTC]; Zincfrin® Ophthalmic [OTC]
Therapeutic Category Ophthalmic Agent, Miscellaneous
Use Soothe, moisturize, and remove redness due to minor eye irritation
Usual Dosage Ophthalmic: Instill 1-2 drops in eye(s) 2-4 times/day as needed
Dosage Forms Solution, ophthalmic: Phenylephrine hydrochloride 0.12% and zinc sulfate
0.25% (15 mL)

phenylephrine hydrochloride (fen ill ef' rin)

Brand Names AK-Dilate® Ophthalmic Solution; AK-Nefrin® Ophthalmic Solution; Alconefrin® Nasal Solution [OTC]; Doktors® Nasal Solution [OTC]; I-Phrine® Ophthalmic Solution; Isopto® Frin Ophthalmic Solution; Mydfrin® Ophthalmic Solution; Neo-Synephrine® Nasal Solution [OTC]; Neo-Synephrine® Ophthalmic Solution; Nostril® Nasal Solution [OTC]; Prefrin™ Ophthalmic Solution; Relief® Ophthalmic Solution; Rhinall® Nasal Solution [OTC]; Sinarest® Nasal Solution [OTC]; St. Joseph® Measured Dose Nasal Solution [OTC]; Vicks Sinex® Nasal Solution [OTC]
Therapeutic Category Adrenergic Agonist Agent; Adrenergic Agonist Agent, Ophthalmic; Alpha-Adrenergic Blocking Agent, Ophthalmic; Nasal Agent, Vasoconstrictor; Ophthalmic Agent, Mydriatic
Use Treatment of hypotension, vascular failure in shock; as a vasoconstrictor in regional analgesia; symptomatic relief of nasal and nasopharyngeal mucosal congestion; as a mydriatic in ophthalmic procedures and treatment of wide-angle glaucoma
Usual Dosage
Ophthalmic procedures:
Infants <1 year: Instill 1 drop of 2.5% 15-30 minutes before procedures
Children and Adults: Instill 1 drop of 2.5% or 10% solution, may repeat in 10-60 minutes as needed

Nasal decongestant:
Children:
2-6 years: Instill 1 drop every 2-4 hours of 0.125% solution as needed
6-12 years: Instill 1-2 sprays or instill 1-2 drops every 4 hours of 0.25% solution as needed
Children >12 years and Adults: Instill 1-2 sprays or instill 1-2 drops every 4 hours of 0.25% to 0.5% solution as needed; 1% solution may be used in adult in cases of extreme nasal congestion; do not use nasal solutions more than 3 days

Hypotension/shock:
Children:
I.M., S.C.: 0.1 mg/kg/dose every 1-2 hours as needed (maximum: 5 mg)
I.V. bolus: 5-20 µg/kg/dose every 10-15 minutes as needed
I.V. infusion: 0.1-0.5 µg/kg/minute; the concentration and rate of infusion can be calculated using the following formulas: Dilute 0.6 mg x weight (kg) to 100 mL; then the dose in µg/kg/minute = 0.1 x the infusion rate in mL/hour
Adults:
I.M., S.C.: 2-5 mg/dose every 1-2 hours as needed (initial dose should not exceed 5 mg)
I.V. bolus: 0.1-0.5 mg/dose every 10-15 minutes as needed (initial dose should not exceed 0.5 mg)
I.V. infusion: 10 mg in 250 mL D$_5$W or NS (1:25,000 dilution) (40 µg/mL); start at 100-180 µg/minute (2-5 mL/minute; 50-90 drops/minute) initially. When blood pressure is stabilized, maintenance rate: 40-60 µg/minute (20-30 drops/minute)

Paroxysmal supraventricular tachycardia: I.V.:
Children: 5-10 µg/kg/dose over 20-30 seconds
Adults: 0.25-0.5 mg/dose over 20-30 seconds

Dosage Forms
Jelly, nasal: 0.5% [5 mg/mL] (18.75 g)
Injection: 1% [10 mg/mL] (1 mL)
Solution:
Nasal:
Drops: 0.125% (15 mL, 30 mL); 0.16% (30 mL); 0.2% (30 mL); 0.25% (15 mL, 30 mL, 473 mL)
Spray: 0.25% (15 mL, 30 mL); 0.5% (15 mL, 30 mL); 1% (15 mL)
Ophthalmic: 0.12% (15 mL); 2.5% (2 mL, 3 mL, 5 mL, 15 mL); 10% (1 mL, 2 mL, 5 mL)

phenylethylmalonylurea see phenobarbital on page 369

Phenylfenesin® L.A. see guaifenesin and phenylpropanolamine on page 219

phenylisohydantoin see pemoline on page 359

phenylpropanolamine and brompheniramine see brompheniramine and phenylpropanolamine on page 59

phenylpropanolamine and caramiphen see caramiphen and phenylpropanolamine on page 72

phenylpropanolamine and chlorpheniramine see chlorpheniramine and phenylpropanolamine on page 93

phenylpropanolamine and guaifenesin see guaifenesin and phenylpropanolamine on page 219

phenylpropanolamine and hydrocodone see hydrocodone and phenylpropanolamine on page 235

phenylpropanolamine hydrochloride (fen ill proe pa nole' a meen)

Brand Names Acutrim® Precision Release® [OTC]; Control® [OTC]; Dex-A-Diet® [OTC]; Dexatrim® [OTC]; Maigret-50; Prolamine® [OTC]; Propadrine; Propagest® [OTC]; Rhindecon®; Stay Trim® Diet Gum [OTC]; Westrim® LA [OTC]
Synonyms dl-norephedrine hydrochloride; PPA
Therapeutic Category Adrenergic Agonist Agent; Anorexiant; Decongestant; Nasal Agent, Vasoconstrictor
Use Anorexiant and nasal decongestant
Usual Dosage Oral:
Children: Decongestant:
2-6 years: 6.25 mg every 4 hours
6-12 years: 12.5 mg every 4 hours not to exceed 75 mg/day

Adults:
Decongestant: 25 mg every 4 hours or 50 mg every 8 hours, not to exceed 150 mg/day
(Continued)

phenylpropanolamine hydrochloride *(Continued)*

Anorexic: 25 mg 3 times/day 30 minutes before meals or 75 mg (timed release) once daily in the morning

Precision release: 75 mg after breakfast

Dosage Forms

Capsule: 37.5 mg

Capsule, timed release: 25 mg, 75 mg

Tablet: 25 mg

Tablet:

Precision release: 75 mg

Timed release: 75 mg

phenyltoloxamine, phenylpropanolamine, and acetaminophen

Brand Names Sinubid®

Therapeutic Category Analgesic, Non-Narcotic; Antihistamine/Decongestant Combination

Use Intermittent symptomatic treatment of nasal congestion in sinus or other frontal headache; allergic rhinitis, vasomotor rhinitis, coryza; facial pain and pressure of acute and chronic sinusitis

Usual Dosage Oral:

Children 6-12 years: $^1/_2$ tablet every 12 hours (twice daily)

Adults: 1 tablet every 12 hours (twice daily)

Dosage Forms Tablet: Phenyltoloxamine citrate 22 mg, phenylpropanolamine hydrochloride 25 mg, and acetaminophen 325 mg

Phenylzin® Ophthalmic [OTC] *see* phenylephrine and zinc sulfate *on page 372*

phenytoin *(fen' i toyn)*

Brand Names Dilantin®; Diphenylan Sodium®

Synonyms diphenylhydantoin; DPH

Therapeutic Category Antiarrhythmic Agent, Class Ib; Anticonvulsant, Hydantoin

Use Management of generalized tonic-clonic (grand mal), simple partial and complex partial seizures; prevention of seizures following head trauma/neurosurgery; ventricular arrhythmias, including those associated with digitalis intoxication; beneficial effects in the treatment of migraine or trigeminal neuralgia in some patients

Usual Dosage

Status epilepticus: I.V.:

Neonates: Loading dose: 15-20 mg/kg in a single or divided dose; maintenance: Initial: 5 mg/kg/day in 2 divided doses; usual dose: 5-8 mg/kg/day in 2 divided doses; some patients may require dosing every 8 hours

Infants and Children: Loading dose: 15-18 mg/kg in a single or divided dose; maintenance: Initial: 5 mg/kg/day in 2 divided doses, usual doses:

6 months to 3 years: 8-10 mg/kg/day

4-6 years: 7.5-9 mg/kg/day

7-9 years: 7-8 mg/kg/day

10-16 years: 6-7 mg/kg/day, some patients may require every 8 hours dosing

Adults: Loading dose: 15-18 mg/kg in a single or divided dose; maintenance: usual: 300 mg/day or 5-6 mg/kg/day in 3 divided doses or 1-2 divided doses using extended release

Anticonvulsant: Children and Adults: Oral: Loading dose: 15-20 mg/kg; based on phenytoin serum concentrations and recent dosing history; administer oral loading dose in 3 divided doses given every 2-4 hours to decrease GI adverse effects and to ensure complete oral absorption; maintenance dose: same as I.V.

Arrhythmias:

Children and Adults: Loading dose: I.V.: 1.25 mg/kg IVP every 5 minutes may repeat up to total loading dose: 15 mg/kg

Children: Maintenance dose: Oral, I.V.: 5-10 mg/kg/day in 2 divided doses

Adults: Maintenance dose: Oral: 250 mg 4 times/day for 1 day, 250 mg twice daily for 2 days, then maintenance at 300-400 mg/day in divided doses 1-4 times/day

Dosage Forms
Capsule, as sodium:
    Extended: 30 mg, 100 mg
    Prompt: 30 mg, 100 mg
Injection, as sodium: 50 mg/mL (2 mL, 5 mL)
Suspension, oral: 30 mg/5 mL (5 mL, 240 mL); 125 mg/5 mL (5 mL, 240 mL)
Tablet, chewable: 50 mg

phenytoin with phenobarbital

Brand Names Dilantin® With Phenobarbital

Therapeutic Category Anticonvulsant, Barbiturate; Anticonvulsant, Hydantoin

Use Management of generalized tonic-clonic (grand mal), simple partial and complex partial seizures

Usual Dosage Children and Adults: Oral: Loading dose: 15-20 mg/kg; based on phenytoin serum concentrations and recent dosing history; administer oral loading dose in 3 divided doses given every 2-4 hours to decrease GI adverse effects and to ensure complete oral absorption

Dosage Forms Capsule: Phenytoin 100 mg and phenobarbital 15 mg; phenytoin 100 mg and phenobarbital 30 mg

Pherazine® VC see promethazine and phenylephrine on page 398

Pherazine® w/DM see promethazine with dextromethorphan on page 399

Pherazine® With Codeine see promethazine and codeine on page 398

Phicon® [OTC] see pramoxine hydrochloride on page 390

Phillips'® LaxCaps® [OTC] see docusate and phenolphthalein on page 158

Phillips'® Milk of Magnesia [OTC] see magnesium hydroxide on page 282

pHisoAc- BP® [OTC] see benzoyl peroxide on page 49

pHisoHex® see hexachlorophene on page 228

Phos-Ex® see calcium acetate on page 65

Phos-Flur® see fluoride on page 201

PhosLo® see calcium acetate on page 65

Phosphaljel® [OTC] see aluminum phosphate on page 17

phosphate, potassium see potassium phosphate on page 388

Phospholine Iodide® Ophthalmic see echothiophate iodide on page 165

phosphonoformic acid see foscarnet on page 206

phosphorated carbohydrate solution

Brand Names Emetrol® [OTC]; Naus-A-Way® [OTC]; Nausetrol® [OTC]

Synonyms dextrose, levulose and phosphoric acid; levulose, dextrose and phosphoric acid; phosphoric acid, levulose and dextrose

Therapeutic Category Antiemetic

Use Relieve nausea associated with upset stomach that occurs with intestinal flu, pregnancy, food indiscretions, and emotional upsets

Usual Dosage
Morning sickness: 15-30 mL on arising; repeat every 3 hours or when nausea threatens

Motion sickness and vomiting due to drug therapy: 5 mL doses for young children; 15 mL doses for older children and adults

Regurgitation in infants: 5 or 10 mL, 10-15 minutes before each feeding; in refractory cases: 10-15 mL, 30 minutes before each feeding

(Continued)

phosphorated carbohydrate solution (Continued)

Vomiting due to psychogenic factors:
  Children: 5-10 mL; repeat dose every 15 minutes until distress subsides; do not take for more than 1 hour
  Adults: 15-30 mL; repeat dose every 15 minutes until distress subsides; do not take for more than 1 hour
Dosage Forms Liquid, oral: Fructose, dextrose, and orthophosphoric acid (120 mL, 480 mL, 4000 mL)

phosphoric acid, levulose and dextrose see phosphorated carbohydrate solution on previous page

Phrenilin® see butalbital compound on page 63

Phrenilin® Forte® see butalbital compound on page 63

p-hydroxyampicillin see amoxicillin trihydrate on page 24

Phyllocontin® see aminophylline on page 19

phylloquinone see phytonadione on this page

physostigmine (fye zoe stig' meen)

Brand Names Antilirium® Injection; Isopto® Eserine Ophthalmic
Synonyms eserine salicylate
Therapeutic Category Antidote, Anticholinergic Agent; Cholinergic Agent; Cholinergic Agent, Ophthalmic
Use Reverse toxic CNS effects caused by anticholinergic drugs; used as miotic in treatment of glaucoma
Usual Dosage
  Children: Reserve for life-threatening situations only: I.V.: 0.01-0.03 mg/kg/dose; may repeat after 15-20 minutes to a maximum total dose of 2 mg
  Adults:
    I.M., I.V., S.C.: 0.5-2 mg to start, repeat every 20 minutes until response occurs or adverse effect occurs
    I.M., I.V. to reverse the anticholinergic effects of atropine or scopolamine given as preanesthetic medications: Give twice the dose, on a weight basis of the anticholinergic drug
    Ophthalmic: 1-2 drops of 0.25% or 0.5% solution every 4-8 hours (up to 4 times/day); the ointment can be instilled at night
Dosage Forms
  Injection, as salicylate: 1 mg/mL (2 mL)
  Ointment, ophthalmic: 0.25% (3.5 g, 3.7 g)
  Solution, ophthalmic: 0.25% (15 mL); 0.5% (2 mL, 15 mL)

phytomenadione see phytonadione on this page

phytonadione (fye toe na dye' one)

Brand Names AquaMEPHYTON® Injection; Konakion® Injection; Mephyton® Oral
Synonyms methylphytyl napthoquinone; phylloquinone; phytomenadione; vitamin K₁
Therapeutic Category Vitamin, Water Soluble
Use Prevention and treatment of hypoprothrombinemia caused by drug-induced or anticoagulant-induced vitamin K deficiency, hemorrhagic disease of the newborn
Usual Dosage I.V. route should be restricted for emergency use only
  Hemorrhagic disease of the newborn:
    Prophylaxis: I.M., S.C.: 0.5-1 mg within 1 hour of birth
    Treatment: I.M., S.C.: 1-2 mg/dose/day
  Oral anticoagulant overdose:
    Infants: I.M., I.V., S.C.: 1-2 mg/dose every 4-8 hours

Children and Adults: Oral, I.M., I.V., S.C.: 2.5-10 mg/dose; rarely up to 25-50 mg has been used; may repeat in 6-8 hours if given by I.M., I.V., S.C. route; may repeat 12-48 hours after oral route

Vitamin K deficiency: Due to drugs, malabsorption or decreased synthesis of vitamin K
Infants and Children:
Oral: 2.5-5 mg/24 hours
I.M., I.V.: 1-2 mg/dose as a single dose
Adults:
Oral: 5-25 mg/24 hours
I.M., I.V.: 10 mg

Minimum daily requirement: Not well established
Infants: 1-5 μg/kg/day
Adults: 0.03 μg/kg/day

Dosage Forms
Injection:
Aqueous colloidal: 2 mg/mL (0.5 mL); 10 mg/mL (1 mL, 2.5 mL, 5 mL)
Aqueous (I.M. only): 2 mg/mL (0.5 mL); 10 mg/mL (1 mL)
Tablet: 5 mg

Pilagan® Ophthalmic *see pilocarpine on this page*

Pilocar® Ophthalmic *see pilocarpine on this page*

pilocarpine (pye loe kar' peen)
Brand Names Adsorbocarpine® Ophthalmic; Akarpine® Ophthalmic; Isopto® Carpine Ophthalmic; Ocu-Carpine® Ophthalmic; Ocusert Pilo-20® Ophthalmic; Ocusert Pilo-40® Ophthalmic; Pilagan® Ophthalmic; Pilocar® Ophthalmic; Pilopine HS® Ophthalmic; Piloptic® Ophthalmic; Pilostat® Ophthalmic
Therapeutic Category Cholinergic Agent, Ophthalmic; Ophthalmic Agent, Miotic
Use Management of chronic simple glaucoma, chronic and acute angle-closure glaucoma; counter effects of cycloplegics
Usual Dosage Ophthalmic:
1-2 drops up to 6 times/day; adjust the concentration and frequency as required to control elevated intraocular pressure
To counteract the mydriatic effects of sympathomimetic agents: 1 drop of a 1% solution in the affected eye
Dosage Forms
Gel, ophthalmic, as hydrochloride (Pilopine HS®): 4% (3.5 g)
Ocular therapeutic system (Ocusert® Pilo): Releases 20 or 40 μg per hour for 1 week (8s)
Solution, ophthalmic, as hydrochloride (Adsorbocarpine®, Akarpine®, Isopto® Carpine® Pilagan®, Pilocar®, Piloptic®, Pilostat®): 0.25% (15 mL); 0.5% (15 mL, 30 mL); 1% (1 mL, 2 mL, 15 mL, 30 mL); 2% (1 mL, 2 mL, 15 mL, 30 mL); 3% (15 mL, 30 mL); 4% (1 mL, 2 mL, 15 mL, 30 mL); 6% (15 mL, 30 mL); 8% (2 mL); 10% (15 mL)
Solution, ophthalmic, as nitrate (Pilagan®): 1% (15 mL); 2% (15 mL); 4% (15 mL)

pilocarpine and epinephrine
Brand Names E-Pilo-x® Ophthalmic; P$_x$E$_x$® Ophthalmic
Therapeutic Category Ophthalmic Agent, Miotic
Use Treatment of glaucoma; counter effect of cycloplegics
Usual Dosage Ophthalmic: Instill 1-2 drops up to 6 times/day
Dosage Forms Solution, ophthalmic: Epinephrine bitartrate 1% and pilocarpine hydrochloride 1%, 2%, 4%, 6% (15 mL)

Pilopine HS® Ophthalmic *see pilocarpine on this page*

Piloptic® Ophthalmic *see pilocarpine on this page*

Pilostat® Ophthalmic *see pilocarpine on this page*

Pima® *see* potassium iodide *on page 387*

pimaricin *see* natamycin *on page 326*

pimozide (pi' moe zide)
Brand Names Orap™
Therapeutic Category Neuroleptic Agent
Use Suppression of severe motor and phonic tics in patients with Tourette's disorder
Usual Dosage Children >12 years and Adults: Oral: Initial: 1-2 mg/day, then increase dosage as needed every other day; range is usually 7-16 mg/day, maximum dose: 20 mg/day or 0.3 mg/kg/day should not be exceeded
Dosage Forms Tablet: 2 mg

pindolol (pin' doe lole)
Brand Names Visken®
Therapeutic Category Beta-Adrenergic Blocker
Use Management of hypertension
Usual Dosage Oral: 5 mg twice daily
Dosage Forms Tablet: 5 mg, 10 mg

Pin-Rid® [OTC] *see* pyrantel pamoate *on page 407*

Pin-X® [OTC] *see* pyrantel pamoate *on page 407*

PIO *see* pemoline *on page 359*

pipecuronium bromide (pi pe kure oh' nee um)
Brand Names Arduan®
Therapeutic Category Neuromuscular Blocker Agent, Nondepolarizing
Use Adjunct to general anesthesia, to provide skeletal muscle relaxation during surgery and to provide skeletal muscle relaxation for endotracheal intubation; recommended only for procedures anticipated to last 90 minutes or longer
Usual Dosage I.V.:
Children:
3 months to 1 year: Adult dosage
1-14 years: May be less sensitive to effects

Adults: Dose is individualized based on ideal body weight, ranges are 85-100 μg/kg initially to a maintenance dose of 5-25 μg/kg
Dosage Forms Injection: 10 mg (10 mL)

piperacillin sodium (pi per' a sill in)
Brand Names Pipracil®
Therapeutic Category Antibiotic, Penicillin
Use Treatment of carbenicillin or ticarcillin-resistant *Pseudomonas aeruginosa* infections in combination with an aminoglycoside which are susceptible to piperacillin
Usual Dosage
Neonates: I.M., I.V.: 100 mg/kg/dose every 12 hours

Infants and Children: I.M., I.V.: 200-300 mg/kg/day in divided doses every 4-6 hours; maximum dose: 24 g/day
Higher doses have been used in cystic fibrosis: 350-500 mg/kg/day in divided doses every 4 hours

Adults:
I.M.: 2-3 g/dose every 6-12 hours I.M.; maximum 24 g/24 hours
I.V.: 3-4 g/dose every 4-6 hours; maximum 24 g/24 hours
Dosage Forms Powder for injection: 2 g, 3 g, 4 g, 40 g

piperacillin sodium and tazobactam sodium

Brand Names Zosyn™

Therapeutic Category Antibiotic, Penicillin

Use Peritonitis, appendicitis, uncomplicated/complicated skin and skin structure, postpartum and pelvic infections and community acquired pneumonia

Usual Dosage

Adults: I.V.: 3.375 g (3 g piperacillin/.375 tazobactam) every 6 hours

Dosing interval in renal impairment:

Cl_{cr} <40 mL/minute: No change

Cl_{cr} 20-40 mL/minute: Administer 2.25 g every 6 hours

Cl_{cr} <20 mL/minute: Administer 2.25 g every 8 hours

Hemodialysis: Administer 2.25 g every 8 hours with an additional dose of 0.75 g after each dialysis

Dosage Forms Injection: Piperacillin sodium 2 g and tazobactam sodium 0.25 g; piperacillin sodium 3 g and tazobactam sodium 0.375 g; piperacillin sodium 4 g and tazobactam sodium 0.5 g

piperazine citrate (pi' per a zeen)

Brand Names Vermizine®

Therapeutic Category Anthelmintic

Use Treatment of pinworm and roundworm infections (used as an alternative to first-line agents, mebendazole, or pyrantel pamoate)

Usual Dosage Oral:

Pinworms:

Children and Adults: 65 mg/kg/day as a single daily dose for 7 days, in severe infections, repeat course after a 1-week interval; not to exceed 2.5 g/day

Roundworms:

Children: 75 mg/kg/day as a single daily dose for 2 days; maximum: 3.5 g/day;

Adults: 3.5 g/day for 2 days (in severe infections, repeat course, after a 1-week interval)

Dosage Forms

Syrup: 500 mg/5 mL (473 mL, 4000 mL)

Tablet: 250 mg

piperazine estrone sulfate *see* estropipate *on page 180*

pipobroman (pi poe broe' man)

Brand Names Vercyte®

Therapeutic Category Antineoplastic Agent, Alkylating Agent

Use Treat polycythemia vera; chronic myelocytic leukemia

Usual Dosage Refer to individual protocols

Children >15 years and Adults: Oral:

Polycythemia: 1 mg/kg/day for 30 days; may increase to 1.5-3 mg/kg until hematocrit reduced to 50% to 55%; maintenance: 0.1-0.2 mg/kg/day

Myelocytic leukemia: 1.5-2.5 mg/kg/day until WBC drops to 10,000 mm^3 then start maintenance 7-175 mg/day; stop if WBC falls below 3000/mm^3 or platelets fall below 150,000/mm^3

Dosage Forms Tablet: 25 mg

Pipracil® *see* piperacillin sodium *on previous page*

pirbuterol acetate (peer byoo' ter ole)

Brand Names Maxair™ Inhalation Aerosol

Therapeutic Category Beta-2-Adrenergic Agonist Agent; Bronchodilator

Use Prevention and treatment of reversible bronchospasm including asthma

(Continued)

pirbuterol acetate (Continued)

Usual Dosage Children >12 years and Adults: 2 inhalations every 4-6 hours for prevention; two inhalations at an interval of at least 1-3 minutes, followed by a third inhalation in treatment of bronchospasm, not to exceed 12 inhalations/day

Dosage Forms Aerosol, oral: 0.2 mg/actuation (25.6 g)

piroxicam (peer ox' i kam)

Brand Names Feldene®

Therapeutic Category Analgesic, Non-Narcotic; Anti-inflammatory Agent; Nonsteroidal Anti-Inflammatory Agent (NSAID), Oral

Use Management of inflammatory disorders; symptomatic treatment of acute and chronic rheumatoid arthritis, osteoarthritis, and ankylosing spondylitis

Usual Dosage Oral:

Children: 0.2-0.3 mg/kg/day once daily; maximum dose: 15 mg/day

Adults: 10-20 mg/day once daily; although associated with increases in GI adverse effects, doses >20 mg/day have been used (ie, 30-40 mg/day)

Therapeutic efficacy of the drug should not be assessed for at least two weeks after initiation of therapy or adjustment of dosage

Dosage Forms Capsule: 10 mg, 20 mg

p-isobutylhydratropic acid see ibuprofen on page 245

PIT see oxytocin on page 352

Pitocin® Injection see oxytocin on page 352

Pitressin® Injection see vasopressin on page 492

pix carbonis see coal tar on page 110

Placidyl® see ethchlorvynol on page 181

plague vaccine

Therapeutic Category Vaccine, Inactivated Bacteria

Use Vaccination of persons at high risk exposure to plaque

Usual Dosage Three I.M. doses: First dose 1 mL, second dose (0.2 mL) 1 month later, third dose (0.2 mL) 5 months after the second dose; booster doses (0.2 mL) at 1- to 2-year intervals if exposure continues

Dosage Forms Injection: 2 mL, 20 mL

plantago seed see psyllium on page 407

plantain seed see psyllium on page 407

Plaquenil® see hydroxychloroquine sulfate on page 240

Plasbumin® see albumin human on page 10

Plasmanate® see plasma protein fraction on this page

Plasma-Plex® see plasma protein fraction on this page

plasma protein fraction

Brand Names Plasmanate®; Plasma-Plex®; Plasmatein®; Protenate®

Therapeutic Category Blood Product Derivative

Use Plasma volume expansion and maintenance of cardiac output in the treatment of certain types of shock or impending shock

Usual Dosage I.V.: 250-1500 mL/day

Dosage Forms Injection: 5% (50 mL, 250 mL, 500 mL)

Plasmatein® see plasma protein fraction on this page

Platinol® *see* cisplatin *on page 103*

Platinol®-AQ *see* cisplatin *on page 103*

Plendil® *see* felodipine *on page 191*

plicamycin (plye kay mye' sin)
Brand Names Mithracin®
Synonyms mithramycin
Therapeutic Category Antidote, Hypercalcemia; Antineoplastic Agent, Antibiotic
Use Malignant testicular tumors, in the treatment of hypercalcemia and hypercalciuria of malignancy; Paget's disease
Usual Dosage Refer to individual protocols
Adults: I.V. (dose based on ideal body weight):
Testicular cancer: 25-50 μg/kg/day or every other day for 5-10 days

Blastic chronic granulocytic leukemia: 25 μg/kg over 2-4 hours every other day for 3 weeks

Hypercalcemia: 15-25 μg/kg/day once daily for 3-4 days or 25 μg/kg every 48-72 hours; additional courses of therapy may be given at intervals of 1 week or more if the initial course is unsuccessful. Reduce dose to 12.5 μg/kg in patients with pre-existing hepatic or renal impairment

Paget's disease: 15 μg/kg/day once daily for 10 days
Dosage Forms Powder for injection: 2.5 mg

pneumococcal vaccine, polyvalent
Brand Names Pneumovax® 23; Pnu-Imune® 23
Therapeutic Category Vaccine, Inactivated Bacteria
Use Immunity to pneumococcal lobar pneumonia and bacteremia in individuals $\geq$2 years of age who are at high risk of morbidity and mortality from pneumococcal infection
Usual Dosage Children >2 years and Adults: I.M., S.C.: 0.5 mL
Revaccination should be considered if $\geq$6 years since initial vaccination; revaccination is recommended in patients who received 14-valent pneumococcal vaccine and are at highest risk (asplenic) for fatal infection, or at $\geq$6 years in patients with nephrotic syndrome, renal failure, or transplant recipients, or 3-5 years in children with nephrotic syndrome, asplenia or sickle cell disease
Dosage Forms Injection: 25 μg each of 23 polysaccharide isolates/0.5 mL dose (0.5 mL, 1 mL, 5 mL)

Pneumomist® *see* guaifenesin *on page 217*

Pneumovax® 23 *see* pneumococcal vaccine, polyvalent *on this page*

Pnu-Imune® 23 *see* pneumococcal vaccine, polyvalent *on this page*

Pod-Ben-25® *see* podophyllum resin *on next page*

Podocon-25® *see* podophyllum resin *on next page*

podofilox (po do fil' ox)
Brand Names Condylox®
Therapeutic Category Keratolytic Agent
Use Treatment of external genital warts
Usual Dosage Adults: Apply twice daily (morning and evening) for 3 consecutive days, then withhold use for 4 consecutive days; repeat this cycle may be repeated up to 4 times until there is no visible wart tissue
Dosage Forms Solution, topical: 0.5% (3.5 mL)

Podofin® *see* podophyllum resin *on next page*

podophyllin and salicylic acid
Brand Names Verrex-C&M®
Synonyms salicylic acid and podophyllin
Therapeutic Category Keratolytic Agent
Use Topical treatment of benign growths including external genital and perianal warts, papillomas, fibroids
Usual Dosage Topical: Apply daily with applicator, allow to dry; remove necrotic tissue before each application
Dosage Forms Solution, topical: Podophyllum 10% and salicylic acid 30% with penederm 0.5% (7.5 mL)

podophyllum resin po dof' fill um)
Brand Names Pod-Ben-25®; Podocon-25®; Podofin®
Synonyms mandrake; may apple
Therapeutic Category Keratolytic Agent
Use Topical treatment of benign growths including external genital and perianal warts, papillomas, fibroids
Usual Dosage Topical:
Children and Adults: 10% to 25% solution in compound benzoin tincture; apply drug to dry surface, use 1 drop at a time allowing drying between drops until area is covered; total volume should be limited to <0.5 mL per treatment session

Condylomata acuminatum: 25% solution is applied daily; use a 10% solution when applied to or near mucous membranes

Verrucae: 25% solution is applied 3-5 times/day directly to the wart
Dosage Forms Liquid, topical: 25% in benzoin (5 mL, 7.5 mL, 30 mL)

Point-Two® *see* fluoride *on page 201*
Poladex® *see* dexchlorpheniramine maleate *on page 134*
Polaramine® *see* dexchlorpheniramine maleate *on page 134*
Polargen® *see* dexchlorpheniramine maleate *on page 134*
poliomyelitis vaccine *see* poliovirus vaccine, inactivated *on this page*

poliovirus vaccine, inactivated
Brand Names IPOL™
Synonyms IPV; poliomyelitis vaccine; Salk
Therapeutic Category Vaccine, Live Virus and Inactivated Virus
Use Active immunization for the prevention of poliomyelitis
Usual Dosage
S.C.: 3 doses of 0.5 mL; the first 2 doses should be administered at an interval of 8 weeks; the third dose should be given at least 6 and preferably 12 months after the second dose
Booster dose: All children who have received the 3 dose primary series in infancy and early childhood should receive a booster dose of 0.5 mL before entering school. However, if the third dose of the primary series is administered on or after the fourth birthday, a fourth (booster) dose is not required at school entry.
Dosage Forms Injection: Suspension of three types of poliovirus (Types 1, 2 and 3) grown in human diploid cell cultures (0.5 mL)

poliovirus vaccine, live, trivalent, oral
Brand Names Orimune®
Synonyms OPV; Sabin; TOPV
Therapeutic Category Vaccine, Live Virus
Use Poliovirus immunization

Usual Dosage Oral:

Infants: 0.5 mL dose at age 2 months, 4 months, and 18 months; optional dose may be given at 6 months in areas where poliomyelitis is endemic

Older Children, Adolescents and Adults: Two 0.5 mL doses 8 weeks apart; third dose of 0.5 mL 6-12 months after second dose; a reinforcing dose of 0.5 mL should be given before entry to school, in children who received the third primary dose before their fourth birthday

Dosage Forms Solution, oral: Mixture of type 1, 2, and 3 viruses in monkey kidney tissue (0.5 mL)

Polocaine® Injection see mepivacaine hydrochloride on page 293

Polycillin® see ampicillin on page 26

Polycillin-N® see ampicillin on page 26

Polycillin-PRB® see ampicillin and probenecid on page 26

Polycitra® see sodium citrate and potassium citrate mixture on page 436

Polycitra®-K see potassium citrate and citric acid on page 386

Polycose® [OTC] see glucose polymers on page 213

polyestradiol phosphate (pol ee ess tra dye' ole)
Brand Names Estradurin®
Therapeutic Category Estrogen Derivative
Use Palliative treatment of advanced, inoperable carcinoma of the prostate
Usual Dosage Adults: I.M.: 40 mg every 2-4 weeks or less frequently
Dosage Forms Powder for injection: 40 mg

polyethylene glycol-electrolyte solution (pol ee eth' i leen gly' kol)
Brand Names Co-Lav®; Colovage®; CoLyte®; Go-Evac®; GoLYTELY®; NuLYTELY®; OCL®
Synonyms electrolyte lavage solution; PEG-ES
Therapeutic Category Laxative, Bowel Evacuant
Use For bowel cleansing prior to GI examination
Usual Dosage The recommended dose for adults is 4 L of solution prior to gastrointestinal examination, as ingestion of this dose produces a satisfactory preparation in >95% of patients. Ideally the patient should fast for approximately 3-4 hours prior to administration, but in no case should solid food be given for at least 2 hours before the solution is given. The solution is usually administered orally, but may be given via nasogastric tube to patients who are unwilling or unable to drink the solution.

Children: Oral administration: 25-40 mL/kg/hour for 4-10 hours

Adults:

Oral administration: At a rate of 240 mL (8 oz) every 10 minutes, until 4 liters are consumed or the rectal effluent is clear; rapid drinking of each portion is preferred to drinking small amounts continuously

Nasogastric tube administration: At the rate of 20-30 mL/minute (1.2-1.8 L/hour); the first bowel movement should occur approximately one hour after the start of administration

Dosage Forms Powder, for oral solution: PEG 3350 236 g, sodium sulfate 22.74 g, sodium bicarbonate 6.74 g, sodium chloride 5.86 g and potassium chloride 2.97 g (2000 mL, 4000 mL, 4800 mL, 6000 mL)

Polyflex® see chlorzoxazone on page 99

Polygam® see immune globulin, intravenous on page 247

Poly-Histine CS® see brompheniramine, phenylpropanolamine, and codeine on page 60

Polymox® see amoxicillin trihydrate on page 24

polymyxin b and hydrocortisone
Brand Names Otobiotic® Otic; Pyocidin-Otic®
Therapeutic Category Antibacterial, Otic; Corticosteroid, Otic
Use Treatment of superficial bacterial infections of external ear canal
Usual Dosage Otic: Instill 4 drops 3-4 times/day
Dosage Forms Solution, otic: Polymyxin b sulfate 10,000 units and hydrocortisone 0.5% [5 mg/mL] per mL (10 mL, 15 mL)

polymyxin b and neomycin *see* neomycin and polymyxin b *on page 328*

polymyxin b and oxytetracycline *see* oxytetracycline and polymyxin b *on page 351*

polymyxin b and trimethoprim *see* trimethoprim and polymyxin b *on page 480*

polymyxin b sulfate (pol i mix' in)
Brand Names Aerosporin® Injection
Therapeutic Category Antibiotic, Ophthalmic; Antibiotic, Topical
Use
Topical: Wound irrigation and bladder instillation against *Pseudomonas aeruginosa*; used occasionally for gut decontamination
Parenteral: Has mainly been replaced by less toxic antibiotics; reserved for life-threatening infections caused by organisms resistant to the preferred drugs
Usual Dosage
Infants <2 years:
I.M.: 25,000-40,000 units/kg/day divided every 6 hours
I.V.: 15,000-45,000 units/kg/day by continuous I.V. infusion or divided every 12 hours
Children ≥2 years and Adults:
I.M.: 25,000-30,000 units/kg/day divided every 4-6 hours
I.V.: 15,000-25,000 units/kg/day divided every 12 hours or by continuous infusion
Total daily dose should not exceed 2,000,000 units/day
Bladder irrigation: Continuous irrigant or rinse in the urinary bladder for up to 10 days using 20 mg (equal to 200,000 units) added to 1 L of normal saline; usually no more than 1 L of irrigant is used per day unless urine flow rate is high; administration rate is adjusted to patient's urine output
Topical irrigation or topical solution: 0.1% to 0.3% solution used to irrigate infected wounds; should not exceed 2 million units/day in adults
Gut sterilization: Oral: 100,000-200,000 units/kg/day divided every 6-8 hours
Ophthalmic: A concentration of 0.1% to 0.25% is administered as 1-3 drops every hour, then increasing the interval as response indicates
Dosage Forms
Injection: 500,000 units
Powder for ophthalmic solution: 500,000 units

polymyxin e *see* colistin sulfate *on page 114*

Poly-Pred® Liquifilm® Ophthalmic *see* neomycin, polymyxin b, and prednisolone *on page 329*

polysaccharide-iron complex
Brand Names Hytinic® [OTC]; Niferex® [OTC]; Nu-Iron® [OTC]
Therapeutic Category Iron Salt
Use Prevention and treatment of iron deficiency anemias
Usual Dosage
Children: 3 mg/kg 3 times/day
Adults: 200 mg 3-4 times/day
Dosage Forms
Capsule: Elemental iron 150 mg
Elixir: Elemental iron 100 mg/5 mL (240 mL)

Tablet: Elemental iron 50 mg

Polysporin® Ophthalmic *see* bacitracin and polymyxin b *on page 42*

Polysporin® Topical *see* bacitracin and polymyxin b *on page 42*

Polytar® [OTC] *see* coal tar *on page 110*

polythiazide (pol i thye' a zide)
Brand Names Renese®
Therapeutic Category Diuretic, Thiazide
Use Adjunctive therapy in treatment of edema and hypertension
Usual Dosage Adults: Oral: 1-4 mg/day
Dosage Forms Tablet: 1 mg, 2 mg, 4 mg

Polytrim® Ophthalmic *see* trimethoprim and polymyxin b *on page 480*

Poly-Vi-Flor® Chewable Tablet *see* vitamin, multiple (pediatric) *on page 499*

Poly-Vi-Flor® Drops *see* vitamin, multiple (pediatric) *on page 499*

polyvinyl alcohol *see* artificial tears *on page 33*

Poly-Vi-Sol® Chewable Tablet [OTC] *see* vitamin, multiple (pediatric) *on page 499*

Poly-Vi-Sol® Drops [OTC] *see* vitamin, multiple (pediatric) *on page 499*

Pondimin® *see* fenfluramine hydrochloride *on page 192*

Ponstel® *see* mefenamic acid *on page 290*

Pontocaine® Injection *see* tetracaine hydrochloride *on page 457*

Pontocaine® Topical *see* tetracaine hydrochloride *on page 457*

Pontocaine® With Dextrose Injection *see* tetracaine with dextrose *on page 458*

Porcelana® Topical [OTC] *see* hydroquinone *on page 239*

Pork NPH Iletin® II *see* insulin preparations *on page 250*

Pork Regular Iletin® II *see* insulin preparations *on page 250*

Posture® [OTC] *see* calcium phosphate, dibasic *on page 69*

Potasalan® *see* potassium chloride *on next page*

potassium acetate
Therapeutic Category Electrolyte Supplement, Parenteral; Potassium Salt
Use Potassium deficiency, hypokalemia; to avoid chloride when high concentration of potassium is needed
Usual Dosage I.V. infusion:
Children: Not to exceed 3 mEq/kg/day

Adults: Up to 150 mEq/day administered at a rate up to 20 mEq/hour; maximum concentration: 40 mEq/L
Dosage Forms Injection: 2 mEq/mL (20 mL, 50 mL, 100 mL); 4 mEq/mL (50 mL)

potassium acid phosphate
Brand Names K-Phos® Original
Therapeutic Category Electrolyte Supplement, Oral; Potassium Salt; Urinary Acidifying Agent
Use To acidify the urine and lower urinary calcium concentration; reduces odor and rash caused by ammoniacal urine
Usual Dosage Adults: Oral: 1000 mg dissolved in 6-8 oz of water 4 times/day with meals and at bedtime
Dosage Forms Tablet, sodium free: 500 mg [potassium 3.67 mEq]

potassium bicarbonate and potassium citrate, effervescent
Brand Names Effer-K™; K-Ide®; Klor-con®/EF; K-Lyte®; K-Vescent®
Synonyms potassium citrate and potassium bicarbonate, effervescent
Therapeutic Category Electrolyte Supplement, Oral; Potassium Salt
Use Treatment or prevention of hypokalemia
Usual Dosage Oral:
Children: 1-4 mEq/kg/24 hours as required to maintain normal serum potassium
Adults:
Prevention: 16-24 mEq/day in 2-4 divided doses
Treatment: 40-100 mEq/day in 2-4 divided doses
Dosage Forms
Capsule, extended release: 8 mEq, 10 mEq
Powder for oral solution: 15 mEq/packet; 20 mEq/packet; 25 mEq/packet
Tablet, effervescent: 25 mEq, 50 mEq

potassium chloride
Brand Names Cena-K®; Gen-K®; Kaochlor® S-F; Kaon-CL®; Kato®; K-Dur®; K-Lor™; Klor-con®; Klorvess®; Klotrix®; K-Lyte/CL®; K-Tab®; Micro-K®; Potasalan®; Rum-K®; Slow-K®
Synonyms KCl
Therapeutic Category Electrolyte Supplement, Oral; Electrolyte Supplement, Parenteral; Potassium Salt
Use Treatment or prevention of hypokalemia
Usual Dosage I.V. doses should be incorporated into the patient's maintenance I.V. fluids, intermittent I.V. potassium administration should be reserved for severe depletion situations in patients undergoing EKG monitoring

Normal daily requirement: Oral, I.V.:
Newborns: 2-6 mEq/kg/day
Children: 2-3 mEq/kg/day
Adults: 40-80 mEq/day

Prevention during diuretic therapy: Oral:
Children: 1-2 mEq/kg/day in 1-2 divided doses
Adults: 20-40 mEq/day in 1-2 divided doses

Treatment: Oral, I.V.:
Children: 2-3 mEq/kg/day
Adults: 40-100 mEq/day

I.V. intermittent infusion:
Children: Dose should not exceed 0.5 mEq/kg/hour, not to exceed 20 mEq/hour
Adults: 10-20 mEq/hour, not to exceed 40 mEq/hour and 150 mEq/day
Dosage Forms
Capsule, controlled release, micro encapsulated (Micro-K®): 600 mg [8 mEq]; 750 mg [10 mEq]
Injection: 1.5 mEq/mL, 2 mEq/mL, 3 mEq/mL
Liquid, oral: 10 mEq/15 mL, 15 mEq/15 mL, 20 mEq/15 mL, 30 mEq/15 mL, 40 mEq/15 mL, 45 mEq/15 mL
Powder, oral: 15 mEq, 20 mEq, 25 mEq packet
Tablet:
Effervescent, as potassium chloride: 25 mEq
Effervescent, as potassium bicarbonate: 20 mEq, 25 mEq, 50 mEq
Sustained release, microcrystalloids (K-Dur®): 750 mg [10 mEq]; 1500 mg [20 mEq]
Wax matrix:
Kaon-Cl®: 500 mg [6.7 mEq]
Slow-K®: 600 mg [8 mEq]; 750 mg [10 mEq]

potassium citrate and citric acid
Brand Names Polycitra®-K
Therapeutic Category Electrolyte Supplement, Oral; Potassium Salt
Use Treatment of metabolic acidosis; alkalinizing agent in conditions where long-term maintenance of an alkaline urine is desirable

Dosage Forms
Crystals for reconstitution: Potassium citrate 3300 mg and citric acid 1002 mg per packet
Solution, oral: Potassium citrate 1100 mg and citric acid 334 mg per 5 mL

potassium citrate and potassium bicarbonate, effervescent *see* potassium bicarbonate and potassium citrate, effervescent *on previous page*

potassium gluconate
Brand Names Kaon®; Kolyum®
Therapeutic Category Electrolyte Supplement, Oral; Potassium Salt
Use Potassium deficiency, hypopotassemia
Usual Dosage Oral:
Normal daily requirement:
Children: 2-3 mEq/kg/day
Adults: 40-80 mEq/day

Prevention during diuretic therapy:
Children: 1-2 mEq/kg/day in 1-2 divided doses
Adults: 20-40 mEq/kg/day in 1-2 divided doses

Treatment of hypokalemia:
Children: 2-3 mEq/kg/day in 2-4 divided doses
Adults: 40-100 mEq/day in 2-4 divided doses
Dosage Forms
Liquid, sugar free (Kaon®): 20 mEq/15 mL
Powder (Kolyum®): Potassium 20 mEq and chloride 3.4 mEq (potassium gluconate and potassium chloride combination) per packet
Tablet: 500 mg, 595 mg

potassium iodide
Brand Names Pima®; Potassium Iodide Enseals®; SSKI®; Thyro-Block®
Synonyms KI; Lugol's solution; strong iodine solution
Therapeutic Category Antithyroid Agent; Expectorant
Use Facilitate bronchial drainage and cough; to reduce thyroid vascularity prior to thyroidectomy and management of thyrotoxic crisis; block thyroidal uptake of radioactive isotopes of iodine in a radiation emergency
Usual Dosage Oral:
Adults RDA: 130 μg

Expectorant:
Children: 60-250 mg every 6-8 hours; maximum single dose: 500 mg
Adults: 300-1000 mg 2-3 times/day, may increase to 1-1.5 g 3 times/day

Preoperative thyroidectomy: Children and Adults: 50-250 mg 3 times/day (2-6 drops strong iodine solution); give for 10 days before surgery

Thyrotoxic crisis:
Infants <1 year: $\frac{1}{2}$ adult dosage
Children and Adults: 300 mg = 6 drops SSKI® every 8 hours

Graves' disease in neonates: 1 drop of Lugol's solution every 8 hours

Sporotrichosis:
Oral: Initial:
Preschool: 50 mg/dose 3 times/day
Children: 250 mg/dose 3 times/day
Adults: 500 mg/dose 3 times/day
Oral increase 50 mg/dose daily
Maximum dose:
Preschool: 500 mg/dose 3 times/day
(Continued)

potassium iodide *(Continued)*
Children and Adults: 1-2 g/dose 3 times/day
Continue treatment for 4-6 weeks after lesions have completely healed
Dosage Forms
Solution, oral:
SSKI®: 1 g/mL (30 mL, 240 mL, 473 mL)
Lugol's solution, strong iodine: 100 mg/mL with iodine 50 mg/mL (120 mL)
Syrup: 325 mg/5 mL
Tablet: 130 mg

Potassium Iodide Enseals® *see* potassium iodide *on previous page*

potassium perchlorate *see* radiological/contrast media (ionic) *on page 413*

potassium phosphate
Brand Names Neutra-Phos®-K
Synonyms phosphate, potassium
Therapeutic Category Electrolyte Supplement, Oral; Electrolyte Supplement, Parenteral; Phosphate Salt; Potassium Salt
Use Source of potassium and phosphorus in parenteral nutrition and large volume I.V. fluids; treatment of conditions associated with excessive renal phosphate and potassium loss, inadequate GI absorption of these electrolytes, or inadequate phosphate and potassium in the diet
Usual Dosage I.V. doses should be incorporated into the patient's maintenance I.V. fluids; intermittent I.V. infusion should be reserved for severe depletion situations in patients undergoing continuous EKG monitoring. It is difficult to determine total body phosphorus deficit, the following dosages are empiric guidelines:

Normal requirements elemental phosphorus: Oral:
0-6 months: 240 mg
6-12 months: 360 mg
1-10 years: 800 mg
>10 years: 1200 mg
Pregnancy lactation: Additional 400 mg/day

Adults RDA: 800 mg
Dosage Forms
Capsule (Neutra-Phos®-K): Potassium 556 mg (14.25 mEq) and phosphorus 250 mg (8 mmol) per capsule
Injection: Potassium 4.4 mEq and phosphate 3 mmol per mL (15 mL)

potassium phosphate and sodium phosphate
Brand Names K-Phos® Neutral; Neutra-Phos®; Uro-KP-Neutral®
Synonyms sodium phosphate and potassium phosphate
Therapeutic Category Electrolyte Supplement, Oral; Phosphate Salt; Potassium Salt
Use Treatment of conditions associated with excessive renal phosphate loss or inadequate GI absorption of phosphate
Usual Dosage All dosage forms to be mixed in 6-8 oz of water prior to administration

Children: 2-3 mmol phosphate/kg/24 hours given 4 times/day
Adults: 100-150 mmol phosphate/24 hours in divided doses after meals and at bedtime; 1-8 tablets or capsules/day, given 4 times/day
Dosage Forms
Capsule: Phosphate 8 mmol, sodium 7.125 mEq, and potassium 7.125 mEq (250 mg of phosphorus)
Powder, concentrate: Phosphate 8 mmol, sodium 7.125 mEq, and potassium 7.125 mEq per 75 mL when reconstituted
Tablet: Phosphate 8 mmol, sodium 13 mEq, and potassium 1.1 mEq (114 mg of phosphorus)

povidone-iodine (poe' vi done)
Brand Names Betadine® [OTC]; Efodine® [OTC]; Iodex® Regular; Isodine® [OTC]
Therapeutic Category Antibacterial, Topical
Use External antiseptic with broad microbicidal spectrum against bacteria, fungi, viruses, protozoa, and yeasts
Usual Dosage Apply as needed for treatment and prevention of susceptible microbicidal infections
Dosage Forms
Aerosol: 5% (90 mL)
Cleanser, topical: 7.5% (30 mL, 120 mL)
Concentrate:
Whirlpool: 10% (3840 mL)
Perineal wash: 10% (240 mL)
Douche: 10% (0.5 oz/packet 240 mL)
Foam, topical: 10% (250 g)
Gel, vaginal: 10% (3 oz)
Mouthwash: 0.5% (180 mL)
Ointment, topical: 10% (0.9 g foil packet, 0.94 g, 28 g, 480 g)
Pads, antiseptic gauze: 10% (3" x 9", 5" x 9")
Scrub, surgical: 7.5% (480 mL, 946 mL)
Shampoo: 7.5% (120 mL)
Solution:
Swab aid: 10% (100s)
Swabsticks, 4": 10%
Topical: 10% (240 mL, 480 mL, 946 mL)
Suppository, vaginal: 10%

PPA *see* phenylpropanolamine hydrochloride *on page 373*
PPD *see* tuberculin tests *on page 484*
PPL *see* benzylpenicilloyl-polylysine *on page 51*

pralidoxime chloride (pra li dox' eem)
Brand Names Protopam®
Synonyms 2-PAM; 2-pyridine aldoxime methochloride
Therapeutic Category Antidote, Anticholinesterase; Antidote, Organophosphate Poisoning
Use Reverse muscle paralysis with toxic exposure to organophosphate anticholinesterase pesticides and chemicals; control of overdose of drugs used to treat myasthenia gravis
Usual Dosage Poisoning: I.V.:
Children: 20-50 mg/kg/dose; repeat in 1-2 hours if muscle weakness has not been relieved, then at 10- to 12-hour intervals if cholinergic signs recur
Adults: 1-2 g; repeat in 1-2 hours if muscle weakness has not been relieved, then at 10- to 12-hour intervals if cholinergic signs recur
Dosage Forms Injection: 20 mL vial containing 1 g pralidoxime chloride with one 20 mL ampul diluent, disposable syringe, needle, and alcohol swab

PrameGel® [OTC] *see* pramoxine hydrochloride *on next page*
Pramet® FA *see* vitamin, multiple (prenatal) *on page 499*
Pramilet® FA *see* vitamin, multiple (prenatal) *on page 499*
Pramosone® *see* pramoxine and hydrocortisone *on this page*

pramoxine and hydrocortisone
Brand Names Enzone®; Pramosone®; Proctofoam®-HC; Zone-A Forte®
Synonyms hydrocortisone and pramoxine
Therapeutic Category Anti-inflammatory Agent; Corticosteroid, Topical (Low Potency); Local Anesthetic, Topical
(Continued)
389

pramoxine and hydrocortisone *(Continued)*
Use Treatment of severe anorectal or perianal inflammation
Usual Dosage Apply to affected areas 3-4 times/day
Dosage Forms
Cream, topical: Pramoxine hydrochloride 1% and hydrocortisone acetate 0.5% (30 g); pramoxine hydrochloride 1% and hydrocortisone acetate 1%
Foam, rectal: Pramoxine hydrochloride 1% and hydrocortisone acetate 1% (10 g)
Lotion, topical: Pramoxine hydrochloride 1% and hydrocortisone 0.25%; pramoxine hydrochloride 1% and hydrocortisone 2.5%; pramoxine hydrochloride 2.5% and hydrocortisone 1% (37.5 mL, 120 mL, 240 mL)

pramoxine hydrochloride (pra mox' een)
Brand Names Itch-X® [OTC]; Phicon® [OTC]; PrameGel® [OTC]; Prax® [OTC]; Proctofoam® [OTC]; Tronolane® [OTC]; Tronothane® [OTC]
Therapeutic Category Local Anesthetic, Topical
Use Temporary relief of pain and itching associated with anogenital pruritus or irritation; dermatosis, minor burns or hemorrhoids
Usual Dosage Apply as directed, usually every 3-4 hours
Dosage Forms
Aerosol foam: 1% in an anesthetic mucoadhesive foam base (15 g)
Cream: 0.5% (30 g, 60 g); 1% (28.4 g, 113.4 g)
Gel, topical: 1% (37.5 g)
Liquid, topical: 1% (118 mL)
Lotion: 1% (15 mL, 20 mL, 240 mL)

Pravachol® *see* pravastatin sodium *on this page*

pravastatin sodium (pra' va stat in)
Brand Names Pravachol®
Therapeutic Category Antilipemic Agent; HMG-COA Reductase Inhibitor
Use Adjunct to diet for the reduction of elevated total and LDL-cholesterol levels in patients with hypercholesterolemia (Type IIa and IIb)
Usual Dosage Adults: Oral: 10-20 mg once daily at bedtime
Dosage Forms Tablet: 10 mg, 20 mg

Prax® [OTC] *see* pramoxine hydrochloride *on this page*

prazepam (pra' ze pam)
Brand Names Centrax®
Therapeutic Category Antianxiety Agent; Anticonvulsant, Benzodiazepine; Benzodiazepine
Use Treatment of anxiety and management of alcohol withdrawal; may also be used as an anticonvulsant in management of simple partial seizures
Usual Dosage Adults: Oral: 30 mg/day in divided doses
Dosage Forms
Capsule: 5 mg, 10 mg, 20 mg
Tablet: 5 mg, 10 mg

praziquantel (pray zi kwon' tel)
Brand Names Biltricide®
Therapeutic Category Anthelmintic
Use Treatment of all stages of schistosomiasis caused by all *Schistosoma* species pathogenic to humans; also active in the treatment of clonorchiasis, opisthorchiasis, cysticercosis, and many intestinal tapeworms

Usual Dosage Children and Adults: Oral:
Schistosomiasis: 20 mg/kg/dose 2-3 times/day for 1 day at 4- to 6-hour intervals

Flukes: 25 mg/kg/dose every 8 hours for 1-2 days

Cysticercosis: 50 mg/kg/day divided every 8 hours for 14 days

Tapeworms: 10-20 mg/kg as a single dose (25 mg/kg for *H. nana*)
Dosage Forms Tablet, tri-scored: 600 mg

prazosin and polythiazide
Brand Names Minizide®
Therapeutic Category Antihypertensive, Combination
Use Management of mild to moderate hypertension
Usual Dosage Adults: Oral: 1 capsule 2-3 times/day
Dosage Forms Capsule:
1: Prazosin 1 mg and polythiazide 0.5 mg
2: Prazosin 2 mg and polythiazide 0.5 mg
5: Prazosin 5 mg and polythiazide 0.5 mg

prazosin hydrochloride (pra' zoe sin)
Brand Names Minipress®
Synonyms furazosin
Therapeutic Category Alpha-Adrenergic Blocking Agent, Oral; Antihypertensive; Vasodilator, Coronary
Use Hypertension, severe congestive heart failure (in conjunction with diuretics and cardiac glycosides)
Usual Dosage Oral:
Children: Initial: 5 µg/kg/dose (to assess hypotensive effects); usual dosing interval every 6 hours; increase dosage gradually up to maintenance of 25-150 µg/kg/day divided every 6 hours

Adults: Initial: 1 mg/dose 2-3 times/day; usual maintenance dose: 3-15 mg/day in divided doses 2-4 times/day; maximum daily dose: 20 mg
Dosage Forms Capsule: 1 mg, 2 mg, 5 mg

Predaject® Injection *see* prednisolone *on this page*
Predalone Injection *see* prednisolone *on this page*
Predalone T.B.A.® Injection *see* prednisolone *on this page*
Predcor® Injection *see* prednisolone *on this page*
Predcor-TBA® Injection *see* prednisolone *on this page*
Pred Forte® Ophthalmic *see* prednisolone *on this page*
Pred-G® Ophthalmic *see* prednisolone and gentamicin *on next page*
Predicort® Injection *see* prednisolone *on this page*
Pred Mild® Ophthalmic *see* prednisolone *on this page*
Prednicen-M® Oral *see* prednisone *on page 393*

prednisolone (pred niss' oh lone)
Brand Names AK-Pred® Ophthalmic; Articulose-50® Injection; Delta-Cortef® Oral; Econopred® Ophthalmic; Econopred® Plus Ophthalmic; Hydeltrasol® Injection; Hydeltra-T.B.A.® Injection; Inflamase® Mild Ophthalmic; Inflamase® Ophthalmic; Key-Pred® Injection; Key-Pred-SP® Injection; Metreton® Ophthalmic; Pediapred® Oral; Predaject® Injection; Predalone Injection; Predalone T.B.A.® Injection; Predcor® Injection; Predcor-TBA® Injection; Pred Forte® Ophthalmic; Predicort® Injection; Pred Mild® Ophthalmic; Prednisol® TBA Injection; Prelone® Oral
(Continued)

prednisolone *(Continued)*

Synonyms deltahydrocortisone; metacortandralone

Therapeutic Category Adrenal Corticosteroid; Anti-inflammatory Agent; Corticosteroid, Ophthalmic; Corticosteroid, Systemic

Use Treatment of palpebral and bulbar conjunctivitis; corneal injury from chemical, radiation, thermal burns, or foreign body penetration; endocrine disorders, rheumatic disorders, collagen diseases, dermatologic diseases, allergic states, ophthalmic diseases, respiratory diseases, hematologic disorders, neoplastic diseases, edematous states, and gastrointestinal diseases; useful in patients with inability to activate prednisone (liver disease)

Usual Dosage Dose depends upon condition being treated and response of patient; dosage for infants and children should be based on severity of the disease and response of the patient rather than on strict adherence to dosage indicated by age, weight, or body surface area. Consider alternate day therapy for long-term therapy. Discontinuation of long-term therapy requires gradual withdrawal by tapering the dose.

Children:
  Acute asthma:
    Oral: 1-2 mg/kg/day in divided doses 1-2 times/day for 3-5 days
    I.V.: 2-4 mg/kg/day divided 3-4 times/day
  Anti-inflammatory or immunosuppressive dose: Oral, I.V.: 0.1-2 mg/kg/day in divided doses 1-4 times/day
  Nephrotic syndrome: Oral: Initial: 2 mg/kg/day (maximum: 80 mg/day) in divided doses 3-4 times/day until urine is protein free for 5 days (maximum: 28 days); if proteinuria persists, use 4 mg/kg/dose every other day for an additional 28 days (maximum: 120 mg/day); maintenance: 2 mg/kg/dose every other day for 28 days (maximum: 80 mg/dose); then taper over 4-6 weeks

Adults:
  Oral, I.V.: 5-60 mg/day
  Ophthalmic suspension: 1-2 drops into conjunctival sac every hour during day, every 2 hours at night until favorable response is obtained, then use 1 drop every 4 hours

Dosage Forms

Injection, as acetate: 25 mg/mL (10 mL, 30 mL); 50 mg/mL (10 mL, 30 mL); 100 mg/mL (10 ` mL)

Injection, as sodium phosphate: 20 mg/mL (2 mL, 5 mL, 10 mL)

Injection, as tebutate: 20 mg/mL (1 mL, 5 mL, 10 mL)

Liquid, oral, as sodium phosphate: 5 mg/5 mL (120 mL)

Solution, ophthalmic, as sodium phosphate: 0.125% (5 mL, 10 mL, 15 mL); 0.5% (5 mL)

Suspension, ophthalmic, as acetate: 0.12% (5 mL, 10 mL); 0.125% (5 mL, 10 mL); 1% (1 mL, 5 mL, 10 mL, 15 mL)

Syrup: 15 mg/5 mL (240 mL)

Tablet: 5 mg

prednisolone acetate and sodium sulfacetamide *see* sodium sulfacetamide and prednisolone *on page 439*

prednisolone and gentamicin

Brand Names Pred-G® Ophthalmic

Synonyms gentamicin and prednisolone

Therapeutic Category Antibiotic, Ophthalmic; Corticosteroid, Ophthalmic

Use Treatment of steroid responsive inflammatory conditions and superficial ocular infections due to strains of microorganisms susceptible to gentamicin

Usual Dosage Children and Adults: Ophthalmic: 1 drop 2-4 times/day; during the initial 24-48 hours, the dosing frequency may be increased if necessary

Dosage Forms

Ointment, ophthalmic: Prednisolone acetate 0.6% and gentamicin sulfate 0.3% (3.5 g)

Suspension, ophthalmic: Prednisolone acetate 1% and gentamicin sulfate 0.3% (5 mL)

Prednisol® TBA Injection *see* prednisolone *on page 391*

prednisone (pred' ni sone)
Brand Names Deltasone® Oral; Liquid Pred® Oral; Meticorten® Oral; Orasone® Oral; Prednicen-M® Oral; Sterapred® Oral
Synonyms deltacortisone; deltadehydrocortisone
Therapeutic Category Adrenal Corticosteroid; Anti-inflammatory Agent; Corticosteroid, Systemic
Use Treatment of a variety of diseases including adrenocortical insufficiency, hypercalcemia, rheumatic and collagen disorders, dermatologic, ocular, respiratory, gastrointestinal and neoplastic diseases, organ transplantation and a variety of diseases including those of hematologic, allergic, inflammatory, and autoimmune in origin
Usual Dosage Dose depends upon condition being treated and response of patient; dosage for infants and children should be based on severity of the disease and response of the patient rather than on strict adherence to dosage indicated by age, weight, or body surface area. Consider alternate day therapy for long-term therapy. Discontinuation of long-term therapy requires gradual withdrawal by tapering the dose.

Children: Oral: 0.05-2 mg/kg/day (anti-inflammatory or immunosuppressive dose) divided 1-4 times/day
  Acute asthma: Oral: 1-2 mg/kg/day in divided doses 1-2 times/day for 3-5 days
  Nephrotic syndrome: Oral: Initial: 2 mg/kg/day (maximum: of 80 mg/day) in divided doses 3-4 times/day until urine is protein free for 5 days (maximum: 28 days); if proteinuria persists, use 4 mg/kg/dose every other day (maximum: 120 mg/day) for an additional 28 days; maintenance: 2 mg/kg/dose every other day for 28 days (maximum: 80 mg/day); then taper over 4-6 weeks

Children and Adults: Physiologic replacement: 4-5 mg/m^2/day
Adults: Oral: 5-60 mg/day in divided doses 1-4 times/day
Dosage Forms
Solution:
  Concentrate: 5 mg/mL (5 mL, 30 mL)
  Oral: 5 mg/5 mL (10 mL, 20 mL, 500 mL)
Syrup: 5 mg/5 mL (120 mL, 240 mL)
Tablet: 1 mg, 2.5 mg, 5 mg, 10 mg, 20 mg, 50 mg

Prefrin™ Ophthalmic Solution *see* phenylephrine hydrochloride *on page 372*

pregnancy tests *see* diagnostic aids (*in vitro*), urine *on page 139*

pregnenedione *see* progesterone *on page 397*

Pregnosis® *see* diagnostic aids (*in vitro*), urine *on page 139*

Pregnospia® II *see* diagnostic aids (*in vitro*), urine *on page 139*

Pregnosticon® Dri-Dot® *see* diagnostic aids (*in vitro*), urine *on page 139*

Pregnyl® *see* chorionic gonadotropin *on page 101*

Prehist® *see* chlorpheniramine and phenylephrine *on page 93*

Prelone® Oral *see* prednisolone *on page 391*

Premarin® Injection *see* estrogens, conjugated *on page 179*

Premarin® Oral *see* estrogens, conjugated *on page 179*

Premarin® Vaginal *see* estrogens, conjugated *on page 179*

Premarin® With Methyltestosterone Oral *see* estrogens with methyltestosterone *on page 180*

prenatal vitamins *see* vitamin, multiple (prenatal) *on page 499*

Prenavite® [OTC] *see* vitamin, multiple (prenatal) *on page 499*

Prepcat® *see* radiological/contrast media (ionic) *on page 413*

Pre-Pen® *see* benzylpenicilloyl-polylysine *on page 51*

Prepidil® Vaginal Gel *see* dinoprostone *on page 151*
Pretz-D® [OTC] *see* ephedrine sulfate *on page 170*
Prevident® *see* fluoride *on page 201*
Prilosec™ *see* omeprazole *on page 343*
primaclone *see* primidone *on this page*
Primacor® *see* milrinone lactate *on page 313*
primaquine and chloroquine *see* chloroquine and primaquine *on page 91*

primaquine phosphate (prim' a kween)
Synonyms prymaccone
Therapeutic Category Antimalarial Agent
Use Provide radical cure of *P. vivax* or *P. ovale* malaria after a clinical attack has been confirmed by blood smear or serologic titer and postexposure prophylaxis
Usual Dosage Oral:
  Children: 0.3 mg base/kg/day once daily for 14 days not to exceed 15 mg/day or 0.9 mg base/kg once weekly for 8 weeks not to exceed 45 mg base/week
  Adults: 15 mg/day (base) once daily for 14 days or 45 mg base once weekly for 8 weeks
Dosage Forms Tablet: 26.3 mg [15 mg base]

Primatene® Inhalation Aerosol [OTC] *see* epinephrine *on page 171*
Primaxin® *see* imipenem/cilastatin *on page 246*

primidone (pri' mi done)
Brand Names Mysoline®
Synonyms desoxyphenobarbital; primaclone
Therapeutic Category Anticonvulsant, Barbiturate
Use Prophylactic management of partial seizures with complex symptomatology (psychomotor seizures), generalized tonic-clonic, and akinetic seizure
Usual Dosage Oral:
  Children: 0.3 mg base/kg/day once daily for 14 days (not to exceed 15 mg/day) or 0.9 mg base/kg once weekly for 8 weeks not to exceed 45 mg base/week
  Adults: 15 mg/day (base) once daily for 14 days or 45 mg base once weekly for 8 weeks
Dosage Forms
  Suspension, oral: 250 mg/5 mL (240 mL)
  Tablet: 50 mg, 250 mg

Principen® *see* ampicillin *on page 26*
Prinivil® *see* lisinopril *on page 275*
Priscoline® Injection *see* tolazoline hydrochloride *on page 471*
Privine® Nasal [OTC] *see* naphazoline hydrochloride *on page 325*
Proampacin® *see* ampicillin and probenecid *on page 26*
Proaqua® *see* benzthiazide *on page 50*
Probalan® *see* probenecid *on this page*
Pro-Banthine® *see* propantheline bromide *on page 400*
Proben-C® *see* colchicine and probenecid *on page 113*

probenecid (proe ben' e sid)
Brand Names Benemid®; Probalan®
Therapeutic Category Adjuvant Therapy, Penicillin Level Prolongation; Uric Acid Lowering Agent

Use Prevention of gouty arthritis; hyperuricemia; prolong serum levels of penicillin/ cephalosporin

Usual Dosage Oral:

Children:

<2 years: Not recommended

2-14 years: Prolong penicillin serum levels: 25 mg/kg starting dose, then 40 mg/kg/day given 4 times/day

Gonorrhea: <45 kg: 25 mg/kg x 1 (maximum: 1 g/dose) 30 minutes before penicillin, ampicillin or amoxicillin

Adults:

Hyperuricemia with gout: 250 mg twice daily for one week; increase to 500 mg 2 times/ day; may increase by 500 mg/month, if needed, to maximum of 2-3 g/day (dosages may be decreased by 500 mg every 6 months if serum urate concentrations are controlled)

Prolong penicillin serum levels: 500 mg 4 times/day

Gonorrhea: 1 g 30 minutes before penicillin, ampicillin or amoxicillin

Dosage Forms Tablet: 500 mg

probenecid and colchicine see colchicine and probenecid on page 113

probucol (proe' byoo kole)

Brand Names Lorelco®

Synonyms biphenabid

Therapeutic Category Antilipemic Agent

Use Adjunct to dietary therapy to decrease elevated serum total and LDL cholesterol concentrations in primary hypercholesterolemia

Usual Dosage Oral:

Children:

<27 kg: 250 mg twice daily with meals

>27 kg: 500 mg twice daily with meals

Adults: 500 mg twice daily administered with the morning and evening meals

Dosage Forms Tablet: 250 mg, 500 mg

procainamide hydrochloride (proe kane a' mide)

Brand Names Procan® SR; Pronestyl®; Pronestyl-SR®

Synonyms procaine amide hydrochloride

Therapeutic Category Antiarrhythmic Agent, Class la

Use Ventricular tachycardia, premature ventricular contractions, paroxysmal atrial tachycardia, and atrial fibrillation; to prevent recurrence of ventricular tachycardia, paroxysmal supraventricular tachycardia, atrial fibrillation or flutter

Usual Dosage Must be titrated to patient's response

Children:

Oral: 15-50 mg/kg/24 hours divided every 3-6 hours; maximum 4 g/24 hours

I.M.: 20-30 mg/kg/24 hours divided every 4-6 hours in divided doses; maximum 4 g/24 hours

I.V.: Load: 3-6 mg/kg/dose over 5 minutes not to exceed 100 mg/dose; may repeat every 5-10 minutes to maximum of 15 mg/kg/load; maintenance as continuous I.V. infusion: 20-80 μg/kg/minute; maximum: 2 g/24 hours

Adults:

Oral: 250-500 mg/dose every 3-6 hours or 500 mg to 1 g every 6 hours sustained release; usual dose: 50 mg/kg/24 hours or 2-4 g/24 hours

I.V.: Load: 50-100 mg/dose, repeated every 5-10 minutes until patient controlled; or load with 15-18 mg/kg, maximum loading dose: 1-1.5 g; maintenance: 2-6 mg/ minute continuous I.V. infusion, usual maintenance: 3-4 mg/minute

Dosage Forms

Capsule: 250 mg, 375 mg, 500 mg

(Continued)

395

procainamide hydrochloride *(Continued)*
Injection: 100 mg/mL (10 mL); 500 mg/mL (2 mL)
Tablet: 250 mg, 375 mg, 500 mg
Tablet, sustained release: 250 mg, 500 mg, 750 mg, 1000 mg

procaine amide hydrochloride *see* procainamide hydrochloride *on previous page*

procaine benzylpenicillin *see* penicillin g procaine, aqueous *on page 362*

procaine hydrochloride
Brand Names Novocain® Injection
Therapeutic Category Local Anesthetic, Injectable
Use Produce spinal anesthesia and epidural and peripheral nerve block by injection and infiltration methods
Usual Dosage Dose varies with procedure, desired depth, and duration of anesthesia, desired muscle relaxation, vascularity of tissues, physical condition, and age of patient
Dosage Forms Injection: 1% [10 mg/mL] (2 mL, 6 mL, 30 mL, 100 mL); 2% [20 mg/mL] (30 mL, 100 mL); 10% (2 mL)

procaine penicillin g *see* penicillin g procaine, aqueous *on page 362*

Pro-Cal-Sof® [OTC] *see* docusate *on page 157*

Procan® SR *see* procainamide hydrochloride *on previous page*

procarbazine hydrochloride (proe kar' ba zeen)
Brand Names Matulane®
Synonyms ibenzmethyzin; MIH; n-methylhydrazine
Therapeutic Category Antineoplastic Agent, Miscellaneous
Use Treatment of Hodgkin's disease, non-Hodgkin's lymphoma, brain tumor, bronchogenic carcinoma
Usual Dosage Refer to individual protocols
Oral:
Children: 50-100 mg/m^2/day once daily; doses as high as 100-200 mg/m^2/day once daily have been used for neuroblastoma and medulloblastoma

Adults: Initial: 2-4 mg/kg/day in single or divided doses for 7 days then increase dose to 4-6 mg/kg/day until response is obtained or leukocyte count decreased <4000/mm^3 or the platelet count decreased <100,000/mm^3; maintenance: 1-2 mg/kg/day
Dose reductions are necessary in patients with reduced renal function, reduced hepatic function, and/or bone marrow disorders
Dosage Forms Capsule: 50 mg

Procardia® *see* nifedipine *on page 334*

Procardia XL® *see* nifedipine *on page 334*

prochlorperazine (proe klor per' a zeen)
Brand Names Compazine® Injection; Compazine® Oral; Compazine® Rectal
Synonyms prochlorperazine edisylate; prochlorperazine maleate
Therapeutic Category Antiemetic; Antipsychotic Agent; Phenothiazine Derivative
Use Management of nausea and vomiting; acute and chronic psychosis
Usual Dosage
Children: Oral, rectal:
>10 kg: 0.4 mg/kg/24 hours in 3-4 divided doses; **or**
9-14 kg: 2.5 mg every 12-24 hours as needed; maximum: 7.5 mg/day
14-18 kg: 2.5 mg every 8-12 hours as needed; maximum: 10 mg/day
18-39 kg: 2.5 mg every 8 hours or 5 mg every 12 hours as needed; maximum: 15 mg/day

I.M.: 0.1-0.15 mg/kg/dose; usual: 0.13 mg/kg/dose; change to oral as soon as possible
I.V.: Not recommended

Adults:
Oral: 5-10 mg 3-4 times/day; usual maximum: 40 mg/day; doses up to 150 mg/day may be required in some patients
I.M.: 5-10 mg every 3-4 hours; usual maximum: 40 mg/day; doses up to 10-20 mg every 4-6 hours may be required in some patients
I.V.: 2.5-10 mg; maximum 10 mg/dose or 40 mg/day; may repeat dose every 3-4 hours as needed
Rectal: 25 mg twice daily

Dosage Forms
Capsule, sustained action, as maleate: 10 mg, 15 mg, 30 mg
Injection, as edisylate: 5 mg/mL (2 mL, 10 mL)
Suppository, rectal: 2.5 mg, 5 mg, 25 mg (12/box)
Syrup, as edisylate: 5 mg/5 mL (120 mL)
Tablet, as maleate: 5 mg, 10 mg, 25 mg

prochlorperazine edisylate see prochlorperazine on previous page
prochlorperazine maleate see prochlorperazine on previous page
Procrit® see epoetin alfa on page 172
Proctocort™ Rectal see hydrocortisone on page 236
Proctofoam® [OTC] see pramoxine hydrochloride on page 390
Proctofoam®-HC see pramoxine and hydrocortisone on page 389

procyclidine hydrochloride (proe sye' kli deen)
Brand Names Kemadrin®
Therapeutic Category Anticholinergic Agent; Antiparkinson Agent
Use Relieve symptoms of Parkinsonian syndrome and drug-induced extrapyramidal symptoms
Usual Dosage Adults: Oral: 2-2.5 mg 3 times/day after meals; if tolerated, gradually increase dose to 4-5 mg 3 times/day
Dosage Forms Tablet: 5 mg

Pro-Depo® Injection see hydroxyprogesterone caproate on page 240
Prodrox® Injection see hydroxyprogesterone caproate on page 240
Profasi® HP see chorionic gonadotropin on page 101
Profenal® Ophthalmic see suprofen on page 451
Profilate® OSD see antihemophilic factor on page 29
Profilnine® Heat-Treated see factor ix complex (human) on page 189
Progestaject® Injection see progesterone on this page

progesterone (proe jess' ter one)
Brand Names Gesterol® Injection; Progestaject® Injection
Synonyms pregnenedione; progestin
Therapeutic Category Progestin
Use Endometrial carcinoma or renal carcinoma as well as secondary amenorrhea or abnormal uterine bleeding due to hormonal imbalance
Usual Dosage Adults: I.M.: 5-10 mg/day for 6-8 days
Dosage Forms Injection, in oil: 50 mg/mL (10 mL)

progestin see progesterone on this page
Proglycem® Oral see diazoxide on page 142

ProHIBiT® *see* hemophilus b conjugate vaccine *on page 226*
Prokine™ *see* sargramostim *on page 426*
Prolamine® [OTC] *see* phenylpropanolamine hydrochloride *on page 373*
Prolastin® Injection *see* alpha₁-proteinase inhibitor (human) *on page 13*
Proleukin® *see* aldesleukin *on page 11*
Prolixin Decanoate® Injection *see* fluphenazine *on page 203*
Prolixin Enanthate® Injection *see* fluphenazine *on page 203*
Prolixin® Injection *see* fluphenazine *on page 203*
Prolixin® Oral *see* fluphenazine *on page 203*
Proloprim® *see* trimethoprim *on page 480*

promazine hydrochloride (proe' ma zeen)
Brand Names Sparine® Injection; Sparine® Oral
Therapeutic Category Antipsychotic Agent; Phenothiazine Derivative
Use Treatment of psychoses
Usual Dosage Oral, I.M.:
Children >12 years: Antipsychotic: 10-25 mg every 4-6 hours
Adults:
　　Psychosis: 10-200 mg every 4-6 hours not to exceed 1000 mg/day
　　Antiemetic: 25-50 mg every 4-6 hours as needed
Dosage Forms
Injection: 25 mg/mL (10 mL); 50 mg/mL (1 mL, 2 mL, 10 mL)
Tablet: 25 mg, 50 mg, 100 mg

Prometa® Oral *see* metaproterenol sulfate *on page 296*

promethazine and codeine
Brand Names Phenergan® with Codeine; Pherazine® With Codeine; Prothazine-DC®
Therapeutic Category Antihistamine; Antitussive; Cough Preparation
Use Temporary relief of coughs and upper respiratory symptoms associated with allergy or the common cold
Usual Dosage Oral (in terms of codeine):
Children: 1-1.5 mg/kg/day every 4 hours as needed; maximum: 30 mg/day **or**
　　2-6 years: 1.25-2.5 mL every 4-6 hours or 2.5-5 mg/dose every 4-6 hours as needed; maximum: 30 mg codeine/day
　　6-12 years: 2.5-5 mL every 4-6 hours as needed or 5-10 mg/dose every 4-6 hours as needed; maximum: 60 mg codeine/day
Adults: 10-20 mg/dose every 4-6 hours as needed; maximum: 120 mg codeine/day; or 5-10 mL every 4-6 hours as needed
Dosage Forms Syrup: Promethazine hydrochloride 6.25 mg and codeine phosphate 10 mg per 5 mL (120 mL, 180 mL, 473 mL)

promethazine and phenylephrine
Brand Names Phenergan® VC; Pherazine® VC
Therapeutic Category Antihistamine/Decongestant Combination
Use Temporary relief of upper respiratory symptoms associated with allergy or the common cold
Usual Dosage Oral:
Children:
　　2-6 years: 1.25 mL every 4-6 hours, not to exceed 7.5 mL in 24 hours
　　6-12 years: 2.5 mL every 4-6 hours, not to exceed 15 mL in 24 hours
Children >12 years and Adults: 5 mL every 4-6 hours, not to exceed 30 mL in 24 hours
Dosage Forms Liquid: Promethazine hydrochloride 6.25 mg and phenylephrine hydrochloride 5 mg per 5 mL (120 mL, 180 mL, 240 mL, 480 mL, 4000 mL)

promethazine hydrochloride (proe meth' a zeen)
Brand Names Anergan® Injection; Phenameth® Oral; Phenazine® Injection; Phenergan® Injection; Phenergan® Oral; Phenergan® Rectal; Prometh® Injection; Prorex® Injection; Prothazine® Injection; Prothazine® Oral; V-Gan® Injection

Therapeutic Category Antiemetic; Antihistamine; Phenothiazine Derivative; Sedative

Use Symptomatic treatment of various allergic conditions, antiemetic, motion sickness, and as a sedative

Usual Dosage

Children:
Antihistamine: Oral: 0.1 mg/kg/dose every 6 hours during the day and 0.5 mg/kg/dose at bedtime as needed
Antiemetic: Oral, I.M., I.V., rectal: 0.25-1 mg/kg 4-6 times/day as needed
Motion sickness: Oral: 0.5 mg/kg 30 minutes to 1 hour before departure, then every 12 hours as needed
Sedation: Oral, I.M., I.V., rectal: 0.5-1 mg/kg/dose every 6 hours as needed

Adults:
Antihistamine:
Oral: 25 mg at bedtime or 12.5 mg 3 times/day
I.M., I.V., rectal: 25 mg, may repeat in 2 hours
Antiemetic: Oral, I.M., I.V., rectal: 12.5-25 mg every 4 hours as needed
Motion sickness: Oral: 25 mg 30 minutes to 1 hour before departure, then every 12 hours as needed
Sedation: Oral, I.M., I.V., rectal: 25-50 mg/dose

Dosage Forms
Injection: 25 mg/mL (1 mL, 10 mL); 50 mg/mL (1 mL, 10 mL)
Suppository, rectal: 12.5 mg, 25 mg, 50 mg
Syrup: 6.25 mg/5 mL (5 mL, 120 mL, 240 mL, 480 mL, 4000 mL); 25 mg/5mL (120 mL, 480 mL, 4000 mL)
Tablet: 12.5 mg, 25 mg, 50 mg

promethazine, phenylephrine, and codeine
Brand Names Mallergan-VC® With Codeine; Phenergan® VC With Codeine

Therapeutic Category Antihistamine/Decongestant Combination; Antitussive; Cough Preparation

Use Temporary relief of coughs and upper respiratory symptoms including nasal congestion

Usual Dosage Oral:
Children (expressed in terms of codeine dosage): 1-1.5 mg/kg/day every 4 hours, maximum: 30 mg/day **or**
<2 years: Not recommended
2 to 6 years:
Weight 25 lb: 1.25-2.5 mL every 4-6 hours, not to exceed 6 mL/24 hours
Weight 30 lb: 1.25-2.5 mL every 4-6 hours, not to exceed 7 mL/24 hours
Weight 35 lb: 1.25-2.5 mL every 4-6 hours, not to exceed 8 mL/24 hours
Weight 40 lb: 1.25-2.5 mL every 4-6 hours, not to exceed 9 mL/24 hours
6 to <12 years: 2.5-5 mL every 4-6 hours, not to exceed 15 mL/24 hours

Adults: 5 mL every 4-6 hours, not to exceed 30 mL/24 hours

Dosage Forms Liquid: Promethazine hydrochloride 6.25 mg, phenylephrine hydrochloride 5 mg, and codeine phosphate 10 mg per 5 mL with alcohol 7% (120 mL, 240 mL, 480 mL, 4000 mL)

promethazine with dextromethorphan
Brand Names Phenameth® DM; Phenergan® with Dextromethorphan; Pherazine® w/DM

Therapeutic Category Antitussive; Cough Preparation

Use Temporary relief of coughs and upper respiratory symptoms associated with allergy or the common cold

(Continued)

promethazine with dextromethorphan *(Continued)*
Usual Dosage Oral:
Children:
2-6 years: 1.25-2.5 mL every 4-6 hours up to 10 mL in 24 hours
6-12 years: 2.5-5 mL every 4-6 hours up to 20 mL in 24 hours
Adults: 5 mL every 4-6 hours up to 30 mL in 24 hours
Dosage Forms Syrup: Promethazine hydrochloride 6.25 mg and dextromethorphan hydrobromide 15 mg per 5 mL with alcohol 7% (120 mL, 480 mL, 4000 mL)

Prometh® Injection *see* promethazine hydrochloride *on previous page*
Promit® *see* dextran 1 *on page 135*
Pronestyl® *see* procainamide hydrochloride *on page 395*
Pronestyl-SR® *see* procainamide hydrochloride *on page 395*
Propacet® *see* propoxyphene and acetaminophen *on page 402*
Propadrine *see* phenylpropanolamine hydrochloride *on page 373*

propafenone hydrochloride (proe pa feen' one)
Brand Names Rythmol®
Therapeutic Category Antiarrhythmic Agent, Class Ic
Use Life threatening ventricular arrhythmias; an oral sodium channel blocker similar to encainide and flecainide; in clinical trials was used effectively to treat atrial flutter, atrial fibrillation and other arrhythmias, but are not labeled indications; can worsen or even cause new ventricular arrhythmias (proarrhythmic effect)
Usual Dosage Adults: Oral: 150 mg every 8 hours, up to 300 mg every 8 hours
Dosage Forms Tablet: 150 mg, 225 mg, 300 mg

Propagest® [OTC] *see* phenylpropanolamine hydrochloride *on page 373*

propantheline bromide (proe pan' the leen)
Brand Names Pro-Banthine®
Therapeutic Category Antispasmodic Agent, Gastrointestinal
Use Adjunctive treatment of peptic ulcer, irritable bowel syndrome, pancreatitis, ureteral and urinary bladder spasm; to reduce duodenal motility during diagnostic radiologic procedures
Usual Dosage Oral:
Antisecretory:
Children: 1-2 mg/kg/day in 3-4 divided doses
Adults: 15 mg 3 times/day before meals or food and 30 mg at bedtime
Elderly: 7.5 mg 3 times/day before meals and at bedtime
Antispasmodic:
Children: 2-3 mg/kg/day in divided doses every 4-6 hours and at bedtime
Adults: 15 mg 3 times/day before meals or food and 30 mg at bedtime
Dosage Forms Tablet: 7.5 mg, 15 mg

proparacaine and fluorescein
Brand Names Fluoracaine® Ophthalmic
Therapeutic Category Diagnostic Agent, Ophthalmic Dye; Local Anesthetic, Ophthalmic
Use Anesthesia for tonometry, gonioscopy; suture removal from cornea; removal of corneal foreign body; cataract extraction, glaucoma surgery
Usual Dosage
Tonometry, gonioscopy, suture removal: Adults: Instill 1-2 drops 0.5% solution in eye just prior to procedure
Ophthalmic surgery: Children and Adults: Instill 1 drop of 0.5% solution in eye every 5-10 minutes for 5-7 doses

Dosage Forms Solution: Proparacaine hydrochloride 0.5% and fluorescein sodium 0.25% (2 mL, 5 mL)

proparacaine hydrochloride (proe par' a kane)
Brand Names AK-Taine® Ophthalmic; Alcaine® Ophthalmic; I-Paracaine® Ophthalmic; Ophthaine® Ophthalmic; Ophthetic® Ophthalmic
Synonyms proxymetacaine
Therapeutic Category Local Anesthetic, Ophthalmic
Use Anesthesia for tonometry, gonioscopy; suture removal from cornea; removal of corneal foreign body; cataract extraction, glaucoma surgery; short operative procedure involving the cornea and conjunctiva
Usual Dosage Children and Adults:
Ophthalmic surgery: Instill 1 drop of 0.5% solution in eye every 5-10 minutes for 5-7 doses

Tonometry, gonioscopy, suture removal: Instill 1-2 drops 0.5% solution in eye just prior to procedure
Dosage Forms Ophthalmic, solution: 0.5% (2 mL, 15 mL)

Propine® Ophthalmic see dipivefrin hydrochloride on page 154

propiomazine hydrochloride (proe pee oh' ma zeen)
Brand Names Largon® Injection
Therapeutic Category Antianxiety Agent; Antiemetic; Phenothiazine Derivative; Sedative
Use Relief of restlessness, nausea and apprehension before and during surgery or during labor
Usual Dosage I.M., I.V.:
Children: 0.55-1.1 mg/kg

Adults: 10-40 mg prior to procedure, additional may be repeated at 3-hour intervals
Dosage Forms Injection: 20 mg/mL (1 mL)

Proplex® SX-T see factor ix complex (human) on page 189
Proplex® T see factor ix complex (human) on page 189

propofol (proe' po fole)
Brand Names Diprivan® Injection
Therapeutic Category General Anesthetic
Use Induction or maintenance of anesthesia for inpatient or outpatient surgery
Usual Dosage Dosage must be individualized and titrated to the desired clinical effect; however, as a general guideline:

No pediatric dose has been established

Induction: I.V.:
Adults ≤55 years, and/or ASA I or II patients: 2-2.5 mg/kg of body weight (approximately 40 mg every 10 seconds until onset of induction)
Elderly, debilitated, hypovolemic, and/or ASA III or IV patients: 1-1.5 mg/kg of body weight (approximately 20 mg every 10 seconds until onset of induction)

Maintenance: I.V. infusion:
Adults ≤55 years, and/or ASA I or II patients: 0.1-0.2 mg/kg of body weight/minute (6-12 mg/kg of body weight/hour)
Elderly, debilitated, hypovolemic, and/or ASA III or IV patients: 0.05-0.1 mg/kg of body weight/minute (3-6 mg/kg of body weight/hour)

I.V. intermittent: 25-50 mg increments, as needed
Dosage Forms Injection: 10 mg/mL (20 mL)

propoxyphene (proe pox' i feen)
Brand Names Darvon®; Darvon-N®; Dolene®
Synonyms dextropropoxyphene
Therapeutic Category Analgesic, Narcotic
Use Management of mild to moderate pain
Usual Dosage Adults: Oral:
Hydrochloride: 65 mg every 3-4 hours as needed for pain; maximum: 390 mg/day
Napsylate: 100 mg every 4 hours as needed for pain; maximum: 600 mg/day
Dosage Forms
Capsule, as hydrochloride: 32 mg, 65 mg
Suspension, oral, as napsylate: 50 mg/5 mL (480 mL)
Tablet, as napsylate: 100 mg

propoxyphene and acetaminophen
Brand Names Darvocet-N®; Darvocet-N® 100; E-Lor®; Genagesic®; Propacet®; Wygesic®
Synonyms propoxyphene hydrochloride and acetaminophen; propoxyphene napsylate and acetaminophen
Therapeutic Category Analgesic, Narcotic
Use Management of mild to moderate pain
Usual Dosage Adults:
Darvocet-N®: 1-2 tablets every 4 hours as needed; maximum: 600 mg propoxyphene napsylate/day
Darvocet-N® 100: 1 tablet every 4 hours as needed; maximum: 600 mg propoxyphene napsylate/day
Dosage Forms Tablet:
Darvocet-N®: Propoxyphene napsylate 50 mg and acetaminophen 325 mg
Darvocet-N® 100: Propoxyphene napsylate 100 mg and acetaminophen 650 mg
E-Lor®, Genagesic®, Wygesic®: Propoxyphene hydrochloride 65 mg and acetaminophen 650 mg

propoxyphene and aspirin
Brand Names Bexophene®; Darvon® Compound-65 Pulvules®
Synonyms propoxyphene hydrochloride and aspirin; propoxyphene napsylate and aspirin
Therapeutic Category Analgesic, Narcotic
Use Management of mild to moderate pain
Usual Dosage Oral: 1-2 capsules every 4 hours as needed
Dosage Forms Capsule: Propoxyphene hydrochloride 65 mg and aspirin 389 mg with caffeine 32.4 mg

propoxyphene hydrochloride and acetaminophen see propoxyphene and acetaminophen on this page

propoxyphene hydrochloride and aspirin see propoxyphene and aspirin on this page

propoxyphene napsylate and acetaminophen see propoxyphene and acetaminophen on this page

propoxyphene napsylate and aspirin see propoxyphene and aspirin on this page

propranolol and hydrochlorothiazide
Brand Names Inderide®
Therapeutic Category Antihypertensive, Combination
Use Management of hypertension
Usual Dosage Dose is individualized
Dosage Forms
Capsule, long acting (Inderide® LA):
80/50 Propranolol hydrochloride 80 mg and hydrochlorothiazide 50 mg

120/50 Propranolol hydrochloride 120 mg and hydrochlorothiazide 50 mg
160/50 Propranolol hydrochloride 160 mg and hydrochlorothiazide 50 mg
Tablet (Inderide®):
40/25 Propranolol hydrochloride 40 mg and hydrochlorothiazide 25 mg
80/25 Propranolol hydrochloride 80 mg and hydrochlorothiazide 25 mg

propranolol hydrochloride (proe pran' oh lole)
Brand Names Inderal®; Inderal® LA
Therapeutic Category Antianginal Agent; Antiarrhythmic Agent, Class Ib; Antiarrhythmic Agent, Class II; Beta-Adrenergic Blocker
Use Management of hypertension, angina pectoris, pheochromocytoma, essential tremor, tetralogy of Fallot cyanotic spells, and arrhythmias (such as atrial fibrillation and flutter, A-V nodal re-entrant tachycardias, and catecholamine-induced arrhythmias); prevention of myocardial infarction, migraine headache; symptomatic treatment of hypertrophic subaortic stenosis
Usual Dosage
Tachyarrhythmias:
Oral:
Children: Initial: 0.5-1 mg/kg/day in divided doses every 6-8 hours; titrate dosage upward every 3-7 days; usual dose: 2-4 mg/kg/day; higher doses may be needed; do not exceed 16 mg/kg/day or 60 mg/day
Adults: 10-80 mg/dose every 6-8 hours
I.V.:
Children: 0.01-0.1 mg/kg slow IVP over 10 minutes; maximum dose: 1 mg
Adults: 1 mg/dose slow IVP; repeat every 5 minutes up to a total of 5 mg

Hypertension: Oral:
Children: Initial: 0.5-1 mg/kg/day in divided doses every 6-12 hours; increase gradually every 3-7 days; maximum: 2 mg/kg/24 hours
Adults: Initial: 40 mg twice daily or 60-80 mg once daily as sustained release capsules; increase dosage every 3-7 days; usual dose: ≤320 mg divided in 2-3 doses/day or once daily as sustained release; maximum daily dose: 640 mg

Migraine headache prophylaxis: Oral:
Children: 0.6-1.5 mg/kg/day **or**
≤35 kg: 10-20 mg 3 times/day
>35 kg: 20-40 mg 3 times/day
Adults: Initial: 80 mg/day divided every 6-8 hours; increase by 20-40 mg/dose every 3-4 weeks to a maximum of 160-240 mg/day given in divided doses every 6-8 hours; if satisfactory response not achieved within 6 weeks of starting therapy, drug should be withdrawn gradually over several weeks

Tetralogy spells: Children: Oral: 1-2 mg/kg/day every 6 hours as needed, may increase by 1 mg/kg/day to a maximum of 5 mg/kg/day, or if refractory may increase slowly to a maximum of 10-15 mg/kg/day

Thyrotoxicosis:
Neonates: Oral: 2 mg/kg/day in divided doses every 6-12 hours; occasionally higher doses may be required
Adolescents and Adults: Oral: 10-40 mg/dose every 6 hours
Adults: I.V.: 1-3 mg/dose slow IVP as a single dose

Adults: Oral:
Angina: 80-320 mg/day in doses divided 2-4 times/day or 80-160 mg of sustained release once daily
Pheochromocytoma: 30-60 mg/day in divided doses
Myocardial infarction prophylaxis: 180-240 mg/day in 3-4 divided doses
Hypertrophic subaortic stenosis: 20-40 mg 3-4 times/day
Essential tremor: 40 mg twice daily initially; maintenance doses: usually 120-320 mg/day
Dosage Forms
Capsule, sustained action: 60 mg, 80 mg, 120 mg, 160 mg
(Continued)
403

propranolol hydrochloride *(Continued)*
Injection: 1 mg/mL (1 mL)
Solution, oral (strawberry-mint flavor): 4 mg/mL (5 mL, 500 mL); 8 mg/mL (5 mL, 500 mL)
Solution, oral, concentrate: 80 mg/mL (30 mL)
Tablet: 10 mg, 20 mg, 40 mg, 60 mg, 80 mg, 90 mg

Propulsid® *see* cisapride *on page 103*

propylene glycol and salicylic acid *see* salicylic acid and propylene glycol *on page 425*

propylhexedrine (proe pill hex' e dreen)
Brand Names Benzedrex® [OTC]
Therapeutic Category Decongestant
Use Topical nasal decongestant
Usual Dosage Inhale through each nostril while blocking the other
Dosage Forms Inhaler: 250 mg

propyliodone *see* radiological/contrast media (ionic) *on page 413*

2-propylpentanoic acid *see* valproic acid and derivatives *on page 490*

propylthiouracil (proe pill thye oh yoor' a sill)
Synonyms PTU
Therapeutic Category Antithyroid Agent
Use Palliative treatment of hyperthyroidism as an adjunct to ameliorate hyperthyroidism in preparation for surgical treatment or radioactive iodine therapy and in the management of thyrotoxic crisis
Usual Dosage Oral:
Neonates: 5-10 mg/kg/day in divided doses every 8 hours

Children: Initial: 5-7 mg/kg/day in divided doses every 8 hours or
6-10 years: 50-150 mg/day
>10 years: 150-300 mg/day
Maintenance: $\frac{1}{3}$ to $\frac{2}{3}$ of the initial dose in divided doses every 8-12 hours

Adults: Initial: 300-450 mg/day in divided doses every 8 hours; maintenance: 100-150 mg/day in divided doses every 8-12 hours
Dosage Forms Tablet: 50 mg

2-propylvaleric acid *see* valproic acid and derivatives *on page 490*

Prorex® Injection *see* promethazine hydrochloride *on page 399*

Proscar® Oral *see* finasteride *on page 196*

Pro-Sof® [OTC] *see* docusate *on page 157*

Pro-Sof® Plus [OTC] *see* docusate and casanthranol *on page 158*

ProSom™ *see* estazolam *on page 177*

prostaglandin E$_1$ *see* alprostadil *on page 13*

prostaglandin E$_2$ *see* dinoprostone *on page 151*

Prostaphlin® Injection *see* oxacillin sodium *on page 347*

Prostaphlin® Oral *see* oxacillin sodium *on page 347*

ProStep® Patch *see* nicotine *on page 334*

Prostigmin® Injection *see* neostigmine *on page 330*

Prostigmin® Oral *see* neostigmine *on page 330*

Prostin/15M® *see* carboprost tromethamine *on page 75*

Prostin E₂® Vaginal Suppository *see* dinoprostone *on page 151*

Prostin VR Pediatric® Injection *see* alprostadil *on page 13*

protamine sulfate (proe' ta meen)
Therapeutic Category Antidote, Heparin
Use Treatment of heparin overdosage; neutralize heparin during surgery or dialysis procedures
Usual Dosage Children and Adults: I.V.: 1 mg of protamine neutralizes, 90 USP units of heparin (lung) and 115 USP units of heparin (intestinal); heparin neutralization occurs within 5 minutes following I.V. injection; administer 1 mg for each 100 units of heparin given in preceding 3-4 hours up to a maximum dose of 50 mg
Dosage Forms Injection: 10 mg/mL (5 mL, 10 mL, 25 mL)

Protenate® *see* plasma protein fraction *on page 380*

Prothazine-DC® *see* promethazine and codeine *on page 398*

Prothazine® Injection *see* promethazine hydrochloride *on page 399*

Prothazine® Oral *see* promethazine hydrochloride *on page 399*

Protilase® *see* pancrelipase *on page 354*

protirelin (proe tye' re lin)
Brand Names Relefact® TRH Injection; Thypinone® Injection
Synonyms lopremone
Therapeutic Category Diagnostic Agent, Thyroid Function
Use Adjunct in the diagnostic assessment of thyroid function, and an adjunct to other diagnostic procedures in assessment of patients with pituitary or hypothalamic dysfunction; also causes release of prolactin from the pituitary and is used to detect defective control of prolactin secretion.
Usual Dosage I.V.:
  Children: 7 μg/kg to a maximum dose of 500 μg

  Adults: 500 μg (range: 200-500 μg)
Dosage Forms Injection: 500 μg/mL (1 mL)

Protopam® *see* pralidoxime chloride *on page 389*

Protostat® Oral *see* metronidazole *on page 309*

protriptyline hydrochloride (proe trip' ti leen)
Brand Names Vivactil®
Therapeutic Category Antidepressant, Tricyclic
Use Treatment of various forms of depression, often in conjunction with psychotherapy
Usual Dosage Oral:
  Adolescents: 15-20 mg/day
  Adults: 15-60 mg in 3-4 divided doses
  Elderly: 15-20 mg/day
Dosage Forms Tablet: 5 mg, 10 mg

Protropin® Injection *see* human growth hormone *on page 230*

Provatene® [OTC] *see* beta-carotene *on page 52*

Proventil® *see* albuterol *on page 10*

Provera® Oral *see* medroxyprogesterone acetate *on page 289*

Provocholine® *see* methacholine chloride *on page 297*

Proxigel® Oral [OTC] *see* carbamide peroxide *on page 73*

proxymetacaine *see* proparacaine hydrochloride *on page 401*

Prozac® *see* fluoxetine hydrochloride *on page 203*

PRP-D *see* hemophilus b conjugate vaccine *on page 226*

Prulet® [OTC] *see* phenolphthalein *on page 370*

prymaccone *see* primaquine phosphate *on page 394*

Pseudo-Car® DM *see* carbinoxamine, pseudoephedrine, and dextromethorphan *on page 74*

Pseudo-Chlor® [OTC] *see* chlorpheniramine and pseudoephedrine *on page 94*

pseudoephedrine (soo doe e fed' rin)
Brand Names Afrinol® [OTC]; Cenafed® [OTC]; Decofed® Syrup [OTC]; Drixoral® Non-Drowsy [OTC]; Neofed® [OTC]; Novafed®; PediaCare® Oral; Sudafed® [OTC]; Sudafed® 12 Hour [OTC]; Sufedrin® [OTC]
Synonyms *d*-isoephedrine hydrochloride
Therapeutic Category Adrenergic Agonist Agent; Decongestant
Use Temporary symptomatic relief of nasal congestion due to common cold, upper respiratory allergies, and sinusitis; also promotes nasal or sinus drainage
Usual Dosage Oral:
Children:
    <2 years: 4 mg/kg/day in divided doses every 6 hours
    2-5 years: 15 mg every 6 hours; maximum: 60 mg/24 hours
    6-12 years: 30 mg every 6 hours; maximum: 120 mg/24 hours
Adults: 60 mg every 6 hours; maximum: 240 mg/24 hours
Dosage Forms
Capsule: 60 mg
Capsule, timed release, as hydrochloride: 120 mg
Drops, oral, as hydrochloride: 7.5 mg/0.8 mL (15 mL)
Liquid, as hydrochloride: 15 mg/5 mL (120 mL); 30 mg/5 mL (120 mL, 240 mL, 473 mL)
Tablet, as hydrochloride: 30 mg, 60 mg
Tablet:
    Timed release, as hydrochloride: 120 mg
    Extended release, as sulfate: 120 mg

pseudoephedrine and azatadine *see* azatadine and pseudoephedrine *on page 40*

pseudoephedrine and chlorpheniramine *see* chlorpheniramine and pseudoephedrine *on page 94*

pseudoephedrine and dexbrompheniramine *see* dexbrompheniramine and pseudoephedrine *on page 134*

pseudoephedrine and guaifenesin *see* guaifenesin and pseudoephedrine *on page 220*

pseudoephedrine and triprolidine *see* triprolidine and pseudoephedrine *on page 482*

Pseudo-gest Plus® [OTC] *see* chlorpheniramine and pseudoephedrine *on page 94*

pseudomonic acid A *see* mupirocin *on page 319*

Psorcon™ Topical *see* diflorasone diacetate *on page 146*

psoriGel® [OTC] *see* coal tar *on page 110*

Psorion® Topical *see* betamethasone *on page 52*

psp *see* phenolsulfonphthalein *on page 370*

P&S® Shampoo [OTC] *see* salicylic acid *on page 424*

psyllium (sill' i yum)
Brand Names Effer-Syllium® [OTC]; Fiberall® Powder [OTC]; Fiberall® Wafer [OTC]; Hydrocil® [OTC]; Konsyl® [OTC]; Konsyl-D® [OTC]; Metamucil® [OTC]; Metamucil® Instant Mix [OTC]; Modane® Bulk [OTC]; Perdiem® Plain [OTC]; Reguloid® [OTC]; Serutan® [OTC]; Siblin® [OTC]; Syllact® [OTC]; V-Lax® [OTC]
Synonyms plantago seed; plantain seed
Therapeutic Category Laxative, Bulk-Producing
Use Treatment of chronic atonic or spastic constipation and in constipation associated with rectal disorders; management of irritable bowel syndrome
Usual Dosage Oral:
Children 6-11 years: $1/2$ to 1 rounded teaspoonful 1-3 times/day
Adults: 1-2 rounded teaspoonfuls or 1-2 packets 1-4 times/day
Dosage Forms
Granules: 4.03 g per rounded teaspoon (100 g, 250 g); 2.5 g per rounded teaspoon
Powder: Psyllium 50% and dextrose 50% (6.5 g, 325 g, 420 g, 480 g, 500 g)
Powder:
Effervescent: 3 g/dose (270 g, 480 g); 3.4 g/dose (single-dose packets)
Psyllium hydrophilic: 3.4 g/per rounded teaspoon (210 g, 300 g, 420 g, 630 g)
Squares, chewable: 1.7 g, 3.4 g
Wafers: 3.4 g

P.T.E.-4® *see* trace metals *on page 472*

P.T.E.-5® *see* trace metals *on page 472*

pteroylglutamic acid *see* folic acid *on page 205*

PTU *see* propylthiouracil *on page 404*

Pulmozyme® *see* dornase alfa *on page 159*

Purge® [OTC] *see* castor oil *on page 77*

Puri-Clens™ [OTC] *see* methylbenzethonium chloride *on page 304*

purified protein derivative *see* tuberculin tests *on page 484*

Purinethol® *see* mercaptopurine *on page 294*

P-V-Tussin® *see* hydrocodone, phenylephrine, pyrilamine, phenindamine, chlorpheniramine, and ammonium chloride *on page 236*

P$_x$E$_x$® Ophthalmic *see* pilocarpine and epinephrine *on page 377*

Pyocidin-Otic® *see* polymyxin b and hydrocortisone *on page 384*

pyrantel pamoate (pi ran' tel pam' oh ate)
Brand Names Antiminth® [OTC]; Pin-Rid® [OTC]; Pin-X® [OTC]; Reese's® Pinworm Medicine [OTC]
Therapeutic Category Anthelmintic
Use Roundworm, pinworm, and hookworm infestations, and trichostrongyliasis
Usual Dosage Children and Adults: Oral:
Roundworm, pinworm, or trichostrongyliasis: 11 mg/kg administered as a single dose; maximum dose is 1 g; dosage should be repeated in 2 weeks for pinworm infection
Hookworm: 11 mg/kg/day once daily for 3 days
Dosage Forms
Capsule: 180 mg
Liquid: 50 mg/mL (30 mL); 144 mg/mL (30 mL)
Suspension, oral (caramel-currant flavor): 50 mg/mL (60 mL)

pyrazinamide (peer a zin' a mide)
Synonyms pyrazinoic acid amide
Therapeutic Category Antitubercular Agent
Use Adjunctive treatment of tuberculosis when primary and secondary agents cannot be used or have failed
(Continued)

pyrazinamide *(Continued)*
Usual Dosage Oral:
Children: 15-30 mg/kg/day in divided doses every 12-24 hours; daily dose not to exceed 2 g

Adults: 15-30 mg/kg/day in 3-4 divided doses; maximum daily dose: 2 g/day
Dosage Forms Tablet: 500 mg

pyrazinoic acid amide *see* pyrazinamide *on previous page*

pyrethrins (pye ree' thrins)
Brand Names A-200™ Pyrinate [OTC]; End Lice® [OTC]; Lice-Enz® [OTC]; Pyrinyl II® [OTC]; RID® [OTC]; Tisit® [OTC]
Therapeutic Category Antiparasitic Agent, Topical; Pediculocide
Use Treatment of *Pediculus humanus* infestations
Usual Dosage Application of pyrethrins:
Apply enough solution to completely wet infested area, including hair
Allow to remain on area for 10 minutes
Wash and rinse with large amounts of warm water
Use fine-toothed comb to remove lice and eggs from hair
Shampoo hair to restore body and luster
Treatment may be repeated if necessary once in a 24-hours period
Repeat treatment in 7-10 days to kill newly hatched lice
Dosage Forms
Gel, topical: 0.3% (30 g, 480 g)
Liquid, topical: 0.18% (60 mL); 0.2% (60 mL, 120 mL); 0.3% (60 mL, 120 mL, 240 mL)
Shampoo: 0.3% (60 mL, 118 mL); 0.33% (60 mL, 120 mL)

pyribenzamine® *see* tripelennamine *on page 481*
Pyridiate® *see* phenazopyridine hydrochloride *on page 368*
2-pyridine aldoxime methochloride *see* pralidoxime chloride *on page 389*
Pyridium® *see* phenazopyridine hydrochloride *on page 368*

pyridostigmine bromide (peer id oh stig' meen)
Brand Names Mestinon® Injection; Mestinon® Oral; Regonol® Injection
Therapeutic Category Antidote, Neuromuscular Blocking Agent; Cholinergic Agent
Use Symptomatic treatment of myasthenia gravis; also used as an antidote for nondepolarizing neuromuscular blockers
Usual Dosage Normally, sustained release dosage form is used at bedtime for patients who complain of morning weakness

Myasthenia gravis:
Oral:
Children: 7 mg/kg/day in 5-6 divided doses
Adults: Initial: 60 mg 3 times/day with maintenance dose ranging from 60 mg to 1.5 g/day; sustained release formulation should be dosed at least every 6 hours (usually 12-24 hours)
I.M., I.V.:
Children: 0.05-0.15 mg/kg/dose (maximum single dose: 10 mg)
Adults: 2 mg every 2-3 hours or 1/30th of oral dose

Reversal of nondepolarizing neuromuscular blocker: I.M., I.V.:
Children: 0.1-0.25 mg/kg/dose preceded by atropine
Adults: 10-20 mg preceded by atropine
Dosage Forms
Injection: 5 mg/mL (2 mL, 5 mL)
Syrup (raspberry flavor): 60 mg/5 mL (480 mL)
Tablet: 60 mg
Tablet, sustained release: 180 mg

pyridoxine hydrochloride (peer i dox' een)
Brand Names Beesix®; Nestrex®
Synonyms vitamin B$_6$
Therapeutic Category Antidote, Cycloserine Toxicity; Antidote, Hydralazine Toxicity; Antidote, Isoniazid Toxicity; Vitamin, Water Soluble
Use Prevent and treat vitamin B$_6$ deficiency, pyridoxine-dependent seizures in infants, adjunct to treatment of acute toxicity from isoniazid, cycloserine, or hydralazine overdose
Usual Dosage
Pyridoxine-dependent Infants:
Oral: 2-100 mg/day
I.M., I.V.: 10-100 mg

Dietary deficiency: Oral:
Children: 5-10 mg/24 hours for 3 weeks
Adults: 10-20 mg/day for 3 weeks

Drug induced neuritis (eg, isoniazid, hydralazine, penicillamine, cycloserine): Oral treatment:
Children: 10-50 mg/24 hours; prophylaxis: 1-2 mg/kg/24 hours
Adults: 100-200 mg/24 hours; prophylaxis: 10-100 mg/24 hours

For the treatment of seizures and/or coma from acute isoniazid toxicity, a dose of pyridoxine hydrochloride equal to the amount of INH ingested can be given I.M./I.V. in divided doses together with other anticonvulsants
Dosage Forms
Injection: 100 mg/mL (10 mL, 30 mL)
Tablet: 25 mg, 50 mg, 100 mg
Tablet, extended release: 100 mg

pyrimethamine (peer i meth' a meen)
Brand Names Daraprim®
Therapeutic Category Antimalarial Agent
Use Prophylaxis of malaria due to susceptible strains of plasmodia; used in conjunction with quinine and sulfadiazine for the treatment of uncomplicated attacks of chloroquine-resistant *P. falciparum* malaria; used in conjunction with fast-acting schizonticide to initiate transmission control and suppression cure; synergistic combination with sulfonamide in treatment of toxoplasmosis
Usual Dosage Oral:
Malaria chemoprophylaxis:
Children: 0.5 mg/kg once weekly; not to exceed 25 mg/dose **or**
Children:
<4 years: 6.25 mg once weekly
4-10 years: 12.5 mg once weekly
Children >10 years and Adults: 25 mg once weekly
Dosage should be continued for all age groups for at least 6-10 weeks after leaving endemic areas

Chloroquine-resistant *P. falciparum* malaria (when used in conjunction with quinine and sulfadiazine):
Children:
<10 kg: 6.25 mg/day once daily for 3 days
10-20 kg: 12.5 mg/day once daily for 3 days
20-40 kg: 25 mg/day once daily for 3 days
Adults: 25 mg twice daily for 3 days

Toxoplasmosis (with sulfadiazine or trisulfapyrimidines):
Children: 1 mg/kg/day divided into 2 equal daily doses; decrease dose after 2-4 days by 50%, continue for about 1 month; used with 100 mg sulfadiazine/kg/day divided every 6 hours; **or** 2 mg/kg/day divided every 12 hours for 3 days followed by 1 mg/kg/day once daily for 4 weeks
Adults: 50-75 mg/day together with 1-4 g of a sulfonamide for 1-3 weeks depending on patient's tolerance and response
Dosage Forms Tablet: 25 mg

Pyrinyl II® [OTC] *see* pyrethrins *on page 408*

pyrithione zinc (peer i thye' one)
Brand Names Danex® [OTC]; DHS Zinc® [OTC]; Head & Shoulders® [OTC]; Sebulon® [OTC]; Theraplex Z® [OTC]; Zincon® Shampoo [OTC]; ZNP® Bar [OTC]
Therapeutic Category Antiseborrheic Agent, Topical
Use Relieves the itching, irritation and scalp flaking associated with dandruff and/or seborrheal dermatitis of the scalp
Usual Dosage Shampoo hair twice weekly, wet hair, apply to scalp and massage vigorously, rinse and repeat
Dosage Forms
Bar: 2% (119 g)
Shampoo: 1% (120 mL); 2% (120 mL, 180 mL, 240 mL, 360 mL)

Quadra-Hist® *see* chlorpheniramine, phenyltoloxamine, phenylpropanolamine, and phenylephrine *on page 96*

quazepam (kway' ze pam)
Brand Names Doral®
Therapeutic Category Benzodiazepine; Hypnotic; Sedative
Use Short-term treatment of insomnia
Usual Dosage Adults: Oral: Initial: 15 mg at bedtime, in some patients the dose may be reduced to 7.5 mg after a few nights
Dosage Forms Tablet: 7.5 mg, 15 mg

Quelicin® Injection *see* succinylcholine chloride *on page 445*

Queltuss® [OTC] *see* guaifenesin and dextromethorphan *on page 218*

Questran® *see* cholestyramine resin *on page 100*

Questran® Light *see* cholestyramine resin *on page 100*

Quibron® *see* theophylline and guaifenesin *on page 461*

Quibron®-T *see* theophylline *on page 460*

Quibron®-T/SR *see* theophylline *on page 460*

Quiess® Injection *see* hydroxyzine *on page 241*

quinacrine hydrochloride (kwin' a kreen)
Brand Names Atabrine®
Synonyms mepacrine hydrochloride
Therapeutic Category Anthelmintic; Antimalarial Agent
Use Treatment of giardiasis and cestodiasis (tapeworm); reserve agent for suppression and chemoprophylaxis of malaria
Usual Dosage Oral (normally an enema is given before treatment to reduce amount of stool that requires examination after treatment):
Children:
Dwarf tapeworm:
4-8 years: 200 mg stat, 100 mg before breakfast for 3 days
8-10 years: 300 mg stat, 100 mg twice daily for 3 days
11-14 years: 400 mg stat, 100 mg 3 times/day for 3 days
Tapeworm (beef, pork, or fish):
5-10 years: 100 mg every 10 minutes for 4 doses, give 300 mg sodium bicarbonate with each dose
11-14 years: 200 mg every 10 minutes for 3 doses, give 300 mg sodium bicarbonate with each dose

Giardiasis: 7 mg/kg/day in 3 divided doses for 5-7 days; maximum dose: 300 mg/day
Malaria treatment:
    1-4 years: 100 mg 3 times/day for one day then 100 mg/day for 6 days
    4-8 years: 200 mg 3 times/day for one day then 100 mg 2 times/day for 6 days
    Children >8 years and Adults: 200 mg and 1 g sodium bicarbonate every 6 hours for
        5 doses, then 100 mg 3 times/day for 6 days
Malaria suppression: 50 mg/day for 1-3 months
Adults:
    Dwarf tapeworm: 900 mg in 3 portions 20 minutes apart, then 100 mg 3 times/day for
        3 days
    Tapeworm (beef, pork, or fish): 200 mg every 10 minutes for 4 doses with 600 mg sodi-
        um bicarbonate with each dose
    Giardiasis: 100 mg 3 times/day for 5-7 days
    Suppression of malaria: 100 mg/day, continue for 1-3 months; for endemic areas, drug
        therapy should be started 2 weeks before arrival and continued for 3-4 weeks after
        departure
Dosage Forms Tablet: 100 mg

Quinaglute® Dura-Tabs® *see* quinidine *on this page*

Quinalan® Oral *see* quinidine *on this page*

quinalbarbitone sodium *see* secobarbital sodium *on page 427*

Quinamm® *see* quinine sulfate *on next page*

quinapril hydrochloride (kwin' a pril)
Brand Names Accupril®
Therapeutic Category Angiotensin Converting Enzyme (ACE) Inhibitors
Use Treatment of hypertension, either alone or in combination with other antihypertensive agents
Usual Dosage Adults: Oral: Initial: 10 mg once daily, adjust according to blood pressure response at peak and trough blood levels; in general, the normal dosage range is 40-80 mg/day
Dosage Forms Tablet: 5 mg, 10 mg, 20 mg, 40 mg

quinestrol (kwin ess' trole)
Brand Names Estrovis®
Therapeutic Category Estrogen Derivative
Use Atrophic vaginitis; hypogonadism; primary ovarian failure; vasomotor symptoms of menopause; prostatic carcinoma; osteoporosis prophylactic
Usual Dosage Adults: Oral: 100 µg once daily for 7 days; followed by 100 µg/week beginning 2 weeks after inception of treatment; may increase to 200 µg/week if necessary
Dosage Forms Tablet: 100 µg

quinethazone (kwin eth' a zone)
Brand Names Hydromox®
Therapeutic Category Diuretic, Thiazide
Use Adjunctive therapy in treatment of edema and hypertension
Usual Dosage Adults: Oral: 50-100 mg once daily up to a maximum of 200 mg daily
Dosage Forms Tablet: 50 mg

Quinidex® Extentabs® *see* quinidine *on this page*

quinidine (kwin' i deen)
Brand Names Cardioquin® Oral; Quinaglute® Dura-Tabs®; Quinalan® Oral; Quinidex® Extentabs®; Quinora® Oral
Synonyms quinidine gluconate; quinidine polygalacturonate; quinidine sulfate
(Continued)

quinidine *(Continued)*
Therapeutic Category Antiarrhythmic Agent, Class Ia
Use Prophylaxis after cardioversion of atrial fibrillation and/or flutter to maintain normal sinus rhythm; also used to prevent reoccurrence of paroxysmal supraventricular tachycardia, paroxysmal A-V junctional rhythm, paroxysmal ventricular tachycardia, paroxysmal atrial fibrillation, and atrial or ventricular premature contractions; also has activity against *Plasmodium falciparum* malaria
Usual Dosage Note: Dosage expressed in terms of the salt: 267 mg of quinidine gluconate = 275 mg of quinidine polygalacturonate = 200 mg of quinidine sulfate

Children: Test dose for idiosyncratic reaction (sulfate, oral or gluconate, I.M.): 2 mg/kg or 60 mg/m^2
   Oral (quinidine sulfate): 15-60 mg/kg/day in 4-5 divided doses or 6 mg/kg every 4-6 hours (AMA 1991); usual 30 mg/kg/day or 900 mg/m^2/day given in 5 daily doses
   I.V. **not** recommended (quinidine gluconate): 2-10 mg/kg/dose every 3-6 hours as needed

Adults: Test dose: 200 mg administered several hours before full dosage (to determine possibility of idiosyncratic reaction)
   Oral (sulfate): 100-600 mg/dose every 4-6 hours; begin at 200 mg/dose and titrate to desired effect
   Oral (gluconate): 324-972 mg every 8-12 hours
   Oral (polygalacturonate): 275 mg every 8-12 hours
   I.M.: 400 mg/dose every 4-6 hours
   I.V.: 200-400 mg/dose diluted and given at a rate ≤10 mg/minute
Dosage Forms
Injection, as gluconate: 80 mg/mL (10 mL)
Tablet, as polygalacturonate: 275 mg
Tablet, as sulfate: 200 mg, 300 mg
Tablet:
   Sustained action, as sulfate: 300 mg
   Sustained release, as gluconate: 324 mg

quinidine gluconate *see* quinidine *on previous page*
quinidine polygalacturonate *see* quinidine *on previous page*
quinidine sulfate *see* quinidine *on previous page*

quinine sulfate *(kwye' nine)*
Brand Names Legatrin® [OTC]; Quinamm®; Quiphile®; Q-vel®
Therapeutic Category Antimalarial Agent; Skeletal Muscle Relaxant
Use Suppression or treatment of chloroquine-resistant *P. falciparum* malaria; treatment of *Babesia microti* infection; prevention and treatment of nocturnal recumbency leg muscle cramps
Usual Dosage Oral (parenteral dosage form may be obtained from Centers for Disease Control if needed):

Children: Chloroquine-resistant malaria and babesiosis: 25 mg/kg/day in divided doses every 8 hours for 7 days; maximum: 650 mg/dose

Adults:
   Chloroquine-resistant malaria: 650 mg every 8 hours for 7 days in conjunction with another agent
   Babesiosis: 650 mg every 6-8 hours for 7 days
   Leg cramps: 200-300 mg at bedtime
Dosage Forms
Capsule: 64.8 mg, 65 mg, 200 mg, 300 mg, 325 mg
Tablet: 162.5 mg, 260 mg

Quinora® Oral *see* quinidine *on previous page*

Quinsana® Plus Topical [OTC] *see* undecylenic acid and derivatives *on page 486*

Quiphile® *see* quinine sulfate *on previous page*

Q-vel® *see* quinine sulfate *on previous page*

rabies immune globulin, human
Brand Names Hyperab®; Imogam®
Synonyms RIG
Therapeutic Category Immune Globulin
Use Passive immunity to rabies for postexposure prophylaxis of individuals exposed to the virus
Usual Dosage Children and Adults: I.M.: 20 units/kg in a single dose (RIG should always be administered in conjunction with rabies vaccine (HDCV)) (Infiltrate $\frac{1}{2}$ of the dose locally around the wound; give the remainder I.M.)
Dosage Forms Injection: 150 units/mL (2 mL, 10 mL)

rabies virus vaccine, human diploid
Brand Names Imovax® Rabies I.D. Vaccine; Imovax® Rabies Vaccine
Synonyms HDCV; HDRS
Therapeutic Category Vaccine, Inactivated Virus
Use Pre-exposure rabies immunization for high risk persons; postexposure antirabies immunization along with local treatment and immune globulin
Usual Dosage
Pre-exposure prophylaxis: Two 1 mL doses I.M. or I.D. 1 week apart, third dose 3 weeks after second. If exposure continues, booster doses can be given every 2 years, or an antibody titer determined and a booster dose given if the titer is inadequate.

Postexposure prophylaxis: All postexposure treatment should begin with immediate cleansing of the wound with soap and water. Persons not previously immunized as above: Rabies immune globulin 20 units/kg body weight, half infiltrated at bite site if possible, remainder I.M.; and 5 doses of rabies vaccine, 1 mL I.M., one each on days 0, 3, 7, 14, 28.

Persons who have previously received postexposure prophylaxis with rabies vaccine, received a recommended I.M. or I.D. pre-exposure series of rabies vaccine or have a previously documented rabies antibody titer considered adequate: Two doses of rabies vaccine, 1 mL I.M., one each on days 0 and 3
Dosage Forms Injection:
I.M. (HDCV): Rabies antigen 2.5 units/mL (1 mL)
Intradermal: Rabies antigen 0.25 units/mL (1 mL)

racemic amphetamine sulfate *see* amphetamine sulfate *on page 24*

racemic epinephrine *see* epinephrine *on page 171*

Racet® Topical *see* clioquinol and hydrocortisone *on page 106*

radiological/contrast media (ionic)
Brand Names Anatrast®; Angio Conray®; Angiovist®; Baricon®; Barobag®; Baro-CAT®; Baroflave®; Barosperse®; Bar-Test®; Bilopaque®; Cholebrine®; Cholografin® Meglumine; Conray®; Cystografin®; Dionosil Oily®; Enecat®; Entrobar®; Epi-C®; Ethiodol®; Flo-Coat®; Gastrografin®; HD 85®; HD 200 Plus®; Hexabrix™; Hypaque-Cysto®; Hypaque® Meglumine; Hypaque® Sodium; Liquid Barosperse®; Liquipake®; Lymphazurin®; Magnevist®; MD-Gastroview®; Oragrafin® Calcium; Oragrafin® Sodium; Perchloracap®; Prepcat®; Reno-M-30®; Reno-M-60®; Reno-M-Dip®; Renovue®-65; Renovue®-DIP; Sinografin®; Telepaque®; Tomocat®; Tonopaque®; Urovist Cysto®; Urovist® Meglumine; Urovist® Sodium 300; Vascoray®
Synonyms barium sulfate; diatrizoate meglumine; diatrizoate meglumine and diatrizoate sodium; diatrizoate meglumine and iodipamide meglumine; diatrizoate sodium; ethiodized
(Continued)

radiological/contrast media (ionic) *(Continued)*

oil; gadopentetate dimeglumine; iocetamic acid; iodamide meglumine; iodipamide meglumine; iopanoic acid; iothalamate meglumine and iothalamate sodium; iothalamate sodium; ipodate calcium; ipodate sodium; isosulfan blue; potassium perchlorate; propyliodone; tyropanoate sodium

Dosage Forms

Oral cholecystographic agents:

Iocetamic Acid
Tablet (Cholebrine®): 750 mg

Iopanoic Acid
Tablet (Telepaque®): 500 mg

Ipodate Calcium
Granules for oral suspension (Oragrafin® Calcium): 3 g

Ipodate Sodium
Capsule (Bilivist®, Oragrafin® Sodium): 500 mg

Tyropanoate Sodium
Capsule (Bilopaque®): 750 mg

GI Contrast Agents: **Barium Sulfate**
Paste (Anatrast®): 100% (500 g)
Powder:
Baroflave®: 100%
Baricon®, HD 200 Plus®: 98%
Barosperse®, Tonopaque®: 95%
Suspension:
Baro-CAT®, Prepcat®: 1.5%
Enecat®, Tomocat®: 5%
Entrobar®: 50%
Liquid Barasperse®: 60%
HD 85®: 85%
Barobag®: 97%
Flo-Coat®, Liquipake®: 100%
Epi-C®: 150%
Tablet (Bar-Test®): 650 mg

Parenteral agents: Injection:

Diatrizoate meglumine:
Hypaque® Meglumine
Reno-M-DIP®
Urovist® Meglumine
Angiovist® 282
Hypaque® Meglumine
Reno-M-60®

Diatrizoate sodium:
Hypaque® Sodium
Hypaque® Sodium
Urovist® Sodium 300

Gadopentetate dimeglumine:
Magnevist®

Iodamide meglumine:
Renovue®-DIP
Renovue®-65

Iodipamide meglumine:
Cholografin® Meglumine

Iothalamate meglumine:
Conray® 30
Conray® 43
Conray®

Iothalamate sodium
Angio Conray®
Conray® 325

ALPHABETICAL LISTING OF DRUGS

Conray® 400
Diatrizoate meglumine and diatrizoate sodium
Angiovist® 292
Angiovist® 370
Hypaque-76®
Hypaque-M®, 75%
Hypaque-M®, 90%
MD-60®
MD-76®
Renografin-60®
Renografin-76®
Renovist® II
Renovist®
Iothalamate meglumine and iothalamate sodium:
Vascoray®
Hexabrix™
Miscellaneous agents: (**NOT** for intravascular use, for instillation into various cavities)
Diatrizoate meglumine:
Urogenital solution, sterile:
Crystografin®
Crystografin® Dilute
Hypaque-Cysto®
Reno-M-30®
Urovist Cysto®
Diatrizoate meglumine and diatrizoate sodium
Solution, Oral or Rectal:
Gastrografin®
MD-Gastroview®
Diatrizoate sodium:
Solution, oral or rectal (Hypaque® Sodium Oral)
Solution, urogenital (Hypaque® Sodium 20%)
Iothalamate meglumine:
Solution, urogenital:
Cysto-Conray®
Cysto-Conray® II
Diatrizoate meglumine and iodipamide meglumine
Injection, urogenital for intrauterine instillation (Sinografin®)
Ethiodized oil
Injection (Ethiodol®)
Propyliodone
Suspension (Dionosil Oily®)
Isosulfan blue
Injection (Lymphazurin® 1%)
Potassium perchlorate
Capsule (Perchloracap®): 200 mg

radiological/contrast media (non-ionic)
Brand Names Amnipaque®; Isovue®; Omnipaque®; Optiray®
Synonyms iohexol; iopamidol; ioversol; metrizamide
Dosage Forms
Parenteral Agents: Injection:
Iohexol: Omnipaque®: 140 mg/mL; 180 mg/mL; 210 mg/mL; 240 mg/mL; 300 mg/mL; 350 mg/mL
Iopamidol
Isovue-128®
Isovue-200®
Isovue-M 200®
Isovue-300®
(Continued)   415

radiological/contrast media (non-ionic) *(Continued)*
Isovue-M 300®
Isovue-370®
Ioversol
Optiray® 160
Optiray® 240
Optiray® 320
Metrizamide
Amnipaque®

ramipril (ra mi' prill)
Brand Names Altace™ Oral
Therapeutic Category Angiotensin Converting Enzyme (ACE) Inhibitors
Use Treatment of hypertension, alone or in combination with thiazide diuretics
Usual Dosage Adults: Oral: 2.5-5 mg once daily
Dosage Forms Capsule: 1.25 mg, 2.5 mg, 5 mg, 10 mg

RAMP® Urine hCG *see* diagnostic aids (*in vitro*), urine *on page 139*

Ramses® [OTC] *see* nonoxynol 9 *on page 338*

ranitidine hydrochloride (ra nye' te deen)
Brand Names Zantac® Injection; Zantac® Oral
Therapeutic Category Histamine-2 Antagonist
Use Short-term treatment of active duodenal ulcers and benign gastric ulcers; long-term prophylaxis of duodenal ulcer and gastric hypersecretory states, gastroesophageal reflux, recurrent postoperative ulcer, upper GI bleeding, prevention of acid-aspiration pneumonitis during surgery, and prevention of stress-induced ulcers
Usual Dosage
Children:
Oral: 1.5-2 mg/kg/dose every 12 hours
I.M., I.V.: 0.75-1.5 mg/kg/dose every 6-8 hours, maximum daily dose: 400 mg
Continuous infusion: 0.1-0.25 mg/kg/hour (preferred for stress ulcer prophylaxis in patients with concurrent maintenance I.V.s or TPNs)
Adults:
Short-term treatment of ulceration: 150 mg/dose twice daily or 300 mg at bedtime
Prophylaxis of recurrent duodenal ulcer: 150 mg at bedtime
Gastric hypersecretory conditions: Oral: 150 mg twice daily, up to 6 g/day
I.M., I.V.: 50 mg/dose every 6-8 hours (dose not to exceed 400 mg/day)
Dosage Forms
Infusion, preservative free, in NaCl 0.45%: 0.5 mg/mL (100 mL)
Injection: 25 mg/mL (2 mL, 10 mL, 40 mL)
Syrup (peppermint flavor): 15 mg/mL (473 mL)
Tablet: 150 mg, 300 mg

RapidTest® Strep *see* diagnostic aids (*in vitro*), other *on page 138*

Raudixin® *see* rauwolfia serpentina *on this page*

Rauverid® *see* rauwolfia serpentina *on this page*

rauwolfia serpentina (rah wool' fee a)
Brand Names Raudixin®; Rauverid®; Wolfina®
Synonyms whole root rauwolfia
Therapeutic Category Antihypertensive; Rauwolfia Alkaloid
Use Mild essential hypertension; relief of agitated psychotic states
Usual Dosage Adults: Oral: 200-400 mg/day in 2 divided doses
Dosage Forms Tablet: 50 mg, 100 mg

rauwolfia serpentina and bendroflumethiazide
Brand Names Rauzide®
Therapeutic Category Antihypertensive, Combination
Use Mild essential hypertension
Usual Dosage Dose is individualized
Dosage Forms Tablet: Rauwolfia serpentina 50 mg and bendroflumethiazide 4 mg

Rauzide® *see* rauwolfia serpentina and bendroflumethiazide *on this page*

Rea-Lo® [OTC] *see* urea *on page 487*

Recombigen® HIV-1 LA *see* diagnostic aids (*in vitro*), blood *on page 137*

recombinant human deoxyribonuclease I *see* dornase alfa *on page 159*

Recombivax HB® *see* hepatitis b vaccine *on page 228*

Redisol® *see* cyanocobalamin *on page 120*

Redutemp® [OTC] *see* acetaminophen *on page 2*

Reese's® Pinworm Medicine [OTC] *see* pyrantel pamoate *on page 407*

Regitine® *see* phentolamine mesylate *on page 371*

Reglan® *see* metoclopramide *on page 308*

Regonol® Injection *see* pyridostigmine bromide *on page 408*

Regulace® [OTC] *see* docusate and casanthranol *on page 158*

Regular [Concentrated] Iletin® II U-500 *see* insulin preparations *on page 250*

Regular Iletin® I *see* insulin preparations *on page 250*

Regulax SS® [OTC] *see* docusate *on page 157*

Reguloid® [OTC] *see* psyllium *on page 407*

Regutol® [OTC] *see* docusate *on page 157*

Rela® *see* carisoprodol *on page 76*

Relafen® *see* nabumetone *on page 321*

Relaxadon® *see* hyoscyamine, atropine, scopolamine, and phenobarbital *on page 242*

Relefact® TRH Injection *see* protirelin *on page 405*

Relief® Ophthalmic Solution *see* phenylephrine hydrochloride *on page 372*

Remular-S® *see* chlorzoxazone *on page 99*

Renacidin® *see* citric acid bladder mixture *on page 103*

Renese® *see* polythiazide *on page 385*

Reno-M-30® *see* radiological/contrast media (ionic) *on page 413*

Reno-M-60® *see* radiological/contrast media (ionic) *on page 413*

Reno-M-Dip® *see* radiological/contrast media (ionic) *on page 413*

Renoquid® *see* sulfacytine *on page 447*

Renovue®-65 *see* radiological/contrast media (ionic) *on page 413*

Renovue®-DIP *see* radiological/contrast media (ionic) *on page 413*

Rentamine® *see* chlorpheniramine, ephedrine, phenylephrine, and carbetapentane *on page 94*

Repan *see* butalbital compound *on page 63*

Reposans-10® Oral *see* chlordiazepoxide *on page 89*

Rep-Pred® Injection *see* methylprednisolone *on page 306*

Resaid® *see* chlorpheniramine and phenylpropanolamine *on page 93*

Rescaps-D® S.R. Capsule *see* caramiphen and phenylpropanolamine *on page 72*

Rescon *see* chlorpheniramine and pseudoephedrine *on page 94*

Rescon-ED® *see* chlorpheniramine and pseudoephedrine *on page 94*

Rescon Jr *see* chlorpheniramine and pseudoephedrine *on page 94*

Rescon Liquid [OTC] *see* chlorpheniramine and phenylpropanolamine *on page 93*

Resectisol® Irrigation Solution *see* mannitol *on page 285*

reserpine (re ser' peen)
    Brand Names Serpalan®; Serpasil®
    Therapeutic Category Rauwolfia Alkaloid
    Use Management of mild to moderate hypertension
    Usual Dosage Adults: Oral: 0.1-0.5 mg/day in 1-2 doses
    Dosage Forms Tablet: 0.1 mg, 0.25 mg, 1 mg

reserpine and chlorothiazide *see* chlorothiazide and reserpine *on page 92*

reserpine and hydrochlorothiazide *see* hydrochlorothiazide and reserpine *on page 233*

Respaire®-60 SR *see* guaifenesin and pseudoephedrine *on page 220*

Respaire®-120 SR *see* guaifenesin and pseudoephedrine *on page 220*

Respbid® *see* theophylline *on page 460*

Respinol-G® *see* guaifenesin, phenylpropanolamine, and phenylephrine *on page 221*

Respiracult-Strep® *see* diagnostic aids (*in vitro*), other *on page 138*

Respiralex® *see* diagnostic aids (*in vitro*), other *on page 138*

Resporal® [OTC] *see* dexbrompheniramine and pseudoephedrine *on page 134*

Restoril® *see* temazepam *on page 453*

Retin-A™ Topical *see* tretinoin *on page 474*

retinoic acid *see* tretinoin *on page 474*

Retrovir® Injection *see* zidovudine *on page 503*

Retrovir® Oral *see* zidovudine *on page 503*

Reversol® Injection *see* edrophonium chloride *on page 167*

Rev-Eyes™ *see* dapiprazole hydrochloride *on page 126*

R-Gen® *see* iodinated glycerol *on page 253*

R-Gene® 10 *see* arginine hydrochloride *on page 32*

RGM-CSF *see* sargramostim *on page 426*

Rheaban® [OTC] *see* attapulgite *on page 38*

Rheomacrodex® *see* dextran *on page 135*

Rhesonativ® *see* Rh$_o$(D) immune globulin *on next page*

Rheumanosticon® Dri-Dot® *see* diagnostic aids (*in vitro*), blood *on page 137*

Rheumatrex® Oral *see* methotrexate *on page 301*

Rhinall® Nasal Solution [OTC] *see* phenylephrine hydrochloride *on page 372*

Rhindecon® *see* phenylpropanolamine hydrochloride *on page 373*

Rhinolar-EX® 12 *see* chlorpheniramine and phenylpropanolamine *on page 93*

Rhinosyn-DMX® [OTC] *see* guaifenesin and dextromethorphan *on page 218*

Rh$_o$(D) immune globulin

Brand Names HypRho®-D; HypRho®-D Mini-Dose; MICRhoGAM™; Mini-Gamulin® Rh; Rhesonativ®; RhoGAM™

Therapeutic Category Immune Globulin

Use To prevent isoimmunization in Rh-negative individuals exposed to Rh-positive blood during delivery of an Rh-positive infant, as a result of an abortion, following amniocentesis or abdominal trauma, or following a transfusion accident; to prevent hemolytic disease of the newborn if there is a subsequent pregnancy with an Rh-positive fetus

Usual Dosage Adults: I.M.:

Obstetrical usage: 1 vial (300 μg) prevents maternal sensitization if fetal packed red blood cell volume that has entered the circulation is <15 mL; if it is more, give additional vials. The number of vials = RBC volume of the calculated fetomaternal hemorrhage divided by 15 mL

Postpartum prophylaxis: 300 μg within 72 hours of delivery

Antepartum prophylaxis: 300 μg at approximately 26-28 weeks gestation; followed by 300 μg within 72 hours of delivery if infant is Rh-positive

Following miscarriage, abortion, or termination of ectopic pregnancy at up to 13 weeks of gestation: 50 μg ideally within 3 hours, but may be given up to 72 hours after; if pregnancy has been terminated at 13 or more weeks of gestation, administer 300 μg

Dosage Forms

Injection: Each package contains one single dose 300 μg of Rh$_o$ (D) immune globulin

Injection, microdose: Each package contains one single dose of microdose, 50 μg of Rh$_o$ (D) immune globulin

RhoGAM™ *see* Rh$_o$(D) immune globulin *on this page*
rHuEPO-α *see* epoetin alfa *on page 172*
Rhulicaine® [OTC] *see* benzocaine *on page 48*

ribavirin (rye ba vye' rin)

Brand Names Virazole® Aerosol

Synonyms RTCA; tribavirin

Therapeutic Category Antiviral Agent, Inhalation Therapy

Use Treatment of patients with respiratory syncytial virus (RSV) infections; may also be used in other viral infections including influenza A and B and adenovirus; specially indicated for treatment of severe lower respiratory tract RSV infections in patients with an underlying compromising condition (prematurity, bronchopulmonary dysplasia, congenital heart disease, immunodeficiency, and immunosuppression)

Usual Dosage Infants, Children, and Adults: Aerosol inhalation:

Use with Viratek® small particle aerosol generator (SPAG-2) at a concentration of 20 mg/mL (6 g reconstituted with 300 mL of sterile water without preservatives)

Aerosol only: 12-18 hours/day for 3 days, up to 7 days in length

Dosage Forms Powder for aerosol: 6 g (100 mL)

riboflavin (rye' boe flay vin)

Brand Names Riobin®

Synonyms lactoflavin; vitamin B$_2$; vitamin G

Therapeutic Category Vitamin, Water Soluble

Use Prevent riboflavin deficiency and treat ariboflavinosis; dietary sources include liver, kidney, dairy products, green vegetables, eggs, whole grain cereals, yeast, mushrooms

Usual Dosage Oral:

Riboflavin deficiency:
Children: 2.5-10 mg/day in divided doses
Adults: 5-30 mg/day in divided doses

Required daily allowance: Adults:
Male: 1.4-4.8 mg
Female: 1.2-1.3 mg

Dosage Forms Tablet: 25 mg, 50 mg, 100 mg

RID® [OTC] *see* pyrethrins *on page 408*
Rid-A-Pain® [OTC] *see* benzocaine *on page 48*
Ridaura® *see* auranofin *on page 39*

rifabutin (rif a bu' tin)
Brand Names Mycobutin® Oral
Synonyms ansamycin
Therapeutic Category Antibiotic, Miscellaneous; Antitubercular Agent
Use Prevention of disseminated *Mycobacterium avium* complex (MAC) in patients with advanced HIV infection
Usual Dosage Oral:
   Children: Efficacy and safety of rifabutin have not been established in children; a limited number of HIV-positive children with MAC (n=22) have been given rifabutin for MAC prophylaxis; doses of 5 mg/kg/day have been useful

   Adults: 300 mg once daily; for patients who experience gastrointestinal upset, rifabutin can be administered 150 mg twice daily with food
Dosage Forms Capsule: 150 mg

Rifadin® Injection *see* rifampin *on this page*
Rifadin® Oral *see* rifampin *on this page*
rifampicin *see* rifampin *on this page*

rifampin (rif' am pin)
Brand Names Rifadin® Injection; Rifadin® Oral; Rimactane® Oral
Synonyms rifampicin
Therapeutic Category Antibiotic, Miscellaneous; Antitubercular Agent
Use Management of active tuberculosis; eliminate meningococci from asymptomatic carriers; prophylaxis of *Haemophilus influenzae* type B infection
Usual Dosage I.V. infusion dose is the same as for the oral route
   Tuberculosis: Oral:
      Children: 10-20 mg/kg/day in divided doses every 12-24 hours
      Adults: 10 mg/kg/day; maximum: 600 mg/day

   American Thoracic Society and CDC currently recommend twice weekly therapy as part of a short-course regimen which follows 1-2 months of daily treatment of uncomplicated pulmonary tuberculosis in the compliant patient
      Children: 10-20 mg/kg/dose (up to 600 mg) twice weekly under supervision to ensure compliance
      Adults: 10 mg/kg (up to 600 mg) twice weekly

   H. influenza prophylaxis:
      Infants and Children: 20 mg/kg/day every 24 hours for 4 days
      Adults: 600 mg every 24 hours for 4 days

   Meningococcal prophylaxis:
      <1 month: 10 mg/kg/day in divided doses every 12 hours
      Infants and Children: 20 mg/kg/day in divided doses every 12 hours for 2 days
      Adults: 600 mg every 12 hours for 2 days

   Nasal carriers of *Staphylococcus aureus*: Adults: 600 mg/day for 5-10 days in combination with other antibiotics
Dosage Forms
   Capsule: 150 mg, 300 mg
   Powder for injection: 600 mg (contains a sulfite)

rIFN-A *see* interferon alfa-2a *on page 252*
RIG *see* rabies immune globulin, human *on page 413*

Rimactane® Oral *see* rifampin *on previous page*

rimantadine hydrochloride (ri man' to deen)
Brand Names Flumadine® Oral
Therapeutic Category Antiviral Agent, Oral
Use Prophylaxis (adults and children) and treatment (adults) of influenza A viral infection
Usual Dosage Oral:
Prophylaxis:
Children (<10 years of age): 5 mg/kg give once daily
Children (>10 years of age) and Adults: 100 mg twice/day

Treatment:
Adults: 100 mg twice/day
Dosage Forms
Syrup: 50 mg/5 mL (60 mL, 240 mL, 480 mL)
Tablet: 100 mg

Rimso®-50 *see* dimethyl sulfoxide *on page 151*
Riobin® *see* riboflavin *on page 419*
Riopan® [OTC] *see* magaldrate *on page 281*
Riopan Plus® [OTC] *see* magaldrate and simethicone *on page 281*
Risperdal® Oral *see* risperidone *on this page*

risperidone (ris per' i done)
Brand Names Risperdal® Oral
Therapeutic Category Antipsychotic Agent
Use Management of psychotic disorders (eg, schizophrenia)
Usual Dosage
Recommended starting dose: 1 mg twice daily; slowly increase to the optimum range of 4-8 mg/day; daily dosages >10 mg does not appear to confer any additional benefit, and the incidence of extrapyramidal reactions is higher than with lower doses

Dosing adjustment in renal, hepatic impairment, and elderly: Starting dose of 0.5 mg twice daily is advisable
Dosage Forms Tablet: 1 mg, 2 mg, 3 mg, 4 mg

Ritalin® *see* methylphenidate hydrochloride *on page 305*
Ritalin-SR® *see* methylphenidate hydrochloride *on page 305*

ritodrine hydrochloride (ri' toe dreen)
Brand Names Yutopar® Oral
Therapeutic Category Adrenergic Agonist Agent; Beta-2-Adrenergic Agonist Agent; Tocolytic Agent
Use Inhibit uterine contraction in preterm labor
Usual Dosage Adults:
Oral: Start 30 minutes before stopping I.V. infusion; 10 mg every 2 hours for 24 hours, then 10-20 mg every 4-6 hours up to 120 mg/day. Continue treatment as long as it is desirable to prolong pregnancy.
I.V.: 50-100 µg/minute; increase by 50 µg/minute every 10 minutes; continue for 12 hours after contractions have stopped
Dosage Forms
Injection: 10 mg/mL (5 mL); 15 mg/mL (10 mL)
Tablet: 10 mg

rLFN-α2 *see* interferon alfa-2b *on page 252*

rIFN-b *see* interferon beta-1b *on page 253*

RMS® Rectal *see* morphine sulfate *on page 318*

Robafen® CF [OTC] *see* guaifenesin, phenylpropanolamine, and dextromethorphan *on page 220*

Robaxin® *see* methocarbamol *on page 300*

Robaxisal® *see* methocarbamol and aspirin *on page 301*

Robicillin® VK Oral *see* penicillin V potassium *on page 362*

Robinul® *see* glycopyrrolate *on page 214*

Robinul® Forte *see* glycopyrrolate *on page 214*

Robitet® Oral *see* tetracycline *on page 458*

Robitussin® [OTC] *see* guaifenesin *on page 217*

Robitussin® A-C *see* guaifenesin and codeine *on page 218*

Robitussin-CF® [OTC] *see* guaifenesin, phenylpropanolamine, and dextromethorphan *on page 220*

Robitussin® Cough Calmers [OTC] *see* dextromethorphan hydrobromide *on page 136*

Robitussin®-DAC *see* guaifenesin, pseudoephedrine, and codeine *on page 221*

Robitussin®-DM [OTC] *see* guaifenesin and dextromethorphan *on page 218*

Robitussin-PE® [OTC] *see* guaifenesin and pseudoephedrine *on page 220*

Robitussin® Pediatric [OTC] *see* dextromethorphan hydrobromide *on page 136*

Robomol® *see* methocarbamol *on page 300*

Rocaltrol® *see* calcitriol *on page 65*

Rocephin® *see* ceftriaxone sodium *on page 82*

rocky mountain spotted fever vaccine
Therapeutic Category Vaccine, Live Bacteria
Dosage Forms Injection: 3 mL

Roferon-A® *see* interferon alfa-2a *on page 252*

Rogaine® Topical *see* minoxidil *on page 314*

Rolaids® [OTC] *see* dihydroxyaluminum sodium carbonate *on page 149*

Rolaids® Calcium Rich [OTC] *see* calcium carbonate *on page 65*

Romazicon™ Injection *see* flumazenil *on page 199*

Ronase® *see* tolazamide *on page 470*

Rondamine-DM® Drops *see* carbinoxamine, pseudoephedrine, and dextromethorphan *on page 74*

Rondec®-DM *see* carbinoxamine, pseudoephedrine, and dextromethorphan *on page 74*

Rondec® Drops *see* carbinoxamine and pseudoephedrine *on page 74*

Rondec® Filmtab® *see* carbinoxamine and pseudoephedrine *on page 74*

Rondec® Syrup *see* carbinoxamine and pseudoephedrine *on page 74*

Rondec-TR® *see* carbinoxamine and pseudoephedrine *on page 74*

Rotalex® *see* diagnostic aids (*in vitro*), feces *on page 138*

Rowasa® Rectal *see* mesalamine *on page 294*

Roxanol™ Oral *see* morphine sulfate *on page 318*

Roxanol SR™ Oral *see* morphine sulfate *on page 318*

Roxicet® 5/500 *see* oxycodone and acetaminophen *on page 349*

Roxicodone™ *see* oxycodone hydrochloride *on page 350*

Roxilox® *see* oxycodone and acetaminophen *on page 349*

Roxiprin® *see* oxycodone and aspirin *on page 350*

RTCA *see* ribavirin *on page 419*

Rubacell® II *see* diagnostic aids (*in vitro*), blood *on page 137*

Rubazyme® *see* diagnostic aids (*in vitro*), blood *on page 137*

rubella and measles vaccines, combined *see* measles and rubella vaccines, combined *on page 286*

rubella and mumps vaccines, combined
Brand Names Biavax®ᵢᵢ
Therapeutic Category Vaccine, Live Virus
Use Promote active immunity to rubella and mumps by inducing production of antibodies
Usual Dosage Children >12 months and Adults: 1 vial in outer aspect of the upper arm
Dosage Forms Injection (mixture of 2 viruses):
  1. Wistar RA 27/3 strain of rubella virus
  2. Jeryl Lynn (B level) mumps strain grown cell cultures of chick embryo

rubella, measles and mumps vaccines, combined *see* measles, mumps and rubella vaccines, combined *on page 287*

rubella virus vaccine, live
Brand Names Meruvax® II
Synonyms german measles vaccine
Therapeutic Category Vaccine, Live Virus
Use Provide vaccine-induced immunity to rubella
Usual Dosage S.C.: 1000 TCID$_{50}$ of rubella
Dosage Forms Injection, single dose: 1000 TCID$_{50}$ (Wistar RA 27/3 Strain)

rubeola vaccine *see* measles virus vaccine, live, attenuated *on page 287*

Rubex® *see* doxorubicin hydrochloride *on page 161*

rubidomycin hydrochloride *see* daunorubicin hydrochloride *on page 127*

Rubramin-PC® *see* cyanocobalamin *on page 120*

Rufen® *see* ibuprofen *on page 245*

Rum-K® *see* potassium chloride *on page 386*

Ru-Tuss® DE *see* guaifenesin and pseudoephedrine *on page 220*

Ru-Tuss II® *see* chlorpheniramine and phenylpropanolamine *on page 93*

Ru-Tuss® Liquid *see* chlorpheniramine and phenylephrine *on page 93*

Ru-Vert-M® *see* meclizine hydrochloride *on page 288*

Rymed® *see* guaifenesin and pseudoephedrine *on page 220*

Rymed-TR® *see* guaifenesin and phenylpropanolamine *on page 219*

Ryna-C® Liquid *see* chlorpheniramine, pseudoephedrine, and codeine *on page 97*

Ryna-CX® *see* guaifenesin, pseudoephedrine, and codeine *on page 221*

Rynatan® Pediatric Suspension *see* chlorpheniramine, pyrilamine, and phenylephrine *on page 97*

Rynatuss® Pediatric Suspension *see* chlorpheniramine, ephedrine, phenylephrine, and carbetapentane *on page 94*

Rythmol® *see* propafenone hydrochloride *on page 400*

S-2® Inhalation Solution [OTC] *see* epinephrine *on page 171*

Sabin *see* poliovirus vaccine, live, trivalent, oral *on page 382*

Salacid® Ointment *see* salicylic acid *on this page*

Sal-Acid® Plaster *see* salicylic acid *on this page*

salbutamol *see* albuterol *on page 10*

Saleto-200® [OTC] *see* ibuprofen *on page 245*

Saleto-400® *see* ibuprofen *on page 245*

Salflex® *see* salsalate *on next page*

Salgesic® *see* salsalate *on next page*

salicylazosulfapyridine *see* sulfasalazine *on page 448*

salicylic acid (sal i sil' ik)

Brand Names Clear Away® Disc [OTC]; Freezone® Solution [OTC]; Gordofilm® Liquid; Hydrisalic™ Gel; Lactisol® Liquid; Mediplast® Plaster [OTC]; Occlusal-HP Liquid; Panscol® Lotion [OTC]; Panscol® Ointment [OTC]; Paplex® Solution; Paplex® Ultra Solution; Pedia-Patch Transdermal Patch [OTC]; P&S® Shampoo [OTC]; Salacid® Ointment; Sal-Acid® Plaster; Trans-Plantar® Transdermal Patch [OTC]; Trans-Ver-Sal® Transdermal Patch [OTC] Verukan® Solution; Vergogel® Gel [OTC]

Therapeutic Category Keratolytic Agent

Use Topically for its keratolytic effect in controlling seborrheic dermatitis or psoriasis of body and scalp, dandruff, and other scaling dermatoses; also used to remove warts, corns and calluses

Usual Dosage
Shampoo: Apply to scalp and allow to remain for a few minutes, then rinse, initially use every day or every other day; 2 treatments/week are usually sufficient to maintain control

Topical: Apply to affected area and place under occlusion at night; hydrate skin for at least 5 minutes before use

Dosage Forms
Cream: 2% (30 g); 2.5% (30 g); 10% (60 g)
Disc: 40% in a rubber-based vehicle
Gel: 5% (60 g); 6% (30 g); 17% (7.5 g)
Liquid: 13.6% (9.3 mL); 17% (9.3 mL, 13.5 mL, 15 mL); 16.7% (15 mL)
Lotion: 2% (177 mL)
Ointment: 25% (60 g, 454 g); 40% (454 g); 60% (60 g)
Patch, transdermal: 15% (20 mm)
Plaster: 15% (6 mm, 12 mm); 40%
Pledgets: 0.5%; 2%
Shampoo: 2% (120 mL, 240 mL); 4% (120 mL)

salicylic acid and benzoic acid *see* benzoic acid and salicylic acid
on page 49

salicylic acid and lactic acid

Brand Names Duofilm® Solution

Synonyms lactic acid and salicylic acid

Therapeutic Category Keratolytic Agent

Use Treatment of benign epithelial tumors such as warts

Usual Dosage Topical: Apply a thin layer directly to wart once daily (may be useful to apply at bedtime and wash off in morning)

Dosage Forms Solution, topical: Salicylic acid 16.7% and lactic acid 16.7% in flexible collodion (15 mL)

salicylic acid and podophyllin *see* podophyllin and salicylic acid *on page 382*

salicylic acid and propylene glycol
Brand Names Keralyt® Gel
Synonyms propylene glycol and salicylic acid
Therapeutic Category Keratolytic Agent
Use Removal of excessive keratin in hyperkeratotic skin disorders, including various ichthyosis, keratosis palmaris and plantaris and psoriasis; may be used to remove excessive keratin in dorsal and plantar hyperkeratotic lesions
Usual Dosage Apply to area at night after soaking region for at least 5 minutes to hydrate area, and place under occlusion; medication is washed off in morning
Dosage Forms Gel, topical: Salicylic acid 6% and propylene glycol 60% in ethyl alcohol 19.4% with hydroxypropyl methylcellulose and water (30 g)

salicylic acid and sulfur *see* sulfur and salicylic acid *on page 450*

Salivart® [OTC] *see* saliva substitute *on this page*

saliva substitute
Brand Names Moi-Stir® [OTC]; Orex® [OTC]; Salivart® [OTC]; Xero-Lube® [OTC]
Therapeutic Category Gastrointestinal Agent, Miscellaneous
Use Relief of dry mouth and throat in xerostomia
Usual Dosage Use as needed
Dosage Forms
Solution: 60 mL, 75 mL, 120 mL, 180 mL
Swabstix: 300s

Salk *see* poliovirus vaccine, inactivated *on page 382*

salsalate (sal' sa late)
Brand Names Argesic®-SA; Artha-G®; Disalcid®; Marthritic®; Mono-Gesic®; Salflex®; Salgesic®; Salsitab®
Synonyms disalicylic acid
Therapeutic Category Analgesic, Non-Narcotic; Anti-inflammatory Agent; Antipyretic; Nonsteroidal Anti-Inflammatory Agent (NSAID), Oral; Salicylate
Use Treatment of minor pain or fever; rheumatoid arthritis, osteoarthritis, and related inflammatory conditions
Usual Dosage Adults: Oral: 1 g 2-4 times/day
Dosage Forms
Capsule: 500 mg
Tablet: 500 mg, 750 mg

Salsitab® *see* salsalate *on this page*

salt *see* sodium chloride *on page 434*

salt poor albumin *see* albumin human *on page 10*

Saluron® *see* hydroflumethiazide *on page 238*

Salutensin® *see* hydroflumethiazide and reserpine *on page 238*

Salutensin-Demi® *see* hydroflumethiazide and reserpine *on page 238*

Sandimmune® Injection *see* cyclosporine *on page 122*

Sandimmune® Oral *see* cyclosporine *on page 122*

Sandoglobulin® *see* immune globulin, intravenous *on page 247*

Sandostatin® *see* octreotide acetate *on page 342*

Sani-Supp® Suppository [OTC] *see* glycerin *on page 214*

Sansert® *see* methysergide maleate *on page 307*

Santyl® *see* collagenase *on page 114*

sargramostim (sar gram' oh stim)
Brand Names Leukine™; Prokine™
Synonyms GM-CSF; granulocyte-macrophage colony stimulating factor; RGM-CSF
Therapeutic Category Colony Stimulating Factor
Use Myeloid reconstitution after autologous bone marrow transplantation; to accelerate myeloid recovery in patients with non-Hodgkin's lymphoma, acute lymphoblastic leukemia, and Hodgkin's lymphoma undergoing autologous BMT; to accelerate myeloid engraftment following chemotherapy
Usual Dosage
Children and Adults (may also administer S.C.):
Bone marrow transplant: I.V.: 250 $\mu g/m^2$/day over at least 2 hours to begin 2-4 hours after the marrow infusion on day 0 of autologous bone marrow transplant or not <24 hours after chemotherapy or 12 hours after last dose of radiotherapy. If significant adverse effects or "first dose" reaction is seen at this dose, discontinue the drug until toxicity resolves, then restart at a reduced dose of 125 $\mu g/m^2$/day
Cancer chemotherapy recovery: I.V.: 3-15 $\mu g/kg$/day over at least 2 hours for 14-21 days; maximum daily dose is 15 $\mu g/kg$/day due to dose-related adverse effects
Discontinue therapy if the ANC count is >20,000/mm^3.

Excessive blood counts return to normal or baseline levels within 3-7 days following cessation of therapy.

Length of therapy: Bone marrow transplant patients: GM-CSF should be administered daily for up to 30 days or until the ANC has reached 1000/mm^3 for 3 consecutive days following the expected chemotherapy-induced neutrophil-nadir.
Dosage Forms Injection: 250 μg, 500 μg

Sarna [OTC] *see* camphor, menthol and phenol *on page 70*

Sastid® Plain Therapeutic Shampoo and Acne Wash [OTC] *see* sulfur and salicylic acid *on page 450*

Scabene® Lotion *see* lindane *on page 274*

Scabene® Shampoo *see* lindane *on page 274*

Scalpicin® Topical *see* hydrocortisone *on page 236*

Scleromate® *see* morrhuate sodium *on page 318*

scopolamine (skoe pol' a meen)
Brand Names Isopto® Hyoscine Ophthalmic; Transderm Scop® Patch
Synonyms hyoscine
Therapeutic Category Anticholinergic Agent; Anticholinergic Agent, Ophthalmic; Anticholinergic Agent, Transdermal; Ophthalmic Agent, Mydriatic
Use Preoperative medication to produce amnesia and decrease salivation and respiratory secretions to produce cycloplegia and mydriasis; treatment of iridocyclitis, prevention of nausea and vomiting by motion
Usual Dosage
Preoperatively:
Children: I.M., S.C.: 6 $\mu g/kg$/dose (maximum: 0.3 mg/dose) or 0.2 mg/m^2 may be repeated every 6-8 hours **or** alternatively:
4-7 months: 0.1 mg
7 months to 3 years: 0.15 mg
3-8 years: 0.2 mg
8-12 years: 0.3 mg

Adults: I.M., I.V., S.C.: 0.3-0.65 mg; may be repeated every 4-6 hours

Motion sickness: Transdermal: Children >12 years and Adults: Apply 1 disc behind the ear at least 4 hours prior to exposure and every 3 days as needed

Ophthalmic:
  Refraction:
    Children: Instill 1 drop of 0.25% to eye(s) twice daily for 2 days before procedure
    Adults: Instill 1-2 drops of 0.25% to eye(s) 1 hour before procedure
  Iridocyclitis:
    Children: Instill 1 drop of 0.25% to eye(s) up to 3 times/day
    Adults: Instill 1-2 drops of 0.25% to eye(s) up to 4 times/day

Dosage Forms
Disc, transdermal: 1.5 mg/disc (4s)
Injection, as hydrobromide: 0.3 mg/mL (1 mL); 0.4 mg/mL (0.5 mL, 1 mL); 0.86 mg/mL (0.5 mL); 1 mg/mL (1 mL)
Solution, ophthalmic, as hydrobromide: 0.25% (5 mL, 15 mL)

scopolamine and phenylephrine *see* phenylephrine and scopolamine *on page 372*

Scot-Tussin® [OTC] *see* guaifenesin *on page 217*

Scot-Tussin DM® Cough Chasers [OTC] *see* dextromethorphan hydrobromide *on page 136*

Sebulex® [OTC] *see* sulfur and salicylic acid *on page 450*

Sebulon® [OTC] *see* pyrithione zinc *on page 410*

secobarbital and amobarbital *see* amobarbital and secobarbital *on page 23*

secobarbital sodium (see koe bar' bi tal)
Brand Names Seconal™ Injection; Seconal™ Oral
Synonyms quinalbarbitone sodium
Therapeutic Category Barbiturate; Hypnotic; Sedative
Use Short-term treatment of insomnia and as preanesthetic agent
Usual Dosage
Children:
  Hypnotic: I.M.: 3-5 mg/kg/dose; maximum: 100 mg/dose
  Sedation: Oral: 6 mg/kg/day divided every 8 hours
Adults:
  Hypnotic:
    Oral, I.M.: 100-200 mg/dose
    I.V.: 50-250 mg/dose
  Sedation: Oral: 20-40 mg/dose 2-3 times/day or 200-300 mg/dose 2-3 hours before surgery
Dosage Forms
Capsule: 100 mg
Injection: 50 mg/mL (2 mL)
Injection, rectal: 50 mg/mL (20 mL)
Tablet: 100 mg

Seconal™ Injection *see* secobarbital sodium *on this page*

Seconal™ Oral *see* secobarbital sodium *on this page*

Secran® *see* vitamin, multiple (prenatal) *on page 499*

secretin (see' cre tin)
Brand Names Secretin-Ferring Injection
Therapeutic Category Diagnostic Agent, Pancreatic Exocrine Insufficiency; Diagnostic Agent, Zollinger-Ellison Syndrome and Pancreatic Exocrine Disease
(Continued)

secretin (Continued)

Use Diagnosis of Zollinger-Ellison syndrome and pancreatic exocrine disease, and some hepatobiliary disease such as obstructive jaundice

Usual Dosage I.V.:
Pancreatic function: 1 CU/kg slow I.V. injection over 1 minute
Zollinger-Ellison: 2 CU/kg slow I.V. injection over 1 minute

Dosage Forms Powder for injection: 75 CU (10 mL)

Secretin-Ferring Injection see secretin on previous page

Sectral® see acebutolol hydrochloride on page 2

Sedapap-10® see butalbital compound on page 63

Seldane® see terfenadine on page 455

Seldane-D® see terfenadine and pseudoephedrine on page 455

selegiline hydrochloride (seh ledge' ah leen)

Brand Names Eldepryl®

Synonyms deprenyl; L-deprenyl

Therapeutic Category Antiparkinson Agent

Use Adjunct in the management of Parkinsonian patients in which levodopa/carbidopa therapy is deteriorating. Unlabeled uses: Early Parkinson's disease; Alzheimer's disease

Usual Dosage Adults: Oral: 5 mg twice daily

Dosage Forms Tablet: 5 mg

selenium injection see trace metals on page 472

selenium sulfide (se lee' nee um)

Brand Names Exsel® Shampoo; Selsun Blue® Shampoo [OTC]; Selsun® Shampoo

Therapeutic Category Shampoos

Use Treat itching and flaking of the scalp associated with dandruff, to control scalp seborrheic dermatitis; treatment of tinea versicolor

Usual Dosage Topical:
Dandruff, seborrhea: Massage 5-10 mL into wet scalp, leave on scalp 2-3 minutes, rinse thoroughly and repeat application; shampoo twice weekly for 2 weeks initially, then use once every 1-4 weeks as indicated depending upon control

Tinea versicolor: Apply the 2.5% lotion to affected area and lather with small amounts of water; leave on skin for 10 minutes, then rinse thoroughly; apply every day for 7 days

Dosage Forms Shampoo: 1% (120 mL, 210 mL, 240 mL, 330 mL); 2.5% (120 mL)

Sele-Pak® see trace metals on page 472

Selepen® see trace metals on page 472

Selestoject® Injection see betamethasone on page 52

Selsun Blue® Shampoo [OTC] see selenium sulfide on this page

Selsun® Shampoo see selenium sulfide on this page

Semicid® [OTC] see nonoxynol 9 on page 338

Semilente see insulin preparations on page 250

Semilente® Iletin® I see insulin preparations on page 250

senna

Brand Names Black Draught® [OTC]; Senna-Gen® [OTC]; Senokot® [OTC]; Senolax® [OTC]; X-Prep® Liquid [OTC]

Therapeutic Category Laxative, Stimulant

Use Short-term treatment of constipation; evacuate the colon for bowel or rectal examinations
Usual Dosage
Children:
Oral:
>6 years: 10-20 mg/kg/dose at bedtime; maximum daily dose: 872 mg
6-12 years, >27 kg: 1 tablet at bedtime, up to 4 tablets/day **or** ½ teaspoonful of granules (326 mg/tsp) at bedtime (up to 2 teaspoonfuls/day)
Liquid:
2-5 years: 5-10 mL at bedtime
6-15 years: 10-15 mL at bedtime
Suppository: ½ at bedtime
Syrup:
1 month to 1 year: 1.25-2.5 mL at bedtime up to 5 mL/day
1-5 years: 2.5-5 mL at bedtime up to 10 mL/day
5-10 years: 5-10 mL at bedtime up to 20 mL/day
Adults:
Granules (326 mg/teaspoon): 1 teaspoonful at bedtime, not to exceed 2 teaspoonfuls twice daily
Liquid: 15-30 mL with meals and at bedtime
Suppository: 1 at bedtime, may repeat once in 2 hours
Syrup: 2-3 teaspoonfuls at bedtime, not to exceed 30 mL/day
Tablet: 187 mg: 2 tablets at bedtime, not to exceed 8 tablets/day
Tablet: 374 mg: 1 at bedtime, up to 4/day; 600 mg: 2 tablets at bedtime, up to 3 tablets/day
Dosage Forms
Granules: 326 mg/teaspoonful
Liquid: 7% [70 mg/mL] (130 mL, 360 mL); 6.5% [65 mg/mL] (75 mL, 150 mL)
Suppository, rectal: 652 mg
Syrup: 218 mg/5 mL (60 mL, 240 mL)
Tablet: 187 mg, 217 mg, 600 mg

Senna-Gen® [OTC] *see* senna *on previous page*
Senokot® [OTC] *see* senna *on previous page*
Senolax® [OTC] *see* senna *on previous page*
Sensorcaine® *see* bupivacaine hydrochloride *on page 61*
Septa® Topical Ointment [OTC] *see* bacitracin, neomycin, and polymyxin b *on page 43*
Septisol® *see* hexachlorophene *on page 228*
Septra® *see* co-trimoxazole *on page 118*
Septra® DS *see* co-trimoxazole *on page 118*
Ser-A-Gen® *see* hydralazine, hydrochlorothiazide, and reserpine *on page 232*
Ser-Ap-Es® *see* hydralazine, hydrochlorothiazide, and reserpine *on page 232*
Serathide® *see* hydralazine, hydrochlorothiazide, and reserpine *on page 232*
Serax® *see* oxazepam *on page 348*
Serentil® *see* mesoridazine besylate *on page 295*

sermorelin acetate (ser moe rel' in)
Brand Names Geref® Injection
Therapeutic Category Diagnostic Agent, Pituitary Function
Use Evaluate ability of the somatotroph of the pituitary gland to secrete growth hormone
Usual Dosage I.V.: In a single dose in the morning following an overnight fast:
Children or subjects <50 kg: Draw venous blood samples for GH determinations 15 minutes before and immediately prior to administration, then administer 1 μg/kg followed by a 3 mL normal saline flush, draw blood samples again for GH determinations
(Continued)

sermorelin acetate *(Continued)*

Adults or subjects >50 kg: Determine the number of ampules needed based on a dose of 1 µg/kg, draw venous blood samples for GH determinations 15 minutes before and immediately prior to administration, then administer 1 µg/kg followed by a 3 mL normal saline flush, draw blood samples again for GH determinations

Dosage Forms Powder for injection, lyophilized: 50 µg

Seromycin® Pulvules® *see* cycloserine *on page 122*

Serophene® *see* clomiphene citrate *on page 108*

Serpalan® *see* reserpine *on page 418*

Serpasil® *see* reserpine *on page 418*

sertraline hydrochloride (ser' tra leen)

Brand Names Zoloft™

Therapeutic Category Antidepressant; Serotonin Antagonist

Use Treatment of major depression; also being studied for use in obesity and obsessive-compulsive disorder

Usual Dosage Oral: Initial: 50 mg/day as a single dose, dosage may be increased at intervals of at least 1 week to a maximum recommended dosage of 200 mg/day

Dosage Forms Tablet: 50 mg, 100 mg

Serutan® [OTC] *see* psyllium *on page 407*

Shohl's solution *see* sodium citrate and citric acid *on page 435*

Shur-Seal® [OTC] *see* nonoxynol 9 *on page 338*

Siblin® [OTC] *see* psyllium *on page 407*

Sickledex™ *see* diagnostic aids (*in vitro*), blood *on page 137*

Silain® [OTC] *see* simethicone *on next page*

Silphen® Cough [OTC] *see* diphenhydramine hydrochloride *on page 152*

Silvadene® Topical *see* silver sulfadiazine *on next page*

silver nitrate

Brand Names Dey-Drop® Ophthalmic Solution

Synonyms AgNO$_3$

Therapeutic Category Topical Skin Product

Use Prevention of gonococcal ophthalmia neonatorum; cauterization of wounds and sluggish ulcers, removal of granulation tissue and warts; aseptic prophylaxis of burns

Usual Dosage

Neonates: Ophthalmic: Instill 2 drops immediately after birth into conjunctival sac of each eye as a single dose; do not irrigate eyes following instillation of eye drops

Children and Adults:

Sticks: Apply to mucous membranes and other moist skin surfaces only on area to be treated 2-3 times/week for 2-3 weeks

Topical solution: Apply a cotton applicator dipped in solution on the affected area 2-3 times/week for 2-3 weeks

Dosage Forms

Applicator, topical: 75% with potassium nitrate 25% (6")

Ointment, topical: 10% (30 g)

Solution:

Ophthalmic: 1% (wax ampuls)

Topical: 10% (30 mL); 25% (30 mL); 50% (30 mL)

silver protein, mild
Brand Names Argyrol® S.S. 10% [OTC]
Therapeutic Category Antibiotic, Topical
Use Stain and coagulate mucus in eye surgery which is then removed by irrigation; eye infections
Usual Dosage
Preop in eye surgery: Place 2-3 drops into eye(s), then rinse out with sterile irrigating solution

Eye infections: 1-3 drops into the affected eye(s) every 3-4 hours for several days
Dosage Forms Solution, ophthalmic: 10% (15 mL, 30 mL)

silver sulfadiazine (sul fa dye' a zeen)
Brand Names Silvadene® Topical; SSD® AF Topical; SSD® Cream; Thermazene® Topical
Therapeutic Category Antibacterial, Topical
Use Adjunct in the prevention and treatment of infection in second and third degree burns
Usual Dosage Children and Adults: Topical: Apply once or twice daily with a sterile gloved hand; apply to a thickness of $^1/_{16}$"; burned area should be covered with cream at all times
Dosage Forms Cream, topical: 1% [10 mg/g] (20 g, 50 g, 100 g, 400 g, 1000 g)

simethicone (sye meth' i kone)
Brand Names Flatulex [OTC]; Gas-X® [OTC]; Mylanta Gas® [OTC]; Mylicon® [OTC]; Phazyme® [OTC]; Silain® [OTC]
Synonyms activated dimethicone; activated methylpolysiloxane
Therapeutic Category Antiflatulent
Use Relieve flatulence and functional gastric bloating, and postoperative gas pains
Usual Dosage Oral:
Infants: 20 mg 4 times/day

Children <12 years: 40 mg 4 times/day

Children >12 years and Adults: 40-120 mg after meals and at bedtime as needed, not to exceed 500 mg/day
Dosage Forms
Capsule: 125 mg
Drops, oral: 40 mg/0.6 mL (30 mL)
Tablet: 50 mg, 60 mg, 95 mg
Tablet, chewable: 40 mg, 80 mg, 125 mg

simethicone and calcium carbonate *see* calcium carbonate and simethicone *on page 66*
simethicone and magaldrate *see* magaldrate and simethicone *on page 281*
Simron® [OTC] *see* ferrous gluconate *on page 194*

simvastatin (sim' va stat in)
Brand Names Zocor™
Therapeutic Category Antilipemic Agent; HMG-COA Reductase Inhibitor
Use Adjunct to dietary therapy to decrease elevated serum total and LDL cholesterol concentrations in primary hypercholesterolemia
Usual Dosage Adults: Oral: 20-40 mg once or twice daily
Dosage Forms Tablet: 5 mg, 10 mg, 20 mg, 40 mg

Sinarest® 12 Hour Nasal Solution *see* oxymetazoline hydrochloride *on page 350*
Sinarest® Nasal Solution [OTC] *see* phenylephrine hydrochloride *on page 372*

sincalide (sin' ka lide)
Brand Names Kinevac®
Synonyms C8-CCK; OP-CCK
Therapeutic Category Diagnostic Agent, Gallbladder Function
Use Postevacuation cholecystography; gallbladder bile sampling; stimulate pancreatic secretion for analysis
Usual Dosage Adults: I.V.:
Contraction of gallbladder: 0.02 µg/kg over 30 seconds to 1 minute, may repeat in 15 minutes a 0.04 µg/kg dose

Pancreatic function: 0.02 µg/kg over 30 minutes
Dosage Forms Injection: 5 µg

Sinemet® *see* levodopa and carbidopa *on page 270*

Sinequan® *see* doxepin hydrochloride *on page 160*

Sinografin® *see* radiological/contrast media (ionic) *on page 413*

Sinubid® *see* phenyltoloxamine, phenylpropanolamine, and acetaminophen *on page 374*

Sinufed® Timecelles® *see* guaifenesin and pseudoephedrine *on page 220*

Sinumist®-SR Capsulets® [OTC] *see* guaifenesin *on page 217*

Sinusol-B® Injection *see* brompheniramine maleate *on page 59*

Sinutab® [OTC] *see* acetaminophen, chlorpheniramine, and pseudoephedrine *on page 4*

sk *see* streptokinase *on page 443*

Skelaxin® *see* metaxalone *on page 297*

Skelex® *see* chlorzoxazone *on page 99*

skin test antigens, multiple
Brand Names Multitest CMI®
Therapeutic Category Diagnostic Agent, Skin Test
Use Detection of nonresponsiveness to antigens by means of delayed hypersensitivity skin testing
Usual Dosage Select only test sites that permit sufficient surface area and subcutaneous tissue to allow adequate penetration of all 8 points, avoid hairy areas

Press loaded unit into the skin with sufficient pressure to puncture the skin and allow adequate penetration of all points, maintain firm contact for at least five seconds, during application the device should not be "rocked" back and forth and side to side without removing any of the test heads from the skin sites
If adequate pressure is applied it will be possible to observe:
1. The puncture marks of the nine tines on each of the eight test heads
2. An imprint of the circular platform surrounding each test head
3. Residual antigen and glycerin at each of the eight sites
If any of the above three criteria are not fully followed, the test results may not be reliable
Reading should be done in good light, read the test sites at both 24 and 48 hours, the largest reaction recorded from the two readings at each test site should be used; if two readings are not possible, a single 48 hour is recommended
A positive reaction from any of the seven delayed hypersensitivity skin test antigens is **induration of ≥2 mm** providing there is no induration at the negative control site; the size of the induration reactions with this test may be smaller than those obtained with other intradermal procedures
Dosage Forms Individual carton containing one preloaded skin test antigen for cellular hypersensitivity

Sleep-eze 3® Oral [OTC] *see* diphenhydramine hydrochloride *on page 152*

Sleepinal® [OTC] *see* diphenhydramine hydrochloride *on page 152*

Slo-bid™ *see* theophylline *on page 460*

Slo-Niacin® [OTC] *see* niacin *on page 332*

Slo-Phyllin® *see* theophylline *on page 460*

Slo-Phyllin GG® *see* theophylline and guaifenesin *on page 461*

Slow FE® [OTC] *see* ferrous sulfate *on page 194*

Slow-K® *see* potassium chloride *on page 386*

Slow-Mag® [OTC] *see* magnesium chloride *on page 281*

SMX-TMP *see* co-trimoxazole *on page 118*

snake (pit vipers) antivenin *see* antivenin (crotalidae) polyvalent *on page 31*

Snaplets-EX® [OTC] *see* guaifenesin and phenylpropanolamine *on page 219*

Snaplets-FR® Granules [OTC] *see* acetaminophen *on page 2*

sodium 2-mercaptoethane sulfonate *see* mesna *on page 295*

sodium acetate
Therapeutic Category Alkalinizing Agent, Parenteral; Electrolyte Supplement, Parenteral; Sodium Salt
Use Sodium source in large volume I.V. fluids to prevent or correct hyponatremia in patients with restricted intake; used to counter acidosis
Usual Dosage Sodium acetate is metabolized to bicarbonate on an equimolar basis outside the liver; administer in large volume I.V. fluids as a sodium source. Refer to sodium bicarbonate monograph.

Maintenance electrolyte requirements of sodium in parenteral nutrition solutions:
Daily requirements: 3-4 mEq/kg/24 hours or 25-40 mEq/1000 kcal/24 hours
Maximum: 100-150 mEq/24 hours
Dosage Forms Injection: 2 mEq/mL (20 mL, 50 mL); 4 mEq/mL (50 mL)

sodium acid carbonate *see* sodium bicarbonate *on next page*

sodium ascorbate
Brand Names Cenolate®
Therapeutic Category Urinary Acidifying Agent; Vitamin, Water Soluble
Use Prevention and treatment of scurvy and to acidify the urine; large doses may decrease the severity of "colds"
Usual Dosage Oral, I.V.:
Children:
Scurvy: 100-300 mg/day in divided doses for at least 2 weeks
Urinary acidification: 500 mg every 6-8 hours
Dietary supplement: 35-45 mg/day

Adults:
Scurvy: 100-250 mg 1-2 times/day for at least 2 weeks
Urinary acidification: 4-12 g/day in divided doses
Dietary supplement: 50-60 mg/day
Prevention and treatment of cold: 1-3 g/day
Dosage Forms
Crystals: 1020 mg per $\frac{1}{4}$ teaspoonful [ascorbic acid 900 mg]
Injection: 250 mg/mL [ascorbic acid 222 mg/mL] (30 mL); 562.5 mg/mL [ascorbic acid 500 mg/mL] (1 mL, 2 mL)
Tablet: 585 mg [ascorbic acid 500 mg]

sodium bicarbonate

Brand Names Neut® Injection
Synonyms baking soda; NaHCO₃; sodium acid carbonate; sodium hydrogen carbonate
Therapeutic Category Alkalinizing Agent Oral; Alkalinizing Agent, Parenteral; Antacid; Electrolyte Supplement, Oral; Electrolyte Supplement, Parenteral; Sodium Salt
Use Management of metabolic acidosis; antacid; alkalinize urine; severe diarrhea
Usual Dosage

Cardiac arrest (patient should be adequately ventilated before administering $NaHCO_3$):
Infants: Use 1:1 dilution of 1 mEq/mL $NaHCO_3$ or use 0.5 mEq/mL $NaHCO_3$ at a dose of 1 mEq/kg slow IVP initially; may repeat with 0.5 mEq/kg in 10 minutes one time or as indicated by the patient's acid-base status. Rate of administration should not exceed 10 mEq/minute.
Children and Adults: IVP: 1 mEq/kg initially; may repeat with 0.5 mEq/kg in 10 minutes one time or as indicated by the patient's acid-base status

Metabolic acidosis: Dosage should be based on the following formula if blood gases and pH measurements are available:
Infants and Children: $HCO_3\text{-}(mEq) = 0.3 \times$ weight (kg) $\times$ base deficit (mEq/L) **or** $HCO_3\text{-}(mEq) = 0.5 \times$ weight (kg) $\times$ (24 - serum $HCO_3\text{-}$) (mEq/L)

Adults: $HCO_3\text{-}(mEq) = 0.2 \times$ weight (kg) $\times$ base deficit (mEq/L) **or** $HCO_3\text{-}(mEq) = 0.5 \times$ weight (kg) $\times$ (24 - serum $HCO_3\text{-}$) (mEq/L)
If acid-base status is not available: Dose for older Children and Adults: 2-5 mEq/kg I.V. infusion over 4-8 hours; subsequent doses should be based on patient's acid-base status

Chronic renal failure: Oral: Children: 1-3 mEq/kg/day

Renal tubular acidosis: Oral:
Distal:
Children: 2-3 mEq/kg/day
Adults: 1 mEq/kg/day
Proximal: Children: Initial: 5-10 mEq/kg/day; maintenance: Increase as required to maintain serum bicarbonate in the normal range

Urine alkalinization: Oral:
Children: 1-10 mEq (84-840 mg)/kg/day in divided doses; dose should be titrated to desired urinary pH
Adults: Initial: 48 mEq (4 g), then 12-24 mEq (1-2 g) every 4 hours; dose should be titrated to desired urinary pH; doses up to 16 g/day have been used

Dosage Forms

Injection: 4% [40 mg/mL = 2.4 mEq/5 mL] (5 mL); 4.2% [42 mg/mL = 5 mEq/10 mL] (10 mL); 7.5% [75 mg/mL = 8.92 mEq/10 mL] (10 mL, 50 mL); 8.4% [84 mg/mL = 10 mEq/10 mL] (10 mL, 50 mL)
Tablet: 300 mg [3.6 mEq]; 325 mg [3.8 mEq]; 520 mg [6.3 mEq]; 600 mg [7.3 mEq]; 650 mg [7.6 mEq]

sodium cellulose phosphate see cellulose sodium phosphate on page 83

sodium chloride

Brand Names Adsorbonac® Ophthalmic [OTC]; Ayr® Nasal [OTC]; Muro 128® Ophthalmic [OTC]; Ocean Nasal Mist [OTC]
Synonyms NaCl; normal saline; salt
Therapeutic Category Electrolyte Supplement, Oral; Electrolyte Supplement, Parenteral; Lubricant, Ocular; Sodium Salt
Use Prevention of muscle cramps and heat prostration; restoration of sodium ion in hyponatremia; induce abortion; restore moisture to nasal membranes; GU irrigant; reduction of corneal edema; source of electrolytes and water for expansion of the extracellular fluid compartment
Usual Dosage

Newborn electrolyte requirement:
Premature: 2-8 mEq/kg/24 hours

Term:
   0-48 hours: 0-2 mEq/kg/24 hours
   >48 hours: 1-4 mEq/kg/24 hours
Children: I.V.: Hypertonic solutions (>0.9%) should only be used for the initial treatment of acute serious symptomatic hyponatremia; maintenance: 3-4 mEq/kg/day; maximum: 100-150 mEq/day; dosage varies widely depending on clinical condition
   Replacement: Determined by laboratory determinations mEq
      Sodium deficiency (mEq/kg) = [% dehydration (L/kg)/100 x 70 (mEq/L) = [0.6 (L/kg) x (140 - serum sodium) (mEq/L)]
   Nasal: Use as often as needed
Adults:
   GI irrigant: 1-3 L/day by intermittent irrigation
   Heat cramps: Oral: 0.5-1 g with full glass of water, up to 4.8 g/day
   Replacement I.V.: Determined by laboratory determinations mEq
      Sodium deficiency (mEq/kg) = [% dehydration (L/kg)/100 x 70 (mEq/L)] + [0.6 (L/kg) x (140 - Serum sodium) (mEq/L)]

To correct acute, serious hyponatremia: mEq sodium = (desired sodium (mEq/L) - actual sodium (mEq/L) x 0.6 x wt (kg)); for acute correction use 125 mEq/L as the desired serum sodium; acutely correct serum sodium in 5 mEq/L/dose increments; more gradual correction in increments of 10 mEq/L/day is indicated in the asymptomatic patient
   Chloride maintenance electrolyte requirement in parenteral nutrition: 2-4 mEq/kg/24 hours or 25-40 mEq/1000 kcals/24 hours; maximum: 100-150 mEq/24 hours
   Sodium maintenance electrolyte requirement in parenteral nutrition: 3-4 mEq/kg/24 hours or 25-40 mEq/1000 kcals/24 hours; maximum: 100-150 mEq/24 hours.
   Nasal: Use as often as needed
   Ophthalmic:
      Ointment: Apply once daily or more often
      Solution: Instill 1-2 drops into affected eye(s) every 3-4 hours
   Abortifacient: 20% (250 mL) administered by transabdominal intra-amniotic instillation
Dosage Forms
Drops, nasal: 0.9% with dropper
Injection: 0.45% [4.5 mg/mL] (500 mL, 1000 mL); 0.9% [9 mg/mL] (10 mL, 20 mL, 50 mL, 100 mL, 150 mL, 250 mL, 500 mL, 1000 mL); 3% [30 mg/mL] (500 mL); 5% [50 mg/mL] (500 mL); 14.6% [146 mg/mL] , 20% [200 mg/mL] (250 mL); 23.4% [234 mg/mL] (30 mL, 100 mL)
Injection:
   Admixtures: 50 mEq, 100 mEq, 625 mEq
   Bacteriostatic: 0.9% [9 mg/mL] (30 mL)
Irrigation: 0.9% [9 mg/mL] (250 mL, 500 mL, 1000 mL, 3000 mL)
Ointment, ophthalmic (Muro 128®): 5% (3.5 g)
Solution:
   Nasal: 0.65% (45 mL)
   Ophthalmic (Adsorbonac®): 2% (15 mL); 5% (15 mL)
Tablet: 650 mg, 1 g
Tablet, enteric coated: 1 g

sodium citrate and citric acid
Brand Names Bicitra®; Oracit®
Synonyms modified Shohl's solution; Shohl's solution
Therapeutic Category Alkalinizing Agent Oral
Use Treatment of metabolic acidosis; alkalinizing agent in conditions where long-term maintenance of an alkaline urine is desirable
Usual Dosage Oral:
   Infants and Children: 2-3 mEq/kg/day in divided doses 3-4 times/day **or** 5-15 mL with water after meals and at bedtime
   Adults: 15-30 mL with water after meals and at bedtime
Dosage Forms Solution, oral:
   Bicitra®: Sodium citrate 500 mg and citric acid 334 mg per 5 mL (15 mL unit dose, 480 mL)

(Continued)

sodium citrate and citric acid *(Continued)*
Oracit®: Sodium citrate 490 mg and citric acid 640 mg per 5 mL
Polycitra®: Sodium citrate 500 mg and citric acid 334 mg with potassium citrate 550 mg per 5 mL

sodium citrate and potassium citrate mixture
Brand Names Polycitra®
Therapeutic Category Alkalinizing Agent Oral
Use Conditions where long-term maintenance of an alkaline urine is desirable as in control and dissolution of uric acid and cystine calculi of the urinary tract
Usual Dosage Oral:
Children: 5-15 mL diluted in water after meals and at bedtime
Adults: 15-30 mL diluted in water after meals and at bedtime
Dosage Forms Syrup: Sodium citrate 500 mg, potassium citrate 550 mg, with citric acid 334 mg per 5 mL [sodium 1 mEq, potassium 1 mEq, bicarbonate 2 mEq]

sodium edetate *see* edetate disodium *on page 167*

sodium ethacrynate *see* ethacrynic acid *on page 180*

sodium etidronate *see* etidronate disodium *on page 187*

sodium fluoride *see* fluoride *on page 201*

sodium hyaluronate (hye al yoor on' nate)
Brand Names Amvisc® Injection; Healon® Injection
Synonyms hyaluronic acid
Therapeutic Category Ophthalmic Agent, Viscoeleastic
Use Surgical aid in cataract extraction, intraocular implantation, corneal transplant, glaucoma filtration, and retinal attachment surgery
Usual Dosage Depends upon procedure (slowly introduce a sufficient quantity into eye)
Dosage Forms Injection, intraocular: 10 mg/mL (0.25 mL, 0.4 mL, 0.5 mL, 0.75 mL, 0.8 mL, 2 mL, 4 mL); 16 mg/mL (0.25 mL, 0.5 mL, 8 mL)

sodium hyaluronate-chrondroitin sulfate *see* chondroitin sulfate-sodium hyaluronate *on page 101*

sodium hydrogen carbonate *see* sodium bicarbonate *on page 434*

sodium hypochlorite solution (hye poe klor' ite)
Synonyms modified Dakin's solution
Therapeutic Category Disinfectant
Use Treatment of athlete's foot (0.5%); wound irrigation (0.5%); to disinfect utensils and equipment (5%)
Dosage Forms
Solution: 5% (4000 mL)
Solution (modified Dakin's solution):
Full strength: 0.5% (1000 mL)
Half strength: 0.25% (1000 mL)
Quarter strength: 0.125% (1000 mL)

sodium lactate
Synonyms 1/6 molar sodium lactate
Therapeutic Category Alkalinizing Agent, Parenteral
Use Source of bicarbonate for prevention and treatment of mild to moderate metabolic acidosis

Usual Dosage Dosage depends on degree of acidosis
Dosage Forms Injection:
1.87 g/100 mL [sodium 16.7 mEq and lactate 16.7 mEq per 100 mL] (1000 mL)
560 mg/mL [sodium 5 mEq sodium and lactate 5 mEq per mL] (10 mL)

sodium *L*-tri-iodothyronine *see* liothyronine sodium *on page 274*

sodium methicillin *see* methicillin sodium *on page 299*

sodium nafcillin *see* nafcillin sodium *on page 322*

sodium nitroferricyanide *see* nitroprusside sodium *on page 337*

sodium nitroprusside *see* nitroprusside sodium *on page 337*

sodium oxacillin *see* oxacillin sodium *on page 347*

Sodium P.A.S. *see* aminosalicylate sodium *on page 20*

sodium-PCA and lactic acid *see* lactic acid and sodium-PCA *on page 266*

sodium phenylacetate and sodium benzoate
Brand Names Ucephan® Oral
Therapeutic Category Hyperammonemia Agent
Use Adjunctive therapy to prevent/treat hyperammonemia in patients with urea cycle enzymopathy (UCE) involving partial or complete deficiencies of carbamoylphosphate synthetase, ornithine transcarbamylase or argininosuccinate synthetase
Usual Dosage Infants and Children: Oral: 2.5 mL (250 mg sodium benzoate and 250 mg sodium phenylacetate)/kg/day divided 3-6 times/day; total daily dose should not exceed 100 mL
Dosage Forms Solution: Sodium phenylacetate 100 mg and sodium benzoate 100 mg per mL (100 mL)

sodium phosphate
Brand Names Fleet® Enema [OTC]; Fleet® Phospho®-Soda [OTC]
Therapeutic Category Electrolyte Supplement, Parenteral; Laxative, Saline; Phosphate Salt; Sodium Salt
Use Source of phosphate in large volume I.V. fluids; short-term treatment of constipation and to evacuate the colon for rectal and bowel exams; source of sodium and phosphorus in parenteral nutrition
Usual Dosage
Normal requirements elemental phosphate: Oral:
0-6 months: 240 mg
6-12 months: 360 mg
1-10 years: 800 mg
>10 years: 1200 mg
Pregnancy lactation: Additional 400 mg/day

Treatment:
It is difficult to provide concrete guidelines for the treatment of severe hypophosphatemia because the extent of total body deficits and response to therapy are difficult to predict. Aggressive doses of phosphate may result in a transient serum elevation followed by redistribution into intracellular compartments or bone tissue. It is recommended that repletion of severe hypophosphatemia (<1 mg/dL in adults) be done I.V. because large doses of oral phosphate may cause diarrhea and intestinal absorption may be unreliable
Pediatric I.V. phosphate repletion:
Neonates: 0.5 mmol/kg/dose up to 1-2 mmol/kg/day
Children: 0.25-0.5 mmol/kg **administer over 4-6 hours and repeat if symptomatic hypophosphatemia persists**; to assess the need for further phosphate administration: obtain serum inorganic phosphate after administration of the first dose and base further doses on serum levels and clinical status

(Continued)

sodium phosphate *(Continued)*

Adult I.V. phosphate repletion:
Initial dose: 0.08 mmol/kg if recent uncomplicated hypophosphatemia
Initial dose: 0.16 mmol/kg if prolonged hypophosphatemia with presumed total body deficits; increase dose by 25% to 50% if patient symptomatic with severe hypophosphatemia
Severe hypophosphatemia:
High-dose = 0.36 mmol/kg over 6 hours; use if serum PO_4 <0.5 mg/dL
Adults: 0.15-0.3 mmol/kg/dose over 12 hours, may repeat as needed to achieve desired serum level

With orders for I.V. phosphate, there is considerable confusion associated with the use of millimoles (mmol) versus milliequivalents (mEq) to express the phosphate requirement. Because inorganic phosphate exists as monobasic and dibasic anions, with the mixture of valences is dependent on pH, ordering by mEq amounts is unreliable and may lead to large dosing errors. In addition, I.V. phosphate is available in the sodium and potassium salt; therefore, the content of these cations must be considered when ordering phosphate. The most reliable method of ordering I.V. phosphate is by millimoles, then specifying the potassium or sodium salt. For example, an order for 15 mmol of phosphate as potassium phosphate in one liter of normal saline would also provide 22 mEq of potassium.

Phosphate maintenance electrolyte requirement in parenteral nutrition: 2 mmol/kg/24 hours or 35 mmol/kcal/24 hours; Maximum: 15-30 mmol/24 hours

Maintenance:
Children: 0.5-1.5 mmol/kg/24 hours I.V. **or** 2-3 mmol/kg/24 hours orally in divided doses
Adults: 15-30 mmol/24 hours I.V. **or** 50-150 mmol/24 hours orally in divided doses

Laxative (Fleet®): Rectal:
Children 2-12 years: 67.5 mL ($^1/_2$ bottle) as a single dose, may repeat
Children ≥12 years and Adults: 133 mL enema as a single dose, may repeat

Laxative (Fleet® Phospho®-Soda): Oral:
Children:
5-9 years: 5 mL as a single dose
10-12 years: 10 mL as a single dose
Children ≥12 years and Adults: 20-30 mL as a single dose

Dosage Forms
Enema: Sodium phosphate 6 g and sodium biphosphate 16 g per 100 mL (135 mL adult enema unit, 67.5 mL pediatric enema unit)
Injection: Phosphate 3 mmol and sodium 4 mEq sodium per mL (15 mL)
Solution, oral: Sodium phosphate 18 g and sodium biphosphate 48 g per 100 mL (30 mL, 45 mL, 90 mL, 237 mL)

sodium phosphate and potassium phosphate *see* potassium phosphate and sodium phosphate *on page 388*

sodium polystyrene sulfonate (pol ee stye' reen)

Brand Names Kayexalate®; SPS®
Therapeutic Category Antidote, Hyperkalemia; Antidote, Potassium
Use Treatment of hyperkalemia
Usual Dosage
Children:
Oral: 1 g/kg/dose every 6 hours
Rectal: 1 g/kg/dose every 2-6 hours (In small children and infants employ lower doses by using the practical exchange ratio of 1 mEq potassium/g of resin as the basis for calculation)

Adults:
Oral: 15 g (60 mL) 1-4 times/day
Rectal: 30-50 g every 6 hours

Dosage Forms Oral or rectal:
Powder for suspension: 454 g
Suspension: 1.25 g/5 mL with sorbitol 33% and alcohol 0.3% (60 mL, 120 mL, 200 mL, 500 mL)

sodium salicylate
Brand Names Uracel®
Therapeutic Category Analgesic, Non-Narcotic
Use Treatment of minor pain or fever; arthritis
Usual Dosage Adults: Oral: 325-650 mg every 4 hours
Dosage Forms Tablet, enteric coated: 325 mg, 650 mg

Sodium Sulamyd® Ophthalmic *see* sodium sulfacetamide *on this page*

sodium sulfacetamide (sul fa see' ta mide)
Brand Names AK-Sulf® Ophthalmic; Bleph®-10 Ophthalmic; Cetamide® Ophthalmic; I-Sulfacet® Ophthalmic; Ophthacet® Ophthalmic; Sodium Sulamyd® Ophthalmic; Sulf-10® Ophthalmic; Sulfair® Ophthalmic
Synonyms sulfacetamide sodium
Therapeutic Category Antibiotic, Ophthalmic
Use Treatment and prophylaxis of conjunctivitis due to susceptible organisms; corneal ulcers; adjunctive treatment with systemic sulfonamides for therapy of trachoma
Usual Dosage Children >2 months and Adults: Ophthalmic:
Ointment: Apply to lower conjunctival sac 1-4 times/day and at bedtime
Solution: 1-2 drops every 2-3 hours in the lower conjunctival sac during the waking hours and less frequently at night
Dosage Forms Ophthalmic:
Ointment: 10% (3.5 g)
Solution: 10% (1 mL, 2 mL, 3.75 mL, 5 mL, 15 mL); 15% (2 mL, 15 mL); 30% (5 mL, 15 mL)

sodium sulfacetamide and phenylephrine
Brand Names Vasosulf® Ophthalmic
Therapeutic Category Antibiotic, Ophthalmic; Ophthalmic Agent, Vasoconstrictor
Usual Dosage Ophthalmic: Instill 1-3 drops in lower conjunctival sac every 3-4 hours
Dosage Forms Solution, ophthalmic: Sodium sulfacetamide 15% and phenylephrine hydrochloride 0.125% (5 mL, 15 mL)

sodium sulfacetamide and prednisolone
Brand Names Blephamide® Ophthalmic; Cetapred® Ophthalmic; Metimyd® Ophthalmic; Vasocidin® Ophthalmic
Synonyms prednisolone acetate and sodium sulfacetamide
Therapeutic Category Antibiotic, Ophthalmic; Corticosteroid, Ophthalmic
Use Steroid-responsive inflammatory ocular conditions where infection is present or there is a risk of infection; ophthalmic suspension may be used as an otic preparation
Usual Dosage Children >2 and Adults: Ophthalmic:
Ointment: Apply to lower conjunctival sac 1-4 times/day
Solution: Instill 1-3 drops every 2-3 hours while awake
Dosage Forms
Ointment, ophthalmic: Sodium sulfacetamide 10% and prednisolone acetate 0.2% (3.5 g)
Ointment, ophthalmic:
Cetapred®: Sodium sulfacetamide 10% and prednisolone acetate 0.25% (3.5 g)
Metimyd®: Sodium sulfacetamide 10% and prednisolone acetate 0.5% (3.5 g)
Suspension, ophthalmic: Sodium sulfacetamide 10% and prednisolone sodium phosphate 0.5% (5 mL)
Suspension, ophthalmic:
Blephamide®: Sodium sulfacetamide 10% and prednisolone acetate 0.2% (2.5 mL, 5 mL, 10 mL)
(Continued)

sodium sulfacetamide and prednisolone *(Continued)*
Vasocidin®: Sodium sulfacetamide 10% and prednisolone acetate 0.25% (5 mL, 10 mL)

sodium sulfacetamide and sulfur *see* sulfur and sodium sulfacetamide
on page 450

sodium tetradecyl sulfate
Brand Names Sotradecol® Injection
Therapeutic Category Sclerosing Agent
Use Treatment of small, uncomplicated varicose veins of the lower extremities; endoscopic sclerotherapy in the management of bleeding esophageal varices
Usual Dosage I.V.: 0.5-2 mL of 1% (5-20 mg) for small veins; 0.5-2 mL of 3% (15-60 mg) for medium or large veins
Dosage Forms Injection: 1% [10 mg/mL] (2 mL); 3% [30 mg/mL] (2 mL)

sodium thiosulfate *(thye oh sul' fate)*
Therapeutic Category Antidote, Cyanide; Antifungal Agent, Topical
Use Alone or with sodium nitrite or amyl nitrite in cyanide poisoning; used to reduce the risk of nephrotoxicity associated with cisplatin therapy; used topically in the treatment of tinea versicolor
Usual Dosage I.V.:
Cyanide and nitroprusside antidote:
Children <25 kg: 50 mg/kg after receiving 4.5-10 mg/kg sodium nitrite; a half dose of each may be repeated if necessary
Children >25 kg and Adults: 12.5 g after 300 mg of sodium nitrite; a half dose of each may be repeated if necessary
Cyanide poisoning: Dose should be based on determination as with nitrite, at rate of 2.5-5 mL/minute to maximum of 50 mL.
Dosage Forms Injection: 10% [100 mg/mL] (10 mL); 25% [250 mg/mL] (50 mL)

Sodol® *see* carisoprodol *on page 76*
Sofarin® *see* warfarin sodium *on page 500*
Solaquin Forte® Topical *see* hydroquinone *on page 239*
Solaquin® Topical [OTC] *see* hydroquinone *on page 239*
Solarcaine® [OTC] *see* benzocaine *on page 48*
Solarcaine® Topical *see* lidocaine hydrochloride *on page 273*
Solatene® *see* beta-carotene *on page 52*
Solfoton® *see* phenobarbital *on page 369*
Solganal® *see* aurothioglucose *on page 39*
soluble fluorescein *see* fluorescein sodium *on page 200*
Solu-Cortef® Injection *see* hydrocortisone *on page 236*
Solu-Medrol® Injection *see* methylprednisolone *on page 306*
Solurex® Injection *see* dexamethasone *on page 132*
Solurex L.A.® Injection *see* dexamethasone *on page 132*
Soma® *see* carisoprodol *on page 76*
Soma® Compound *see* carisoprodol *on page 76*
somatrem *see* human growth hormone *on page 230*
somatropin *see* human growth hormone *on page 230*
Sominex® Oral [OTC] *see* diphenhydramine hydrochloride *on page 152*
Soothe® Ophthalmic [OTC] *see* tetrahydrozoline hydrochloride *on page 459*

Soprodol® *see* carisoprodol *on page 76*

sorbitol (sor' bi tole)
Synonyms D-sorbitol
Therapeutic Category Genitourinary Irrigant
Use Genitourinary irrigant in transurethral prostatic resection or other transurethral resection or other transurethral surgical procedures; diuretic; humectant; sweetening agent; hyperosmotic laxative; facilitate the passage of sodium polystyrene sulfonate through the intestinal tract
Usual Dosage Hyperosmotic laxative (as single dose, at infrequent intervals):
Children 2-11 years:
Oral: 2 mL/kg (as 70% solution)
Rectal enema: 30-60 mL as 25% to 30% solution

Children >12 years and Adults:
Oral: 30-150 mL (as 70% solution)
Rectal enema: 120 mL as 25% to 30% solution
Adjunct to sodium polystyrene sulfonate: 15 mL as 70% solution orally until diarrhea occurs (10-20 mL/2 hours) or 20-100 mL as an oral vehicle for the sodium polystyrene sulfonate resin

When administered with charcoal: Oral:
Children: 4.3 mL/kg of 35% sorbitol with 1 g/kg of activated charcoal
Adults: 4.3 mL/kg of 70% sorbitol with 1 g/kg of activated charcoal
Dosage Forms
Powder: 500 g
Solution, oral: 70% [700 mg/mL] (480 mL)

Sorbitrate® *see* isosorbide dinitrate *on page 259*

Soridol® *see* carisoprodol *on page 76*

sotalol hydrochloride (soe' ta lole)
Brand Names Betapace® Oral
Therapeutic Category Antiarrhythmic Agent, Class II; Antiarrhythmic Agent, Class III
Use Treatment of ventricular arrhythmias
Usual Dosage Adults: Oral: Initial: 80 mg twice daily; may be increased to 240-320 mg/day and up to 480-640 mg/day in patients with life-threatening refractory ventricular arrhythmias
Dosage Forms Tablet: 80 mg, 160 mg, 240 mg

Sotradecol® Injection *see* sodium tetradecyl sulfate *on previous page*
Span-FF® [OTC] *see* ferrous fumarate *on page 193*
Sparine® Injection *see* promazine hydrochloride *on page 398*
Sparine® Oral *see* promazine hydrochloride *on page 398*
Spaslin® *see* hyoscyamine, atropine, scopolamine, and phenobarbital *on page 242*
Spasmoject® Injection *see* dicyclomine hydrochloride *on page 145*
Spasmolin® *see* hyoscyamine, atropine, scopolamine, and phenobarbital *on page 242*
Spasmophen® *see* hyoscyamine, atropine, scopolamine, and phenobarbital *on page 242*
Spasquid® *see* hyoscyamine, atropine, scopolamine, and phenobarbital *on page 242*
Spectam® Injection *see* spectinomycin hydrochloride *on next page*

Spectazole™ Topical *see* econazole nitrate *on page 166*

spectinomycin hydrochloride (spek ti noe mye' sin)
Brand Names Spectam® Injection; Trobicin® Injection
Therapeutic Category Antibiotic, Miscellaneous
Use Treatment of uncomplicated gonorrhea (ineffective against syphilis)
Usual Dosage I.M.:
Children:
    <45 kg: 40 mg/kg/dose 1 time
    ≥45 kg: See adult dose
    Children >8 years who are allergic to PCNS/cephalosporins may be treated with oral tetracycline

Adults: 2 g deep I.M. or 4 g where antibiotic resistance is prevalent 1 time; 4 g (10 mL) dose should be given as 2-5 mL injections
Dosage Forms Injection: 2 g, 4 g

Spectrobid® *see* bacampicillin hydrochloride *on page 42*

Spherulin® *see* coccidioidin skin test *on page 112*

Spironazide® *see* hydrochlorothiazide and spironolactone *on page 233*

spironolactone (speer on oh lak' tone)
Brand Names Aldactone®
Therapeutic Category Diuretic, Potassium Sparing
Use Management of edema associated with excessive aldosterone excretion; hypertension; primary hyperaldosteronism; hypokalemia; treatment of hirsutism, cirrhosis of the liver accompanied by edema or ascites (unlabeled)
Usual Dosage Oral:
Children: 1.5-3.5 mg/kg/day in divided doses every 6-24 hours
    Diagnosis of primary aldosteronism: 125-375 mg/m^2/day in divided doses
    Vaso-occlusive disease: 7.5 mg/kg/day in divided doses twice daily (non-FDA approved dose)

Adults:
    Edema, hypertension, hypokalemia: 25-200 mg/day in 1-2 divided doses
    Diagnosis of primary aldosteronism: 100-400 mg/day in 1-2 divided doses
Dosage Forms Tablet: 25 mg, 50 mg, 100 mg

spironolactone and hydrochlorothiazide *see* hydrochlorothiazide and spironolactone *on page 233*

Spirozide® *see* hydrochlorothiazide and spironolactone *on page 233*

Sporanox® Oral *see* itraconazole *on page 261*

Sportscreme® [OTC] *see* triethanolamine salicylate *on page 477*

SPS® *see* sodium polystyrene sulfonate *on page 438*

S-P-T *see* thyroid *on page 466*

SRC® Expectorant *see* hydrocodone, pseudoephedrine, and guaifenesin *on page 236*

SSD® AF Topical *see* silver sulfadiazine *on page 431*

SSD® Cream *see* silver sulfadiazine *on page 431*

SSKI® *see* potassium iodide *on page 387*

Stadol® *see* butorphanol tartrate *on page 64*

Stadol® NS *see* butorphanol tartrate *on page 64*

Stagesic® *see* hydrocodone and acetaminophen *on page 234*

stannous fluoride *see* fluoride *on page 201*

stanozolol (stan oh' zoe lole)
Brand Names Winstrol®
Therapeutic Category Anabolic Steroid
Use Prophylactic use against angioedema
Usual Dosage
Children: Acute attacks:
<6 years: 1 mg/day
6-12 years: 2 mg/day

Adults: Oral: Initial: 2 mg 3 times/day, may then reduce to a maintenance dose of 2 mg/day or 2 mg every other day after 1-3 months
Dosage Forms Tablet: 2 mg

Staphcillin® *see* methicillin sodium *on page 299*

Staticin® Topical *see* erythromycin, topical *on page 176*

Stay Trim® Diet Gum [OTC] *see* phenylpropanolamine hydrochloride *on page 373*

S-T Cort® Topical *see* hydrocortisone *on page 236*

Stelazine® Injection *see* trifluoperazine hydrochloride *on page 478*

Stelazine® Oral *see* trifluoperazine hydrochloride *on page 478*

Sterapred® Oral *see* prednisone *on page 393*

stilbestrol *see* diethylstilbestrol *on page 146*

Stilphostrol® Injection *see* diethylstilbestrol *on page 146*

Stilphostrol® Oral *see* diethylstilbestrol *on page 146*

St. Joseph® Cough Suppressant [OTC] *see* dextromethorphan hydrobromide *on page 136*

St. Joseph® Measured Dose Nasal Solution [OTC] *see* phenylephrine hydrochloride *on page 372*

Stop® [OTC] *see* fluoride *on page 201*

Streptase® *see* streptokinase *on this page*

streptokinase (strep toe kye' nase)
Brand Names Kabikinase®; Streptase®
Synonyms sk
Therapeutic Category Thrombolytic Agent
Use Thrombolytic agent used in treatment of recent severe or massive deep vein thrombosis, pulmonary emboli, myocardial infarction, and occluded arteriovenous cannulas
Usual Dosage I.V.:
Children: Safety and efficacy not established; limited studies have used: 3500-4000 units/kg over 30 minutes followed by 1000-1500 units/kg/hour; clotted catheter: 25,000 units, clamp for 2 hours then aspirate contents and flush with normal saline

Adults (best results are realized if used within 5-6 hours of myocardial infarction; antibodies to streptokinase remain for 3-6 months after initial dose, use another thrombolytic enzyme, ie, urokinase, if thrombolytic therapy is indicated):
Guidelines for Acute Myocardial Infarction (AMI):
1.5 million units infused over 60 minutes. Monitor for the first few hours for signs of anaphylaxis or allergic reaction. **Infusion should be slowed if lowering of 25 mm Hg in blood pressure or terminated if asthmatic symptoms appear.** Begin heparin 5000-10,000 unit bolus followed by 1000 unit/hour approximately 3-4 hours after completion of streptokinase infusion or when PTT is <100 seconds.

(Continued)
443

streptokinase *(Continued)*

Guidelines for Acute Pulmonary Embolism (APE):
3 million unit dose; administer 250,000 units over 30 minutes followed by 100,000 units/hour for 24 hours. Monitor for the first few hours for signs of anaphylaxis or allergic reaction. **Infusion should be slowed if blood pressure is lowered by 25 mm Hg or if asthmatic symptoms appear**. Begin heparin 1000 units/hour approximately 3-4 hours after completion of streptokinase infusion or when PTT is <100 seconds.

Thromboses: 250,000 units to start, then 100,000 units/hour for 24-72 hours depending on location

Cannula occlusion: 250,000 units into cannula, clamp for 2 hours, then aspirate contents and flush with normal saline

Dosage Forms Powder for injection: 250,000 units (5 mL, 6.5 mL); 600,000 units (5 mL); 750,000 units (6 mL, 6.5 mL); 1,500,000 units (6.5 mL, 10 mL, 50 mL)

streptomycin sulfate (strep toe mye' sin)

Therapeutic Category Antibiotic, Aminoglycoside; Antitubercular Agent
Use Combination therapy of active tuberculosis; used in combination with other agents for treatment of streptococcal or enterococcal endocarditis, mycobacterial infections, plague, tularemia, and brucellosis
Usual Dosage I.M.:
Infants: 20-30 mg/kg/day in divided doses every 12 hours

Children: Tuberculosis: 20-40 mg/kg/day in divided doses every 12-24 hours, not to exceed 2 g/day; usually discontinued after 2-3 months of therapy or sooner if cultures become negative

Adults:
Tuberculosis: 15 mg/kg/day in divided doses every 12 hours, not to exceed 2 g/day
Enterococcal endocarditis: 1 g every 12 hours for 2 weeks, 500 mg every 12 hours for 4 weeks in combination with penicillin
Streptococcal endocarditis: 1 g every 12 hours for 1 week, 500 mg every 12 hours for 1 week
Tularemia: 1-2 g/day in divided doses for 7-10 days or until patient is afebrile for 5-7 days
Plague: 2-4 g/day in divided doses until the patient is afebrile for at least 3 days
Dosage Forms Injection: 400 mg/mL (12.5 mL)

Streptonase-B® *see* diagnostic aids *(in vitro)*, other *on page 138*
Strepto-Sac® *see* diagnostic aids *(in vitro)*, other *on page 138*

streptozocin (strep toe zoe' sin)

Brand Names Zanosar®
Therapeutic Category Antineoplastic Agent, Alkylating Agent (Nitrosourea)
Use Treat metastatic islet cell carcinoma of the pancreas, carcinoid tumor and syndrome, Hodgkin's disease, palliative treatment of colorectal cancer
Usual Dosage Refer to individual protocols
Children and Adults: I.V.: 500 mg/m^2 for 5 days every 6 weeks until optimal benefit or toxicity occurs; or may be given in single dose 1000 mg/m^2 at weekly intervals for 2 doses, then increased to 1500 mg/m^2 weekly; the median total dose to onset of response is about 2000 mg/m^2 and the median total dose to maximum response is about 4000 mg/m^2
Dosage Forms Injection: 1 g

strong iodine solution *see* potassium iodide *on page 387*

strontium-89 chloride (stron' shee um)

Brand Names Metastron® Injection
Therapeutic Category Radiopharmaceutical
Use Relief of bone pain in patients with skeletal metastases

Usual Dosage Adults: I.V.: 148 megabecquerel (4 millicurie) administered by slow I.V. injection over 1-2 minutes or 1.5-2.2 megabecquerel (40-60 microcurie)/kg; repeated doses are generally not recommended at intervals <90 days
Dosage Forms Injection: 10.9-22.6 mg/mL [148 megabecquerel, 4 millicurie] (10 mL)

Stuartnatal® 1+1 *see* vitamin, multiple (prenatal) *on page 499*

Stuart Prenatal® [OTC] *see* vitamin, multiple (prenatal) *on page 499*

Sublimaze® Injection *see* fentanyl citrate *on page 192*

succimer (sux' sim mer)
Brand Names Chemet® Oral
Therapeutic Category Antidote, Lead Toxicity
Use Treatment of lead poisoning in children with blood levels >45 μg/dL. It is not indicated for prophylaxis of lead poisoning in a lead-containing environment.
Usual Dosage Children and Adults: Oral: 30 mg/kg/day in divided doses every 8 hours for an additional 5 days followed by 20 mg/kg/day for 14 days
Dosage Forms Capsule: 100 mg

succinylcholine chloride (suk sin ill koe' leen)
Brand Names Anectine® Chloride Injection; Anectine® Flo-Pack®; Quelicin® Injection; Sucostrin® Injection
Synonyms suxamethonium chloride
Therapeutic Category Neuromuscular Blocker Agent, Depolarizing; Skeletal Muscle Relaxant
Use Produce skeletal muscle relaxation in procedures of short duration such as endotracheal intubation or endoscopic exams
Usual Dosage I.M., I.V.:
Neonates: Intermittent: Initial: 2 mg/kg/dose one time; maintenance: 0.3-0.6 mg/kg/dose at intervals of 5-10 minutes as necessary

Children: 1-2 mg/kg
Intermittent: Initial: 1 mg/kg/dose one time; maintenance: 0.3-0.6 mg/kg every 5-10 minutes as needed

Adults: 0.6 mg/kg (range: 0.3-1.1 mg/kg) over 10-30 seconds, up to 150 mg total dose
Maintenance: 0.04-0.07 mg/kg every 5-10 minutes as needed
Continuous infusion: 2.5 mg/minute (or 0.5-10 mg/minute); dilute to concentration of 1-2 mg/mL in D_5W or NS

Note: Pretreatment with atropine may reduce occurrence of bradycardia
Dosage Forms
Injection: 20 mg/mL (10 mL); 50 mg/mL (10 mL); 100 mg/mL (5 mL, 10 mL, 20 mL)
Powder for injection: 100 mg, 500 mg, 1 g

Sucostrin® Injection *see* succinylcholine chloride *on this page*

sucralfate (soo kral' fate)
Brand Names Carafate®
Synonyms aluminum sucrose sulfate, basic
Therapeutic Category Gastrointestinal Agent, Miscellaneous
Use Short-term management of duodenal ulcers; maintenance for duodenal ulcers; suspension may be used topically for treatment of stomatitis due to cancer chemotherapy and other causes of esophageal and gastric erosions
Usual Dosage
Children: Dose not established, doses of 40-80 mg/kg/day divided every 6 hours have been used
Stomatitis: Oral: 2.5-5 mL (1 g/15 mL suspension), swish and spit or swish and swallow 4 times/day
(Continued)

445

sucralfate *(Continued)*

Adults:
> Duodenal ulcer treatment: Oral: 1 g 4 times/day, 1 hour before meals or food and at bedtime for 4-8 weeks, or alternatively 2 g twice daily
> Duodenal ulcer maintenance therapy: Oral: 1 g twice daily
> Stomatitis: Oral: 1 g/15 mL suspension, swish and spit or swish and swallow 4 times/day

Dosage Forms Tablet: 1 g

Sucrets® [OTC] *see* dyclonine hydrochloride *on page 165*

Sucrets® Cough Calmers [OTC] *see* dextromethorphan hydrobromide *on page 136*

Sudafed® [OTC] *see* pseudoephedrine *on page 406*

Sudafed® 12 Hour [OTC] *see* pseudoephedrine *on page 406*

Sudafed Plus® Tablet *see* chlorpheniramine and pseudoephedrine *on page 94*

Sufedrin® [OTC] *see* pseudoephedrine *on page 406*

Sufenta® Injection *see* sufentanil citrate *on this page*

sufentanil citrate (soo fen' ta nil)

Brand Names Sufenta® Injection
Therapeutic Category Analgesic, Narcotic
Use Analgesic supplement in maintenance of balanced general anesthesia
Usual Dosage I.V.:
> Children <12 years: 10-25 μg/kg with 100% O_2, maintenance: 25-50 μg as needed (total dose of up to 1-2 μg/kg)

> Adults: Dose should be based on body weight. **Note:** In obese patients (ie, >20% above ideal body weight), use lean body weight to determine dosage
>> 1-2 μg/kg with NO_2/O_2 for endotracheal intubation; maintenance: 10-25 μg as needed
>> 2-8 μg/kg with NO_2/O_2 more complicated major surgical procedures; maintenance: 10-50 μg as needed
>> 8-30 μg/kg with 100% O_2 and muscle relaxant produces sleep; at doses of ≥8 μg/kg maintains a deep level of anesthesia; maintenance: 10-50 μg as needed

Dosage Forms Injection: 50 μg/mL (1 mL, 2 mL, 5 mL)

sulbactam and ampicillin *see* ampicillin sodium and sulbactam sodium *on page 26*

sulconazole nitrate (sul kon' a zole)

Brand Names Exelderm® Topical; Sulcosyn® Topical
Therapeutic Category Antifungal Agent, Topical
Use Treatment of superficial fungal infections of the skin, including tinea cruris, tinea corporis, tinea versicolor and possibly tinea pedis
Usual Dosage Topical: Apply once or twice daily for 4-6 weeks
Dosage Forms
> Cream: 1% (15 g, 30 g, 60 g)
> Solution, topical: 1% (30 mL)

Sulcosyn® Topical *see* sulconazole nitrate *on this page*

Sulf-10® Ophthalmic *see* sodium sulfacetamide *on page 439*

sulfabenzamide, sulfacetamide, and sulfathiazole

Brand Names Gyne-Sulf® Vaginal; Sultrin™ Vaginal; Trysul® Vaginal; Vagilia® Vaginal; V.V.S.® Vaginal
Synonyms triple sulfa

ALPHABETICAL LISTING OF DRUGS

Therapeutic Category Antibiotic, Vaginal
Use Treatment of *Haemophilus vaginalis* vaginitis
Usual Dosage Adults:
Cream: Insert one applicatorful in vagina twice daily for 4-6 days; dosage may then be decreased to $\frac{1}{2}$ to $\frac{1}{4}$ of an applicatorful twice daily
Tablet: Insert one intravaginally twice daily for 10 days
Dosage Forms
Cream, vaginal: Sulfabenzamide 3.7%, sulfacetamide 2.86%, and sulfathiazole 3.42% (78 g with applicator, 90 g, 120 g)
Tablet, vaginal: Sulfabenzamide 184 mg, sulfacetamide 143.75 mg, and sulfathiazole 172.5 mg (20 tablets/box with vaginal applicator)

sulfacetamide sodium *see* sodium sulfacetamide *on page 439*
Sulfacet-R® Topical *see* sulfur and sodium sulfacetamide *on page 450*

sulfacytine (sul fa sye' teen)
Brand Names Renoquid®
Therapeutic Category Antibiotic, Sulfonamide Derivative
Use Treatment of urinary tract infections
Usual Dosage Adults: Oral: Initial: 500 mg, then 250 mg every 4 hours for 10 days
Dosage Forms Tablet: 250 mg

sulfadiazine (sul fa dye' a zeen)
Brand Names Microsulfon®
Therapeutic Category Antibiotic, Sulfonamide Derivative
Use Treatment of urinary tract infections and nocardiosis, rheumatic fever prophylaxis; adjunctive treatment in toxoplasmosis; uncomplicated attack of malaria; asymptomatic meningococcal carriers
Usual Dosage Oral:
Congenital toxoplasmosis:
Newborns and Children <2 months: 100 mg/kg/day divided every 6 hours in conjunction with pyrimethamine 1 mg/kg/day once daily and supplemental folinic acid 5 mg every 3 days for 6 months
Children >2 months: 25-50 mg/kg/dose 4 times/day

Toxoplasmosis:
Children: 120-150 mg/kg/day, maximum dose: 6 g/day; divided every 6 hours in conjunction with pyrimethamine 2 mg/kg/day divided every 12 hours for 3 days followed by 1 mg/kg/day once daily (maximum: 25 mg/day) with supplemental folinic acid
Adults: 2-8 g/day divided every 6 hours in conjunction with pyrimethamine 25 mg/day and with supplemental folinic acid
Dosage Forms Tablet: 500 mg

sulfadoxine and pyrimethamine (sul fa dox' een & peer i meth' a meen)
Brand Names Fansidar®
Therapeutic Category Antimalarial Agent
Use Treatment of *Plasmodium falciparum* malaria in patients in whom chloroquine resistance is suspected; malaria prophylaxis for travelers to areas where chloroquine-resistant malaria is endemic
Usual Dosage Children and Adults: Oral:
Treatment of acute attack of malaria: A single dose of the following number of Fansidar® tablets is used in sequence with quinine or alone:
2-11 months: $\frac{1}{4}$ tablet
1-3 years: $\frac{1}{2}$ tablet
4-8 years: 1 tablet
9-14 years: 2 tablets
>14 years: 2-3 tablets
(Continued)

sulfadoxine and pyrimethamine *(Continued)*

Malaria prophylaxis:
The first dose of Fansidar® should be taken 1-2 days before departure to an endemic area (CDC recommends that therapy be initiated 1-2 weeks before such travel), administration should be continued during the stay and for 4-6 weeks after return. Dose = pyrimethamine 0.5 mg/kg/dose and sulfadoxine 10 mg/kg/dose up to a maximum of 25 mg pyrimethamine and 500 mg sulfadoxine/dose weekly.

2-11 months: $^1/_8$ tablet weekly **or** $^1/_4$ tablet once every 2 weeks
1-3 years: $^1/_4$ tablet once weekly **or** $^1/_2$ tablet once every 2 weeks
4-8 years: $^1/_2$ tablet once weekly **or** 1 tablet once every 2 weeks
9-14 years: $^3/_4$ tablet once weekly **or** $1^1/_2$ tablets once every 2 weeks
>14 years: 1 tablet once weekly **or** 2 tablets once every 2 weeks
Dosage Forms Tablet: Sulfadoxine 500 mg and pyrimethamine 25 mg (25s)

Sulfair® Ophthalmic *see* sodium sulfacetamide *on page 439*
Sulfalax® [OTC] *see* docusate *on page 157*
Sulfamethoprim® *see* co-trimoxazole *on page 118*

sulfamethoxazole *(sul fa meth ox' a zole)*

Brand Names Gantanol®; Urobak®
Therapeutic Category Antibiotic, Sulfonamide Derivative
Use Treatment of urinary tract infections, nocardiosis, toxoplasmosis, acute otitis media, and acute exacerbations of chronic bronchitis due to susceptible organisms
Usual Dosage Oral:
Children >2 months: 50-60 mg/kg/day divided every 12 hours; maximum: 3 g/24 hours or 75 mg/kg/day

Adults: 2 g stat, 1 g 2-3 times/day; maximum: 3 g/24 hours
Dosage Forms
Suspension, oral (cherry flavor): 500 mg/5 mL (480 mL)
Tablet: 500 mg

sulfamethoxazole and phenazopyridine

Brand Names Azo Gantanol®
Therapeutic Category Antibiotic, Sulfonamide Derivative
Use Treatment of urinary tract infections complicated with pain
Usual Dosage Oral: 4 tablets to start, then 2 tablets twice daily for up to 2 days, then switch to sulfamethoxazole only
Dosage Forms Tablet: Sulfamethoxazole 500 mg and phenazopyridine 100 mg

sulfamethoxazole and trimethoprim *see* co-trimoxazole *on page 118*
Sulfamylon® Topical *see* mafenide acetate *on page 281*

sulfanilamide *(sul fa nill' a mide)*

Brand Names AVC™ Vaginal Cream; AVC™ Vaginal Suppository; Vagitrol® Vaginal
Therapeutic Category Antifungal Agent, Vaginal
Use Treatment of vulvovaginitis caused by *Candida albicans*
Usual Dosage One applicatorful once or twice daily continued through 1 complete menstrual cycle
Dosage Forms
Cream, vaginal (AVC™, Vagitrol®): 15% [150 mg/g] (120 g with applicator)
Suppository, vaginal (AVC™): 1.05 g (16s)

sulfasalazine *(sul fa sal' a zeen)*

Brand Names Azulfidine®; Azulfidine® EN-tabs®
Synonyms salicylazosulfapyridine
Therapeutic Category 5-Aminosalicylic Acid Derivative; Anti-inflammatory Agent

Use Management of ulcerative colitis
Usual Dosage Oral:
Children >2 years:
Initial: 40-60 mg/kg/day divided every 4-6 hour
Maintenance dose: 20-30 mg/kg/day divided every 6 hours, up to a maximum of 2 g/day
Adults:
Initial: 3-4 g/day divided every 4-6 hours;
Maintenance dose: 2 g/day divided every 6 hours
Dosage Forms
Suspension, oral: 250 mg/5 mL (480 mL)
Tablet: 500 mg
Tablet, enteric coated: 500 mg

Sulfatrim® *see* co-trimoxazole *on page 118*
Sulfatrim® DS *see* co-trimoxazole *on page 118*

sulfinpyrazone (sul fin peer' a zone)
Brand Names Anturane®
Therapeutic Category Uric Acid Lowering Agent
Use Treatment of chronic gouty arthritis and intermittent gouty arthritis
Usual Dosage Oral: 200 mg twice daily
Dosage Forms
Capsule: 200 mg
Tablet: 100 mg

sulfisoxazole (sul fi sox' a zole)
Brand Names Gantrisin® Ophthalmic; Gantrisin® Oral
Synonyms sulfisoxazole acetyl; sulphafurazole
Therapeutic Category Antibiotic, Sulfonamide Derivative
Use Treatment of urinary tract infections, otitis media, *Chlamydia*; nocardiosis; treatment of acute pelvic inflammatory disease in prepubertal children
Usual Dosage
Children >2 months: Oral: 75 mg/kg stat, 120-150 mg/kg/day in divided doses every 4-6 hours; not to exceed 6 g/day
Pelvic inflammatory disease: 100 mg/kg/day in divided doses every 6 hours; used in combination with ceftriaxone
Chlamydia trachomatis: 100 mg/kg/day divided every 6 hours
Children and Adults: Ophthalmic:
Solution: 1-2 drops to affected eye every 2-3 hours
Ointment: Small amount to affected eye 1-3 times/day and at bedtime
Adults: Oral: 2-4 g stat, 4-8 g/day in divided doses every 4-6 hours
Dosage Forms
Solution, ophthalmic, as diolamine: 4% [40 mg/mL] (15 mL)
Suspension, oral, pediatric, as acetyl (raspberry flavor): 500 mg/5 mL (480 mL)
Syrup, as acetyl (chocolate flavor): 500 mg/5 mL (480 mL)
Tablet: 500 mg

sulfisoxazole acetyl *see* sulfisoxazole *on this page*
sulfisoxazole and erythromycin *see* erythromycin and sulfisoxazole *on page 176*

sulfisoxazole and phenazopyridine
Brand Names Azo Gantrisin®
Therapeutic Category Antibiotic, Sulfonamide Derivative; Local Anesthetic, Urinary
Use Treatment of urinary tract infections and nocardiosis
(Continued)
449

sulfisoxazole and phenazopyridine *(Continued)*
Usual Dosage Oral: 4-6 tablets to start, then 2 tablets 4 times/day for 2 days, then continue with sulfisoxazole only
Dosage Forms Tablet: Sulfisoxazole 500 mg and phenazopyridine 50 mg

sulfur and salicylic acid
Brand Names Aveeno® Cleansing Bar [OTC]; Fostex® [OTC]; Pernox® [OTC]; Sastid® Plain Therapeutic Shampoo and Acne Wash [OTC]; Sebulex® [OTC]
Synonyms salicylic acid and sulfur
Therapeutic Category Antiseborrheic Agent, Topical
Use Therapeutic shampoo for dandruff and seborrheal dermatitis; acne skin cleanser
Usual Dosage Children and Adults:
Shampoo: Initial: Use daily or every other day; 1-2 treatments/week will usually maintain control
Soap: Use daily or every other day
Dosage Forms
Cake: Sulfur 2% and salicylic acid 2% (123 g)
Cleanser: Sulfur 2% and salicylic acid 1.5% (60 mL, 120 mL)
Shampoo: Micropulverized sulfur 2% and salicylic acid 2% (120 mL, 240 mL)
Soap: Micropulverized sulfur 2% and salicylic acid 2% (113 g)
Wash: Sulfur 1.6% and salicylic acid 1.6% (75 mL)

sulfur and sodium sulfacetamide
Brand Names Sulfacet-R® Topical
Synonyms sodium sulfacetamide and sulfur
Therapeutic Category Acne Product
Use Aid in the treatment of acne vulgaris, acne rosacea and seborrheic dermatitis
Usual Dosage Topical: Apply in a thin film 1-3 times/day
Dosage Forms Lotion, topical: Sulfur colloid 5% and sodium sulfacetamide 10% (30 mL)

sulindac (sul in' dak)
Brand Names Clinoril®
Therapeutic Category Analgesic, Non-Narcotic; Anti-inflammatory Agent; Nonsteroidal Anti-Inflammatory Agent (NSAID), Oral
Use Management of inflammatory disease, rheumatoid disorders; acute gouty arthritis; structurally similar to indomethacin but acts like aspirin; safest NSAID for use in mild renal impairment
Usual Dosage Oral:
Children: Dose not established
Adults: 150-200 mg twice daily; not to exceed 400 mg/day
Dosage Forms Tablet: 150 mg, 200 mg

sulphafurazole *see* sulfisoxazole *on previous page*
Sultrin™ Vaginal *see* sulfabenzamide, sulfacetamide, and sulfathiazole *on page 446*
Sumacal® [OTC] *see* glucose polymers *on page 213*

sumatriptan succinate (soo' ma trip tan)
Brand Names Imitrex® Injection
Therapeutic Category Antimigraine Agent
Use Serotonin agonist for acute treatment of migraine
Usual Dosage Adults: S.C.: 6 mg; a second injection may be administered at least 1 hour after the initial dose, but not more than 2 injections in a 24-hour period
Dosage Forms Injection: 12 mg/mL (0.5 mL, 2 mL)

Sumycin® Oral *see* tetracycline *on page 458*

SuperChar® [OTC] *see* charcoal *on page 86*

Supprelin™ Injection *see* histrelin *on page 230*

Suppress® [OTC] *see* dextromethorphan hydrobromide *on page 136*

Suprane® *see* desflurane *on page 130*

Suprax® *see* cefixime *on page 79*

suprofen (soo proe' fen)
Brand Names Profenal® Ophthalmic
Therapeutic Category Nonsteroidal Anti-Inflammatory Agent (NSAID), Ophthalmic
Use Inhibition of intraoperative miosis
Usual Dosage On day of surgery, instill 2 drops in conjunctival sac at 3, 2, and 1 hour prior to surgery; or 2 drops in sac every 4 hours, while awake, the day preceding surgery
Dosage Forms Solution, ophthalmic: 1% (2.5 mL)

Surbex® [OTC] *see* vitamin B complex *on page 498*

Surbex-T® Filmtabs® [OTC] *see* vitamin B complex with vitamin C *on page 498*

Surbex® with C Filmtabs® [OTC] *see* vitamin B complex with vitamin C *on page 498*

Surfak® [OTC] *see* docusate *on page 157*

Surgicel® *see* cellulose, oxidized *on page 83*

Surital® Injection *see* thiamylal sodium *on page 463*

Surmontil® *see* trimipramine maleate *on page 481*

Survanta® *see* beractant *on page 51*

Susano® *see* hyoscyamine, atropine, scopolamine, and phenobarbital *on page 242*

Sus-Phrine® Injection *see* epinephrine *on page 171*

Sustaire® *see* theophylline *on page 460*

sutilains (soo' ti lains)
Brand Names Travase® Topical
Therapeutic Category Enzyme, Topical Debridement
Use To promote debridement of necrotic debris, as an adjunct in the treatment of second and third degree burns, decubitus ulcers
Usual Dosage Thoroughly cleanse and irrigate wound then apply ointment in a thin layer extending $\frac{1}{4}$" to $\frac{1}{2}$" beyond the tissue being debrided; apply loose moist dressing; repeat 3-4 times/day
Dosage Forms Ointment: 82,000 casein units/g (14.2 g)

suxamethonium chloride *see* succinylcholine chloride *on page 445*

Sween Cream® [OTC] *see* methylbenzethonium chloride *on page 304*

Swim-Ear® Otic [OTC] *see* boric acid *on page 56*

Syllact® [OTC] *see* psyllium *on page 407*

Symadine® *see* amantadine hydrochloride *on page 17*

Symmetrel® *see* amantadine hydrochloride *on page 17*

Synacort® Topical *see* hydrocortisone *on page 236*

synacthen *see* cosyntropin *on page 117*

Synalar-HP® Topical *see* fluocinolone acetonide *on page 199*

Synalar®️ Topical *see* fluocinolone acetonide *on page 199*

Synalgos®️ [OTC] *see* aspirin *on page 34*

Synalgos®️-DC *see* dihydrocodeine compound *on page 148*

Synarel®️ *see* nafarelin acetate *on page 322*

Synemol®️ Topical *see* fluocinolone acetonide *on page 199*

Synkayvite®️ *see* menadiol sodium diphosphate *on page 291*

synthetic lung surfactant *see* colfosceril palmitate *on page 114*

Synthroid®️ Injection *see* levothyroxine sodium *on page 271*

Synthroid®️ Oral *see* levothyroxine sodium *on page 271*

Syntocinon®️ Injection *see* oxytocin *on page 352*

Syntocinon®️ Nasal Spray *see* oxytocin *on page 352*

Syprine®️ *see* trientine hydrochloride *on page 477*

Syracol-CF®️ [OTC] *see* guaifenesin and dextromethorphan *on page 218*

Sytobex®️ *see* cyanocobalamin *on page 120*

T_3/T_4 liotrix *see* liotrix *on page 275*

T_3 thyronine sodium *see* liothyronine sodium *on page 274*

T_4 thyroxine sodium *see* levothyroxine sodium *on page 271*

Tac™-3 Injection *see* triamcinolone *on page 474*

Tac™-40 Injection *see* triamcinolone *on page 474*

Tacaryl®️ *see* methdilazine hydrochloride *on page 299*

TACE®️ *see* chlorotrianisene *on page 92*

tacrine hydrochloride (tak' reen)
Brand Names Cognex®️ Oral
Synonyms tetrahydroaminoacrine; THA
Therapeutic Category Cholinergic Agent
Use Treatment of Alzheimer's disease
Usual Dosage Adults: Oral: 40 mg/day
Dosage Forms Capsule: 10 mg, 20 mg, 30 mg, 40 mg

Tagamet®️ *see* cimetidine *on page 102*

Talacen®️ *see* pentazocine compound *on page 364*

Talwin®️ *see* pentazocine *on page 364*

Talwin®️ Compound *see* pentazocine compound *on page 364*

Talwin®️ NX *see* pentazocine *on page 364*

Tambocor®️ *see* flecainide acetate *on page 196*

Tamine®️ [OTC] *see* brompheniramine and phenylpropanolamine *on page 59*

tamoxifen citrate (ta mox' i fen)
Brand Names Nolvadex®️ Oral
Therapeutic Category Antineoplastic Agent, Hormone (Antiestrogen)
Use Palliative or adjunctive treatment of advanced breast cancer in postmenopausal women
Usual Dosage Refer to individual protocols
Oral: 10-20 mg twice daily
Dosage Forms Tablet: 10 mg

Tao®️ *see* troleandomycin *on page 483*

Tapazole® *see* methimazole *on page 300*

Tarabine® PFS *see* cytarabine hydrochloride *on page 123*

Taractan® *see* chlorprothixene *on page 98*

taste function test *see* diagnostic aids (*in vitro*), other *on page 138*

TAT *see* tetanus antitoxin *on page 456*

Tavist® *see* clemastine fumarate *on page 105*

Tavist®-1 [OTC] *see* clemastine fumarate *on page 105*

Tavist-D® *see* clemastine and phenylpropanolamine *on page 105*

Taxol® *see* paclitaxel *on page 352*

Tazicef® *see* ceftazidime *on page 81*

Tazidime® *see* ceftazidime *on page 81*

TCN *see* tetracycline *on page 458*

tD *see* diphtheria and tetanus toxoid *on page 153*

Tearisol® [OTC] *see* artificial tears *on page 33*

Tebamide® Rectal *see* trimethobenzamide hydrochloride *on page 480*

Tedral® *see* theophylline, ephedrine, and phenobarbital *on page 462*

Tega-Vert® Oral *see* dimenhydrinate *on page 150*

Tegison® *see* etretinate *on page 188*

Tegopen® *see* cloxacillin sodium *on page 110*

Tegretol® *see* carbamazepine *on page 72*

Tegrin®-HC Topical [OTC] *see* hydrocortisone *on page 236*

T.E.H.® *see* theophylline, ephedrine, and hydroxyzine *on page 462*

Telachlor® Oral *see* chlorpheniramine maleate *on page 94*

Teladar® Topical *see* betamethasone *on page 52*

Teldrin® Oral [OTC] *see* chlorpheniramine maleate *on page 94*

Telepaque® *see* radiological/contrast media (ionic) *on page 413*

Teline® Oral *see* tetracycline *on page 458*

Temaril® *see* trimeprazine tartrate *on page 479*

temazepam (te maz' e pam)
Brand Names Restoril®
Therapeutic Category Benzodiazepine; Hypnotic; Sedative
Use Treatment of anxiety and as an adjunct in the treatment of depression; also may be used in the management of panic attacks; transient insomnia and sleep latency
Usual Dosage Adults: Oral: 15-30 mg at bedtime
Dosage Forms Capsule: 15 mg, 30 mg

Temovate® Topical *see* clobetasol dipropionate *on page 107*

Tempra® [OTC] *see* acetaminophen *on page 2*

Tencet™ *see* butalbital compound *on page 63*

Tencon® *see* butalbital compound *on page 63*

Tenex® *see* guanfacine hydrochloride *on page 222*

teniposide (ten i poe' side)
Brand Names Vumon Injection
Synonyms EPT; VM-26
Therapeutic Category Antineoplastic Agent, Miscellaneous
(Continued)
453

teniposide *(Continued)*
Use Treatment of Hodgkin's and non-Hodgkin's lymphomas, acute lymphocytic leukemia, bladder carcinoma and neuroblastoma
Usual Dosage Refer to individual protocols
I.V.:
Children: 130 mg/m²/week, increasing to 150 mg/m² after 3 weeks and to 180 mg/m² after 6 weeks
Adults: 50-180 mg/m² once or twice weekly for 4-6 weeks
Dosage Forms Injection: 10 mg/mL (5 mL)

Tenoretic® *see* atenolol and chlorthalidone *on page 36*
Tenormin® *see* atenolol *on page 36*
Tensilon® Injection *see* edrophonium chloride *on page 167*
Tenuate® *see* diethylpropion hydrochloride *on page 146*
Tepanil® *see* diethylpropion hydrochloride *on page 146*
Terazol® Vaginal *see* terconazole *on next page*

terazosin (ter ay' zoe sin)
Brand Names Hytrin®
Therapeutic Category Alpha-Adrenergic Blocking Agent, Oral
Use Management of mild to moderate hypertension; considered a step 2 drug in stepped approach to hypertension; benign prostate hypertrophy
Usual Dosage Adults: Oral: 1 mg; slowly increase dose to achieve desired blood pressure, up to 20 mg/day
Dosage Forms Tablet: 1 mg, 2 mg, 5 mg, 10 mg

terbinafine hydrochloride (ter' bin a feen)
Brand Names Lamisil® Topical
Therapeutic Category Antifungal Agent, Topical
Use Topical antifungal for the treatment of tinea pedis, tinea cruris and tinea corporis
Usual Dosage Adults: Topical:
Athlete's foot: Apply twice daily for at least 1 week, not to exceed 4 weeks
Ringworm and jock itch: Apply once or twice daily for at least 1 week, not to exceed 4 weeks
Dosage Forms Cream: 1% (15 g, 30 g)

terbutaline sulfate (ter byoo' ta leen)
Brand Names Brethaire® Inhalation Areosol; Brethine® Injection; Brethine® Oral; Bricanyl® Injection; Bricanyl® Oral
Therapeutic Category Adrenergic Agonist Agent; Beta-2-Adrenergic Agonist Agent; Bronchodilator; Tocolytic Agent
Use Bronchodilator in reversible airway obstruction and bronchial asthma; management of preterm labor
Usual Dosage
Children <12 years:
Oral: Initial: 0.05 mg/kg/dose 3 times/day, increased gradually as required; maximum: 0.15 mg/kg/dose 3-4 times/day or a total of 5 mg/24 hours
S.C.: 0.005-0.01 mg/kg/dose to a maximum of 0.3 mg/dose every 15-20 minutes for 3 doses
Nebulization: 0.1-0.3 mg/kg/dose up to a maximum of 10 mg/dose every 4-6 hours
Inhalation: 1-2 inhalations every 4-6 hours
Children >12 years and Adults:
Oral:

12-15 years: 2.5 mg every 6 hours 3 times/day; not to exceed 7.5 mg in 24 hours
>15 years: 5 mg/dose every 6 hours 3 times/day; if side effects occur, reduce dose
    to 2.5 mg every 6 hours; not to exceed 15 mg in 24 hours
S.C.: 0.25 mg/dose repeated in 15-30 minutes for one time only; a total dose of 0.5 mg
    should not be exceeded within a 4-hour period
Nebulization: 0.1-0.3 mg/kg/dose every 4-6 hours
Inhalation: 2 inhalations every 4-6 hours; wait 1 minute between inhalations
Dosage Forms
Aerosol, oral: 0.2 mg/actuation (10.5 g)
Injection: 1 mg/mL (1 mL)
Tablet: 2.5 mg, 5 mg

terconazole (ter kone' a zole)
Brand Names Terazol® Vaginal
Synonyms triaconazole
Therapeutic Category Antifungal Agent, Vaginal
Use Local treatment of vulvovaginal candidiasis
Usual Dosage One applicatorful in vagina at bedtime for 7 consecutive days
Dosage Forms
Cream, vaginal: 0.4% (45 g); 0.8% (20 g)
Suppository, vaginal: 80 mg (3s)

terfenadine (ter fen' a deen)
Brand Names Seldane®
Therapeutic Category Antihistamine
Use Perennial and seasonal allergic rhinitis and other allergic symptoms including urticaria
Usual Dosage Oral:
Children:
    3-6 years: 15 mg twice daily
    6-12 years: 30 mg twice daily
Children >12 years and Adults: 60 mg twice daily
Dosage Forms Tablet: 60 mg

terfenadine and pseudoephedrine
Brand Names Seldane-D®
Therapeutic Category Antihistamine/Decongestant Combination
Use Temporary relief of symptoms of seasonal and perennial allergic rhinitis, and vasomotor rhinitis, including nasal obstruction
Usual Dosage Oral: Adults: One tablet every morning and at bedtime
Dosage Forms Tablet: Terfenadine 60 mg and pseudoephedrine hydrochloride 120 mg

teriparatide (ter i par' a tide)
Brand Names Parathar™ Injection
Therapeutic Category Diagnostic Agent, Hypothyroidism
Use Diagnosis of hypocalcemia in either hypoparathyroidism or pseudohypoparathyroidism
Usual Dosage I.V.:
Children ≥3 years: 3 units/kg up to 200 units
Adults: 200 units over 10 minutes
Dosage Forms Powder for injection: 200 units hPTH activity (10 mL)

Terramycin® I.M. Injection *see* oxytetracycline hydrochloride *on page 352*

Terramycin® Ophthalmic Ointment *see* oxytetracycline and polymyxin b *on page 351*

Terramycin® Oral *see* oxytetracycline hydrochloride *on page 352*

ALPHABETICAL LISTING OF DRUGS

Terramycin® w/ Polymyxin B Sulfate Vaginal *see* oxytetracycline and polymyxin b *on page 351*

Teslac® *see* testolactone *on this page*

TESPA *see* thiotepa *on page 465*

Tessalon® Perles *see* benzonatate *on page 49*

Tes-Tape® [OTC] *see* diagnostic aids (*in vitro*), urine *on page 139*

testolactone (tess toe lak' tone)
Brand Names Teslac®
Therapeutic Category Androgen
Use Palliative treatment of advanced disseminated breast carcinoma
Usual Dosage Adults: Females: Oral: 250 mg 4 times/day for at least 3 months; desired response may take as long as 3 months
Dosage Forms Tablet: 50 mg

testosterone (tess toss' ter one)
Brand Names Andro-Cyp® Injection; Andro® Injection; Andro-L.A.® Injection; Andronate® Injection; Andropository® Injection; Delatest® Injection; Delatestryl® Injection; Depotest® Injection; Depo®-Testosterone Injection; Duratest® Injection; Durathate® Injection; Everone® Injection; Histerone® Injection
Synonyms aqueous testosterone
Therapeutic Category Androgen
Use Androgen replacement therapy in the treatment of delayed male puberty; postpartum breast pain and engorgement; inoperable breast cancer; male hypogonadism
Usual Dosage I.M.:
Delayed puberty: Children: 40-50 mg/m^2/dose monthly for 6 months

Male hypogonadism: 50-400 mg every 2-4 weeks
Initiation of pubertal growth: 40-50 mg/m^2/dose monthly until the growth rate falls to prepubertal levels (~5 cm/year)
During terminal growth phase: 100 mg/m^2/dose monthly until growth ceases
Maintenance virilizing dose: 100 mg/m^2/dose twice monthly or 50-400 mg/dose every 2-4 weeks

Inoperable breast cancer: Adults: 200-400 mg every 2-4 weeks
Dosage Forms Injection:
Aqueous suspension: 25 mg/mL (10 mL, 30 mL); 50 mg/mL (10 mL, 30 mL); 100 mg/mL (10 mL, 30 mL)
In oil, as cypionate: 100 mg/mL (1 mL, 10 mL); 200 mg/mL (1 mL, 10 mL)
In oil, as enanthate: 100 mg/mL (5 mL, 10 mL); 200 mg/mL (5 mL, 10 mL)
In oil, as propionate: 50 mg/mL (10 mL, 30 mL); 100 mg/mL (10 mL, 30 mL)

testosterone and estradiol *see* estradiol and testosterone *on page 178*
Testred® *see* methyltestosterone *on page 307*
tetanus and diphtheria toxoid *see* diphtheria and tetanus toxoid *on page 153*

tetanus antitoxin
Synonyms TAT
Therapeutic Category Antitoxin
Use Tetanus prophylaxis or treatment of active tetanus only when tetanus immune globulin (TIG) is not available
Usual Dosage
Prophylaxis: I.M., S.C.:
Children <30 kg: 1500 units
Children and Adults >30 kg: 3000-5000 units

456

Treatment: Children and Adults: Inject 10,000-40,000 units into wound; give 40,000-100,000 units I.V.

Dosage Forms Injection, equine: Not less than 400 units/mL (12.5 mL, 50 mL)

tetanus immune globulin, human
Brand Names Hyper-Tet®
Synonyms TIG
Therapeutic Category Immune Globulin
Use Passive immunization against tetanus; tetanus immune globulin is preferred over tetanus antitoxin for treatment of active tetanus; part of the management of an unclean, non-minor wound in a person whose history of previous receipt of tetanus toxoid is unknown or who has received less than three doses of tetanus toxoid
Usual Dosage I.M.:
Prophylaxis of tetanus:
Children: 4 units/kg; some recommend administering 250 units to small children
Adults: 250 units

Treatment of tetanus:
Children: 500-3000 units; some should infiltrate locally around the wound
Adults: 3000-6000 units
Dosage Forms Injection: 250 units/mL

tetanus toxoid, adsorbed
Therapeutic Category Toxoid
Use Active immunity against tetanus
Usual Dosage Adults: I.M.:
Primary immunization: 0.5 mL; repeat 0.5 mL at 4-8 weeks after first dose and at 6-12 months after second dose
Routine booster doses are recommended only every 5-10 years
Dosage Forms Injection:
Tetanus 5 Lf units/0.5 mL dose (0.5 mL, 5 mL)
Tetanus 10 Lf units/2.5 mL dose (5 mL)

tetanus toxoid, fluid
Synonyms tetanus toxoid plain
Therapeutic Category Toxoid
Use Active immunization against tetanus in adults and children
Usual Dosage Inject 3 doses of 0.5 mL I.M. or S.C. at 4- to 8-week intervals with fourth dose given only 6-12 months after third dose
Dosage Forms Injection:
Tetanus 4 Lf units/0.5 mL dose (7.5 mL)
Tetanus 5 Lf units/0.5 mL dose (0.5 mL, 7.5 mL)

tetanus toxoid plain see tetanus toxoid, fluid *on this page*

tetracaine hydrochloride (tet' ra kane)
Brand Names Pontocaine® Injection; Pontocaine® Topical
Synonyms amethocaine hydrochloride
Therapeutic Category Local Anesthetic, Injectable; Local Anesthetic, Ophthalmic; Local Anesthetic, Oral; Local Anesthetic, Topical
Use Spinal anesthesia; local anesthesia in the eye for various diagnostic and examination purposes; topically applied to nose and throat for various diagnostic procedures
Usual Dosage
Children: Safety and efficacy have not been established

Adults:
Ophthalmic (not for prolonged use):
Ointment: Apply $\frac{1}{2}$" to 1" to lower conjunctival fornix
(Continued)

tetracaine hydrochloride *(Continued)*
Solution: Instill 1-2 drops
Spinal anesthesia 1% solution:
Subarachnoid injection: 5-20 mg
Saddle block: 2-5 mg; a 1% solution should be diluted with equal volume of CSF before administration
Topical mucous membranes (2% solution): Apply as needed; dose should not exceed 20 mg
Topical for skin: Apply to affected areas as needed
Dosage Forms
Cream: 1% (28 g)
Injection: 1% [10 mg/mL] (2 mL)
Injection, with dextrose 6%: 0.2% [2 mg/mL] (2 mL); 0.3% [3 mg/mL] (5 mL)
Ointment:
Ophthalmic: 0.5% [5 mg/mL] (3.75 g)
Topical: 0.5% [5 mg/mL] (28 g)
Solution:
Ophthalmic: 0.5% [5 mg/mL] (1 mL, 2 mL, 15 mL, 59 mL)
Topical: 2% [20 mg/mL] (30 mL, 118 mL)

tetracaine hydrochloride, benzocaine butyl aminobenzoate and benzalkonium chloride *see* benzocaine, butyl aminobenzoate, tetracaine, and benzalkonium chloride *on page 48*

tetracaine with dextrose
Brand Names Pontocaine® With Dextrose Injection
Therapeutic Category Local Anesthetic, Injectable
Use Spinal anesthesia (saddle block)
Usual Dosage Dose varies with procedure, depth of anesthesia, duration desired and physical condition of patient
Dosage Forms Injection: Tetracaine hydrochloride 0.2% with dextrose 6% (2 mL); tetracaine hydrochloride 0.3% with dextrose 6% (5 mL)

Tetracap® Oral *see* tetracycline *on this page*

tetracosactide *see* cosyntropin *on page 117*

tetracycline (tet ra sye' kleen)
Brand Names Achromycin® Ophthalmic; Achromycin® Topical; Achromycin® V Oral; Ala-Tet® Oral; Nor-tet® Oral; Panmycin® Oral; Robitet® Oral; Sumycin® Oral; Teline® Oral; Tetracap® Oral; Tetralan® Oral; Tetram® Oral; Topicycline® Topical
Synonyms TCN
Therapeutic Category Acne Product; Antibiotic, Ophthalmic; Antibiotic, Tetracycline Derivative; Antibiotic, Topical
Use Treatment of susceptible bacterial infections of both gram-positive and gram-negative organisms; also some unusual organisms including *Mycoplasma*, *Chlamydia*, and *Rickettsia*; may also be used for acne, exacerbations of chronic bronchitis, and treatment of gonorrhea and syphilis in patients that are allergic to penicillin
Usual Dosage
Children >8 years:
Oral: 25-50 mg/kg/day in divided doses every 6 hours; not to exceed 3 g/day
Ophthalmic:
Suspension: Instill 1-2 drops 2-4 times/day or more often as needed
Ointment: Instill every 2-12 hours

Adults:
Oral: 250-500 mg/dose every 6 hours

Ophthalmic:
  Suspension: Instill 1-2 drops 2-4 times/day or more often as needed
  Ointment: Instill every 2-12 hours
  Topical: Apply to affected areas 1-4 times/day
Dosage Forms
  Capsule: 100 mg, 250 mg, 500 mg
  Ointment:
    Ophthalmic: 1% [10 mg/mL] (3.5 g)
    Topical: 3% [30 mg/mL] (14.2 g, 30 g)
  Solution, topical: 2.2 mg/mL (70 mL)
  Suspension:
    Ophthalmic: 1% [10 mg/mL] (0.5 mL, 1 mL, 4 mL)
    Oral: 125 mg/5 mL (60 mL, 480 mL)
  Tablet: 250 mg, 500 mg

tetrahydroaminoacrine *see* tacrine hydrochloride *on page 452*

tetrahydrocannabinol *see* dronabinol *on page 162*

tetrahydrozoline hydrochloride (tet ra hye drozz' a leen)
Brand Names Collyrium Fresh® Ophthalmic [OTC]; Eyesine® Ophthalmic [OTC]; Eye-Zine® Ophthalmic [OTC]; Mallazine® Eye Drops [OTC]; Murine® Plus Ophthalmic [OTC]; Optigene® Ophthalmic [OTC]; Soothe® Ophthalmic [OTC]; Tetra-Ide® Ophthalmic [OTC]; Tyzine® Nasal; Visine® Ophthalmic [OTC]
Synonyms tetryzoline
Therapeutic Category Adrenergic Agonist Agent; Adrenergic Agonist Agent, Ophthalmic; Nasal Agent, Vasoconstrictor; Ophthalmic Agent, Vasoconstrictor
Use Symptomatic relief of nasal congestion and conjunctival congestion
Usual Dosage
  Nasal congestion:
    Children 2-6 years: Instill 2-3 drops of 0.05% solution every 4-6 hours as needed
    Children >6 years and Adults: Instill 2-4 drops or 0.1% spray nasal mucosa every 4-6 hours as needed

  Conjunctival congestion: Adults: Instill 1-2 drops in each eye 2-3 times/day
Dosage Forms Solution:
  Nasal: 0.05% (15 mL), 0.1% (30 mL, 473 mL)
  Ophthalmic: 0.05% (15 mL, 22.5 mL, 30 mL)

Tetra-Ide® Ophthalmic [OTC] *see* tetrahydrozoline hydrochloride *on this page*

Tetralan® Oral *see* tetracycline *on previous page*

Tetram® Oral *see* tetracycline *on previous page*

Tetramune® *see* diphtheria, tetanus toxoids, and whole-cell pertussis vaccine and hemophilus b conjugate vaccine *on page 154*

tetryzoline *see* tetrahydrozoline hydrochloride *on this page*

Texacort® Topical *see* hydrocortisone *on page 236*

TG *see* thioguanine *on page 464*

6-TG *see* thioguanine *on page 464*

T/Gel® [OTC] *see* coal tar *on page 110*

T-Gen® Rectal *see* trimethobenzamide hydrochloride *on page 480*

T-Gesic® *see* hydrocodone and acetaminophen *on page 234*

THA *see* tacrine hydrochloride *on page 452*

Thalitone® *see* chlorthalidone *on page 99*

THAM-E® Injection *see* tromethamine *on page 483*

THAM® **Injection** *see* tromethamine *on page 483*

THC *see* dronabinol *on page 162*

Theelin® **Injection** *see* estrone *on page 180*

Theo-24® *see* theophylline *on this page*

Theobid® *see* theophylline *on this page*

Theochron® *see* theophylline *on this page*

Theoclear® L.A. *see* theophylline *on this page*

Theo-Dur® *see* theophylline *on this page*

Theo-G® *see* theophylline and guaifenesin *on next page*

Theolair™ *see* theophylline *on this page*

Theolate® *see* theophylline and guaifenesin *on next page*

theophylline (thee off' i lin)

Brand Names Aerolate®; Aerolate III®; Aerolate JR®; Aerolate SR® S; Aquaphyllin®; As-malix®; Bronkodyl®; Constant-T®; Elixicon®; Elixophyllin®; Elixophyllin® SR; Quibron®-T; Quibron®-T/SR; Respbid®; Slo-bid™; Slo-Phyllin®; Sustaire®; Theo-24®; Theobid®; Theochron®; Theoclear® L.A.; Theo-Dur®; Theolair™; Theospan®-SR; Theovent®; Theox®; Uniphyl®

Synonyms theophylline anhydrous

Therapeutic Category Antiasthmatic; Bronchodilator; Theophylline Derivative

Use Bronchodilator in reversible airway obstruction due to asthma or COPD; for neonatal apnea/bradycardia

Usual Dosage

Neonatal apnea:

Loading dose: 5 mg/kg

Maintenance dose: 1-3 mg/kg every 8-12 hours depending on age

Asthma: Loading dose: Dependent on pretherapy theophylline serum level (**loading dose (boluses) are given as aminophylline because of product availability**):

>10 μg/mL: Do not give load dose

Continuous infusion (begin when bolus is infused): See table.

Guidelines for Drawing Theophylline Serum Levels

Dosage Form	Time to Draw Level
I.V. bolus	30 min after end of 30 min infusion
I.V. continuous infusion	12–24 h after initiation of infusion
P.O. liquid, fast–release tab	Peak: 1 h post a dose after at least 1 day of therapy Trough: Just before a dose after at least 1 day of therapy
P.O. slow–release product	Peak: 4 h post a dose after at least 1 day of therapy Trough: Just before a dose after at least 1 day of therapy

Once a loading dose achieves a therapeutic level, draw the next serum concentration 5-6 hours after this last level.

Dosage Forms

Capsule:

Immediate release (Bronkodyl®, Elixophyllin®): 100 mg, 200 mg

Timed release:

8-12 hours (Aerolate®): 65 mg [III]; 130 mg [JR], 260 mg [SR]

8-12 hours (Elixophyllin SR®): 125 mg, 250 mg

8-12 hours (Slo-Bid™): 50 mg, 75 mg, 100 mg, 125 mg, 200 mg, 300 mg

8-12 hours (Slo-Phyllin® Gyrocaps®): 60 mg, 125 mg, 250 mg
12 hours (Theobid® Jr. Duracaps®): 130 mg
12 hours (Theobid® Duracaps®): 260 mg
12 hours (Theoclear® L.A.): 130 mg, 260 mg
12 hours (Theo-Dur® Sprinkle®): 50 mg, 75 mg, 125 mg, 200 mg
12 hours (Theospan®-SR): 130 mg, 260 mg
12 hours (Theovent®): 125 mg, 250 mg
24 hours (Theo-24®): 100 mg, 200 mg, 300 mg

Elixir (Asmalix®, Elixomin®, Elixophyllin®, Lanophyllin®): 80 mg/15 mL (15 mL, 30 mL, 480 mL, 4000 mL)

Infusion, in D₅W: 0.4 mg/mL (1000 mL); 0.8 mg/mL (500 mL, 1000 mL); 1.6 mg/mL (250 mL, 500 mL); 2 mg/mL (100 mL); 3.2 mg/mL (250 mL); 4 mg/mL (50 mL, 100 mL);

Solution, oral:
Theolair™: 80 mg/15 mL (15 mL, 18.75 mL, 30 mL, 480 mL)
Aerolate®: 150 mg/15 mL (480 mL)

Syrup:
Aquaphyllin®, Slo-Phyllin®, Theoclear-80®, Theostat-80®: 80 mg/15 mL (15 mL, 30 mL, 500 mL)
Accurbron®: 150 mg/15 mL (480 mL)

Tablet: Immediate release:
Slo-Phyllin®: 100 mg, 200 mg
Theolair™: 125 mg, 250 mg
Quibron®-T: 300 mg

Tablet:
Controlled release (Theox®): 100 mg, 200 mg, 300 mg
Timed release:
12-24 hours: 100 mg, 200 mg, 300 mg
8-12 hours (Constant-T®): 200 mg, 300 mg
8-12 hours (Quibron®-T/SR): 300 mg
8-12 hours (Respbid®): 250 mg, 500 mg
8-12 hours (Sustaire®): 100 mg, 300 mg
8-12 hours (T-Phyl®): 200 mg
12-24 hours (Theochron®): 100 mg, 200 mg, 300 mg
8-24 hours (Theo-Dur®): 100 mg, 200 mg, 300 mg, 450 mg
8-24 hours (Theo-Sav®): 100 mg, 200 mg, 300 mg
24 hours (Theolair™-SR): 200 mg, 250 mg, 300 mg, 500 mg
24 hours (Uniphyl®): 400 mg

theophylline and guaifenesin

Brand Names Bronchial®; Glycerol-T®; Lanophyllin-GG®; Quibron®; Slo-Phyllin GG®; Theo-G®; Theolate®

Therapeutic Category Antiasthmatic; Bronchodilator; Expectorant; Theophylline Derivative

Use Symptomatic treatment of bronchospasm associated with bronchial asthma, chronic bronchitis and pulmonary emphysema

Usual Dosage Adults: Oral: 1 or 2 capsules every 6-8 hours

Dosage Forms
Capsule: Theophylline 150 mg and guaifenesin 90 mg; theophylline 300 mg and guaifenesin 180 mg
Elixir: Theophylline 150 mg and guaifenesin 90 mg per 15 mL (480 mL)

theophylline anhydrous see theophylline on previous page

theophylline, ephedrine, and hydroxyzine
Brand Names Hydrophen®; Marax®; T.E.H.®
Therapeutic Category Antiasthmatic; Bronchodilator; Theophylline Derivative
Use Possibly effective for controlling bronchospastic disorders
Usual Dosage
Children:
2-5 years: ½ tablet 2-4 times/day or 2.5 mL 3-4 times/day
>5 years: ½ tablet 2-4 times/day or 5 mL 3-4 times/day

Adults: 1 tablet 2-4 times/day
Dosage Forms
Syrup, dye free: Theophylline 32.5 mg, ephedrine 6.25 mg, and hydroxyzine 2.5 mg per 5 mL
Tablet: Theophylline 130 mg, ephedrine 25 mg, and hydroxyzine 10 mg

theophylline, ephedrine, and phenobarbital
Brand Names Tedral®
Synonyms ephedrine, theophylline and phenobarbital
Therapeutic Category Antiasthmatic; Bronchodilator; Theophylline Derivative
Use Prevention and symptomatic treatment of bronchial asthma; relief of asthmatic bronchitis and other bronchospastic disorders
Usual Dosage
Children >60 lb: 1 tablet or 5 mL every 4 hours
Adults: 1-2 tablets or 10-20 mL every 4 hours
Dosage Forms
Suspension: Theophylline 65 mg, ephedrine sulfate 12 mg, and phenobarbital 4 mg per 5 mL
Tablet: Theophylline 118 mg, ephedrine sulfate 25 mg, and phenobarbital 11 mg; theophylline 130 mg, ephedrine sulfate 24 mg, and phenobarbital 8 mg

theophylline ethylenediamine *see* aminophylline *on page 19*

Theospan®-SR *see* theophylline *on page 460*

Theovent® *see* theophylline *on page 460*

Theox® *see* theophylline *on page 460*

Thera-Combex® H-P Kapseals® [OTC] *see* vitamin B complex with vitamin C *on page 498*

TheraCys™ *see* BCG *on page 44*

Theramin® Expectorant [OTC] *see* guaifenesin and phenylpropanolamine *on page 219*

Theraplex Z® [OTC] *see* pyrithione zinc *on page 410*

Thermazene® Topical *see* silver sulfadiazine *on page 431*

Theroxide® *see* benzoyl peroxide *on page 49*

thiabendazole (thye a ben' da zole)
Brand Names Mintezol®
Synonyms tiabendazole
Therapeutic Category Anthelmintic
Use Treatment of strongyloidiasis, cutaneous larva migrans, visceral larva migrans, dracunculiasis, trichinosis, and mixed helminthic infections
Usual Dosage Oral:
Children and Adults: 50 mg/kg/day divided every 12 hours (maximum dose: 3 g/day)
Strongyloidiasis: For 2 consecutive days
Cutaneous larva migrans: For 2-5 consecutive days
Visceral larva migrans: For 5-7 consecutive days
Trichinosis: For 2-4 consecutive days
Dracunculosis: 50-75 mg/kg/day divided every 12 hours for 3 days

Dosage Forms
Suspension, oral: 500 mg/5 mL (120 mL)
Tablet, chewable (orange flavor): 500 mg

thiamazole *see* methimazole *on page 300*

thiamine hydrochloride (thye' a min)
Brand Names Betalin®S; Biamine®
Synonyms aneurine hydrochloride; thiaminium chloride hydrochloride; vitamin B₁
Therapeutic Category Vitamin, Water Soluble
Use Treatment of thiamine deficiency including beriberi, Wernicke's encephalopathy syndrome, and peripheral neuritis associated with pellagra, alcoholic patients with altered sensorium; various genetic metabolic disorders
Usual Dosage Dietary supplement (depends on caloric or carbohydrate content of the diet):
Infants: 0.3-0.5 mg/day
Children: 0.5-1 mg/day
Adults: 1-2 mg/day
Note: The above doses can be found as a combination in multivitamin preparations
Children:
Noncritically ill thiamine deficiency: Oral: 10-50 mg/day in divided doses every day for 2 weeks followed by 5-10 mg/day for one month
Beriberi: I.M.: 10-25 mg/day for 2 weeks, then 5-10 mg orally every day for one month (oral as therapeutic multivitamin)
Adults:
Wernicke's encephalopathy: I.M., I.V.: 50 mg as a single dose, then 50 mg I.M. every day until normal diet resumed
Noncritically ill thiamine deficiency: Oral: 10-50 mg/day in divided doses
Beriberi: I.M., I.V.: 10-30 mg 3 times/day for 2 weeks, then switch to 5-10 mg orally every day for one month (oral as therapeutic multivitamin)
Dosage Forms
Injection: 100 mg/mL (1 mL, 2 mL, 10 mL, 30 mL); 200 mg/mL (30 mL)
Tablet: 50 mg, 100 mg, 250 mg, 500 mg
Tablet, enteric coated: 20 mg

thiaminium chloride hydrochloride *see* thiamine hydrochloride *on this page*

thiamylal sodium (thye am' i lal)
Brand Names Surital® Injection
Therapeutic Category Barbiturate; General Anesthetic
Use Induction of anesthesia; maintenance of anesthesia; agent for inducing a hypnotic state
Usual Dosage Adults: I.V.:
Induction: 2.5% of intermittent injection
Maintenance: 0.3% intermittent injection or drip
Dosage Forms Injection: 1 g, 5 g, 10 g

thiethylperazine maleate (thye eth il per' a zeen)
Brand Names Torecan® Injection; Torecan® Oral; Torecan® Rectal
Therapeutic Category Antiemetic
Use Relief of nausea and vomiting
Usual Dosage Children >12 years and Adults:
Oral, I.M., rectal: 10 mg 1-3 times/day as needed
I.V. and S.C. routes of administration are not recommended
Dosage Forms
Injection: 5 mg/mL (2 mL)
Suppository, rectal: 10 mg
(Continued)

463

thiethylperazine maleate *(Continued)*
Tablet: 10 mg

thimerosal (thye mer' oh sal)
Brand Names Aeroaid® [OTC]; Mersol® [OTC]
Therapeutic Category Antibacterial, Topical
Use Organomercurial antiseptic with sustained bacteriostatic and fungistatic activity
Usual Dosage Apply 1-3 times/day
Dosage Forms
Ointment, ophthalmic: 0.02% [0.2 mg/mL] (3.5 g)
Solution, topical: 0.1% [1 mg/mL = 1:1000] (120 mL, 480 mL, 4000 mL)
Spray, antiseptic: 0.1% [1 mg/mL = 1:1000] with alcohol 2% (90 mL)
Tincture: 0.1% [1 mg/mL = 1:1000] with alcohol 50% (120 mL, 480 mL, 4000 mL)

thioguanine (thye oh gwah' neen)
Synonyms 2-amino-6-mercaptopurine; TG; 6-TG; 6-thioguanine; tioguanine
Therapeutic Category Antineoplastic Agent, Antimetabolite
Use Remission induction consolidation and maintenance therapy of acute nonlymphocytic leukemia; treatment of chronic myelogenous leukemia
Usual Dosage Refer to individual protocols
Oral:
Infants <3 years: Combination drug therapy for acute nonlymphocytic leukemia: 3.3 mg/kg/day in divided doses twice daily for 4 days

Children and Adults: 2-3 mg/kg/day calculated to nearest 20 mg or 75-200 mg/m^2/day in 1-2 divided doses for 5-7 days or until remission is attained
Dosage Forms Tablet, scored: 40 mg

6-thioguanine *see* thioguanine *on this page*

thiopental sodium (thye oh pen' tal)
Brand Names Pentothal® Sodium
Therapeutic Category Barbiturate; General Anesthetic; Sedative
Use Induction of anesthesia; adjunct for intubation in head injury patients; control of convulsive states; treatment of elevated intracranial pressure
Usual Dosage I.V.:
Induction anesthesia:
Neonates: 3-4 mg/kg
Infants: 5-8 mg/kg
Children 1-12 years: 5-6 mg/kg
Adults: 3-5 mg/kg

Maintenance anesthesia:
Children: 1 mg/kg as needed
Adults: 25-100 mg as needed

Increased intracranial pressure: Children and Adults: 1.5-5 mg/kg/dose; repeat as needed to control intracranial pressure

Seizures:
Children: 2-3 mg/kg/dose, repeat as needed
Adults: 75-250 mg/dose, repeat as needed

Rectal administration: (Patient should be NPO for no less than 3 hours prior to administration)
Suggested initial doses of thiopental rectal suspension are:
<3 months: 15 mg/kg/dose
>3 months: 25 mg/kg/dose
Note: The age of a premature infant should be adjusted to reflect the age that the infant would have been if full-term (eg, an infant, now age 4 months, who was 2 months premature should be considered to be a 2-month old infant).

Doses should be rounded downward to the nearest 50 mg increment to allow for accurate measurement of the dose

Inactive or debilitated patients and patients recently medicated with other sedatives, (eg, chloral hydrate, meperidine, chlorpromazine, and promethazine), may require smaller doses than usual

If the patient is not sedated within 15-20 minutes, a single repeat dose of thiopental can be given. The single repeat doses are:
<3 months of age: <7.5 mg/kg/dose
>3 months of age: 15 mg/kg/dose
Adults weighing >90 kg should not receive >3 g as a total dose (initial plus repeat doses)
Children weighing >34 kg should not receive >1 g as a total dose (initial plus repeat doses)
Neither adults nor children should receive more than one course of thiopental rectal suspension (initial dose plus repeat dose) per 24-hour period

Dosage Forms
Injection: 250 mg, 400 mg, 500 mg, 1 g, 2.5 g, 5 g
Suspension, rectal: 400 mg/g (2 g)

thioridazine (thye oh rid' a zeen)
Brand Names Mellaril®; Mellaril-S®
Synonyms thioridazine hydrochloride
Therapeutic Category Antipsychotic Agent; Phenothiazine Derivative
Use Management of manifestations of psychotic disorders; depressive neurosis; alcohol withdrawal; dementia in elderly; behavioral problems in children
Usual Dosage Oral:
Children >2 years: Range: 0.5-3 mg/kg/day in 2-3 divided doses; usual: 1 mg/kg/day; maximum: 3 mg/kg/day
Behavior problems: Initial: 10 mg 2-3 times/day, increase gradually
Severe psychoses: Initial: 25 mg 2-3 times/day, increase gradually

Adults:
Psychoses: Initial: 50-100 mg 3 times/day with gradual increments as needed and tolerated; maximum daily dose: 800 mg/day in 2-4 divided doses
Depressive disorders, dementia: Initial: 25 mg 3 times/day; maintenance dose: 20-200 mg/day

Dosage Forms
Concentrate, oral: 30 mg/mL (120 mL); 100 mg/mL (3.4 mL, 120 mL)
Suspension, oral: 25 mg/5 mL (480 mL); 100 mg/5 mL (480 mL)
Tablet: 10 mg, 15 mg, 25 mg, 50 mg, 100 mg, 150 mg, 200 mg

thioridazine hydrochloride see thioridazine on this page

thiotepa (thye oh tep' a)
Synonyms TESPA; triethylenethiophosphoramide; TSPA
Therapeutic Category Antineoplastic Agent, Alkylating Agent
Use Treatment of superficial tumors of the bladder; palliative treatment of adenocarcinoma of breast or ovary; lymphomas and sarcomas; controlling intracavitary effusions caused by metastatic tumors
Usual Dosage Refer to individual protocols
Children: Sarcomas: I.V.: 25-65 mg/m^2 as a single dose every 21 days

Adults:
I.M., I.V., S.C.: 8 mg/m^2 daily for 5 days or 30-60 mg/m^2 once per week
High dose therapy for bone marrow transplant: I.V.: 500 mg/m^2
Intracavitary: 0.6-0.8 mg/kg or 60 mg in 60 mL SWI instilled into the bladder at 1- to 4-week intervals
(Continued)

465

thiotepa (Continued)

Intrathecal: Doses of 1-10 mg/m^2 administered 1-2 times/week in concentrations of 1 mg/mL diluted with preservative free sterile water for injection

Dosage Forms Powder for injection: 15 mg

thiothixene (thye oh thix' een)

Brand Names Navane®
Synonyms tiotixene
Therapeutic Category Antipsychotic Agent; Phenothiazine Derivative
Use Management of psychotic disorders
Usual Dosage
Children <12 years: Oral: Not well established; 0.25 mg/kg/24 hours in divided doses
Children >12 years and Adults:
Oral: Initial: 2 mg 3 times/day, up to 20-30 mg/day; maximum: 60 mg/day
I.M. (give undiluted injection): 4 mg 2-4 times/day, increase dose gradually; usual: 16-20 mg/day; maximum: 30 mg/day; change to oral dose as soon as able
Dosage Forms
Capsule: 1 mg, 2 mg, 5 mg, 10 mg, 20 mg
Concentrate, oral, as hydrochloride: 5 mg/mL (30 mL, 120 mL)
Injection, as hydrochloride: 2 mg/mL (2 mL)
Powder for injection, as hydrochloride: 5 mg/mL (2 mL)

Thorazine® see chlorpromazine hydrochloride on page 97
Thrombate® III see antithrombin III on page 30
Thrombinar® see thrombin, topical on this page

thrombin, topical

Brand Names Thrombinar®; Thrombogen®; Thrombostat®
Therapeutic Category Hemostatic Agent
Use Hemostasis whenever minor bleeding from capillaries and small venules is accessible
Usual Dosage Use 1000-2000 units/mL of solution where bleeding is profuse; apply powder directly to the site of bleeding or on oozing surfaces; use 100 units/mL for bleeding from skin or mucosal surfaces
Dosage Forms Powder: 1000 units, 5000 units, 10,000 units, 20,000 units, 50,000 units

Thrombogen® see thrombin, topical on this page
Thrombostat® see thrombin, topical on this page

thymopentin (thye' moe pen tin)

Brand Names Timunox®
Synonyms thymopoietin; tp5
Therapeutic Category Immune Modulator
Use Immunomodulator
Dosage Forms Injection: 10 mg/mL (10 mL)

thymopoietin see thymopentin on this page
Thypinone® Injection see protirelin on page 405
Thyrar® see thyroid on this page
Thyro-Block® see potassium iodide on page 387

thyroid (thye' roid)

Brand Names Armour® Thyroid; S-P-T; Thyrar®; Westhroid®
Synonyms desiccated thyroid; thyroid extract
Therapeutic Category Thyroid Product

Use Replacement or supplemental therapy in hypothyroidism

Usual Dosage Oral: Adults: Start at 30 mg/day and titrate by 30 mg/day in increments of 2- to 3-week intervals; usual maintenance dose: 60-120 mg/day

Dosage Forms
Capsule; 60 mg, 120 mg, 180 mg, 300 mg
Tablet: 15 mg, 30 mg, 60 mg, 90 mg, 120 mg, 180 mg, 240 mg, 300 mg

thyroid extract *see* thyroid *on previous page*

thyroid-stimulating hormone *see* thyrotropin *on this page*

Thyrolar® *see* liotrix *on page 275*

thyrotropin (thye roe troe' pin)
Brand Names Thytropar®
Synonyms thyroid-stimulating hormone; TSH
Therapeutic Category Diagnostic Agent, Hypothyroidism; Diagnostic Agent, Thyroid Function
Use Diagnostic aid to determine subclinical hypothyroidism or decreased thyroid reserve, to differentiate between primary and secondary hypothyroidism and between primary hypothyroidism and euthyroidism in patients receiving thyroid replacement
Usual Dosage I.M., S.C.: 10 units/day for 1-3 days; follow by a radioiodine study 24 hours past last injection, no response in thyroid failure, substantial response in pituitary failure
Dosage Forms Injection: 10 units

Thytropar® *see* thyrotropin *on this page*

tiabendazole *see* thiabendazole *on page 462*

Ticar® *see* ticarcillin disodium *on this page*

ticarcillin and clavulanate potassium
Brand Names Timentin®
Synonyms ticarcillin and clavulanic acid
Therapeutic Category Antibiotic, Penicillin
Use Treat infections of lower respiratory tract, urinary tract, skin and skin structures, bone and joint, and septicemia caused by susceptible organisms. Clavulanate expands activity of ticarcillin to include beta-lactamase producing strains of *S. aureus, H. influenzae, Enterobacteriaceae, Pseudomonas, Klebsiella, Citrobacter,* and *Serratia*
Usual Dosage I.V.:
Children: 200-300 mg of ticarcillin/kg/day in divided doses every 4-6 hours

Adults: 3.1 g (ticarcillin 3 g plus clavulanic acid 0.1 g) every 4-6 hours; maximum: 18-24 g/day; for urinary tract infections: 3.1 g every 6-8 hours
Dosage Forms
Infusion, premixed (frozen): Ticarcillin disodium 3 g and clavulanic acid 0.1 g (100 mL)
Powder for injection: Ticarcillin disodium 3 g and clavulanic acid 0.1 g (3.1 g, 31 g)

ticarcillin and clavulanic acid *see* ticarcillin and clavulanate potassium *on this page*

ticarcillin disodium (tye kar sill' in)
Brand Names Ticar®
Therapeutic Category Antibiotic, Penicillin
Use Treatment of susceptible infections such as septicemia, acute and chronic respiratory tract infections, skin and soft tissue infections, and urinary tract infections due to susceptible strains of *Pseudomonas, Proteus,* and *Escherichia coli* and *Enterobacter*
Usual Dosage I.V. (ticarcillin is generally given I.M. only for the treatment of uncomplicated urinary tract infections):
(Continued)

ticarcillin disodium *(Continued)*
Neonates:
Postnatal age <7 days:
<2000 g: 150 mg/kg/day in divided doses every 12 hours
>2000 g: 225 mg/kg/day in divided doses every 8 hours
Postnatal age >7 days:
<1200 g: 150 mg/kg/day in divided doses every 12 hours
1200-2000 g: 225 mg/kg/day in divided doses every 8 hours
>2000 g: 300 mg/kg/day in divided doses every 6 hours
Infants and Children: 200-300 mg/kg/day in divided doses every 4-6 hours; maximum dose: 24 g/day
Adults: 1-4 g every 4-6 hours
Dosage Forms Powder for injection: 1 g, 3 g, 6 g, 20 g, 30 g

TICE® BCG *see BCG on page 44*
Ticlid® *see ticlopidine hydrochloride on this page*

ticlopidine hydrochloride (tye kloe' pi deen)
Brand Names Ticlid®
Therapeutic Category Antiplatelet Agent
Use Platelet aggregation inhibitor that reduces the risk of thrombotic stroke in patients who have had a stroke or stroke precursors
Usual Dosage Adults: Oral: 1 tablet twice daily with food
Dosage Forms Tablet: 250 mg

Ticon® Injection *see trimethobenzamide hydrochloride on page 480*
TIG *see tetanus immune globulin, human on page 457*
Tigan® Injection *see trimethobenzamide hydrochloride on page 480*
Tigan® Oral *see trimethobenzamide hydrochloride on page 480*
Tigan® Rectal *see trimethobenzamide hydrochloride on page 480*
Tiject® Injection *see trimethobenzamide hydrochloride on page 480*
Tilade® Inhalation Aerosol *see nedocromil sodium on page 327*
Timentin® *see ticarcillin and clavulanate potassium on previous page*

timolol maleate (tye' moe lole)
Brand Names Blocadren® Oral; Timoptic® Ophthalmic
Therapeutic Category Beta-Adrenergic Blocker; Beta-Adrenergic Blocker, Ophthalmic
Use Ophthalmic dosage form used to treat elevated intraocular pressure such as glaucoma or ocular hypertension; orally for treatment of hypertension and angina and reduce mortality following myocardial infarction and prophylaxis of migraine
Usual Dosage
Children and Adults:
Ophthalmic: Initial: 0.25% solution, instill 1 drop twice daily; increase to 0.5% solution if response not adequate; decrease to 1 drop/day if controlled; do not exceed 1 drop twice daily of 0.5% solution
Adults: Oral:
Hypertension: Initial: 10 mg twice daily, increase gradually every 7 days, usual dosage: 20-40 mg/day in 2 divided doses; maximum: 60 mg/day
Prevention of myocardial infarction: 10 mg twice daily initiated within 1-4 weeks after infarction
Migraine headache: Initial: 10 mg twice daily, increase to maximum of 30 mg/day
Dosage Forms
Solution, ophthalmic (Timoptic®): 0.25% (2.5 mL, 5 mL, 10 mL, 15 mL); 0.5% (2.5 mL, 5 mL, 10 mL, 15 mL)

Solution, ophthalmic, preservative free, single use (Timoptic® OcuDose®): 0.25%, 0.5%
Tablet (Blocadren®): 5 mg, 10 mg, 20 mg

Timoptic® Ophthalmic see timolol maleate *on previous page*
Timunox® see thymopentin *on page 466*
Tinactin® [OTC] see tolnaftate *on page 471*
TinBen® [OTC] see benzoin *on page 49*
TinCoBen® [OTC] see benzoin *on page 49*
Tindal® see acetophenazine maleate *on page 5*

tioconazole (tye oh kone' a zole)
Brand Names Vagistat® Vaginal
Therapeutic Category Antifungal Agent, Vaginal
Use Local treatment of vulvovaginal candidiasis
Usual Dosage Vaginal: Insert 1 applicatorful in vagina, just prior to bedtime, as a single
dose
Dosage Forms Cream, vaginal: 6.5% with applicator (4.6 g)

tioguanine see thioguanine *on page 464*
tiotixene see thiothixene *on page 466*
Tisit® [OTC] see pyrethrins *on page 408*
tissue plasminogen activator, recombinant see alteplase, recombinant
on page 14
Titralac® Plus Liquid [OTC] see calcium carbonate and simethicone
on page 66
TMP see trimethoprim *on page 480*
TMP-SMX see co-trimoxazole *on page 118*
TobraDex® Ophthalmic see tobramycin and dexamethasone *on next page*

tobramycin (toe bra mye' sin)
Brand Names Nebcin® Injection; Tobrex® Ophthalmic
Therapeutic Category Antibiotic, Aminoglycoside; Antibiotic, Ophthalmic
Use Treatment of documented or suspected *Pseudomonas aeruginosa* infection; infection
with a nonpseudomonal enteric bacillus which is more sensitive to tobramycin than gen-
tamicin based on susceptibility tests; susceptible organisms in lower respiratory tract in-
fections, CNS infections, intra-abdominal, skin, bone, and urinary tract infections; empiric
therapy in cystic fibrosis and immunocompromised patients; topically used to treat superficial ophthalmic infections caused by susceptible bacteria
Usual Dosage Dosage should be based on an estimate of ideal body weight
Neonates: I.M., I.V.:
Postnatal age <7 days:
<1000 g, <28 weeks gestational age: 3 mg/kg/dose every 24 hours
<1500 g, <34 weeks gestational age: 2.5 mg/kg/dose every 18 hours
>1500 g, >34 weeks gestational age: 2.5 mg/kg/dose every 12 hours
Postnatal age >7 days:
<2000 g: 2.5 mg/kg/dose every 12 hours
>2000 g: 2.5 mg/kg/dose every 8 hours

Infants and Children: I.M., I.V.: 2.5 mg/kg/dose every 8 hours
Note: Some patients may require larger or more frequent doses if serum levels document the need (ie, cystic fibrosis or febrile granulocytopenic patients)

Adults: I.M., I.V.: 3-5 mg/kg/day in 3 divided doses

Children and Adults: Renal dysfunction: 2.5 mg/kg (2-3 serum level measurements should
be obtained after the initial dose to measure the half-life in order to determine the frequency of subsequent doses)
(Continued)

tobramycin *(Continued)*
Children and Adults: Ophthalmic: 1-2 drops every 4 hours; apply ointment 2-3 times/day; for severe infections apply ointment every 3-4 hours, or 2 drops every 30-60 minutes initially, then reduce to less frequent intervals
Dosage Forms
Injection, as sulfate: 10 mg/mL (2 mL); 40 mg/mL (1.5 mL, 2 mL)
Ointment, ophthalmic: 0.3% [3 mg/mL] (3.5 g)
Powder for injection: 40 mg/mL (1.2 g vials)
Solution, ophthalmic: 0.3% [3 mg/mL] (5 mL)

tobramycin and dexamethasone
Brand Names TobraDex® Ophthalmic
Synonyms dexamethasone and tobramycin
Therapeutic Category Antibiotic, Ophthalmic; Corticosteroid, Ophthalmic
Use Treatment of external ocular infection caused by susceptible gram-negative bacteria and steroid responsive inflammatory conditions of the palpebral and bulbar conjunctiva, lid, cornea, and anterior segment of the globe
Usual Dosage Ophthalmic: Adults:
Suspension: Instill 1-2 drops every 4-6 hours (first 24-48 hours may increase frequency to every 2 hours until signs of clinical improvement are seen); apply every 30-60 minutes for severe infections
Ointment: Apply 1.25 cm (½") every 3-4 hours to 2-3 times/day
Dosage Forms
Ointment, ophthalmic: Tobramycin 0.3% and dexamethasone 0.1% (3.5 g)
Suspension, ophthalmic: Tobramycin 0.3% and dexamethasone 0.1% (2.5 mL, 5 mL)

Tobrex® Ophthalmic *see* tobramycin *on previous page*

tocainide hydrochloride (toe kay' nide)
Brand Names Tonocard®
Therapeutic Category Antiarrhythmic Agent, Class Ib
Use Suppress and prevent symptomatic ventricular arrhythmias
Usual Dosage Adults: Oral: 1200-1800 mg/day in 3 divided doses
Dosage Forms Tablet: 400 mg, 600 mg

tocophersolan (toe koff er soe' lan)
Brand Names Liqui-E®
Synonyms tpgs
Therapeutic Category Vitamin, Fat Soluble
Use Approved for the treatment of vitamin E deficiency resulting from malabsorption due to prolonged cholestatic hepatobiliary disease.
Usual Dosage Dietary supplement: Oral: 15 mg (400 units) every day
Dosage Forms Liquid: 26.6 units/mL

Tofranil® Injection *see* imipramine *on page 247*
Tofranil® Oral *see* imipramine *on page 247*
Tofranil-PM® Oral *see* imipramine *on page 247*

tolazamide (tole az' a mide)
Brand Names Ronase®; Tolinase®
Therapeutic Category Antidiabetic Agent; Hypoglycemic Agent, Oral; Sulfonylurea Agent
Use Adjunct to diet for the management of mild to moderately severe, stable, noninsulin-dependent (type II) diabetes mellitus
Usual Dosage Adults: Oral: 100-1000 mg/day
Dosage Forms Tablet: 100 mg, 250 mg, 500 mg

tolazoline hydrochloride (tole az' oh leen)
Brand Names Priscoline® Injection
Synonyms benzazoline hydrochloride
Therapeutic Category Alpha-Adrenergic Blocking Agent, Parenteral; Vasodilator, Coronary
Use Persistent pulmonary vasoconstriction and hypertension of the newborn (persistent fetal circulation), peripheral vasospastic disorders
Usual Dosage
Neonates: Initial: I.V.: 1-2 mg/kg over 10-15 minutes via scalp vein or upper extremity; maintenance: 1-2 mg/kg/hour; use lower maintenance doses in patients with decreased renal function. Also used in neonates for acute vasospasm "cath toes" at 0.25 mg/kg/hour (no load)

Adults: Peripheral vasospastic disorder: I.M., I.V., S.C.: 10-50 mg 4 times/day
Dosage Forms Injection: 25 mg/mL (4 mL)

tolbutamide (tole byoo' ta mide)
Brand Names Orinase® Diagnostic Injection; Orinase® Oral
Therapeutic Category Antidiabetic Agent; Hypoglycemic Agent, Oral; Sulfonylurea Agent
Use Adjunct to diet for the management of mild to moderately severe, stable, noninsulin-dependent (type II) diabetes mellitus
Usual Dosage Adults:
Oral: 250-2000 mg/day
I.V. bolus: 20 mg/kg
Dosage Forms
Injection, diagnostic, as sodium: 1 g (20 mL)
Tablet: 250 mg, 500 mg

Tolectin® *see* tolmetin sodium *on this page*

Tolinase® *see* tolazamide *on previous page*

tolmetin sodium (tole' met in)
Brand Names Tolectin®
Therapeutic Category Analgesic, Non-Narcotic; Nonsteroidal Anti-Inflammatory Agent (NSAID), Oral
Use Treatment of rheumatoid arthritis and osteoarthritis, juvenile rheumatoid arthritis
Usual Dosage Oral:
Children ≥2 years: Anti-inflammatory: Initial: 20 mg/kg/day in 3 divided doses, then 15-30 mg/kg/day in 3 divided doses; maximum dose: 30 mg/kg/day

Adults: 400 mg 3 times/day; usual dose: 600-1.8 g/day; maximum: 2 g/day
Dosage Forms
Capsule: 400 mg
Tablet: 200 mg, 600 mg

tolnaftate (tole naf' tate)
Brand Names Absorbine® Antifungal [OTC]; Absorbine® Jock Itch [OTC]; Absorbine Jr.® Antifungal [OTC]; Aftate® [OTC]; Desenex® [OTC]; Genaspor® [OTC]; NP-27® [OTC]; Tinactin® [OTC]; Zeasorb-AF® [OTC]
Therapeutic Category Antifungal Agent, Topical
Use Treatment of tinea pedis, tinea cruris, tinea corporis; due to *Trichophyton rubrum, T. mentagrophytes, T. tonsurans, Microsporum canis, M. audouinii,* and *Epidermophyton floccosum,* and for tinea versicolor due to *Malassezia furfur*
Usual Dosage Children and Adults: Topical: Wash and dry affected area; apply 1-2 drops of solution or a small amount of cream or powder and rub into the affected areas twice daily for 2-4 weeks
(Continued)

471

tolnaftate *(Continued)*
Dosage Forms
Aerosol, topical:
Liquid: 1% (59.2 mL, 90 mL, 120 mL)
Powder: 1% (56.7 g, 100 g, 105 g, 150 g)
Cream: 1% (0.7 g, 15 g, 21.3 g, 30 g)
Gel, topical: 1% (15 g)
Powder, topical: 1% (45 g, 90 g)
Solution, topical: 1% (10 mL)

Tolu-Sed® DM [OTC] *see* guaifenesin and dextromethorphan *on page 218*
Tomocat® *see* radiological/contrast media (ionic) *on page 413*
Tonocard® *see* tocainide hydrochloride *on page 470*
Tonopaque® *see* radiological/contrast media (ionic) *on page 413*
Topicort® *see* desoximetasone *on page 132*
Topicort®-LP *see* desoximetasone *on page 132*
Topicycline® Topical *see* tetracycline *on page 458*
Toprol XL® *see* metoprolol *on page 309*
TOPV *see* poliovirus vaccine, live, trivalent, oral *on page 382*
Toradol® Injection *see* ketorolac tromethamine *on page 264*
Toradol® Oral *see* ketorolac tromethamine *on page 264*
Torecan® Injection *see* thiethylperazine maleate *on page 463*
Torecan® Oral *see* thiethylperazine maleate *on page 463*
Torecan® Rectal *see* thiethylperazine maleate *on page 463*
Tornalate® *see* bitolterol mesylate *on page 56*

torsemide
Brand Names Demadex® Injection; Demadex® Oral
Therapeutic Category Diuretic, Loop
Use Management of edema associated with congestive heart failure and hepatic or renal disease; used alone or in combination with antihypertensives in treatment of hypertension
Dosage Forms
Injection: 10 mg/mL (2 mL, 5 mL)
Tablet: 5 mg, 10 mg, 20 mg, 100 mg

Totacillin® *see* ampicillin *on page 26*
Totacillin®-N *see* ampicillin *on page 26*
Touro LA® *see* guaifenesin and pseudoephedrine *on page 220*
tp5 *see* thymopentin *on page 466*
t-PA *see* alteplase, recombinant *on page 14*
tpgs *see* tocophersolan *on page 470*
TPM® Test *see* diagnostic aids (*in vitro*), blood *on page 137*
Trace-4® *see* trace metals *on this page*

trace metals
Brand Names Chroma-Pak®; Iodopen®; Molypen®; M.T.E.-4®; M.T.E.-5®; M.T.E.-6®; Multe-Pak-4®; Neotrace-4®; Pedte-Pak-5®; Pedtrace-4®; P.T.E.-4®; P.T.E.-5®; Sele-Pak®; Sele-pen®; Trace-4®; Zinca-Pak®
Synonyms chromium injection; copper injection; iodine injection; manganese injection; molybdenum injection; neonatal trace metals; selenium injection; zinc injection

Therapeutic Category Trace Element, Parenteral
Use Supplement to TPN solutions
Dosage Forms
Chromium: Injection: 4 μg/mL, 20 μg/mL
Copper: Injection: 0.4 mg/mL, 2 mg/mL
Manganese: Injection: 0.1 mg/mL (as chloride or sulfate salt)
Molybdenum: Injection: 25 μg/mL
Selenium: Injection: 40 μg/mL
Zinc: Injection: 1 mg/mL (sulfate); 1 mg/mL (chloride); 5 mg/mL (sulfate)

Tracer bG®️ [OTC] see diagnostic aids (in vitro), blood on page 137
Tracrium®️ see atracurium besylate on page 37
Trandate®️ Injection see labetalol hydrochloride on page 265
Trandate®️ Oral see labetalol hydrochloride on page 265

tranexamic acid (tran ex am' ik)
Brand Names Cyklokapron®️ Injection; Cyklokapron®️ Oral
Therapeutic Category Antihemophilic Agent
Use Short-term use (2-8 days) in hemophilia patients during and following tooth extraction to reduce or prevent hemorrhage
Usual Dosage Children and Adults: I.V.: 10 mg/kg immediately before surgery, then 25 mg/kg/dose orally 3-4 times/day for 2-8 days

Alternatively:
Oral: 25 mg/kg 3-4 times/day beginning 1 day prior to surgery
I.V.: 10 mg/kg 3-4 times/day in patients who are unable to take oral
Dosage Forms
Injection: 100 mg/mL (10 mL)
Tablet: 500 mg

transamine sulphate see tranylcypromine sulfate on this page
Transdermal-NTG®️ Patch see nitroglycerin on page 336
Transderm-Nitro®️ Patch see nitroglycerin on page 336
Transderm Scop®️ Patch see scopolamine on page 426
Trans-Plantar®️ Transdermal Patch [OTC] see salicylic acid on page 424
Trans-Ver-Sal®️ Transdermal Patch [OTC] see salicylic acid on page 424

Tranxene®️ see clorazepate dipotassium on page 109

tranylcypromine sulfate (tran ill sip' roe meen)
Brand Names Parnate®️
Synonyms transamine sulphate
Therapeutic Category Antidepressant, Monoamine Oxidase Inhibitor
Use Symptomatic treatment of depressed patients refractory to or intolerant to tricyclic antidepressants or electroconvulsive therapy; has a more rapid onset of therapeutic effect than other MAO inhibitors, but causes more severe hypertensive reactions
Usual Dosage Adults: Oral: 10 mg twice daily, increase by 10 mg increments at 1- to 3-week intervals; maximum: 60 mg/day
Dosage Forms Tablet: 10 mg

Travase®️ Topical see sutilains on page 451

trazodone hydrochloride (traz' oh done)
Brand Names Desyrel®
Therapeutic Category Antidepressant
Use Treatment of depression
Usual Dosage Oral:
Adolescents: Initial: 25-50 mg/day; increase to 100-150 mg/day in divided doses

Adults: Initial: 150 mg/day in 3 divided doses (may increase by 50 mg/day every 3-7 days); maximum: 600 mg/day
Dosage Forms Tablet: 50 mg, 100 mg, 150 mg, 300 mg

Trecator®-SC see ethionamide on page 185

Trendar® [OTC] see ibuprofen on page 245

Trental® see pentoxifylline on page 365

tretinoin (tret' i noyn)
Brand Names Retin-A™ Topical
Synonyms retinoic acid; vitamin A acid
Therapeutic Category Acne Product; Retinoic Acid Derivative; Vitamin, Topical
Use Treatment of acne vulgaris, photodamaged skin, and some skin cancers
Usual Dosage Children >12 years and Adults: Topical: Apply once daily before retiring; if stinging or irritation develop, decrease frequency of application
Dosage Forms
Cream: 0.025% (20 g, 45 g); 0.05% (20 g, 45 g); 0.1% (20 g, 45 g)
Gel, topical: 0.01% (15 g, 45 g); 0.025% (15 g, 45 g)
Liquid, topical: 0.05% (28 mL)

Trexan™ Oral see naltrexone hydrochloride on page 324

triacetin (trye a see' tin)
Brand Names Fungoid® Topical; Ony-Clear® Nail Topical
Synonyms glycerol triacetate
Therapeutic Category Antifungal Agent, Topical
Use Fungistat for athlete's foot and other superficial fungal infections
Usual Dosage Apply twice daily, cleanse areas with dilute alcohol or mild soap and water before application; continue treatment for 7 days after symptoms have disappeared
Dosage Forms
Cream: With cetylpyridinium chloride and chloroxylenol (30 g)
Liquid: With cetylpyridinium chloride and chloroxylenol (30 mL)
Solution: With cetylpyridinium chloride, chloroxylenol, and benzalkonium chloride in an oil base (15 mL)
Spray, aerosol: With cetylpyridinium chloride, chloroxylenol, and benzalkonium chloride (45 mL, 60 mL)

Triacet® Topical see triamcinolone on this page

triacetyloleandomycin see troleandomycin on page 483

Triacin-C® see triprolidine, pseudoephedrine, and codeine on page 482

triaconazole see terconazole on page 455

Triad® see butalbital compound on page 63

Triam-A® Injection see triamcinolone on this page

triamcinolone (trye am sin' oh lone)
Brand Names Amcort® Injection; Aristocort® A Topical; Aristocort® Forte Injection; Aristocort® Intralesional Injection; Aristocort® Oral; Aristocort® Topical; Aristospan® Intra-articular Injection; Aristospan® Intralesional Injection; Articulose L.A.® Injection; Atolone®

Oral; Azmacort™ Oral Inhaler; Cenocort® A Injection; Cenocort® Forte Injection; Cinonide® Injection; Delta-Tritex® Topical; Flutex® Topical; Kenacort® Oral; Kenaject® Injection; Kenalog® Injection; Kenalog® in Orabase®; Kenalog® Topical; Kenonel® Topical; Nasacort®; Tac™-3 Injection; Tac™-40 Injection; Triacet® Topical; Triam-A® Injection; Triam Forte® Injection; Triamolone® Injection; Triamonide® Injection; Tri-Kort® Injection; Trilog® Injection; Trilone® Injection; Trisoject® Injection

Therapeutic Category Anti-inflammatory Agent; Corticosteroid, Inhalant; Corticosteroid, Systemic; Corticosteroid, Topical (Medium Potency)

Use For severe inflammation or immunosuppression

Usual Dosage In general, single I.M. dose of 4-7 times oral dose will control patient from 4-7 days up to 3-4 weeks.

Children 6-12 years:
Inhalation: 1-2 inhalations 3-4 times/day, not to exceed 12 inhalations/day
I.M.: Acetonide or hexacetonide: 0.03-0.2 mg/kg at 1- to 7-day intervals

Children >12 years and Adults:
Intranasal: 2 sprays in each nostril once daily; may increase after 4-7 days up to 4 sprays once daily or 1 spray 4 times/day in each nostril
Topical: Apply a thin film 2-3 times/day
Oral: 4-100 mg/day
I.M.: Acetonide or hexacetonide: 60 mg (of 40 mg/mL), additional 20-100 mg doses (usual: 40-80 mg) may be given when signs and symptoms recur, best at 6-week intervals to minimize HPA suppression
Oral inhalation: 2 inhalations 3-4 times/day, not to exceed 16 inhalations/day
Intra-articularly, intrasynovially, intralesionally: 2.5-40 mg as diacetate salt or acetonide salt, dose may be repeated when signs and symptoms recur
Intra-articularly: Hexacetonide: 2-20 mg every 3-4 weeks as hexacetonide salt
Intralesional (use 10 mg/mL): Diacetate or acetonide: 1 mg/injection site, may be repeated one or more times/week depending upon patients response; maximum; 30 mg at any one time; may use multiple injections if they are more than 1 cm apart
Intra-articular, intrasynovial, and soft-tissue injection (use 10 mg/mL or 40 mg/mL): Diacetate or acetonide: 2.5-40 mg depending upon location, size of joints, and degree of inflammation; repeat when signs and symptoms recur
Sublesionally (as acetonide): Up to 1 mg per injection site and may be repeated one or more times weekly; multiple sites may be injected if they are 1 cm or more apart, not to exceed 30 mg

Dosage Forms
Aerosol:
Oral inhalation: 100 μg/metered spray (2 oz)
Nasal: 55 μg per actuation (15 mL)
Topical, as acetonide: 0.2 mg/2 second spray (23 g, 63 g)
Cream, as acetonide: 0.025% (15 g, 60 g, 80 g, 240 g, 454 g); 0.1% (15 g, 30 g, 60 g, 80 g, 90 g, 120 g, 240 g); 0.5% (15 g, 20 g, 30 g, 240 g)
Injection, as acetonide: 10 mg/mL (5 mL); 40 mg/mL (1 mL, 5 mL, 10 mL)
Injection, as diacetate: 25 mg/mL (5 mL); 40 mg/mL (1 mL, 5 mL, 10 mL)
Injection, as hexacetonide: 5 mg/mL (5 mL); 20 mg/mL (1 mL, 5 mL)
Lotion, as acetonide: 0.025% (60 mL); 0.1% (15 mL, 60 mL)
Ointment:
Oral: 0.1% (5 g)
Topical, as acetonide: 0.025% (15 g, 30 g, 60 g, 80 g, 120 g, 454 g); 0.1% (15 g, 30 g, 60 g, 80 g, 120 g, 240 g, 454 g); 0.5% (15 g, 20 g, 30 g, 240 g)
Syrup: 2 mg/5 mL (120 mL); 4 mg/5 mL (120 mL)
Tablet: 1 mg, 2 mg, 4 mg, 8 mg

triamcinolone and nystatin see nystatin and triamcinolone on page 342

Triam Forte® Injection see triamcinolone on previous page

Triaminic-12® [OTC] see chlorpheniramine and phenylpropanolamine on page 93

Triaminic® Expectorant [OTC] *see* guaifenesin and phenylpropanolamine *on page 219*

Triaminicol® Multi-Symptom Cold Syrup [OTC] *see* chlorpheniramine, phenylpropanolamine, and dextromethorphan *on page 96*

Triaminic® Oral Infant Drops *see* pheniramine, phenylpropanolamine, and pyrilamine *on page 369*

Triaminic® Syrup [OTC] *see* chlorpheniramine and phenylpropanolamine *on page 93*

Triamolone® Injection *see* triamcinolone *on page 474*

Triamonide® Injection *see* triamcinolone *on page 474*

triamterene (trye am' ter een)
Brand Names Dyrenium®
Therapeutic Category Diuretic, Potassium Sparing
Use Used alone or in combination with other diuretics to treat edema and hypertension; decreases potassium excretion caused by kaliuretic diuretics
Usual Dosage Oral:
    Children: 2-4 mg/kg/day in 1-2 divided doses; maximum: 300 mg/day
    Adults: 100-300 mg/day in 1-2 divided doses; maximum dose: 300 mg/day
Dosage Forms Capsule: 50 mg, 100 mg

triamterene and hydrochlorothiazide *see* hydrochlorothiazide and triamterene *on page 234*

Triaprin® *see* butalbital compound *on page 63*

Triavil® *see* amitriptyline and perphenazine *on page 21*

triazolam (trye ay' zoe lam)
Brand Names Halcion®
Therapeutic Category Benzodiazepine; Hypnotic; Sedative
Use Short-term treatment of insomnia
Usual Dosage Oral (onset of action is rapid, patient should be in bed when taking medication):
    Children <18 years: Dosage not established
    Adults: 0.125-0.25 mg at bedtime
Dosage Forms Tablet: 0.125 mg, 0.25 mg

Triban® *see* trimethobenzamide hydrochloride *on page 480*

tribavirin *see* ribavirin *on page 419*

trichlormethiazide (trye klor meth eye' a zide)
Brand Names Metahydrin®; Naqua®
Therapeutic Category Diuretic, Thiazide
Use Management of mild to moderate hypertension; treatment of edema in congestive heart failure and nephrotic syndrome
Usual Dosage Oral:
    Children >6 months: 0.07 mg/kg/24 hours or 2 mg/m^2/24 hours
    Adults: 1-4 mg/day
Dosage Forms Tablet: 2 mg, 4 mg

trichloroacetaldehyde monohydrate *see* chloral hydrate *on page 87*

Trichophyton skin test (try ko fi' ton)
Brand Names Dermatophytin®
Therapeutic Category Diagnostic Agent, Skin Test
Use Assess cell-mediated immunity
Usual Dosage 0.1 mL intradermally, examine reaction site in 24-48 hours; induration of $\geq$5 mm in diameter is a positive reaction
Dosage Forms Injection: 1:30 (5 mL)

Tri-Clear® Expectorant [OTC] *see* guaifenesin and phenylpropanolamine *on page 219*
Tricosal® *see* choline magnesium trisalicylate *on page 100*
Tridesilon® Topical *see* desonide *on page 131*

tridihexethyl chloride (trye dye hex e' thill)
Brand Names Pathilon®
Therapeutic Category Anticholinergic Agent; Antispasmodic Agent, Gastrointestinal
Use Adjunctive therapy in peptic ulcer treatment
Usual Dosage Adults: Oral: 1-2 tablets 3-4 times/day before meals and 2 tablets at bedtime
Dosage Forms Tablet: 25 mg

Tridil® Injection *see* nitroglycerin *on page 336*
Tridione® *see* trimethadione *on page 479*

trientine hydrochloride (trye' en teen)
Brand Names Syprine®
Therapeutic Category Antidote, Copper Toxicity; Chelating Agent, Oral
Use Treatment of Wilson's disease in patients intolerant to penicillamine
Usual Dosage Oral (administer on an empty stomach):
Children <12 years: 500-750 mg/day in divided doses 2-4 times/day; maximum: 1.5 g/day
Adults: 750-1250 mg/day in divided doses 2-4 times/day; maximum daily dose: 2 g
Dosage Forms Capsule: 250 mg

triethanolamine polypeptide oleate-condensate
(trye eth a nole' a meen)
Brand Names Cerumenex® Otic
Therapeutic Category Otic Agent, Cerumenolytic
Use Removal of ear wax (cerumen)
Usual Dosage Children and Adults: Otic: Fill ear canal, insert cotton plug; allow to remain 15-30 minutes; flush ear with lukewarm water
Dosage Forms Solution, otic: 6 mL, 12 mL

triethanolamine salicylate
Brand Names Myoflex® [OTC]; Sportscreme® [OTC]
Therapeutic Category Analgesic, Topical
Use Relief of pain of muscular aches, rheumatism, neuralgia, sprains, arthritis on intact skin
Usual Dosage Apply to area as needed
Dosage Forms Cream: 10% in a nongreasy base

triethylenethiophosphoramide *see* thiotepa *on page 465*
Trifed® [OTC] *see* triprolidine and pseudoephedrine *on page 482*
Trifed-C® *see* triprolidine, pseudoephedrine, and codeine *on page 482*

trifluoperazine hydrochloride (trye floo oh per' a zeen)
Brand Names Stelazine® Injection; Stelazine® Oral
Therapeutic Category Antianxiety Agent; Antipsychotic Agent; Phenothiazine Derivative
Use Treatment of psychoses and management of anxiety
Usual Dosage

Children 6-12 years: Psychoses:

Oral: Hospitalized or well supervised patients: Initial dose: 1 mg 1-2 times/day, gradually increase until symptoms are controlled or adverse effects become troublesome; maximum: 15 mg/day

I.M.: 1 mg twice daily

Adults:

Psychoses:

Outpatients: Oral: 1-2 mg twice daily

Hospitalized or well supervised patients: Initial dose: 2-5 mg twice daily with optimum response in the 15-20 mg/day range; do not exceed 40 mg/day

I.M.: 1-2 mg every 4-6 hours as needed up to 10 mg/24 hours maximum

Nonpsychotic anxiety: Oral: 1-2 mg twice daily; maximum: 6 mg/day; therapy for anxiety should not exceed 12 weeks; do not exceed 6 mg/day for longer than 12 weeks when treating anxiety; agitation, jitteriness or insomnia may be confused with original neurotic or psychotic symptoms

Dosage Forms
Concentrate, oral: 10 mg/mL (60 mL)
Injection: 2 mg/mL (10 mL)
Tablet: 1 mg, 2 mg, 5 mg, 10 mg

trifluorothymidine *see* trifluridine *on this page*

trifluridine (trye flure' i deen)
Brand Names Viroptic® Ophthalmic
Synonyms F_3T; trifluorothymidine
Therapeutic Category Antiviral Agent, Ophthalmic
Use Treatment of primary keratoconjunctivitis and recurrent epithelial keratitis caused by herpes simplex virus types I and II
Usual Dosage Adults: Instill 1 drop into affected eye every 2 hours while awake, to a maximum of 9 drops/day, until re-epithelialization of corneal ulcer occurs; then use 1 drop every 4 hours for another 7 days; do **not** exceed 21 days of treatment
Dosage Forms Solution, ophthalmic: 1% (7.5 mL)

triglycerides, medium chain *see* medium chain triglycerides *on page 289*
Trihexy® *see* trihexyphenidyl hydrochloride *on this page*

trihexyphenidyl hydrochloride (trye hex ee fen' i dill)
Brand Names Artane®; Trihexy®
Synonyms benzhexol hydrochloride
Therapeutic Category Anticholinergic Agent; Antiparkinson Agent
Use Adjunctive treatment of Parkinson's disease; also used in treatment of drug-induced extrapyramidal effects and acute dystonic reactions
Usual Dosage

Parkinsonism: Initial: Administer 1-2 mg the first day; increase by 2 mg increments at intervals of 3-5 days, until a total of 6-10 mg is given daily. Many patients derive maximum benefit from a total daily dose of 6-10 mg; however, postencephalitic patients may require a total daily dose of 12-15 mg in 3-4 divided doses

Concomitant use with levodopa: 3-6 mg/day in divided doses is usually adequate

Drug-induced extrapyramidal disorders: Start with a single 1 mg dose; daily dosage usually ranges between 5-15 mg in 3-4 divided doses

Dosage Forms
Capsule, sustained release: 5 mg
Elixir: 2 mg/5 mL (480 mL)
Tablet: 2 mg, 5 mg

Tri-Hydroserpine® *see* hydralazine, hydrochlorothiazide, and reserpine *on page 232*

Tri-Immunol® *see* diphtheria and tetanus toxoids and pertussis vaccine, adsorbed *on page 153*

Tri-Kort® Injection *see* triamcinolone *on page 474*

Trilafon® *see* perphenazine *on page 367*

Tri-Levlen® *see* ethinyl estradiol and levonorgestrel *on page 183*

Trilisate® *see* choline magnesium trisalicylate *on page 100*

Trilog® Injection *see* triamcinolone *on page 474*

Trilone® Injection *see* triamcinolone *on page 474*

Trimazide® Oral *see* trimethobenzamide hydrochloride *on next page*

Trimazide® Rectal *see* trimethobenzamide hydrochloride *on next page*

trimeprazine tartrate (trye mep' ra zeen)
Brand Names Temaril®
Synonyms alimenazine tartrate
Therapeutic Category Antihistamine; Phenothiazine Derivative
Use Perennial and seasonal allergic rhinitis and other allergic symptoms including urticaria
Usual Dosage Oral:
Children:
6 months to 3 years: 1.25 mg at bedtime or 3 times/day if needed
>3 years: 2.5 mg at bedtime or 3 times/day if needed
>6 years: Sustained release: 5 mg/day

Adults: 2.5 mg 4 times/day (5 mg every 12-hour sustained release)
Dosage Forms
Capsule, extended release: 5 mg
Syrup: 2.5 mg/5 mL
Tablet: 2.5 mg

trimetaphan camsilate *see* trimethaphan camsylate *on next page*

trimethadione (trye meth a dye' one)
Brand Names Tridione®
Synonyms troxidone
Therapeutic Category Anticonvulsant, Oxazolidinedione
Use To control absence (petit mal) seizures refractory to other drugs
Usual Dosage Oral:
Children: Initial: 25-50 mg/kg/24 hours in 3-4 equally divided doses every 6-8 hours

Adults: Initial: 900 mg/day in 3-4 equally divided doses, increase by 300 mg/day at weekly intervals until therapeutic results or toxic symptoms appear
Dosage Forms
Capsule: 300 mg
Solution: 40 mg/mL (473 mL)
Tablet, chewable: 150 mg

trimethaphan camphorsulfonate *see* trimethaphan camsylate *on next page*

479

trimethaphan camsylate (trye meth' a fan)
Brand Names Arfonad® Injection
Synonyms trimetaphan camsilate; trimethaphan camphorsulfonate
Therapeutic Category Adrenergic Blocking Agent; Anticholinergic Agent; Ganglionic Blocking Agent
Use Immediate and temporary reduction of blood pressure in patients with hypertensive emergencies; controlled hypotension during surgery
Usual Dosage I.V.:
Children: 50-150 µg/kg/minute
Adults: Initial: 0.5-2 mg/minute; titrate to effect; usual dose: 0.3-6 mg/minute
Dosage Forms Injection: 50 mg/mL (10 mL)

trimethobenzamide hydrochloride (trye meth oh ben' za mide)
Brand Names Arrestin® Injection; Tebamide® Rectal; T-Gen® Rectal; Ticon® Injection; Tigan® Injection; Tigan® Oral; Tigan® Rectal; Tiject® Injection; Triban®; Trimazide® Oral; Trimazide® Rectal
Therapeutic Category Antiemetic
Use Control of nausea and vomiting (especially for long-term antiemetic therapy)
Usual Dosage Rectal use: Contraindicated in neonates and premature infants
Children:
Oral, rectal: 15-20 mg/kg/day or 400-500 mg/m²/day divided into 3-4 doses
I.M.: Not recommended

Adults:
Oral: 250 mg 3-4 times/day
I.M., rectal: 200 mg 3-4 times/day
Dosage Forms
Capsule: 100 mg, 250 mg
Injection: 100 mg/mL (2 mL, 20 mL)
Suppository, rectal: 100 mg, 200 mg

trimethoprim (trye meth' oh prim)
Brand Names Proloprim®; Trimpex®
Synonyms TMP
Therapeutic Category Antibiotic, Miscellaneous
Use Treatment of urinary tract infections; acute otitis media in children; acute exacerbations of chronic bronchitis in adults
Usual Dosage Adults: Oral: 100 mg every 12 hours or 200 mg every 24 hours
Dosage Forms Tablet: 100 mg, 200 mg

trimethoprim and polymyxin b
Brand Names Polytrim® Ophthalmic
Synonyms polymyxin b and trimethoprim
Therapeutic Category Antibiotic, Ophthalmic
Use Treatment of surface ocular bacterial conjunctivitis and blepharoconjunctivitis
Usual Dosage Ophthalmic: Instill 1-2 drops in eye(s) every 4-6 hours
Dosage Forms Solution, ophthalmic: Trimethoprim sulfate 1 mg and polymyxin b sulfate 10,000 units per mL (10 mL)

trimethoprim and sulfamethoxazole *see co-trimoxazole on page 118*
trimethylpsoralen *see trioxsalen on next page*

trimetrexate glucuronate (tri me trex' ate glue cur ron' ate)
Brand Names Neutrexin™ Injection
Therapeutic Category Folic Acid Antagonist
Use Alternative therapy for the treatment of moderate-to-severe *Pneumocystis carinii* pneumonia (PCP) in immunocomprised patients, including patients with acquired immunodefi-

ciency syndrome (AIDS), who are intolerant of, or are refractory to co-trimoxazole therapy or for whom co-trimoxazole is contraindicated
Usual Dosage Adults: I.V.: 45 mg/m² once daily over 60 minutes for 21 days
Dosage Forms Injection: 25 mg

trimipramine maleate (trye mi' pra meen)
Brand Names Surmontil®
Therapeutic Category Antidepressant, Tricyclic
Use Treatment of various forms of depression, often in conjunction with psychotherapy
Usual Dosage Oral: 50-150 mg/day as a single bedtime dose
Dosage Forms Capsule: 25 mg, 50 mg, 100 mg

Trimox® *see* amoxicillin trihydrate *on page 24*

Trimpex® *see* trimethoprim *on previous page*

Trinalin® *see* azatadine and pseudoephedrine *on page 40*

Trind® Liquid [OTC] *see* chlorpheniramine and phenylpropanolamine *on page 93*

Tri-Norinyl® *see* ethinyl estradiol and norethindrone *on page 183*

Triofed® [OTC] *see* triprolidine and pseudoephedrine *on next page*

Triostat™ Injection *see* liothyronine sodium *on page 274*

trioxsalen (trye ox' sa len)
Brand Names Trisoralen® Oral
Synonyms trimethylpsoralen
Therapeutic Category Psoralen
Use In conjunction with controlled exposure to ultraviolet light or sunlight for repigmentation of idiopathic vitiligo; increasing tolerance to sunlight with albinism; enhance pigmentation
Usual Dosage Children > 12 years and Adults: Oral: 10 mg/day as a single dose, 2-4 hours before controlled exposure to UVA or sunlight
Dosage Forms Tablet: 5 mg

Tripalgen® Cold [OTC] *see* chlorpheniramine and phenylpropanolamine *on page 93*

Tripedia® *see* diphtheria, tetanus toxoids, and acellular pertussis vaccine *on page 154*

tripelennamine (tri pel enn' a meen)
Brand Names PBZ®; PBZ-SR®
Synonyms pyribenzamine®; tripelennamine citrate; tripelennamine hydrochloride
Therapeutic Category Antihistamine
Use Perennial and seasonal allergic rhinitis and other allergic symptoms including urticaria
Usual Dosage Oral:
Infants and Children: 5 mg/kg/day in 4-6 divided doses, up to 300 mg/day maximum

Adults: 25-50 mg every 4-6 hours, extended release tablets 100 mg morning and evening up to 100 mg every 8 hours
Dosage Forms
Elixir, as citrate: 37.5 mg/5 mL (473 mL)
Tablet, as hydrochloride: 25 mg, 50 mg
Tablet, extended release, as hydrochloride: 100 mg

tripelennamine citrate *see* tripelennamine *on this page*
tripelennamine hydrochloride *see* tripelennamine *on this page*

Triphasil® *see* ethinyl estradiol and levonorgestrel *on page 183*

Tri-Phen-Chlor® *see* chlorpheniramine, phenyltoloxamine, phenylpropanolamine, and phenylephrine *on page 96*

Triphenyl® Expectorant [OTC] *see* guaifenesin and phenylpropanolamine *on page 219*

Triphenyl® Syrup [OTC] *see* chlorpheniramine and phenylpropanolamine *on page 93*

Triple Antibiotic® Topical *see* bacitracin, neomycin, and polymyxin b *on page 43*

triple sulfa *see* sulfabenzamide, sulfacetamide, and sulfathiazole *on page 446*

Triposed® [OTC] *see* triprolidine and pseudoephedrine *on this page*

triprolidine and pseudoephedrine (trye proe' li deen)

Brand Names Actagen® [OTC]; Actifed® [OTC]; Allerfrin® [OTC]; Allerphed [OTC]; Aprodine® [OTC]; Cenafed® Plus [OTC]; Genac® [OTC]; Trifed® [OTC]; Triofed® [OTC]; Triposed® [OTC]

Synonyms pseudoephedrine and triprolidine

Therapeutic Category Antihistamine/Decongestant Combination

Use Temporary relief of nasal congestion, running nose, sneezing, itching of nose or throat and itchy, watery eyes due to common cold, hay fever or other upper respiratory allergies

Usual Dosage May dose according to **pseudoephedrine** component (4 mg/kg/day in divided doses 3-4 times/day) Oral:

Children:
    4 months to 2 years: 1.25 mL 3-4 times/day
    2-4 years: 2.5 mL 3-4 times/day
    4-6 years: 3.75 mL 3-4 times/day
    6-12 years: 5 mL or ½ tablet 3-4 times/day, not to exceed 2 tablets/day

Children >12 years and Adults: 10 mL or 1 tablet 3-4 times/day, not to exceed 4 tablets/day

Dosage Forms
Capsule: Triprolidine hydrochloride 2.5 mg and pseudoephedrine hydrochloride 60 mg
Capsule, extended release: Triprolidine hydrochloride 5 mg and pseudoephedrine hydrochloride 120 mg
Syrup: Triprolidine hydrochloride 1.25 mg and pseudoephedrine hydrochloride 30 mg per 5 mL
Tablet: Triprolidine hydrochloride 2.5 mg and pseudoephedrine hydrochloride 60 mg

triprolidine, pseudoephedrine, and codeine

Brand Names Actagen-C®; Actifed® With Codeine; Allerfrin® w/Codeine; Aprodine® w/C; Triacin-C®; Trifed-C®

Therapeutic Category Antihistamine/Decongestant Combination; Cough Preparation

Use Symptomatic relief of cough

Usual Dosage Oral:
Children:
    2-6 years: 2.5 mL 4 times/day
    7-12 years: 5 mL 4 times/day

Children >12 years and Adults: 10 mL 4 times/day

Dosage Forms Syrup: Triprolidine hydrochloride 1.25 mg, pseudoephedrine hydrochloride 30 mg, and codeine phosphate 10 mg per 5 mL with alcohol 4.3%

TripTone® Caplets® [OTC] *see* dimenhydrinate *on page 150*

tris buffer *see* tromethamine *on next page*

tris(hydroxymethyl)aminomethane *see* tromethamine *on next page*

Trisoject® Injection *see* triamcinolone *on page 474*

Trisoralen® Oral *see* trioxsalen *on page 481*

Tri-Statin® II Topical *see* nystatin and triamcinolone *on page 342*

Tritan® *see* chlorpheniramine, pyrilamine, and phenylephrine *on page 97*

Tri-Tannate Plus® *see* chlorpheniramine, ephedrine, phenylephrine, and carbetapentane *on page 94*

Tritann® Pediatric *see* chlorpheniramine, pyrilamine, and phenylephrine *on page 97*

Tri-Thalmic® Ophthalmic Solution *see* neomycin, polymyxin b, and gramicidin *on page 329*

Tri-Vi-Flor® Chewable Tablet *see* vitamin, multiple (pediatric) *on page 499*

Tri-Vi-Flor® Drops *see* vitamin, multiple (pediatric) *on page 499*

Tri-Vi-Sol® Chewable Tablet [OTC] *see* vitamin, multiple (pediatric) *on page 499*

Tri-Vi-Sol® Drops [OTC] *see* vitamin, multiple (pediatric) *on page 499*

Trobicin® Injection *see* spectinomycin hydrochloride *on page 442*

Trocal® [OTC] *see* dextromethorphan hydrobromide *on page 136*

troleandomycin (troe lee an doe mye' sin)
Brand Names Tao®
Synonyms triacetyloleandomycin
Therapeutic Category Antibiotic, Macrolide
Use Adjunct in the treatment of corticosteroid-dependent asthma due to its steroid sparing properties; obsolete antibiotic with spectrum of activity similar to erythromycin
Usual Dosage Oral:
Children: 25-40 mg/kg/day divided every 6 hours
Adjunct in corticosteroid-dependent asthma: 14 mg/kg/day in divided doses every 6-12 hours not to exceed 250 mg every 6 hours; dose is tapered to once daily then alternate day dosing

Adults: 250-500 mg 4 times/day
Dosage Forms Capsule: 250 mg

tromethamine (troe meth' a meen)
Brand Names THAM-E® Injection; THAM® Injection
Synonyms tris buffer; tris(hydroxymethyl)aminomethane
Therapeutic Category Alkalinizing Agent, Parenteral
Use Correction of metabolic acidosis associated with cardiac bypass surgery or cardiac arrest; to correct excess acidity of stored blood that is preserved with acid citrate dextrose; to prime the pump-oxygenator during cardiac bypass surgery; indicated in infants needing alkalinization after receiving maximum sodium bicarbonate (8-10 mEq/kg/24 hours); (advantage of THAM® is that it alkalinizes without increasing pCO_2 and sodium)
Usual Dosage Dose depends on buffer base deficit; when deficit is known: tromethamine mL of 0.3 M solution = body weight (kg) x base deficit (mEq/L); when base deficit is not known: 3-6 mL/kg/dose I.V. (1-2 mEq/kg/dose)

Metabolic acidosis with cardiac arrest:
I.V.: 3.5-6 mL/kg (1-2 mEq/kg/dose) into large peripheral vein
I.V.: 500-1000 mL if needed in adults
I.V. continuous drip: Infuse slowly by syringe pump over 3-6 hours

Excess acidity of ACD priming blood: 14-70 mL of 0.3 molar solution added to each 500 mL of blood
Dosage Forms Injection:
THAM®: 18 g [0.3 molar] (500 mL)
THAM-E®: 36 g with sodium 30 mEq, potassium 5 mEq, and chloride 35 mEq (1000 mL)

Tronolane® **[OTC]** *see* pramoxine hydrochloride *on page 390*
Tronothane® **[OTC]** *see* pramoxine hydrochloride *on page 390*
Tropicacyl® Ophthalmic *see* tropicamide *on this page*

tropicamide (troe pik' a mide)
Brand Names I-Picamide® Ophthalmic; Mydriacyl® Ophthalmic; Tropicacyl® Ophthalmic
Synonyms bistropamide
Therapeutic Category Ophthalmic Agent, Mydriatic
Use Short-acting mydriatic used in diagnostic procedures; as well as preoperatively and postoperatively; treatment of some cases of acute iritis, iridocyclitis, and keratitis
Usual Dosage Children and Adults:
Cycloplegia: 1-2 drops (1%); may repeat in 5 minutes
Mydriasis: 1-2 drops (0.5%) 15-20 minutes before exam; may repeat every 30 minutes as needed
Dosage Forms Solution, ophthalmic: 0.5% (2 mL, 15 mL); 1% (2 mL, 3 mL, 15 mL)

troxidone *see* trimethadione *on page 479*
Truphylline® *see* aminophylline *on page 19*

trypsin, balsam peru, and castor oil
Brand Names Granulex
Therapeutic Category Protectant, Topical; Topical Skin Product
Use Treatment of decubitus ulcers, varicose ulcers, debridement of eschar, dehiscent wounds and sunburn
Usual Dosage Topical: Apply a minimum of twice daily or as often as necessary
Dosage Forms Aerosol, topical: Trypsin 0.1 mg, balsam Peru 72.5 mg, and castor oil 650 mg per 0.82 mL (60 g, 120 g)

Trysul® Vaginal *see* sulfabenzamide, sulfacetamide, and sulfathiazole *on page 446*
TSH *see* thyrotropin *on page 467*
TSPA *see* thiotepa *on page 465*
T-Stat® Topical *see* erythromycin, topical *on page 176*

tuberculin tests
Brand Names Aplisol®; Tubersol®
Synonyms Mantoux; old tuberculin; OT; PPD; purified protein derivative
Therapeutic Category Diagnostic Agent, Skin Test
Use Skin test in diagnosis of tuberculosis, to aid in assessment of cell-mediated immunity; routine tuberculin testing is recommended at 12 months of age and at every 1-2 years thereafter, before the measles vaccination
Usual Dosage Children and Adults: Intradermally: 0.1 mL approximately 4" below elbow; use $^1/_4$" to $^1/_2$" or 26- or 27-gauge needle; significant reactions are ≥5 mm in diameter
Dosage Forms Injection:
First test strength: 1 TU/0.1 mL
Intermediate test strength: 5 TU/0.1 mL
Second test strength: 250 TU/0.1 mL
Tine: 5 TU each test

Tubersol® *see* tuberculin tests *on this page*

tubocurarine chloride (too boe kyoor ar' een)
Synonyms *d*-tubocurarine chloride
Therapeutic Category Neuromuscular Blocker Agent, Nondepolarizing; Skeletal Muscle Relaxant

Use Adjunct to anesthesia to induce skeletal muscle relaxation
Usual Dosage I.V.:
Neonates <1 month: 0.3 mg/kg as a single dose; maintenance: 0.15 mg/kg/dose as needed to maintain paralysis
Children and Adults: 0.2-0.4 mg/kg as a single dose; maintenance: 0.04-0.2 mg/kg/dose as needed to maintain paralysis
Alternative adult dose: 6-9 mg once daily, then 3-4.5 mg as needed to maintain paralysis
Dosage Forms Injection: 3 mg/mL [3 units/mL] (5 mL, 10 mL, 20 mL)

Tucks® **[OTC]** *see* witch hazel *on page 501*
Tuinal® *see* amobarbital and secobarbital *on page 23*
Tums® **[OTC]** *see* calcium carbonate *on page 65*
Tums® E-X Extra Strength Tablet [OTC] *see* calcium carbonate *on page 65*
Tums® Extra Strength Liquid [OTC] *see* calcium carbonate *on page 65*
Tussafed® Drops *see* carbinoxamine, pseudoephedrine, and dextromethorphan *on page 74*
Tussafin® Expectorant *see* hydrocodone, pseudoephedrine, and guaifenesin *on page 236*
Tuss-Allergine® Modified T.D. Capsule *see* caramiphen and phenylpropanolamine *on page 72*
Tuss-DM® [OTC] *see* guaifenesin and dextromethorphan *on page 218*
Tuss-Genade® Modified Capsule *see* caramiphen and phenylpropanolamine *on page 72*
Tussigon® *see* hydrocodone and homatropine *on page 235*
Tussionex® *see* hydrocodone and chlorpheniramine *on page 234*
Tussi-Organidin® *see* iodinated glycerol and codeine *on page 254*
Tussi-Organidin® DM *see* iodinated glycerol and dextromethorphan *on page 254*
Tussi-R-Gen® *see* iodinated glycerol and codeine *on page 254*
Tussi-R-Gen DM® *see* iodinated glycerol and dextromethorphan *on page 254*
Tuss-LA® *see* guaifenesin and pseudoephedrine *on page 220*
Tusso-DM® *see* iodinated glycerol and dextromethorphan *on page 254*
Tussogest® Extended Release Capsule *see* caramiphen and phenylpropanolamine *on page 72*
Tuss-Ornade® Liquid *see* caramiphen and phenylpropanolamine *on page 72*
Tuss-Ornade® Spansule® *see* caramiphen and phenylpropanolamine *on page 72*
Tusstat® Syrup *see* diphenhydramine hydrochloride *on page 152*
Twilite® Oral [OTC] *see* diphenhydramine hydrochloride *on page 152*
Two-Dyne® *see* butalbital compound *on page 63*
Tylenol® [OTC] *see* acetaminophen *on page 2*
Tylenol® Cold Effervescent Medication Tablet [OTC] *see* chlorpheniramine, phenylpropanolamine, and acetaminophen *on page 96*
Tylenol® With Codeine *see* acetaminophen and codeine *on page 3*
Tylox® *see* oxycodone and acetaminophen *on page 349*

typhoid vaccine
Brand Names Vivotif Berna™ Oral
Synonyms typhoid vaccine live oral ty21a
Therapeutic Category Vaccine, Inactivated Bacteria
(Continued)
485

typhoid vaccine *(Continued)*

Use Promotes active immunity to typhoid fever for patients exposed to typhoid carrier or foreign travel to typhoid fever endemic area

Usual Dosage

S.C.:
  Children 6 months to 10 years: 0.25 mL; repeat in ≥4 weeks (total immunization is 2 doses)
  Adults and Children >10 years: 0.5 mL; repeat dose in ≥4 weeks (total immunization is 2 doses)
  Booster: 0.25 mL every 3 years for children 6 months to 10 years and 0.5 mL every 3 years for adults and children >10 years

Oral: Adults:
  Primary immunization: 1 capsule on alternate days (day 1, 3, 5, and 7)
  Booster immunization: Repeat full course of primary immunization every 5 years

Dosage Forms

Capsule, enteric coated: Viable *S. typhi* Ty21a Colony-forming units 2-6 x 10^9 and nonviable *S. typhi* Ty21a Colony-forming units 50 x 10^9 with sucrose, ascorbic acid, amino acid mixture, lactose and magnesium stearate
Injection: 1.5 mL

typhoid vaccine live oral ty21a *see* typhoid vaccine *on previous page*

tyropanoate sodium *see* radiological/contrast media (ionic) *on page 413*

Tyzine® Nasal *see* tetrahydrozoline hydrochloride *on page 459*

UAD® Topical *see* clioquinol and hydrocortisone *on page 106* ·

Ucephan® Oral *see* sodium phenylacetate and sodium benzoate *on page 437*

UCG-Slide® Test *see* diagnostic aids (*in vitro*), urine *on page 139*

U-Cort™ Topical *see* hydrocortisone *on page 236*

uk *see* urokinase *on page 488*

ULR® *see* guaifenesin, phenylpropanolamine, and phenylephrine *on page 221*

ULR-LA® *see* guaifenesin and phenylpropanolamine *on page 219*

ULTRAbrom® PD *see* brompheniramine and pseudoephedrine *on page 59*

Ultracef® *see* cefadroxil monohydrate *on page 78*

Ultralente *see* insulin preparations *on page 250*

Ultralente® Iletin® I *see* insulin preparations *on page 250*

Ultra Mide® Topical *see* urea *on next page*

Ultravate™ Topical *see* halobetasol propionate *on page 224*

Unasyn® *see* ampicillin sodium and sulbactam sodium *on page 26*

undecylenic acid and derivatives (un de sill enn' ik)

Brand Names Caldesene® Topical [OTC]; Cruex® Topical [OTC]; Merlenate® Topical [OTC]; Pedi-Dri Topical; Pedi-Pro Topical [OTC]; Quinsana® Plus Topical [OTC]; Undogu-ent® Topical [OTC]

Synonyms calcium undecylenate; zinc undecylenate

Therapeutic Category Antifungal Agent, Topical

Use Antifungal/antibacterial agents for athlete's foot and ringworm exclusive of nails and hairy areas; relief of diaper rash, jock itch, and other minor skin irritation; excessive perspiration and irritation in the groin area

Usual Dosage Children and Adults: Topical: Apply as needed twice daily after cleansing the affected area for 2-4 weeks

Dosage Forms

Cream: Total undecylenate 20% (15 g, 82.5 g)

Foam, topical: Undecylenic acid 10% (42.5 g)
Liquid, topical: Undecylenic acid 10% (42.5 g)
Ointment, topical: Total undecylenate 22% (30 g, 60 g, 454 g); total undecylenate 25% (60 g, 454 g)
Powder, topical: Calcium undecylenate 10% (45 g, 60 g, 120 g); total undecylenate 22% (45 g, 54 g, 81 g, 90 g, 105 g, 165 g, 454 g)

Undoguent® Topical [OTC] *see* undecylenic acid and derivatives *on previous page*

Unguentine® [OTC] *see* benzocaine *on page 48*

Uni-Ace® [OTC] *see* acetaminophen *on page 2*

Uni-Bent® Cough Syrup *see* diphenhydramine hydrochloride *on page 152*

Uni-Decon® *see* chlorpheniramine, phenyltoloxamine, phenylpropanolamine, and phenylephrine *on page 96*

Unilax® [OTC] *see* docusate and phenolphthalein *on page 158*

Unipen® Injection *see* nafcillin sodium *on page 322*

Unipen® Oral *see* nafcillin sodium *on page 322*

Uniphyl® *see* theophylline *on page 460*

Unipres® *see* hydralazine, hydrochlorothiazide, and reserpine *on page 232*

Uni-Pro® [OTC] *see* ibuprofen *on page 245*

Uni-tussin® [OTC] *see* guaifenesin *on page 217*

Uni-tussin® DM [OTC] *see* guaifenesin and dextromethorphan *on page 218*

Unna's boot *see* zinc gelatin *on page 503*

Unna's paste *see* zinc gelatin *on page 503*

Uracel® *see* sodium salicylate *on page 439*

uracil mustard (yoor' a sil)
Therapeutic Category Antineoplastic Agent, Alkylating Agent (Nitrogen Mustard)
Use Palliative treatment in symptomatic chronic lymphocytic leukemia; non-Hodgkin's lymphomas
Usual Dosage Refer to individual protocols
Oral:
Children: 0.3 mg/kg in a single weekly dose for 4 weeks

Adults: 0.15 mg/kg in a single weekly dose for 4 weeks
Thrombocytosis: 1-2 mg/day for 14 days
Dosage Forms Capsule: 1 mg

urea
Brand Names Amino-Cerv™ Vaginal Cream; Aquacare® Topical [OTC]; Carmol® Topical [OTC]; Gormel® Creme [OTC]; Lanaphilic® Topical [OTC]; Nutraplus® Topical [OTC]; Rea-Lo® [OTC]; Ultra Mide® Topical; Ureacin®-20 Topical [OTC]; Ureacin®-40 Topical; Ureaphil® Injection
Synonyms carbamide
Therapeutic Category Diuretic, Osmotic; Topical Skin Product
Use Reduce intracranial pressure and intraocular pressure (30%); promotes hydration and removal of excess keratin in hyperkeratotic conditions and dry skin; mild cervicitis
Usual Dosage
Children: I.V. slow infusion:
<2 years: 0.1-0.5 g/kg
>2 years: 0.5-1.5 g/kg

Adults:
I.V. infusion: 1-1.5 g/kg by slow infusion (1-2$\frac{1}{2}$ hours); maximum: 120 g/24 hours
(Continued)
487

urea *(Continued)*

Topical: Apply 1-3 times/day
Vaginal: 1 applicatorful in vagina at bedtime for 2-4 weeks
Dosage Forms
Cream:
Topical: 2% [20 mg/mL] (75 g); 10% [100 mg/mL] (75 g, 90 g, 454 g); 20% [200 mg/mL] (45 g, 75 g, 90 g, 454 g); 30% [300 mg/mL] (60 g, 454 g); 40% (30 g)
Vaginal: 8.34% [83.4 mg/g] (82.5 g)
Injection: 40 g/150 mL
Lotion: 2% (240 mL); 10% (180 mL, 240 mL, 480 mL); 15% (120 mL, 480 mL); 25% (180 mL)

urea and hydrocortisone

Brand Names Carmol-HC® Topical
Synonyms hydrocortisone and urea
Therapeutic Category Corticosteroid, Topical (Low Potency); Topical Skin Product
Use Inflammation of corticosteroid-responsive dermatoses
Usual Dosage Topical: Apply thin film and rub in well 1-4 times/day
Dosage Forms Cream, topical: Urea 10% and hydrocortisone acetate 1% in a water-washable vanishing cream base (30 g)

Ureacin®-20 Topical [OTC] *see* urea *on previous page*

Ureacin®-40 Topical *see* urea *on previous page*

urea peroxide *see* carbamide peroxide *on page 73*

Ureaphil® Injection *see* urea *on previous page*

Urecholine® *see* bethanechol chloride *on page 53*

Urex® *see* methenamine *on page 299*

Uricult® *see* diagnostic aids (*in vitro*), urine *on page 139*

Urispas® *see* flavoxate hydrochloride *on page 196*

Uristix® *see* diagnostic aids (*in vitro*), urine *on page 139*

Uri-Tet® Oral *see* oxytetracycline hydrochloride *on page 352*

Urobak® *see* sulfamethoxazole *on page 448*

Urodine® *see* phenazopyridine hydrochloride *on page 368*

urofollitropin *(yoor oh fol li troe' pin)*

Brand Names Metrodin® Injection
Therapeutic Category Ovulation Stimulator
Use Induction of ovulation in patients with polycystic ovarian disease and to stimulate the development of multiple oocytes
Usual Dosage Adults: Female: I.M.: 75 units/day for 7-12 days, used with hCG may repeat course of treatment 2 more times
Dosage Forms Injection: 0.83 mg [75 units FSH activity] (2 mL)

urokinase *(yoor oh kin' ase)*

Brand Names Abbokinase® Injection
Synonyms uk
Therapeutic Category Thrombolytic Agent
Use Thrombolytic agent used in treatment of recent severe or massive deep vein thrombosis, pulmonary emboli, myocardial infarction, and occluded arteriovenous cannulas
Usual Dosage
Children and Adults: Deep vein thrombosis: I.V.: Loading: 4400 units/kg over 10 minutes, then 4400 units/kg/hour for 12 hours

Adults:
Myocardial infarction: Intracoronary: 750,000 units over 2 hours (6000 units/minute over up to 2 hours)
Occluded I.V. catheters:
5000 units (use only Abbokinase® Open Cath) in each lumen over 1-2 minutes, leave in lumen for 1-4 hours, then aspirate; may repeat with 10,000 units in each lumen if 5000 units fails to clear the catheter; **do not infuse into the patient**; volume to instill into catheter is equal to the volume of the catheter
I.V. infusion: 200 units/kg/hour in each lumen for 12-48 hours at a rate of at least 20 mL/hour
Dialysis patients: 5000 units is administered in each lumen over 1-2 minutes; leave urokinase in lumen for 1-2 days, then aspirate
Clot lysis (large vessel thrombi): Loading: I.V.: 4400 units/kg over 10 minutes, increase to 6000 units/kg/hour; maintenance: 4400-6000 units/kg/hour adjusted to achieve clot lysis or patency of affected vessel; doses up to 50,000 units/kg/hour have been used. **Note:** Therapy should be initiated as soon as possible after diagnosis of thrombi and continued until clot is dissolved (usually 24-72 hours).
Acute pulmonary embolism: Three treatment alternatives: 3 million unit dosage
Alternative 1: 12-hour infusion: 4400 units/kg (2000 units/lb) bolus over 10 minutes followed by 4400 units/kg/hour (2000 units/lb); begin heparin 1000 units/hour approximately 3-4 hours after completion of urokinase infusion or when PTT is <100 seconds
Alternative 2: 2-hour infusion: 1 million unit bolus over 10 minutes followed by 2 million units over 110 minutes; begin heparin 1000 units/hour approximately 3-4 hours after completion of urokinase infusion or when PTT is <100 seconds
Alternative 3: Bolus dose only: 15,000 units/kg over 10 minutes; begin heparin 1000 units/hour approximately 3-4 hours after completion of urokinase infusion or when PTT is <100 seconds

Dosage Forms
Powder for injection: 250,000 units (5 mL)
Powder for injection, catheter clear: 5000 units (1 mL)

Uro-KP-Neutral® *see* potassium phosphate and sodium phosphate *on page 388*

Urolene Blue® Oral *see* methylene blue *on page 305*

Uroplus® DS *see* co-trimoxazole *on page 118*

Uroplus® SS *see* co-trimoxazole *on page 118*

Urovist Cysto® *see* radiological/contrast media (ionic) *on page 413*

Urovist® Meglumine *see* radiological/contrast media (ionic) *on page 413*

Urovist® Sodium 300 *see* radiological/contrast media (ionic) *on page 413*

ursodeoxycholic acid *see* ursodiol *on this page*

ursodiol (er' soe dye ole)
Brand Names Actigall™
Synonyms ursodeoxycholic acid
Therapeutic Category Gallstone Dissolution Agent
Use Gallbladder stone dissolution
Usual Dosage Oral: 8-10 mg/kg/day in 2-3 divided doses
Dosage Forms Capsule: 300 mg

Uticort® Topical *see* betamethasone *on page 52*

Vagilia® Vaginal *see* sulfabenzamide, sulfacetamide, and sulfathiazole *on page 446*

Vagistat® Vaginal *see* tioconazole *on page 469*

Vagitrol® Vaginal *see* sulfanilamide *on page 448*

Valergen® Injection *see* estradiol *on page 178*

Valertest No.1® Injection *see* estradiol and testosterone *on page 178*

Valisone® Topical *see* betamethasone *on page 52*

Valium® Injection *see* diazepam *on page 142*

Valium® Oral *see* diazepam *on page 142*

Valpin® 50 *see* anisotropine methylbromide *on page 28*

valproic acid and derivatives (val proe' ik)

Brand Names Depakene®; Depakote®

Synonyms dipropylacetic acid; divalproex sodium; DPA; 2-propylpentanoic acid; 2-propylvaleric acid

Therapeutic Category Anticonvulsant, Miscellaneous

Use Management of simple and complex absence seizures; mixed seizure types; myoclonic and generalized tonic-clonic (grand mal) seizures; may be effective in partial seizures and infantile spasms

Usual Dosage Children and Adults:

Oral: Initial: 10-15 mg/kg/day in 1-3 divided doses; increase by 5-10 mg/kg/day at weekly intervals until therapeutic levels are achieved; maintenance: 30-60 mg/kg/day in 2-3 divided doses

Children receiving more than 1 anticonvulsant (ie, polytherapy) may require doses up to 100 mg/kg/day in 3-4 divided doses

Rectal: Dilute syrup 1:1 with water for use as a retention enema; loading dose: 20 mg/kg one time; maintenance: 10-15 mg/kg/dose every 8 hours beginning 8 hours after administration of the loading dose

Dosage Forms

Capsule, sprinkle, as divalproex sodium (Depakote® Sprinkle®): 125 mg

Capsule, as valproic acid (Depakene®): 250 mg

Syrup, as sodium valproate (Depakene®): 250 mg/5mL (5 mL, 50 mL, 480 mL)

Tablet, delayed release, as divalproex sodium (Depakote®): 125 mg, 250 mg, 500 mg

Valrelease® Oral *see* diazepam *on page 142*

Vamate® Oral *see* hydroxyzine *on page 241*

Vancenase® AQ Inhaler *see* beclomethasone dipropionate *on page 45*

Vancenase® Nasal Inhaler *see* beclomethasone dipropionate *on page 45*

Vanceril® Oral Inhaler *see* beclomethasone dipropionate *on page 45*

Vancocin® Injection *see* vancomycin hydrochloride *on this page*

Vancocin® Oral *see* vancomycin hydrochloride *on this page*

Vancoled® Injection *see* vancomycin hydrochloride *on this page*

vancomycin hydrochloride (van koe mye' sin)

Brand Names Lyphocin® Injection; Vancocin® Injection; Vancocin® Oral; Vancoled® Injection

Therapeutic Category Antibiotic, Miscellaneous

Use Used in the treatment of patients with the following infections or conditions: treatment of infections due to documented or suspected methicillin-resistant *S. aureus* or beta-lactam resistant coagulase negative *Staphylococcus*; treatment of serious or life-threatening infections (ie, endocarditis, meningitis) due to documented or suspected staphylococcal or streptococcal infections in patients who are allergic to penicillins and/or cephalosporins; empiric therapy of infections associated with central lines, VP shunts, vascular grafts, prosthetic heart valves; treatment of febrile granulocytopenic patient who has not responded after 48 hours to antibiotic treatment directed at gram-negative rod infections; used orally for staphylococcal enterocolitis or for antibiotic-associated pseudomembranous colitis produced by *C. difficile*

Usual Dosage Initial dosage recommendation: I.V.:
Neonates:
Postnatal age <7 days:
<1200 g: 7.5 mg/kg/dose given every 24 hours
1200-2000 g: 10 mg/kg/dose given every 12 hours
>2000 g: 15 mg/kg/dose given every 12 hours
Postnatal age >7 days:
<1200 g: 7.5 mg/kg/dose given every 24 hours
≥1200 g: 10 mg/kg/dose given every 8 hours

Infants >1 month and Children: 40 mg/kg/day in divided doses every 6 hours

Infants >1 month and Children with staphylococcal central nervous system infection: 60 mg/kg/day in divided doses every 6 hours

Note: Some patients may require larger or more frequent doses if serum levels document the need (ie, febrile granulocytopenic patients)

Adults:
<60 kg: 750 mg every 12 hours
60-100 kg: 1 g every 12 hours
100-120 kg: 1.25 g every 12 hours
>120 kg: 1.5 g every 12 hours

Dosing interval in renal impairment: Following a usual loading dose, dosages and frequency of administration are best determined by measurement of serum levels and assessment of renal insufficiency
Not dialyzable (0% to 5%)

Dosing adjustments/comments in hepatic impairment: Reduce dose by 60%

Intrathecal:
Neonates: 5-10 mg/day
Children: 5-20 mg/day
Adults: 20 mg/day

Oral: Pseudomembranous colitis produced by *C. difficile*:
Neonates: 10 mg/kg/day in divided doses
Children: 40 mg/kg/day in divided doses, added to fluids
Adults: 250-500 mg 3 times/day in divided doses

Dosage Forms
Capsule: 125 mg, 250 mg
Powder for oral solution: 1 g, 10 g
Powder for injection: 500 mg, 1 g, 2 g, 5 g, 10 g

Vanex-LA® *see* guaifenesin and phenylpropanolamine *on page 219*

Vanoxide® [OTC] *see* benzoyl peroxide *on page 49*

Vanoxide-HC® *see* benzoyl peroxide and hydrocortisone *on page 50*

Vansil™ *see* oxamniquine *on page 348*

Vantin® *see* cefpodoxime proxetil *on page 81*

Vaponefrin® Inhalation Solution [OTC] *see* epinephrine *on page 171*

varicella-zoster immune globulin (human) (veer i sel' a- zos' ter)
Synonyms VZIG
Therapeutic Category Immune Globulin
Use Passive immunization of susceptible immunodeficient patients after exposure to varicella; most effective if begun within 96 hours of exposure

VZIG supplies are limited, restrict administration to those meeting the following criteria:
One of the following underlying illnesses or conditions:
Neoplastic disease (eg, leukemia or lymphoma)
Congenital or acquired immunodeficiency

(Continued)
491

varicella-zoster immune globulin (human) *(Continued)*

Immunosuppressive therapy with steroids, antimetabolites or other immunosuppressive treatment regimens

Newborn of mother who had onset of chickenpox within 5 days before delivery or within 48 hours after delivery

Premature (≥28 weeks gestation) whose mother has no history of chickenpox

Premature (<28 weeks gestation or ≤1000 g VZIG) regardless of maternal history

One of the following types of exposure to chickenpox or zoster patient(s):
Continuous household contact

Playmate contact (>1 hour play indoors)

Hospital contact (in same 2-4 bedroom or adjacent beds in a large ward or prolonged face-to-face contact with an infectious staff member or patient)

Susceptible to varicella-zoster

Age of <15 years; administer to immunocompromised adolescents and adults and to other older patients on an individual basis

An acceptable alternative to VZIG prophylaxis is to treat varicella, if it occurs, with high-dose I.V. acyclovir

Usual Dosage High risk susceptible patients who are exposed again more than 3 weeks after a prior dose of VZIG should receive another full dose; there is no evidence VZIG modifies established varicella-zoster infections.

I.M.: Administer by deep injection in the gluteal muscle or in another large muscle mass. Inject 125 units/10 kg (22 lb); maximum dose: 625 units (5 vials); minimum dose: 125 units; do not give fractional doses. Do not inject I.V.

Dosage Forms Injection: 125 units of antibody in single-dose vials

Vascor® *see* bepridil hydrochloride *on page 51*

Vascoray® *see* radiological/contrast media (ionic) *on page 413*

Vaseretic® 10-25 *see* enalapril and hydrochlorothiazide *on page 169*

Vasocidin® Ophthalmic *see* sodium sulfacetamide and prednisolone *on page 439*

VasoClear® Ophthalmic [OTC] *see* naphazoline hydrochloride *on page 325*

Vasocon-A® Ophthalmic *see* naphazoline and antazoline *on page 325*

Vasocon Regular® Ophthalmic *see* naphazoline hydrochloride *on page 325*

Vasodilan® *see* isoxsuprine hydrochloride *on page 260*

vasopressin (vay soe press' in)

Brand Names Pitressin® Injection

Synonyms antidiuretic hormone; 8-arginine vasopressin

Therapeutic Category Antidiuretic Hormone Analog; Hormone, Posterior Pituitary

Use Treatment of diabetes insipidus; prevention and treatment of postoperative abdominal distention; differential diagnosis of diabetes insipidus; [unlabeled] adjunct in the treatment of GI hemorrhage and esophageal varices

Usual Dosage
Diabetes insipidus:
I.M., S.C.:
Children: 2.5-5 units 2-4 times/day as needed
Adults: 5-10 units 2-4 times/day as needed (dosage range 5-60 units/day)
Intranasal: Administer on cotton pledget or nasal spray

Abdominal distention Adults: I.M.: 5 mg stat, 10 mg every 3-4 hours

GI hemorrhage: I.V.: Administer in a peripheral vein; dilute aqueous in NS or D₅W to 0.1-1 unit/mL and infuse at 0.2-0.4 units/minute and progressively increase to 0.9 units/minute if necessary; I.V. infusion administration requires the use of an infusion pump and should be administered in a peripheral line to minimize adverse reactions on coronary arteries

Dosage Forms Injection, aqueous: 20 pressor units/mL (0.5 mL, 1 mL)

Vasosulf® Ophthalmic *see* sodium sulfacetamide and phenylephrine *on page 439*

Vasotec® I.V. *see* enalapril *on page 168*

Vasotec® Oral *see* enalapril *on page 168*

Vasoxyl® *see* methoxamine hydrochloride *on page 302*

V-Cillin K® Oral *see* penicillin V potassium *on page 362*

VCR *see* vincristine sulfate *on page 496*

V-Dec-M® *see* guaifenesin and pseudoephedrine *on page 220*

vecuronium (ve kyoo' roe ni um)
Brand Names Norcuron®
Synonyms ORG NC 45
Therapeutic Category Neuromuscular Blocker Agent, Nondepolarizing; Skeletal Muscle Relaxant
Use Adjunct to anesthesia, to facilitate intubation, and provide skeletal muscle relaxation during surgery or mechanical ventilation
Usual Dosage I.V.:

Infants >7 weeks to 1 year: Initial: 0.08-0.1 mg/kg/dose; maintenance: 0.05-0.1 mg/kg/ every hour as needed

Children >1 year and Adults: Initial: 0.08-0.1 mg/kg/dose; maintenance: 0.05-0.1 mg/kg/ every hour as needed; may be administered as a continuous infusion at 0.1 mg/kg/hour

Note: Children may require slightly higher initial doses and slightly more frequent supplementation
Dosage Forms Powder for injection: 10 mg (5 mL, 10 mL)

Veetids® Oral *see* penicillin V potassium *on page 362*

Velban® Injection *see* vinblastine sulfate *on page 495*

Velosef® *see* cephradine *on page 85*

Velosulin® *see* insulin preparations *on page 250*

Velsar® Injection *see* vinblastine sulfate *on page 495*

Veltane® Tablet *see* brompheniramine maleate *on page 59*

venlafaxine (ven' la fax een)
Brand Names Effexor®
Therapeutic Category Antidepressant
Use Treatment of depression
Usual Dosage Oral: Adults: 75 mg/day, administered in 2 or 3 divided doses, taken with food; dose may be increased to 150 mg/day up to 225-375 mg/day
Dosage Forms Tablet: 25 mg, 37.5 mg, 50 mg, 75 mg, 100 mg

Venoglobulin®-I *see* immune globulin, intravenous *on page 247*

Ventolin® *see* albuterol *on page 10*

VePesid® Injection *see* etoposide *on page 188*

VePesid® Oral *see* etoposide *on page 188*

verapamil hydrochloride (ver ap' a mill)
Brand Names Calan®; Isoptin®; Verelan®
Synonyms iproveratril hydrochloride
Therapeutic Category Antianginal Agent; Antiarrhythmic Agent, Class IV; Calcium Channel Blocker
(Continued)

493

verapamil hydrochloride *(Continued)*

Use Angina, hypertension; I.V. for supraventricular tachyarrhythmias (PSVT, atrial fibrillation, atrial flutter); hypertrophic cardiomyopathy

Usual Dosage

Children: I.V.:
  0-1 year: 0.1-0.2 mg/kg/dose, repeated after 30 minutes as needed
  1-16 years: 0.1-0.3 mg/kg over 2-3 minutes; maximum: 5 mg/dose, may repeat dose once in 30 minutes if adequate response not achieved; maximum for second dose: 10 mg/dose

Children: Oral (dose not well established):
  4-8 mg/kg/day in 3 divided doses **or** 1-5 years: 40-80 mg every 8 hours
  >5 years: 80 mg every 6-8 hours

Adults:
  Oral: 240-480 mg/24 hours divided 3-4 times/day
  I.V.: 5-10 mg (0.075-0.15 mg/kg); may repeat 10 mg (0.15 mg/kg) 15-30 minutes after the initial dose if needed and if patient tolerated initial dose

Dosage Forms

Capsule, sustained release: 120 mg, 180 mg, 240 mg
Injection: 2.5 mg/mL (2 mL, 4 mL)
Tablet: 40 mg, 80 mg, 120 mg
Tablet, sustained release: 120 mg, 180 mg, 240 mg

Verazinc® Oral [OTC] *see* zinc sulfate *on page 504*

Vercyte® *see* pipobroman *on page 379*

Verelan® *see* verapamil hydrochloride *on previous page*

Vergogel® Gel [OTC] *see* salicylic acid *on page 424*

Vergon® [OTC] *see* meclizine hydrochloride *on page 288*

Vermizine® *see* piperazine citrate *on page 379*

Vermox® *see* mebendazole *on page 287*

Verr-Canth™ *see* cantharidin *on page 70*

Verrex-C&M® *see* podophyllin and salicylic acid *on page 382*

Versacaps® *see* guaifenesin and pseudoephedrine *on page 220*

Versed® *see* midazolam hydrochloride *on page 312*

V-Gan® Injection *see* promethazine hydrochloride *on page 399*

Vibramycin® Injection *see* doxycycline *on page 161*

Vibramycin® Oral *see* doxycycline *on page 161*

Vibra-Tabs® *see* doxycycline *on page 161*

Vicks Formula 44® [OTC] *see* dextromethorphan hydrobromide *on page 136*

Vicks Formula 44® Pediatric Formula [OTC] *see* dextromethorphan hydrobromide *on page 136*

Vicks Sinex® Long-Acting Nasal Solution [OTC] *see* oxymetazoline hydrochloride *on page 350*

Vicks Sinex® Nasal Solution [OTC] *see* phenylephrine hydrochloride *on page 372*

Vicks Vatronol® [OTC] *see* ephedrine sulfate *on page 170*

Vicodin® *see* hydrocodone and acetaminophen *on page 234*

Vicodin® ES *see* hydrocodone and acetaminophen *on page 234*

Vicon-C® [OTC] *see* vitamin B complex with vitamin C *on page 498*

vidarabine (vye dare' a been)
Brand Names Vira-A® Injection; Vira-A® Ophthalmic
Synonyms adenine arabinoside; Ara-A
Therapeutic Category Antiviral Agent, Ophthalmic; Antiviral Agent, Parenteral
Use Treatment of acute keratoconjunctivitis and epithelial keratitis due to herpes simplex virus; herpes simplex encephalitis; neonatal herpes simplex virus infections; herpes zoster in immunosuppressed patients; reduces mortality from herpes simplex encephalitis from 70% to 28%; definitive diagnosis of herpes simplex conjunctivitis should be made before instituting ophthalmic therapy
Usual Dosage
Neonates: I.V.: 15-30 mg/kg/day as an 18- to 24-hour infusion

Children and Adults:
I.V.: 10-15 mg/kg/day as a 12-hour or longer infusion
Ophthalmic: Keratoconjunctivitis: 1/2" of ointment in lower conjunctival sac 5 times/day every 3 hours while awake until complete re-epithelialization has occurred, then twice daily for an additional 7 days
Dosage Forms
Injection, suspension: 200 mg/mL [base 187.4 mg] (5 mL)
Ointment, ophthalmic, as monohydrate: 3% [30 mg/mL = 28 mg/mL base] (3.5 g)

Vi-Daylin® ADC Chewable Tablet [OTC] *see* vitamin, multiple (pediatric) *on page 499*
Vi-Daylin® ADC Drops [OTC] *see* vitamin, multiple (pediatric) *on page 499*
Vi-Daylin® Chewable Tablet [OTC] *see* vitamin, multiple (pediatric) *on page 499*
Vi-Daylin® Drops [OTC] *see* vitamin, multiple (pediatric) *on page 499*
Vi-Daylin/F® ADC + Iron Chewable Tablet *see* vitamin, multiple (pediatric) *on page 499*
Vi-Daylin/F® ADC + Iron Drops *see* vitamin, multiple (pediatric) *on page 499*
Vi-Daylin/F® Chewable Tablet *see* vitamin, multiple (pediatric) *on page 499*
Vi-Daylin/F® Drops *see* vitamin, multiple (pediatric) *on page 499*
Videx® Oral *see* didanosine *on page 145*

vinblastine sulfate (vin blas' teen)
Brand Names Alkaban-AQ® Injection; Velban® Injection; Velsar® Injection
Synonyms vincaleukoblastine; VLB
Therapeutic Category Antineoplastic Agent, Miotic Inhibitor
Use Palliative treatment of Hodgkin's disease and other lymphomas; breast cancer, advanced testicular germinal-cell cancers; mycosis fungoides; Kaposi's sarcoma
Usual Dosage Refer to individual protocols
Varies depending upon clinical and hematological response. Give at intervals of at least 7 days and only after leukocyte count has returned to at least 4000/mm³; maintenance therapy should be titrated according to leukocyte count. Dosage should be reduced in patients with recent exposure to radiation therapy or chemotherapy; single doses in these patients should not exceed 5.5 mg/m².

Children and Adults: I.V.: 4-12 mg/m² every 7-10 days **or** 5-day continuous infusion of 1.4-1.8 mg/m²/day **or** 0.1-0.5 mg/kg/week
Dosage Forms
Injection: 1 mg/mL (10 mL)
Powder for injection: 10 mg

vincaleukoblastine *see* vinblastine sulfate *on this page*
Vincasar® PFS Injection *see* vincristine sulfate *on next page*

vincristine sulfate (vin kris' teen)
Brand Names Oncovin® Injection; Vincasar® PFS Injection
Synonyms LCR; leurocristine; VCR
Therapeutic Category Antineoplastic Agent, Miotic Inhibitor
Use Treatment of leukemias, Hodgkin's disease, neuroblastoma, malignant lymphomas, Wilms' tumor, and rhabdomyosarcoma
Usual Dosage Refer to individual protocols
Adjustments are made depending upon clinical and hematological response and upon adverse reactions

Children: I.V.:
≤10 kg or BSA <1 m^2: 0.05 mg/kg once weekly
2 mg/m^2; may repeat every week

Adults: I.V.: 0.4-1.4 mg/m^2, up to 2 mg maximum; may repeat every week
Dosage Forms Injection: 1 mg/mL (1 mL, 2 mL, 5 mL)

Vioform-HC® Topical *see* clioquinol and hydrocortisone *on page 106*

Vioform® Topical [OTC] *see* clioquinol *on page 106*

Viokase® *see* pancrelipase *on page 354*

viosterol *see* ergocalciferol *on page 173*

Vira-A® Injection *see* vidarabine *on previous page*

Vira-A® Ophthalmic *see* vidarabine *on previous page*

Virazole® Aerosol *see* ribavirin *on page 419*

Virilon® *see* methyltestosterone *on page 307*

Virogen® Herpes Slide Test *see* diagnostic aids (*in vitro*), other *on page 138*

Virogen® Rotatest® *see* diagnostic aids (*in vitro*), feces *on page 138*

Virogen® Rubella Microlatex® *see* diagnostic aids (*in vitro*), blood *on page 137*

Virogen® Rubella Slide Test *see* diagnostic aids (*in vitro*), blood *on page 137*

Viroptic® Ophthalmic *see* trifluridine *on page 478*

Viscoat® *see* chondroitin sulfate-sodium hyaluronate *on page 101*

Visidex® II [OTC] *see* diagnostic aids (*in vitro*), blood *on page 137*

Visine® L.R. Ophthalmic [OTC] *see* oxymetazoline hydrochloride *on page 350*

Visine® Ophthalmic [OTC] *see* tetrahydrozoline hydrochloride *on page 459*

Visken® *see* pindolol *on page 378*

Vistacon-50® Injection *see* hydroxyzine *on page 241*

Vistaject-25® Injection *see* hydroxyzine *on page 241*

Vistaject-50® Injection *see* hydroxyzine *on page 241*

Vistaquel® Injection *see* hydroxyzine *on page 241*

Vistaril® Injection *see* hydroxyzine *on page 241*

Vistaril® Oral *see* hydroxyzine *on page 241*

Vistazine® Injection *see* hydroxyzine *on page 241*

Vita-C® [OTC] *see* ascorbic acid *on page 33*

Vitacarn® Oral *see* levocarnitine *on page 270*

vitamin A
Brand Names Aquasol A® Injection; Aquasol A® Oral [OTC]
Synonyms oleovitamin A
Therapeutic Category Vitamin, Fat Soluble

Use Treatment and prevention of vitamin A deficiency

Usual Dosage

RDA:

0-3 years: 400 μg*

4-6 years: 500 μg*

7-10 years: 700 μg*

>10 years: 800-1000 μg*

*μg retinol equivalent (0.3 μg retinol = 1 unit vitamin A)

Supplementation in measles: Children: Oral:

<1 year: 100,000 units/day for 2 days

>1 year: 200,000 units/day for 2 days

Severe deficiency with xerophthalmia:

Children 1-8 years:

Oral: 5000-10,000 units/kg/day for 5 days or until recovery occurs

I.M.: 5000-15,000 units/day for 10 days

Children >8 years and Adults:

Oral: 500,000 units/day for 3 days, then 50,000 units/day for 14 days, then 10,000-20,000 units/day for 2 months

I.M.: 50,000-100,000 units/day for 3 days, 50,000 units/day for 14 days

Deficiency (without corneal changes): Oral:

Infants <1 year: 10,000 units/kg/day for 5 days, then 7500-15,000 units/day for 10 days

Children 1-8 years: 5000-10,000 units/kg/day for 5 days, then 17,000-35,000 units/day for 10 days

Children >8 years and Adults: 100,000 units/day for 3 days then 50,000 units/day for 14 days

Malabsorption syndrome (prophylaxis): Children >8 years and Adults: Oral: 10,000-50,000 units/day of water miscible product

Dietary supplement: Oral:

Infants up to 6 months: 1500 units/day

Children:

6 months to 3 years: 1500-2000 units/day

4-6 years: 2500 units/day

7-10 years: 3300-3500 units/day

Children >10 years and Adults: 4000-5000 units/day

Dosage Forms

Capsule: 10,000 units, 25,000 units, 50,000 units

Drops, oral (water miscible): 5000 units/0.1 mL (30 mL)

Injection: 50,000 units/mL (2 mL)

vitamin A acid see tretinoin on page 474

vitamin A and vitamin D

Brand Names A and D™ Ointment [OTC]

Synonyms cod liver oil

Therapeutic Category Protectant, Topical; Topical Skin Product

Use Temporary relief of discomfort due to chapped skin, diaper rash, minor burns, abrasions, as well as irritations associated with ostomy skin care

Usual Dosage

Oral, oil: Dietary supplement: 2.5 mL/day

Topical: Apply locally with gentle massage as needed

Dosage Forms Ointment, topical: In a lanolin-petrolatum base (60 g)

vitamin B₁ see thiamine hydrochloride on page 463

vitamin B₂ see riboflavin on page 419

vitamin B₃ see niacin on page 332

vitamin B₅ *see* pantothenic acid *on page 355*

vitamin B₆ *see* pyridoxine hydrochloride *on page 409*

vitamin B₁₂ *see* cyanocobalamin *on page 120*

vitamin B₁₂ₐ *see* hydroxocobalamin *on page 240*

vitamin B complex

Brand Names Apatate® [OTC]; Gevrabon® [OTC]; Lederplex® [OTC]; Lipovite® [OTC]; Mega-B® [OTC]; Megaton™ [OTC]; Mucoplex® [OTC]; NeoVadrin® B Complex [OTC]; Orexin® [OTC]; Surbex® [OTC]

Therapeutic Category Vitamin, Water Soluble

Usual Dosage Dosage is usually 1 tablet or capsule/day; please refer to package insert

vitamin B complex with vitamin C

Brand Names Allbee® With C [OTC]; Surbex-T® Filmtabs® [OTC]; Surbex® with C Filmtabs® [OTC]; Thera-Combex® H-P Kapseals® [OTC]; Vicon-C® [OTC]

Therapeutic Category Vitamin, Water Soluble

Use Supportive nutritional supplementation in conditions in which water-soluble vitamins are required like GI disorders, chronic alcoholism, pregnancy, severe burns, and recovery from surgery

Usual Dosage Adults: Oral: 1 every day

vitamin B complex with vitamin C and folic acid

Brand Names Berroca®; Folbesyn®; Nephrocaps® [OTC]

Therapeutic Category Vitamin, Water Soluble

Use Supportive nutritional supplementation in conditions in which water-soluble vitamins are required like GI disorders, chronic alcoholism, pregnancy, severe burns, and recovery from surgery

Usual Dosage Adults: Oral: 1 every day

vitamin C *see* ascorbic acid *on page 33*

vitamin D₂ *see* ergocalciferol *on page 173*

vitamin E

Brand Names Amino-Opti-E® Oral [OTC]; Aquasol E® Oral [OTC]; Vitec® Topical [OTC]

Synonyms *d*-alpha tocopherol; *dl*-alpha tocopherol

Therapeutic Category Vitamin, Fat Soluble

Use Prevention and treatment hemolytic anemia secondary to vitamin E deficiency, dietary supplement

Usual Dosage

RDA: Oral:
  Premature infants ≤3 months: 25 units/day
  Infants:
    ≤6 months: 4.5 units/day
    6-12 months: 6 units/day
  Children:
    1-3 years: 9 units/day
    4-10 years: 10.5 units/day
  Adults >11 years:
    Female: 12 units/day
    Male: 15 units/day

Prevention of vitamin E deficiency: Neonates, premature, low birthweight (results in normal levels within 1 week): Oral: 25-50 units/24 hours until 6-10 weeks of age or 125-150 units/kg total in 4 doses on days 1, 2, 7, and 8 of life

Vitamin E deficiency treatment: Adults: Oral: 50-200 units/24 hours for 2 weeks

Topical: Apply a thin layer over affected areas as needed

Dosage Forms
Capsule: 100 units, 200 units, 400 units, 500 units, 600 units, 1000 units
Capsule, water miscible: 73.5 mg, 147 mg, 165 mg, 330 mg, 400 units
Cream: 50 mg/g (15 g, 30 g, 60 g, 75 g, 120 g, 454 g)
Drops, oral: 50 mg/mL
Liquid, topical: 10 mL, 15 mL, 30 mL, 60 mL
Oil: 15 mL, 30 mL, 60 mL
Ointment, topical: 30 mg/g (45 g, 60 g)
Tablet: 200 units, 400 units

vitamin G see riboflavin *on page 419*

vitamin K$_1$ see phytonadione *on page 376*

vitamin K$_4$ see menadiol sodium diphosphate *on page 291*

vitamin, multiple (injectable)
Brand Names M.V.C.® 9 + 3; M.V.I.®-12; M.V.I.® Concentrate; M.V.I.® Pediatric
Therapeutic Category Vitamin
Usual Dosage
Children:
Oral:
≤2 years: Drops: 1 mL/day (premature infants may get 0.5-1 mL/day)
>2 years: Chew 1 tablet daily
≥4 years: 5 mL/day
I.V.:
≤5 kg: 10 mL/1000 mL TPN (M.V.I.® Pediatric)
5.1 kg to 11 years: 5 mL/one TPN bag/day (M.V.I.® Pediatric)

Adults:
Oral: 1 tablet daily or 5 mL/day
I.V.: >11 years: 5 mL of vials 1 and 2 (M.V.I.®-12)/one TPN bag/day

vitamin, multiple (pediatric)
Brand Names Adeflor® Drops; Adeflor® Tablet; Florvite®; LKV-Drops® [OTC]; Multi Vit® Drops [OTC]; Poly-Vi-Flor® Chewable Tablet; Poly-Vi-Flor® Drops; Poly-Vi-Sol® Chewable Tablet [OTC]; Poly-Vi-Sol® Drops [OTC]; Tri-Vi-Flor® Chewable Tablet; Tri-Vi-Flor® Drops; Tri-Vi-Sol® Chewable Tablet [OTC]; Tri-Vi-Sol® Drops [OTC]; Vi-Daylin® ADC Chewable Tablet [OTC]; Vi-Daylin® ADC Drops [OTC]; Vi-Daylin® Chewable Tablet [OTC]; Vi-Daylin® Drops [OTC]; Vi-Daylin/F® ADC + Iron Chewable Tablet; Vi-Daylin/F® ADC + Iron Drops; Vi-Daylin/F® Chewable Tablet; Vi-Daylin/F® Drops
Synonyms children's vitamins; multivitamins/fluoride
Therapeutic Category Vitamin
Use Nutritional supplement, vitamin deficiency
Usual Dosage Oral: 0.6 mL or 1 mL daily; please refer to package insert

vitamin, multiple (prenatal)
Brand Names Chromagen® OB [OTC]; Filibon® [OTC]; Natabec® [OTC]; Natabec® FA [OTC]; Natabec® Rx; Natalins® [OTC]; Natalins® Rx; NeoVadrin® [OTC]; Niferex®-PN; Pramet® FA; Pramilet® FA; Prenavite® [OTC]; Secran®; Stuartnatal® 1+1; Stuart Prenatal® [OTC]
Synonyms prenatal vitamins
Therapeutic Category Vitamin
Use Nutritional supplement, vitamin deficiency
Usual Dosage Oral: 1 tablet or capsule daily; please refer to package insert

Vitec® Topical [OTC] *see* vitamin E *on page 498*

Vivactil® *see* protriptyline hydrochloride *on page 405*

Vivotif Berna™ Oral *see* typhoid vaccine *on page 485*

V-Lax® [OTC] *see* psyllium *on page 407*

VLB *see* vinblastine sulfate *on page 495*

VM-26 *see* teniposide *on page 453*

Volmax® *see* albuterol *on page 10*

Voltaren® Ophthalmic *see* diclofenac *on page 144*

Voltaren® Oral *see* diclofenac *on page 144*

Vontrol® *see* diphenidol hydrochloride *on page 152*

VoSol® HC Otic *see* acetic acid, propanediol diacetate, and hydrocortisone *on page 5*

VoSol® Otic *see* acetic acid *on page 5*

VP-16 *see* etoposide *on page 188*

Vumon Injection *see* teniposide *on page 453*

V.V.S.® Vaginal *see* sulfabenzamide, sulfacetamide, and sulfathiazole *on page 446*

Vytone® Topical *see* iodoquinol and hydrocortisone *on page 255*

VZIG *see* varicella-zoster immune globulin (human) *on page 491*

warfarin sodium (war' far in)

Brand Names Coumadin®; Panwarfin®; Sofarin®
Therapeutic Category Anticoagulant
Use Prophylaxis and treatment of thromboembolic disorders
Usual Dosage Oral:

Children and Infants: 0.05-0.34 mg/kg/day; infants <12 months old may require doses at or near the high end of this range; consistent anticoagulation may be difficult to maintain in children <5 years of age

Adults: 5-15 mg/day for 2-5 days, then adjust dose according to results of prothrombin time; usual maintenance dose ranges from 2-10 mg/day

Dosage Forms Tablet: 1 mg, 2 mg, 2.5 mg, 5 mg, 7.5 mg, 10 mg

4-Way® Long Acting Nasal Solution [OTC] *see* oxymetazoline hydrochloride *on page 350*

Wehamine® Injection *see* dimenhydrinate *on page 150*

Wehdryl® Injection *see* diphenhydramine hydrochloride *on page 152*

Wellbutrin® *see* bupropion *on page 62*

Wellcovorin® Injection *see* leucovorin calcium *on page 268*

Wellcovorin® Oral *see* leucovorin calcium *on page 268*

Westcort® Topical *see* hydrocortisone *on page 236*

Westhroid® *see* thyroid *on page 466*

Westrim® LA [OTC] *see* phenylpropanolamine hydrochloride *on page 373*

Whitfield's Ointment [OTC] *see* benzoic acid and salicylic acid *on page 49*

whole root rauwolfia *see* rauwolfia serpentina *on page 416*

Wigraine® *see* ergotamine derivatives *on page 174*

Winstrol® *see* stanozolol *on page 443*

witch hazel
Brand Names Tucks® [OTC]
Synonyms hamamelis water
Therapeutic Category Astringent
Use After-stool wipe to remove most causes of local irritation; temporary management of vulvitis, pruritus ani and vulva; help relieve the discomfort of simple hemorrhoids, anorectal surgical wounds, and episiotomies
Usual Dosage Apply to anorectal area as needed
Dosage Forms
Cream: 50% (40 g)
Pads: 50% with glycerine, water and methylparaben (40/jar)

Wolfina® *see* rauwolfia serpentina *on page 416*

wood sugar *see* d-xylose *on page 164*

Wyamine® Sulfate Injection *see* mephentermine sulfate *on page 292*

Wyamycin® S Oral *see* erythromycin *on page 175*

Wycillin® Injection *see* penicillin g procaine, aqueous *on page 362*

Wydase® Injection *see* hyaluronidase *on page 231*

Wygesic® *see* propoxyphene and acetaminophen *on page 402*

Wymox® *see* amoxicillin trihydrate *on page 24*

Wytensin® *see* guanabenz acetate *on page 222*

Xanax® *see* alprazolam *on page 13*

Xerac™ BP [OTC] *see* benzoyl peroxide *on page 49*

Xero-Lube® [OTC] *see* saliva substitute *on page 425*

X-Prep® Liquid [OTC] *see* senna *on page 428*

X-seb® T [OTC] *see* coal tar and salicylic acid *on page 111*

Xylocaine® HCl I.V. Injection for Cardiac Arrhythmias *see* lidocaine hydrochloride *on page 273*

Xylocaine® Oral *see* lidocaine hydrochloride *on page 273*

Xylocaine® Topical Ointment *see* lidocaine hydrochloride *on page 273*

Xylocaine® Topical Solution *see* lidocaine hydrochloride *on page 273*

Xylocaine® Topical Spray *see* lidocaine hydrochloride *on page 273*

Xylocaine® With Epinephrine *see* lidocaine and epinephrine *on page 272*

xylometazoline hydrochloride (zye loe met az' oh leen)
Brand Names Otrivin® Nasal [OTC]
Therapeutic Category Adrenergic Agonist Agent; Nasal Agent, Vasoconstrictor
Use Symptomatic relief of nasal and nasopharyngeal mucosal congestion
Usual Dosage
Children <12 years: 2-3 drops (0.05%) in each nostril every 8-10 hours
Children >12 years and Adults: 2-3 drops or sprays (0.1%) in each nostril every 8-10 hours
Dosage Forms Solution, nasal: 0.05% [0.5 mg/mL] (20 mL); 0.1% [1 mg/mL] (15 mL, 20 mL)

Xylo-Pfan® [OTC] *see* d-xylose *on page 164*

yellow fever vaccine
Brand Names YF-VAX®
Therapeutic Category Vaccine, Live Virus
Use Active immunization against yellow fever
(Continued)

ALPHABETICAL LISTING OF DRUGS

yellow fever vaccine *(Continued)*
Usual Dosage Single-dose S.C.: 0.5 mL
Dosage Forms Injection: Not less than 5.04 Log$_{10}$ Plaque Forming Units (PFU) per 0.5 mL

yellow mercuric oxide *see* mercuric oxide *on page 294*
YF-VAX® *see* yellow fever vaccine *on previous page*
Yocon® *see* yohimbine hydrochloride *on this page*
Yodoxin® *see* iodoquinol *on page 254*

yohimbine hydrochloride *(yo him' bine)*
Brand Names Aphrodyne™; Dayto Himbin®; Yocon®; Yohimex™
Therapeutic Category Miscellaneous Product
Use No FDA sanctioned indications
Usual Dosage Adults: Oral: 1 tablet 3 times/day
Dosage Forms Tablet: 5.4 mg

Yohimex™ *see* yohimbine hydrochloride *on this page*
Yutopar® Oral *see* ritodrine hydrochloride *on page 421*

zalcitabine *(zal site' a been)*
Brand Names Hivid®
Synonyms ddC; dideoxycytidine
Therapeutic Category Antiviral Agent, Oral
Use The FDA has approved zalcitabine for use in the treatment of HIV infections only in combination with zidovudine in adult patients with advanced HIV disease demonstrating a significant clinical or immunological deterioration
Usual Dosage
Safety and efficacy in children <13 years of age has not been established
Adults: Oral (dosed in combination with zidovudine): Daily dose: 0.750 mg every 8 hours, given together with 200 mg of zidovudine (ie, total daily dose: 2.25 mg of zalcitabine and 600 mg of zidovudine).
Dosage Forms Tablet: 0.375 mg, 0.75 mg

Zanosar® *see* streptozocin *on page 444*
Zantac® Injection *see* ranitidine hydrochloride *on page 416*
Zantac® Oral *see* ranitidine hydrochloride *on page 416*
Zantryl® *see* phentermine hydrochloride *on page 371*
Zarontin® *see* ethosuximide *on page 185*
Zaroxolyn® *see* metolazone *on page 309*
Zartan *see* cephalexin monohydrate *on page 84*
Zeasorb-AF® [OTC] *see* tolnaftate *on page 471*
Zebeta® *see* bisoprolol fumarate *on page 55*
Zebrax® *see* clidinium and chlordiazepoxide *on page 105*
Zefazone® *see* cefmetazole sodium *on page 79*
Zephiran® [OTC] *see* benzalkonium chloride *on page 47*
Zephrex® *see* guaifenesin and pseudoephedrine *on page 220*
Zephrex LA® *see* guaifenesin and pseudoephedrine *on page 220*
Zeroxin® *see* benzoyl peroxide *on page 49*
Zestril® *see* lisinopril *on page 275*

Zetar® [OTC] *see* coal tar *on page 110*
Zetran® Injection *see* diazepam *on page 142*

zidovudine (zye doe' vue deen)
Brand Names Retrovir® Injection; Retrovir® Oral
Synonyms azidothymidine; AZT; compound S
Therapeutic Category Antiviral Agent, Oral; Antiviral Agent, Parenteral
Use Management of patients with HIV infections who have had at least one episode of *Pneumocystis carinii* pneumonia or who have CD4 cell counts of ≤500/mm³; patients who have HIV-related symptoms or who are asymptomatic with abnormal laboratory values indicating HIV-related immunosuppression
Usual Dosage
Children 3 months to 12 years:
Oral: 90-180 mg/m²/dose every 6 hours; maximum: 200 mg every 6 hours
I.V. continuous infusion: 0.5-1.8 mg/kg/hour
I.V. intermittent infusion: 100 mg/m²/dose every 6 hours

Adults:
Oral:
Asymptomatic infection: 100 mg every 4 hours while awake (500 mg/day)
Symptomatic HIV infection: Initial: 200 mg every 4 hours (1200 mg/day), then after 1 month, 100 mg every 4 hours (600 mg/day)
I.V.: 1-2 mg/kg/dose every 4 hours
Dosage Forms
Capsule: 100 mg
Injection: 10 mg/mL (20 mL)
Syrup (strawberry flavor): 50 mg/5 mL (240 mL)

Zinacef® Injection *see* cefuroxime *on page 83*
Zinca-Pak® *see* trace metals *on page 472*
Zincate® Oral *see* zinc sulfate *on next page*
Zincfrin® Ophthalmic [OTC] *see* phenylephrine and zinc sulfate *on page 372*

zinc gelatin
Brand Names Gelucast®
Synonyms Unna's boot; Unna's paste
Therapeutic Category Protectant, Topical
Use Protectant and to support varicosities and similar lesions of the lower limbs
Usual Dosage Apply externally as an occlusive boot
Dosage Forms Bandage: 4" x 10 yards

zinc injection *see* trace metals *on page 472*
Zincon® Shampoo [OTC] *see* pyrithione zinc *on page 410*

zinc oxide
Synonyms Lassar's zinc paste
Therapeutic Category Topical Skin Product
Use Protective coating for mild skin irritations and abrasions, soothing and protective ointment to promote healing of chapped skin, diaper rash
Usual Dosage Infants, Children and Adults: Topical: Apply several times daily to affected area
Dosage Forms
Ointment, topical: 20% (30 g, 60 g, 454 g)
Paste, topical: 25% (in white petrolatum)

zinc oxide, cod liver oil, and talc
Brand Names Desitin® Topical [OTC]
Therapeutic Category Protectant, Topical
Use Relief of diaper rash, superficial wounds and burns, and other minor skin irritations
Usual Dosage Apply thin layer as needed
Dosage Forms Ointment, topical: Zinc oxide, cod liver oil, and talc in a petrolatum and lanolin base (30 g)

zinc sulfate
Brand Names Eye-Sed® Ophthalmic [OTC]; Orazinc® Oral [OTC]; Verazinc® Oral [OTC]; Zincate® Oral
Therapeutic Category Mineral, Oral; Trace Element, Parenteral
Use Zinc supplement (oral and parenteral); may improve wound healing in those who are deficient
Usual Dosage
RDA: Oral:
    Birth to 6 months: 3 mg elemental zinc/day
    6-12 months: 5 mg elemental zinc/day
    1-10 years: 10 mg elemental zinc/day
    ≥11 years: 15 mg elemental zinc/day
Zinc deficiency: Oral:
    Infants and Children: 0.5-1 mg elemental zinc/kg/day divided 1-3 times/day; somewhat larger quantities may be needed if there is impaired intestinal absorption or an excessive loss of zinc
    Adults: 110-220 mg zinc sulfate (25-50 mg elemental zinc)/dose 3 times/day
Ophthalmic: Instill 1-2 drops into eye(s) up to 4 times daily
Dosage Forms
Capsule: 110 mg [elemental zinc 25 mg]; 220 mg [elemental zinc 50 mg]
Solution, ophthalmic: 0.25% (15 mL)
Tablet: 66 mg [elemental zinc 15 mg]; 200 mg [elemental zinc 46 mg]

zinc undecylenate *see* undecylenic acid and derivatives *on page 486*

Zithromax™ *see* azithromycin dihydrate *on page 41*

ZNP® Bar [OTC] *see* pyrithione zinc *on page 410*

Zocor™ *see* simvastatin *on page 431*

Zofran® *see* ondansetron hydrochloride *on page 344*

Zoladex® Implant *see* goserelin acetate *on page 216*

Zolicef® *see* cefazolin sodium *on page 79*

Zoloft™ *see* sertraline hydrochloride *on page 430*

zolpidem tartrate (zole pi' dem)
Brand Names Ambien™
Therapeutic Category Hypnotic; Sedative
Use Short-term treatment of insomnia
Usual Dosage Adults: Oral: 10 mg immediately before bedtime
Dosage Forms Tablet: 5 mg, 10 mg

Zolyse® *see* chymotrypsin *on page 101*

Zone-A Forte® *see* pramoxine and hydrocortisone *on page 389*

ZORprin® *see* aspirin *on page 34*

Zostrix® *see* capsaicin *on page 71*

Zosyn™ *see* piperacillin sodium and tazobactam sodium *on page 379*

Zovirax® *see* acyclovir *on page 7*

Zydone® *see* hydrocodone and acetaminophen *on page 234*

Zyloprim® *see* allopurinol *on page 12*

Zymase® *see* pancrelipase *on page 354*

APPENDIX

NORMAL LABORATORY VALUES FOR ADULTS*

CHEMISTRY

Chemistry, Routine

Albumin		3.5-5.0 g/dL
Bilirubin, conjugated		0-0.2 mg/dL
Bilirubin, total		0.2-1.2 mg/dL
Blood urea nitrogen		8-23 mg/dL
Calcium		8.4-10.3 mg/dL
Creatinine		0.5-1.2 mg/dL
Glucose		65-110 mg/dL
Phosphorus		2.8-4.5 mg/dL
Protein, total		6.0-8.0 g/dL
Uric acid	male	3.5-7.2 mg/dL
	female	2.6-6.5 mg/dL

Electrolytes

Chlorides	100-110 mEq/L
CO_2	23-31 mEq/L
Potassium	3.5-5.0 mEq/L
Sodium	136-146 mEq/L
Anion gap	5-14 mEq/L

Enzymes

Alkaline phosphatase	male	34-110 units/L
	female	24-100 units/L
ALT		5-35 units/L
AST		5-35 units/L
CPK	male	0-206 units/L
	female	0-175 units/L
LDH		50-200 units/L

Thyroid Function

FTI (free thyroxine index)	4.5-12.0
T_3 resin uptake	25%-35%
T_3 (tri-iodothyronine) by RIA	70-200 ng/dL
T_4 (thyroxine) by RIA	4.0-11.0 μg/dL

Others

Ammonia, plasma		20-60 μg/dL
Amylase, serum		44-128 units/L
Calcium, ionized		4.6-5.2 mg/dL
Cholesterol		140-230 mg/dL
Iron, serum		50-170 μg/dL
Lactate, serum		1.4-3.9 mEq/L
Lipase		10-208 units/L
Magnesium		1.5-2.5 mg/dL
Oncotic pressure		22-28 mm Hg
Osmolality		280-300 mOsm/kg
Serum ferritin	male	25-400 ng/mL
	female	10-150 ng/mL
TIBC		270-390 μg/dL
Triglycerides		50-150 mg/dL

*The normal ranges for laboratory values vary with different age groups, and may change as new methodologies for the lab tests are used. These values are current for adults (age 17 years or older). **Note:** Normal laboratory values may differ according to laboratory, institution, and analytical technique.

HEMATOLOGY

Hematocrit	male	40%-52%
	female	35%-47%
Hemoglobin	male	13.5-17.5 g/dL
	female	11.5-16.0 g/dL
MCH		27-34 pg
MCV		82-100 fL
Platelet count		150-450 10^3/mm^3
RBC count	male	4.5-5.9 10^6/mm^3
	female	4.0-4.9 10^6/mm^3
Reticulocyte count		0.5%-1.5%
Sed rate (Westergren)	male	0-10 mm/h
	female	0-20 mm/h
WBC count		4.5-11.0 10^3/mm^3
WBC differential		
bands		2%-8%
basophils		0%-2%
eosinophils		0%-4%
lymphocytes		20%-45%
monocytes		2%-8%
neutrophils		40%-70%

BLOOD GASES

	Arterial	Venous
Base excess	-3.0 to +3.0 mEq/L	-5.0 to +5.0 mEq/L
HCO$_3$	18-25 mEq/L	18-25 mEq/L
O$_2$ saturation	90%-98%	60%-85%
pCO$_2$	34-45 mm Hg	35-52 mm Hg
pH	7.35-7.45	7.32-7.42
pO$_2$	80-95 mm Hg	30-48 mm Hg
TCO$_2$	23-29 mEq/L	24-30 mEq/L

Weight/Volume Equivalents

1 mg/dL = 10 μg/mL   1 ppm = 1 mg/L

1 mg/dL = 1 mg%   1 μg/mL = 1 mg/L

NORMAL LABORATORY VALUES FOR CHILDREN

CHEMISTRY

Albumin	0-1 y	2-4 g/dL
	1 y - adult	3.5-5.5 g/dL
Ammonia	newborn	90-150 µg/dL
	child	40-120 µg/dL
	adult	18-54 µg/dL
Amylase	newborn	0-60 units/L
	adult	30-110 units/L
Bilirubin, conjugated, direct	newborn	<1.5 mg/dL
	1 mo - adult	0-0.5 mg/dL
Bilirubin, total	0-3 d	2-10 mg/dL
	1 mo - adult	0-1.5 mg/dL
Bilirubin, unconjugated, indirect		0.6-10.5 mg/dL
Calcium	newborn	7-12 mg/dL
	0-2 y	8.8-11.2 mg/dL
	2 y - adult	9-11 mg/dL
Calcium, ionized, whole blood		4.4-5.4 mg/dL
Carbon dioxide, total		23-33 mEq/L
Chloride		95-105 mEq/L
Cholesterol	newborn	45-170 mg/dL
	0-1 y	65-175 mg/dL
	1-20 y	120-230 mg/dL
Creatinine	0-1 y	≤0.6 mg/dL
	1 y - adult	0.5-1.5 mg/dL
Glucose	newborn	30-90 mg/dL
	0-2 y	60-105 mg/dL
	child - adult	70-110 mg/dL
Iron	newborn	110-270 µg/dL
	infant	30-70 µg/dL
	child	55-120 µg/dL
	adult	70-180 µg/dL
Iron binding	newborn	59-175 µg/dL
	infant	100-400 µg/dL
	adult	250-400 µg/dL
Lactic acid, lactate		2-20 mg/dL
Lead, whole blood		<30 µg/dL
Lipase	child	20-140 units/L
	adult	0-190 units/L
Magnesium		1.5-2.5 mEq/L
Osmolality, serum		275-296 mOsm/kg
Osmolality, urine		50-1400 mOsm/kg

Chemistry *(continued)*

Phosphorus	newborn	4.2-9 mg/dL
	6 wk - 19 mo	3.8-6.7 mg/dL
	18 mo - 3 y	2.9-5.9 mg/dL
	3-15 y	3.6-5.6 mg/dL
	>15 y	2.5-5 mg/dL
Potassium, plasma	newborn	4.5-7.2 mEq/L
	2 d - 3 mo	4-6.2 mEq/L
	3 mo - 1 y	3.7-5.6 mEq/L
	1-16 y	3.5-5 mEq/L
Protein, total	0-2 y	4.2-7.4 g/dL
	>2 y	6-8 g/dL
Sodium		136-145 mEq/L
Triglycerides	infant	0-171 mg/dL
	child	20-130 mg/dL
	adult	30-200 mg/dL
Urea nitrogen, blood	0-2 y	4-15 mg/dL
	2 y - adult	5-20 mg/dL
Uric acid	male	3-7 mg/dL
	female	2-6 mg/dL

ENZYMES

Alanine aminotransferase (ALT) (SGPT)	0-2 mo	8-78 units/L
	>2 mo	8-36 units/L
Alkaline phosphatase (ALKP)	newborn	60-130 units/L
	0-16 y	85-400 units/L
	>16 y	30-115 units/L
Aspartate aminotransferase (AST) (SGOT)	infant	18-74 units/L
	child	15-46 units/L
	adult	5-35 units/L
Creatine kinase (CK)	infant	20-200 units/L
	child	10-90 units/L
	adult male	0-206 units/L
	adult female	0-175 units/L
Lactate dehydrogenase (LDH)	newborn	290-501 units/L
	1 mo - 2 y	110-144 units/L
	>16 y	60-170 units/L

BLOOD GASES

	Arterial	Capillary	Venous
pH	7.35-7.45	7.35-7.45	7.32-7.42
pCO$_2$ (mm Hg)	35-45	35-45	38-52
pO$_2$ (mm Hg)	70-100	60-80	24-48
HCO$_3$ (mEq/L)	19-25	19-25	19-25
TCO$_2$ (mEq/L)	19-29	19-29	23-33
O$_2$ saturation (%)	90-95	90-95	40-70
Base excess (mEq/L)	-5 to +5	-5 to +5	-5 to +5

THYROID FUNCTION TESTS

T$_4$ (thyroxine)
- 1-7 d 10.1-20.9 μg/dL
- 8-14 d 9.8-16.6 μg/dL
- 1 mo - 1 y 5.5-16 μg/dL
- >1 y 4-12 μg/dL

FTI
- 1-3 d 9.3-26.6
- 1-4 wk 7.6-20.8
- 1-4 mo 7.4-17.9
- 4-12 mo 5.1-14.5
- 1-6 y 5.7-13.3
- >6 y 4.8-14

T$_3$ by RIA
- newborns 100-470 ng/dL
- 1-5 y 100-260 ng/dL
- 5-10 y 90-240 ng/dL
- 10 y - adult 70-210 ng/dL

T$_3$ uptake
- 35%-45%

TSH
- cord 3-22 μU/mL
- 1-3 d <40 μU/mL
- 3-7 d <25 μU/mL
- >7 d 0-10 μU/mL

HEMATOLOGY

Complete Blood Count

	Hgb (g/dL)	Hct (%)	MCV (fL)	MCH (pg)	MCHC (%)	RBC (x 10^6/mm^3)	RDW	PLTS (x 10^3/mm^3)
0-3 d	15-20	45-61	95-115	31-37	29-37	4-5.9	<18	250-450
1-2 wk	12.5-18.5	39-57	86-110	28-36	28-38	3.6-5.5	<17	250-450
1-6 mo	10-13	29-42	74-96	25-35	30-36	3.1-4.3	<16.5	300-700
7 mo - 2 y	10.5-13	33-38	70-84	23-30	31-37	3.7-4.9	<16	250-600
2-5 y	11.5-13	34-39	75-87	24-30	31-37	3.9-5	<15	250-550
5-8 y	11.5-14.5	35-42	77-95	25-33	31-37	4-4.9	<15	250-550
13-18 y	12-15.2	36-47	78-96	25-35	31-37	4.5-5.1	<14.5	150-450
Adult male	13.5-16.5	41-50	80-100	26-34	31-37	4.5-5.5	<14.5	150-450
Adult female	12-15	36-44	80-100	26-34	31-37	4-4.9	<14.5	150-450

WBC and Diff

	WBC (x 10³/mm³)	Segmented Neutrophils	Band Neutrophils	Eosinophils	Basophils	Lymphocytes	Atypical Lymphs	Monocytes	# of NRBCs
0-3 d	9-35	32-62	10-18	0-2	0-1	19-29	0-8	5-7	0-2
1-2 wk	5-20	14-34	6-14	0-2	0-1	36-45	0-8	6-10	0
1-6 mo	6-17.5	13-33	4-12	0-3	0-1	41-71	0-8	4-7	0
7 mo - 2 y	6-17	15-35	5-11	0-3	0-1	45-76	0-8	3-6	0
2-5 y	5.5-15.5	23-45	5-11	0-3	0-1	35-65	0-8	3-6	0
5-8 y	5-14.5	32-54	5-11	0-3	0-1	28-48	0-8	3-6	0
13-18 y	4.5-13	34-64	5-11	0-3	0-1	25-45	0-8	3-6	0
Adult	4.5-11	35-66	5-11	0-3	0-1	24-44	0-8	3-6	0

Sedimentation rate, Westergren:
Children: 0-20 mm/hour
Adult male 0-15 mm/hour
Adult female 0-20 mm/hour

Sedimentation rate, Wintrobe:
Children 0-13 mm/hour
Adult male 0-10 mm/hour
Adult female 0-15 mm/hour

Reticulocyte count
Newborn 2-6%
1-6 months 0-2.8%
Adult 0.5-1.5%

APOTHECARY/METRIC CONVERSIONS

Liquid Measures

Basic equivalent: 1 fluid ounce = 30 mL

Examples:

1 gallon	3800 mL	4 fluid ounces	120 mL
1 quart	960 mL	15 minims	1 mL
1 pint	480 mL	10 minims	0.6 mL
8 fluid ounces	240 mL		

1 gallon	128 fluid ounces
1 quart	32 fluid ounces
1 pint	16 fluid ounces

Approximate Household Equivalents

1 teaspoonful . . . .5 mL   1 tablespoonful . . . .15 mL

Weights

Basic equivalents:

1 ounce = 30 g   15 grains = 1 g

Examples:

4 ounces	120 g	1 grain	.60 mg
2 ounces	60 g	$1/100$ grain	600 μg
10 grains	600 mg	$1/150$ grain	400 μg
7 ½ grains	500 mg	$1/200$ grain	300 μg
16 ounces	1 pound		

Metric Conversions

Basic equivalents:

1 g . . . . 1000 mg   1 mg . . . . 1000 μg

Examples:

5 g	5000 mg	5 mg	5000 μg
0.5 g	500 mg	0.5 mg	500 μg
0.05 g	50 mg	0.05 mg	50 μg

Exact Equivalents

1 gram (g) = 15.43 grains	0.1 mg	= 1/600 gr
1 milliliter (mL) = 16.23 minims	0.12 mg	= 1/500 gr
1 minim (℈) = 0.06 milliliter	0.15 mg	= 1/400 gr
1 grain (gr) = 64.8 milligrams	0.2 mg	= 1/300 gr
1 ounce (℥) = 31.1 grams	0.5 mg	= 1/120 gr
1 ounce (oz) = 28.35 grams	0.8 mg	= 1/80 gr
1 pound (lb) = 453.6 grams	1 mg	= 1/65 gr
1 kilogram (kg) = 2.2 pounds		

Solids*

¼ grain = 15 mg
½ grain = 30 mg
1½ grain = 100 mg
5 grains = 300 mg
10 grains = 600 mg

*Use exact equivalents for compounding and calculations requiring a high degree of accuracy.

POUNDS/KILOGRAMS CONVERSION

1 pound = 0.45359 kilograms
1 kilogram = 2.2 pounds

lb	=	kg	lb	=	kg	lb	=	kg
1		0.45	70		31.75	140		63.50
5		2.27	75		34.02	145		65.77
10		4.54	80		36.29	150		68.04
15		6.80	85		38.56	155		70.31
20		9.07	90		40.82	160		72.58
25		11.34	95		43.09	165		74.84
30		13.61	100		45.36	170		77.11
35		15.88	105		47.63	175		79.38
40		18.14	110		49.90	180		81.65
45		20.41	115		52.16	185		83.92
50		22.68	120		54.43	190		86.18
55		24.95	125		56.70	195		88.45
60		27.22	130		58.91	200		90.72
65		29.48	135		61.24			

TEMPERATURE CONVERSION

Centigrade to Fahrenheit = (°C x 9/5) + 32 = °F
Fahrenheit to Centigrade = (°F - 32) x 5/9 = °C

°C	=	°F	°C	=	°F	°C	=	°F
100.0		212.0	39.0		102.2	36.8		98.2
50.0		122.0	38.8		101.8	36.6		97.9
41.0		105.8	38.6		101.5	36.4		97.5
40.8		105.4	38.4		101.1	36.2		97.2
40.6		105.1	38.2		100.8	36.0		96.8
40.4		104.7	38.0		100.4	35.8		96.4
40.2		104.4	37.8		100.1	35.6		96.1
40.0		104.0	37.6		99.7	35.4		95.7
39.8		103.6	37.4		99.3	35.2		95.4
39.6		103.3	37.2		99.0	35.0		95.0
39.4		102.9	37.0		98.6	0		32.0
39.2		102.6						

APPENDIX

ACQUIRED IMMUNODEFICIENCY SYNDROME (AIDS)

This list of tests is not intended in any way to suggest patterns of physician's orders, nor is it complete. These tests may support possible clinical diagnoses or rule out other diagnostic possibilities. Each laboratory test relevant to AIDS is listed and weighted. Two symbols (**) indicate that the test is diagnostic, that is, documents the diagnosis if the expected is found. A single symbol (*) indicates a test frequently used in the diagnosis or management of the disease. The other listed tests are useful on a selective basis with consideration of clinical factors and specific aspects of the case.

Acid-Fast Stain
Acid-Fast Stain, Modified, *Nocardia* Species
Babesiosis Serological Test
Bacteremia Detection, Buffy Coat Micromethod
Beta$_2$-Microglobulin
Biopsy or Body Fluid Anaerobic Bacterial Culture
Biopsy or Body Fluid Fungus Culture
Biopsy or Body Fluid Mycobacteria Culture
Blood and Fluid Precautions, Specimen Collection
Blood Culture, Aerobic and Anaerobic
Blood Fungus Culture
Bronchial Washings Cytology
Bronchoalveolar Lavage
Bronchoalveolar Lavage Cytology
Brushings Cytology
Candida Antigen
Candidiasis Serologic Test
Cerebrospinal Fluid Cytology
Cerebrospinal Fluid Fungus Culture
Cerebrospinal Fluid Mycobacteria Culture
Chromosome Analysis, Blood or Bone Marrow
Complete Blood Count
Cryptococcal Antigen Titer, Serum or Cerebrospinal Fluid
Cryptosporidium Diagnostic Procedures, Stool
Cytomegalic Inclusion Disease Cytology
Cytomegalovirus Antibody
Cytomegalovirus Culture
Cytomegalovirus Isolation, Rapid
Darkfield Examination, Syphilis
Electron Microscopy
Estrogen Receptor Immunocytochemical Assay
Folic Acid, Serum
Hemoglobin A$_2$
Hepatitis B Surface Antigen
Herpes Cytology
Herpes Simplex Virus Antigen Detection
Herpes Simplex Virus Culture
Herpes Simplex Virus Isolation, Rapid
Histopathology
Histoplasmosis Serology
**HIV-1/HIV-2 Serology
HTLV-I/II Antibody
*Human Immunodeficiency Virus Culture
*Human Immunodeficiency Virus DNA Amplification
India Ink Preparation
Inhibitor, Lupus, Phospholipid Type
KOH Preparation
Leishmaniasis Serological Test

515

*Lymphocyte Subset Enumeration
Lymphocyte Transformation Test
Migration Inhibition Test
Mycobacteria by DNA Probe
Neisseria gonorrhoeae Culture
Nocardia Culture, All Sites
*p24 Antigen
Ova and Parasites, Stool
Platelet Count
Pneumocystis carinii Preparation
Pneumocystis Fluorescence
Polymerase Chain Reaction
Red Blood Cell Indices
Risks of Transfusion
Skin Biopsies
Skin Mycobacteria Culture
Skin Test, Tuberculosis
Sputum Culture
Sputum Cytology
Sputum Fungus Culture
Sputum Mycobacteria Culture
Stool Culture
Stool Fungus Culture
Stool Mycobacteria Culture
Susceptibility Testing, Fungi
Susceptibility Testing, Mycobacteria
T- and B-Lymphocyte Subset Assay
Throat Culture
Toxoplasmosis Serology
Urine Culture, Clean Catch
Urine Fungus Culture
VDRL, Serum
Viral Culture
Viral Culture, Blood
Viral Culture, Body Fluid
Viral Culture, Dermatological Symptoms
Viral Culture, Tissue
White Blood Count

Drugs Used in the Treatment of Acquired Immunodeficiency Syndrome (AIDS)

Currently on market:

AS-101
3'azido-2,3'dodeoxyuridine
carbovir
CD4, human recombinant soluble (Receptin®)
CD4, human truncated-369 AA polypeptide (recombinant CHO cells)
cryptosporidium hyperimmune bovine colostrum IgC concentrate
dextran sulfate sodium
didanosine (Videx®)
2'-3'-dideoxyadenosine
2'-3'-dideoxycytidine
2'-3'-dideoxyinosine
diethyldithiocarbamate [DTC] (Imuthiol®)
eflornithine hydrochloride (Orinidyl®)
HIV neutralizing antibodies (Immupath®)
HPA-23

human immunodeficiency virus (HIV-1) immune globulin
human T-lymphotropic virus type III gp160 antigens, recombinant vaccine, alum absorbed (VaxSyn® HIV-1)
interferon beta, recombinant human (Betaseron®)
lactobin
piritrexim isethionate
polyribonucleotide (Ampligen®)
SDZ MSL-109
tumor necrosis factor [TNF] binding protein I
tumor necrosis factor [TNF] binding protein II
zalcitabine (Hivid®)
zidovudine [AZT] (Retrovir®)

AIDS related complex (ARC) therapeutic agents currently on market:

atovaquone (Mepron®)
co-trimoxazole (Bactrim™, Septra®, and others)
fluconazole (Diflucan®)
epoetin alfa (Epogen®, Procrit®)
didanosine (Videx®)
foscarnet (Foscavir®)
interferon alfa-2a (Roferon-A®)
interferon alfa-2b (Intron® A)
pentamidine isethionate (NebuPent™, Pentam-300®)
rifabutin (Mycobutin™)
trimetrexate glucuronate (Neutrexin®)
zidovudine [AZT] (Retrovir®)

AIDS/ARC drugs soon to be released or in development:

acemannan (Carrisyn®)
AL-271
AR-121
AS-101
azidouridine
bropirimine [ABPP]
curdlan sulfate [CRDS]
deoxynojirimycin, n-butyl [DNJ]
fialuridine [FIAU]
filgrastim (Neupogen®) — new indication
FK-565
HIV protease inhibitor (Vertex®)
hypericin (VIMRxyn®)
interleukin-2 (Proleukin®) — new indication
iscador
isoprinosine
lentinan
molgramostim [GM-CSF] (Leucomax®)
muramyl-tripeptide [MTP-PE]
nevirapine
oxothiazolidone carboxylate (Procysteine®)
roquinimex (Linomide®)
stavudine [d4T; didehydrothymidine]
TAT antagonist
thymopentin (Timunox®)
thymostimuline [TP-1]
trichosanthin [GLQ223; compound Q]

APPENDIX

CANCER CHEMOTHERAPY

Acronyms	Used for
7 + 3	Leukemia — acute myeloid leukemia, induction
AC	Sarcoma — bony sarcoma
AC (DC)	Multiple myeloma
ACE	Lung cancer — small cell
ACe	Breast cancer
ABVD	Lymphoma — Hodgkin's
AVDP	Leukemia — acute lymphoblastic, relapse
m-BACOD	Lymphoma — non-Hodgkin's
BACOP	Lymphoma — non-Hodgkin's
BCDT	Malignant melanoma
BCP	Multiple myeloma
BEP	Genitourinary cancer — testicular, induction, good risk
BHD	Malignant melanoma
CAF	Breast cancer
CAMP	Lung cancer — non-small cell
CAP	Genitourinary cancer — bladder
	Head and neck cancer
	Lung cancer — non-small cell
CC	Ovarian cancer — epithelial
CD	Leukemia — acute nonlymphoblastic, consolidation
CDC	Ovarian cancer — epithelial
CF	Head and neck cancer
CFM	Breast cancer
CFPT	Breast cancer
CHAP	Ovarian cancer — epithelial
CHL + PRED	Leukemia — chronic lymphocytic leukemia
CHOP	Lymphoma — non-Hodgkin's
CHOP-Bleo	Lymphoma — non-Hodgkin's
CHOR	Lung cancer — small cell
CISCA	Genitourinary cancer — bladder
Cladribine (2-CdA)	Leukemia — chronic lymphocytic leukemia
CMC-High Dose	Lung cancer — small cell
CMF	Breast cancer
CMFP	Breast cancer
CMFVP (Cooper's)	Breast cancer
CMV	Genitourinary cancer — bladder
COB	Head and neck cancer
COP	Lymphoma — non-Hodgkin's
COP-BLAM	Lymphoma — non-Hodgkin's
COPP (or "C" MOPP)	Lymphoma — non-Hodgkin's
CP	Ovarian cancer — epithelial
CV	Lung cancer — non-small cell
CVI	Lung cancer — non-small cell
CVP	Leukemia — chronic lymphocytic leukemia
	Lymphoma — non-Hodgkin's
CYADIC	Sarcoma — soft tissue
CYVADIC	Sarcoma — bony sarcoma
	Sarcoma — soft tissue
DAT	Leukemia — acute myeloid leukemia, induction
DHAP	Lymphoma — non-Hodgkin's
DMC	Gestational trophoblastic cancer
DTIC-ACTD	Malignant melanoma
DVP	Leukemia — acute lymphoblastic, induction
DVPA	Leukemia — acute lymphoblastic, induction
FAC	Breast cancer
FAM	Gastric cancer
	Lung cancer — non-small cell
	Pancreatic cancer
FAME	Gastric cancer
FAMTX	Gastric cancer
FCE	Gastric cancer
FL	Genitourinary cancer — prostate

Acronyms	Used for
Fludarabine	Leukemia — chronic lymphocytic leukemia
FMS (SMF)	Pancreatic cancer
FMV	Colon cancer
FOMi	Lung cancer — non-small cell
FOMi/CAP	Lung cancer — non-small cell
5FU/LDLF	Colon cancer
FU/LV	Colon cancer
5FU/LV (Weekly)	Colon cancer
HDAC	Leukemia — acute myeloid leukemia, induction
HDMTX	Sarcoma — bony sarcoma
IC	Leukemia — acute myeloid leukemia, induction
ID	Sarcoma — soft tissue
IMAC	Sarcoma — bony sarcoma
IMF	Breast cancer
IMVP-16	Lymphoma — non-Hodgkin's
LDAC	Leukemia — acute myeloid leukemia, induction
L-VAM	Genitourinary cancer — prostate
M-2	Multiple myeloma
MACC	Lung cancer — non-small cell
MACOP-B	Lymphoma — non-Hodgkin's
MAID	Sarcoma — soft tissue
MAP	Head and neck cancer
MBC (MBD)	Head and neck cancer
MC	Leukemia — acute myeloid leukemia, induction
MeCP	Multiple myeloma
MF	Head and neck cancer
MINE	Lymphoma — non-Hodgkin's
MM	Leukemia — acute lymphoblastic, maintenance
MMC (MTX + MP + CTX)	Leukemia — acute lymphoblastic, maintenance
MOPP	Lymphoma — Hodgkin's
MOPP/ABV Hybrid	Lymphoma — Hodgkin's
MP	Multiple myeloma
MV	Leukemia — acute myeloid leukemia, induction
MVAC	Genitourinary cancer — bladder
MVPP	Lymphoma — Hodgkin's
PAC (CAP)	Ovarian cancer — epithelial
PE	Genitourinary cancer — testicular, induction, good risk
	Lung cancer — small cell
PFL	Head and neck cancer
POCC	Lung cancer — small cell
Pro-MACE	Lymphoma — non-Hodgkin's
Pro-MACE-CytaBOM	Lymphoma — non-Hodgkin's
PT	Ovarian cancer — epithelial
SD	Pancreatic cancer
VAB VI	Genitourinary cancer — testicular, induction, salvage
VAC	Ovarian cancer — germ cell
	Sarcoma — soft tissue
VAC (CAV) (Induction)	Lung cancer — small cell
VAD	Multiple myeloma
VADRIAC — High Dose	Sarcoma — bony sarcoma
VAIE	Sarcoma — bony sarcoma
VATH	Breast cancer
VBAP	Multiple myeloma
VBC	Malignant melanoma
VBP (PVB)	Genitourinary cancer — testicular, induction, salvage
VC	Lung cancer — small cell
VCAP	Multiple myeloma
VDP	Malignant melanoma
VIP	Genitourinary cancer — testicular, induction, poor risk
VIP (Einhorn)	Genitourinary cancer — testicular, induction, poor risk
VP	Leukemia — acute lymphoblastic, induction
VP-L-Asparaginase	Leukemia — acute lymphoblastic, induction

CANCER CHEMOTHERAPY REGIMENS

Breast Cancer

ACe
Cyclophosphamide
Doxorubicin (Adriamycin®)

CAF
Cyclophosphamide
Doxorubicin (Adriamycin®)
Fluorouracil
G CSF

CFM
Cyclophosphamide
Fluorouracil
Mitoxantrone

CFPT
Cyclophosphamide
Fluorouracil
Prednisone
Tamoxifen

CMF
Cyclophosphamide
Methotrexate
Fluorouracil

CMFP
Cyclophosphamide
Methotrexate
Fluorouracil
Prednisone

CMFVP (Cooper's)
Cyclophosphamide
Methotrexate
Fluorouracil
Vincristine
Prednisone

FAC
Fluorouracil
Doxorubicin (Adriamycin®)
Cyclophosphamide

IMF
Ifosfamide
Mesna
Methotrexate
Fluorouracil

VATH
Vinblastine
Doxorubicin (Adriamycin®)
Thiotepa
Fluoxymesterone (Halotestin®)

Colon Cancer

FU/LV
Fluorouracil
Leucovorin

5FU/LV (Weekly)
Fluorouracil
Leucovorin

FMV
Fluorouracil
Methyl-CCNU
Vincristine

5FU/LDLF
Fluorouracil
Leucovorin

Gastric Cancer

FAM
Fluorouracil
Doxorubicin (Adriamycin®)
Mitomycin C

FAME
Fluorouracil
Doxorubicin (Adriamycin®)
Methyl-CCNU

FAMTX
Methotrexate
Fluorouracil
Leucovorin
Doxorubicin (Adriamycin®)

FCE
Fluorouracil
Cisplatin
Etoposide

Genitourinary Cancer — Bladder

CAP
Cyclophosphamide
Doxorubicin (Adriamycin®)
Cisplatin (Platinol®)

CISCA
Cisplatin
Cyclophosphamide
Doxorubicin (Adriamycin®)

CMV
Cisplatin
Methotrexate
Vinblastine

MVAC
Methotrexate
Vinblastine
Doxorubicin (Adriamycin®)
Cisplatin

Genitourinary Cancer — Prostate

FL
Flutamide
Leuprolide acetate
Leuprolide acetate depot

L-VAM
Leuprolide acetate
Vinblastine
Doxorubicin (Adriamycin®)
Mitomycin C

Genitourinary Cancer — Testicular, Induction, Good Risk

BEP
Bleomycin
Etoposide
Cisplatin (Platinol®)

PE
Cisplatin (Platinol®)
Etoposide

Genitourinary Cancer — Testicular, Induction, Poor Risk

VIP
Etoposide (VePesid®)
Ifosfamide
Cisplatin (Platinol®)
Mesna

VIP (Einhorn)
Vinblastine
Ifosfamide
Cisplatin (Platinol®)
Mesna

Genitourinary Cancer — Testicular, Induction, Salvage

VAB VI
Vinblastine
Dactinomycin (Actinomycin D)
Bleomycin
Cisplatin
Cyclophosphamide

VBP (PVB)
Vinblastine
Bleomycin
Cisplatin (Platinol®)

Gestational Trophoblastic Cancer

DMC
Dactinomycin
Methotrexate
Cyclophosphamide

Head and Neck Cancer

CAP
Cyclophosphamide
Doxorubicin (Adriamycin®)
Cisplatin (Platinol®)

CF
Cisplatin
Fluorouracil

COB
Cisplatin
Vincristine (Oncovin®)
Bleomycin

MAP
Mitomycin C
Doxorubicin (Adriamycin®)
Cisplatin (Platinol®)

MBC (MBD)
Methotrexate
Bleomycin
Cisplatin

MF
Methotrexate
Fluorouracil
Leucovorin calcium

PFL
Cisplatin (Platinol®)
Fluorouracil
Leucovorin calcium

Leukemia — Acute Lymphoblastic, Induction

DVP
Daunorubicin
Vincristine
Prednisone

DVPA
Daunorubicin
Vincristine
Prednisone
Asparaginase

VP
Vincristine
Prednisone

VP-L-Asparaginase
Vincristine
Prednisone
L-asparaginase

Leukemia — Acute Lymphoblastic, Maintenance

MM
Mercaptopurine
Methotrexate

MMC (MTX + MP + CTX)
Methotrexate
Mercaptopurine
Cyclophosphamide

Leukemia — Acute Lymphoblastic, Relapse

AVDP
Asparaginase
Vincristine
Daunorubicin
Prednisone

Leukemia — Acute Myeloid, Induction

7 + 3
Cytarabine
Daunorubicin

DAT
Daunorubicin
Cytarabine (Ara-C)
Tioguanine

HDAC
Cytarabine

IC
Idarubicin (Idamycin®)
Cytarabine

LDAC
Cytarabine

MC
Mitoxantrone
Cytarabine

MV
Mitoxantrone
Etoposide (VePesid®)

Leukemia — Acute Nonlymphoblastic, Consolidation

CD
Cytarabine
Daunorubicin

Leukemia — Chronic Lymphocytic

CHL + PRED
Chlorambucil
Prednisone

CVP
Cyclophosphamide
Vincristine (Oncovin®)
Prednisone

Fludarabine

Cladribine (2-CdA)

Lung Cancer — Small Cell

ACE
Doxorubicin (Adriamycin®)
Cyclophosphamide
Etoposide

CHOR
Cyclophosphamide
Doxorubicin (Adriamycin®)
Vincristine
Radiation

CMC-High Dose
Cyclophosphamide
Methotrexate
Lomustine (CCNU)

PE
Cisplatin (Platinol®)
Etoposide

POCC
Procarbazine
Vincristine (Oncovin®)
Cyclophosphamide
Lomustine (CCNU)

VAC (CAV) (Induction)
Vincristine
Doxorubicin (Adriamycin®)
Cyclophosphamide

VC
Etoposide (VePesid®)
Carboplatin

Lung Cancer — Non-Small Cell

CAMP
Cyclophosphamide
Doxorubicin (Adriamycin®)
Methotrexate
Procarbazine

CAP
Cyclophosphamide
Doxorubicin (Adriamycin®)
Cisplatin (Platinol®)

CV
Cisplatin
Etoposide (VePesid®)

CVI
Carboplatin
Etoposide (VePesid®)
Ifosfamide
Mesna

FAM
Fluorouracil
Doxorubicin (Adriamycin®)
Mitomycin C

FOMi
Fluorouracil
Vincristine (Oncovin®)
Mitomycin C

FOMi/CAP
Fluorouracil
Vincristine
Mitomycin C
Cyclophosphamide
Doxorubicin (Adriamycin®)
Cisplatin

MACC
Methotrexate
Doxorubicin (Adriamycin®)
Cyclophosphamide
Lomustine

Lymphoma — Hodgkin's

ABVD
Doxorubicin (Adriamycin®)
Bleomycin
Vinblastine
Dacarbazine

MOPP
Mechlorethamine
Vincristine (Oncovin®)
Procarbazine
Prednisone

MOPP/ABV Hybrid
Mechlorethamine
Vincristine (Oncovin®)
Procarbazine
Prednisone
Doxorubicin (Adriamycin®)
Bleomycin
Vinblastine

MVPP
Mechlorethamine
Vinblastine
Procarbazine
Prednisone

Lymphoma — Non-Hodgkin's

BACOP
Bleomycin
Doxorubicin (Adriamycin®)
Cyclophosphamide
Vincristine (Oncovin®)
Prednisone

CHOP
Cyclophosphamide
Doxorubicin (Hydroxydaunomycin)
Vincristine (Oncovin®)
Prednisone

CHOP-Bleo
Cyclophosphamide
Doxorubicin (Hydroxydaunomycin)
Vincristine (Oncovin®)
Prednisone
Bleomycin

COP
Cyclophosphamide
Vincristine (Oncovin®)
Prednisone

COP-BLAM
Cyclophosphamide
Vincristine (Oncovin®)
Prednisone
Bleomycin
Doxorubicin (Adriamycin®)
Procarbazine (Matulane®)

COPP (or "C" MOPP)
Cyclophosphamide
Vincristine (Oncovin®)
Procarbazine
Prednisone

CVP
Cyclophosphamide
Vincristine
Prednisone

DHAP
Dexamethasone (Decadron®)
Cytarabine
Cisplatin

IMVP-16
Ifosfamide
Mesna
Methotrexate
Etoposide (VePesid®)

MACOP-B
Methotrexate
Doxorubicin (Adriamycin®)
Cyclophosphamide
Vincristine (Oncovin®)
Bleomycin
Prednisone
Leucovorin

m-BACOD
Methotrexate
Calcium leucovorin
Bleomycin
Doxorubicin (Adriamycin®)
Cyclophosphamide
Vincristine (Oncovin®)
Dexamethasone

MINE
Mesna
Ifosfamide
Mitoxantrone (Novantrone®)
Etoposide

Pro-MACE
Prednisone
Methotrexate
Calcium leucovorin
Doxorubicin (Adriamycin®)
Cyclophosphamide
Etoposide

Pro-MACE-CytaBOM
Prednisone
Doxorubicin (Adriamycin®)
Cyclophosphamide
Etoposide
Cytarabine
Bleomycin
Vincristine (Oncovin™)
Methotrexate
Leucovorin

Malignant Melanoma

BCDT
Carmustine (BCNU)
Cisplatin
Dacarbazine
Tamoxifen

BHD
Carmustine (BCNU)
Hydroxyurea
Dacarbazine

DTIC-ACTD
Dacarbazine
Dactinomycin

VBC
Vinblastine
Bleomycin
Cisplatin

VDP
Vinblastine
Dacarbazine
Cisplatin (Platinol™)

Multiple Myeloma

AC (DC)
Doxorubicin (Adriamycin®)
Carmustine

BCP
Carmustine (BCNU)
Cyclophosphamide
Prednisone

MeCP
Methyl-CCNU
Cyclophosphamide
Prednisone

MP
Melphalan
Prednisone

M-2
Vincristine
Carmustine
Cyclophosphamide
Melphalan
Prednisone

VAD
Vincristine
Doxorubicin (Adriamycin®)
Dexamethasone

VBAP
Vincristine
Carmustine (BCNU)
Doxorubicin (Adriamycin®)
Prednisone

VCAP
Vincristine
Cyclophosphamide
Doxorubicin (Adriamycin®)
Prednisone

Ovarian Cancer — Epithelial

CC
Carboplatin
Cyclophosphamide

CDC
Carboplatin
Doxorubicin
Cyclophosphamide

CHAP
Cyclophosphamide
Hexamethylmelamine
Doxorubicin (Adriamycin®)
Cisplatin (Platinol®)

CP
Cyclophosphamide
Cisplatin (Platinol®)

PAC (CAP)
Cisplatin (Platinol®)
Doxorubicin (Adriamycin®)
Cyclophosphamide

PT
Cisplatin (Platinol®)
Taxol

Ovarian Cancer — Germ Cell

VAC
Vincristine
Dactinomycin (Actinomycin D)
Cyclophosphamide

Pancreatic Cancer

FAM
Fluorouracil
Doxorubicin (Adriamycin®)
Mitomycin C

FMS (SMF)
Fluorouracil
Mitomycin C
Streptozocin

SD
Streptozocin
Doxorubicin

Sarcoma — Bony Sarcoma

AC
Doxorubicin (Adriamycin®)
Cisplatin

CYVADIC
Cyclophosphamide
Vincristine
Doxorubicin (Adriamycin®)
Dacarbazine (DTIC)

HDMTX
Methotrexate
Calcium leucovorin

IMAC
Ifosfamide
Mesna
Doxorubicin (Adriamycin®)
Cisplatin

VAIE
Vincristine
Doxorubicin (Adriamycin®)
Ifosfamide
Etoposide

VADRIAC — High Dose
Vincristine
Cyclophosphamide
Doxorubicin (Adriamycin®)

Sarcoma — Soft Tissue

CYADIC
Cyclophosphamide
Doxorubicin (Adriamycin®)
Dacarbazine (DTIC)

CYVADIC
Cyclophosphamide
Vincristine
Doxorubicin (Adriamycin®)
Dacarbazine (DTIC)

ID
Ifosfamide
Mesna
Doxorubicin

MAID
Mesna
Doxorubicin (Adriamycin®)
Ifosfamide
Dacarbazine

VAC
Vincristine
Dactinomycin
Cyclophosphamide

WHAT'S NEW

New Drugs Introduced or Approved by the FDA in 1993

Brand Name	Generic Name	Use
Aceon™	perindopril	Hypertension
Alomide™	lodoxamide	Ophthalmic mast cell stabilizer
Ambien™	zolpidem tartrate	Insomnia
Betaseron™	interferon beta-1b	Multiple sclerosis
Claritin™	loratadine	Antihistamine
Cognex™	tacrine	Alzheimer's disease
Daypro™	oxaprozin	Nonsteroidal anti-inflammatory
Dermadex™	torsemide	Loop diuretic
Dermatop™	prednicarbate	Steroid cream
Dovonex™	calcipotriene	Psoriasis
Effexor™	venlafaxine	Depression
Felbatol™	felbamate	Epilepsy
Flumadine™	rimantadine	Antiviral
Imitrex™	sumatriptan succinate	Migraine headaches
Kytril™	granisetron	Antinauseant
Lamisil™	terbinafine hydrochloride	Topical antifungal
Lescol™	fluvastatin	Cholesterol synthesis inhibitor
Leustatin™	cladribine	Hairy cell and chronic lymphocytic leukemia
Lipidil™	fenofibrate	Lower serum triglycerides
Livostin™	levocabastine	Seasonal allergic conjunctivitis
Lovenox™	enoxaparin	Thromboses
Mepron™	atovaquone	AIDS-related
Metastron™	strontium-89	Painful bone metastases
Mycobutin™	rifabutin	*Mycobacterium avium* complex (MAC)
Neurontin™	gabapentin	Epilepsy
Orlaam™	levomethadyl	Narcotic for opiod addiction
Paxil™	paroxetine hydrochloride	Depression
Pulmozyme™	dornase alfa, DNase	Cystic fibrosis
Propulsid™	cisapride	GI stimulant for GERD
Risperdal™	risperidone	Antipsychotic for schizophrenia
Taxol™	paclitaxel	Ovarian cancer
Tilade™	nedocromil sodium	Asthma
Trasylol®	aprotinin	Protease inhibitor to reduce blood loss
Zosyn™	piperacillin/tazobactam	I.V. beta-lactam antibiotic

Pending Drugs

Arasine®	acadesine	Ischemia during bypass surgery
Ethyol™	amifosine	Chemoprotective agent
Fosamax®	alendronate	Osteoporosis
Freedox®	tirilazad	Stroke/head trauma
Immuneron™	interferon gamma	Rheumatoid arthritis
Reactine®	cetrizine	Long-acting antihistamine
Respivir™	RSVIG	Antiviral
Serevent®	salmeterol	Antiasthmatic

INDICATION/THERAPEUTIC
CATEGORY
INDEX

INDICATION/THERAPEUTIC CATEGORY INDEX

INDICATION/THERAPEUTIC CATEGORY INDEX

INDICATION/THERAPEUTIC CATEGORY INDEX

INDICATION/THERAPEUTIC CATEGORY INDEX

541

INDICATION/THERAPEUTIC CATEGORY INDEX

542

ASPERGILLOSIS

Antifungal Agent, Systemic

ASPIRIN POISONING

Alkalinizing Agent Oral

Alkalinizing Agent, Parenteral

ASTHMA

Adrenal Corticosteroid

Adrenergic Agonist Agent

ASTHMA (DIAGNOSTIC)

Diagnostic Agent, Bronchial Airway Hyperactivity

ATELECTASIS

Expectorant

ATROPHIC GASTRITIS

Gastrointestinal Agent, Miscellaneous

ATTENTION DEFICIT HYPERACTIVE DISORDER (ADHD)

Amphetamine

INDICATION/THERAPEUTIC CATEGORY INDEX

Nonsteroidal Anti-Inflammatory Agent (NSAID), Oral

Skeletal Muscle Relaxant

BACTERIURIA (UNSPECIFIC)

Antibiotic, Urinary Irrigation

BACTEROIDES FRAGILIS

Antibiotic, Anaerobic

Antibiotic, Cephalosporin (Second Generation)

Antibiotic, Miscellaneous

Antibiotic, Penicillin

INDICATION/THERAPEUTIC CATEGORY INDEX

554

Antifungal Agent, Ophthalmic
Myprozine® Ophthalmic 326
Natacyn® Ophthalmic 326
natamycin 326

BLEPHAROCONJUNCTIVITIS

Antibiotic, Ophthalmic
Garamycin® Ophthalmic 211
Genoptic® Ophthalmic 211
Genoptic® S.O.P. Ophthalmic
. 211
Gentacidin® Ophthalmic 211
Gent-AK® Ophthalmic 211
gentamicin sulfate 211
Gentrasul® Ophthalmic 211
Polytrim® Ophthalmic 480
trimethoprim and polymyxin b
. 480

BLEPHAROSPASM

Ophthalmic Agent, Toxin
botulinum toxin type A 57
Oculinum® 57

BORRELLA BURGDORFERI

Antibiotic, Cephalosporin (Third Generation)
ceftriaxone sodium 82
Rocephin® 82

Antibiotic, Penicillin
amoxicillin trihydrate 24
Amoxil® .24
ampicillin .26
Beepen-VK® Oral 362
Betapen®-VK Oral 362
Biomox® .24
Ledercillin® VK Oral 362
Marcillin® 26
Omnipen® 26
Omnipen®-N 26
penicillin g, parenteral 361
penicillin V potassium 362
Pen.Vee® K Oral 362
Pfizerpen® Injection 361
Polycillin® 26
Polycillin-N® 26
Polymox® 24
Principen® 26
Robicillin® VK Oral 362
Totacillin® 26
Totacillin®-N 26
Trimox® .24
V-Cillin K® Oral 362
Veetids® Oral 362
Wymox® .24

Antibiotic, Tetracycline Derivative
Bio-Tab® Oral 161
Doryx® Oral 161
Doxychel® Injection 161
Doxychel® Oral 161
doxycycline 161
Doxy® Oral 161
Monodox® Oral 161
Vibramycin® Injection 161
Vibramycin® Oral 161
Vibra-Tabs® 161

BOWEL CLEANSING

Laxative, Bowel Evacuant
Co-Lav® 383
Colovage® 383
CoLyte® 383
Go-Evac® 383
GoLYTELY® 383
NuLYTELY® 383
OCL® 383
polyethylene glycol-electrolyte
solution 383

Laxative, Saline
Citro-Nesia™ [OTC] 282
Evac-Q-Mag® [OTC] 282
Fleet® Enema [OTC] 437
Fleet® Phospho®-Soda [OTC]
. 437
magnesium citrate 282
sodium phosphate 437

Laxative, Stimulant
Alphamul® [OTC] 77
castor oil .77
Emulsoil® [OTC] 77
Fleet® Flavored Castor Oil [OTC]
. 77
Neoloid® [OTC] 77
Purge® [OTC] 77

BOWEL STERILIZATION

Antibiotic, Aminoglycoside
Mycifradin® Sulfate Oral 330
Neo-fradin® Oral 330
neomycin sulfate 330
Neo-Tabs® Oral 330

Antibiotic, Anaerobic
Flagyl® Oral 309
Metizol® Oral 309
metronidazole 309
Protostat® Oral 309

Antibiotic, Macrolide
E.E.S.® Oral 175
E-Mycin® Oral 175
Eryc® Oral 175
EryPed® Oral 175
Ery-Tab® Oral 175
Erythrocin® Oral 175
erythromycin 175
Ilosone® Oral 175
PCE® Oral 175
Wyamycin® S Oral 175

Antibiotic, Tetracycline Derivative
Achromycin® V Oral 458
Ala-Tet® Oral 458
Nor-tet® Oral 458
Panmycin® Oral 458
Robitet® Oral 458
Sumycin® Oral 458
Teline® Oral 458
Tetracap® Oral 458
tetracycline 458
Tetralan® Oral 458
Tetram® Oral 458

BRADYCARDIA

Antibiotic, Cephalosporin (Second Generation)

Antibiotic, Cephalosporin (Third Generation)

Antibiotic, Penicillin

Antibiotic, Sulfonamide Derivative

Antibiotic, Tetracycline Derivative

BRONCHITIS (CHRONIC)

Antibiotic, Cephalosporin (Second Generation)

Antibiotic, Cephalosporin (Third Generation)

Antibiotic, Macrolide

Antibiotic, Miscellaneous

Antibiotic, Penicillin

Antibiotic, Quinolone

Nonsteroidal Anti-Inflammatory Agent (NSAID), Oral

CACHEXIA

Antihistamine

Progestin

CAMPYLOBACTER JEJUNI

Antibiotic, Aminoglycoside

Antibiotic, Macrolide

Antibiotic, Miscellaneous

Antibiotic, Penicillin

Corticosteroid, Systemic
Adlone® Injection . . . 306
A-hydroCort® Injection . . . 236
Amcort® Injection . . . 474
A-methaPred® Injection . . . 306
Aristocort® Forte Injection . . . 474
Aristocort® Intralesional Injection . . . 474
Aristocort® Oral . . . 474
Articulose L.A.® Injection . . . 474
Atolone® Oral . . . 474
Cenocort® A Injection . . . 474
Cenocort® Forte Injection . . . 474
Cetacort® Topical . . . 236
Cinonide® Injection . . . 474
Cortef® Oral . . . 236
Dalalone D.P.® Injection . . . 132
Dalalone® Injection . . . 132
Dalalone L.A.® Injection . . . 132
Decadron®-LA Injection . . . 132
Decadron® Oral . . . 132
Decadron® Phosphate Injection . . . 132
Decaject® Injection . . . 132
Decaject-LA® Injection . . . 132
Dekasol® Injection . . . 132
Dekasol-L.A.® Injection . . . 132
depMedalone® Injection . . . 306
Depoject® Injection . . . 306
Depo-Medrol® Injection . . . 306
Depopred® Injection . . . 306
Dexacen® Injection . . . 132
Dexacen® LA Injection . . . 132
dexamethasone . . . 132
Dexasone® Injection . . . 132
Dexasone® L.A. Injection . . . 132
Dexone® Injection . . . 132
Dexone® LA Injection . . . 132
Dexone® Tablet . . . 132
D-Med® Injection . . . 306
Duralone® Injection . . . 306
Hexadrol® Phosphate Injection . . . 132
Hexadrol® Tablet . . . 132
hydrocortisone . . . 236
Hydrocortone® Acetate Injection . . . 236
Hydrocortone® Oral . . . 236
Hydrocortone® Phosphate Injection . . . 236
Hytone® Topical . . . 236
Kenacort® Oral . . . 474
Kenaject® Injection . . . 474
Kenalog® Injection . . . 474
Medralone® Injection . . . 306
Medrol® Oral . . . 306
methylprednisolone . . . 306
M-Prednisol® Injection . . . 306
Rep-Pred® Injection . . . 306
Solu-Cortef® Injection . . . 236
Solu-Medrol® Injection . . . 306
Solurex® Injection . . . 132
Solurex L.A.® Injection . . . 132
Tac™-3 Injection . . . 474
Tac™-40 Injection . . . 474
Triam-A® Injection . . . 474
triamcinolone . . . 474
Triam Forte® Injection . . . 474
Triamolone® Injection . . . 474
Triamonide® Injection . . . 474
Tri-Kort® Injection . . . 474
Trilog® Injection . . . 474
Trilone® Injection . . . 474
Trisoject® Injection . . . 474

Estrogen and Androgen Combination
Estratest H.S.® Oral . . . 180
Estratest® Oral . . . 180
estrogens with methyltestosterone . . . 180
Premarin® With Methyltestosterone Oral . . . 180

Estrogen Derivative
Delestrogen® Injection . . . 178
depGynogen® Injection . . . 178
Depo®-Estradiol Injection . . . 178
Depogen® Injection . . . 178
diethylstilbestrol . . . 146
Dioval® Injection . . . 178
Dura-Estrin® Injection . . . 178
Duragen® Injection . . . 178
Estrace® Oral . . . 178
Estraderm® Transdermal . . . 178
Estra-D® Injection . . . 178
estradiol . . . 178
Estra-L® Injection . . . 178
Estro-Cyp® Injection . . . 178
estrogens, conjugated . . . 179
Estroject-L.A.® Injection . . . 178
Gynogen L.A.® Injection . . . 178
Premarin® Injection . . . 179
Premarin® Oral . . . 179
Premarin® Vaginal . . . 179
Stilphostrol® Injection . . . 146
Stilphostrol® Oral . . . 146
Valergen® Injection . . . 178

Immune Modulator
Ergamisol® . . . 269
levamisole hydrochloride . . . 269

Progestin
Megace® . . . 290
megestrol acetate . . . 290

CARCINOMA (CERVIX)

Antineoplastic Agent, Alkylating Agent
carboplatin . . . 75
cisplatin . . . 103
Paraplatin® . . . 75
Platinol® . . . 103
Platinol®-AQ . . . 103

Antineoplastic Agent, Antibiotic
Blenoxane® . . . 56
bleomycin sulfate . . . 56
mitomycin . . . 315
Mutamycin® . . . 315

Antineoplastic Agent, Miotic Inhibitor
Oncovin® Injection . . . 496
Vincasar® PFS Injection . . . 496
vincristine sulfate . . . 496

CIRRHOSIS

Antilipemic Agent

Calcium Salt

Immunosuppressant Agent

Vitamin D Analog

Decongestant, Nasal

CONGESTIVE HEART FAILURE

Adrenergic Agonist Agent

Alpha-Adrenergic Blocking Agent, Oral

Angiotensin-Converting Enzyme (ACE) Inhibitors

Antihypertensive, Combination

Cardiac Glycoside

Cardiovascular Agent, Other

CONVULSANT DRUG POISONING

Hypnotic

COPROPORPHYRIA

Beta-Adrenergic Blocker

Blood Modifiers

CORNEAL ULCER

Antibiotic, Ophthalmic

CORYNEBACTERIUM (JK GROUP)

Antibiotic, Aminoglycoside

Antibiotic, Miscellaneous

COUGH

Antihistamine

Antihistamine/Decongestant Combination

Antitussive

INDICATION/THERAPEUTIC CATEGORY INDEX

INDICATION/THERAPEUTIC CATEGORY INDEX

Corticosteroid, Topical (Low Potency)

Corticosteroid, Topical (Medium/High Potency)

Corticosteroid, Topical (Medium Potency)

Dietary Supplement

Phenothiazine Derivative

Topical Skin Product

INDICATION/THERAPEUTIC CATEGORY INDEX

617

GRANULOMATOUS DISEASE, CHRONIC

GROWTH HORMONE DEFICIENCY

GROWTH HORMONE (DIAGNOSTIC)

HACEK GROUP

HAEMOPHILUS INFLUENZAE

Antibiotic, Quinolone

Antibiotic, Sulfonamide Derivative

Vaccine, Inactivated Bacteria

HARTNUP DISEASE

Vitamin, Water Soluble

HASHIMOTO'S THYROIDITIS

Thyroid Hormone

Thyroid Product

HEADACHE (SINUS)

Analgesic, Non-Narcotic

Antihistamine/Decongestant Combination

HEADACHE (TENSION)

Analgesic, Narcotic

Analgesic, Non-Narcotic

Antianxiety Agent

Antimigraine Agent

Barbiturate

Skeletal Muscle Relaxant, Long Acting

HEADACHE (VASCULAR)

Adrenergic Blocking Agent

Analgesic, Non-Narcotic

Corticosteroid, Topical (Low Potency)

Corticosteroid, Topical (Medium/High Potency)

Corticosteroid, Topical (Medium Potency)

MACROGLOBULINEMIA OF WALDENSTRÖM

Antineoplastic Agent, Alkylating Agent (Nitrogen Mustard)

MIOSIS (INOPERATIVE)

Nonsteroidal Anti-Inflammatory Agent (NSAID), Ophthalmic

MITRAL VALVE PROLAPSE

Beta-Adrenergic Blocker

MORAXELLA CATARRHALIS

Antibiotic, Cephalosporin (Second Generation)

Antibiotic, Cephalosporin (Third Generation)

Antibiotic, Penicillin

Antibiotic, Quinolone

Antibiotic, Sulfonamide Derivative

MOTION SICKNESS

Anticholinergic Agent, Transdermal

Antiemetic

Psoralen

MYDRIASIS

Adrenergic Agonist Agent, Ophthalmic

Anticholinergic Agent, Ophthalmic

MYELOMA

Antineoplastic Agent, Alkylating Agent

Antineoplastic Agent, Alkylating Agent (Nitrogen Mustard)

Antineoplastic Agent, Alkylating Agent (Nitrosourea)

Antineoplastic Agent, Antibiotic

Antineoplastic Agent, Miscellaneous

Corticosteroid, Systemic

MYOCARDIAL INFARCTION

Anticoagulant

Antiplatelet Agent

Beta-Adrenergic Blocker

Thrombolytic Agent

Vasodilator, Coronary

MYOCARDIAL ISCHEMIA (PROPHYLAXIS)

Blood Modifiers

MYOCARDIAL REINFARCTION

Analgesic, Non-Narcotic

PANCREATIC EXOCRINE INSUFFICIENCY

Pancreatic Enzyme

PANCREATIC EXOCRINE INSUFFICIENCY (DIAGNOSTIC)

Diagnostic Agent, Pancreatic Exocrine Insufficiency

PANCREATITIS

Antispasmodic Agent, Gastrointestinal

PANIC ATTACKS

Benzodiazepine

PAPILLITIS

Corticosteroid, Systemic

PARACOCCIDIOIDES BRASILIENSIS

Antibiotic, Sulfonamide Derivative

Antifungal Agent, Systemic

PARACOCCIDIOIDOMYCOSIS

Antifungal Agent, Systemic

PARALYTIC ILEUS (PROPHYLAXIS)

Gastrointestinal Agent, Stimulant

PARKINSONISM

Anticholinergic Agent

Antiparkinson Agent

Ergot Alkaloid

PASTEURELLA

Antibiotic, Miscellaneous

Antibiotic, Penicillin

Antibiotic, Tetracycline Derivative

PELLAGRA

Vitamin, Water Soluble

PELVIC INFLAMMATORY DISEASE (PID)

Antibiotic, Aminoglycoside

Antibiotic, Anaerobic

Antibiotic, Cephalosporin (Second Generation)

Antibiotic, Cephalosporin (Third Generation)

Antibiotic, Macrolide

Antibiotic, Penicillin

Antibiotic, Tetracycline Derivative

PEMPHIGUS

PENICILLIN HYPERSENSITIVITY (DIAGNOSTIC)

Diagnostic Agent, Penicillin Allergy Skin Test

PEPTIC ULCER

Antispasmodic Agent, Gastrointestinal

Gastric Acid Secretion Inhibitor

Gastrointestinal Agent, Miscellaneous

Histamine-2 Antagonist

PEPTOSTREPTOCOCCUS

Antibiotic, Cephalosporin (Second Generation)

Antibiotic, Miscellaneous

Antibiotic, Penicillin

PERICARDITIS

Antibiotic, Penicillin

Corticosteroid, Systemic

PERIPHERAL VASCULAR DISEASE (PVD)

Vasodilator, Peripheral

PHARYNGITIS

Antibiotic, Carbacephem

Antibiotic, Cephalosporin (First Generation)

Antibiotic, Cephalosporin (Second Generation)

Antibiotic, Macrolide

Antibiotic, Penicillin

Corticosteroid, Topical (Low Potency)

Corticosteroid, Topical (Medium/ High Potency)

POLIO

Vaccine, Live Virus

Vaccine, Live Virus and Inactivated Virus

POLYCYTHEMIA VERA

Antineoplastic Agent, Alkylating Agent

Antineoplastic Agent, Alkylating Agent (Nitrogen Mustard)

POLYMYOSITIS

Antineoplastic Agent, Alkylating Agent (Nitrogen Mustard)

Antineoplastic Agent, Antimetabolite

Corticosteroid, Systemic

Corticosteroid, Topical (High Potency)

Corticosteroid, Topical (Low Potency)

Corticosteroid, Topical (Medium/High Potency)

PUBERTY (DELAYED)

Androgen

PUBERTY (PRECOCIOUS)

Gonadotropin Releasing Hormone Analog

Hormone, Posterior Pituitary

PULMONARY EMBOLISM

Anticoagulant

Plasma Volume Expander

Thrombolytic Agent

PURPURA (HENOCH-SCHÖNLEIN)

Corticosteroid, Systemic

RESPIRATORY DISTRESS SYNDROME

Lung Surfactant

RESPIRATORY SYNCYTIAL VIRUS

Antiviral Agent, Inhalation Therapy

RETINOBLASTOMA

Antineoplastic Agent, Alkylating Agent (Nitrogen Mustard)

Antineoplastic Agent, Antibiotic

REYE'S SYNDROME

Corticosteroid, Systemic

Corticosteroid, Inhalant

Decongestant, Nasal

Inhalation, Miscellaneous

RICKETS

Vitamin D Analog

ROCKY MOUNTAIN SPOTTED FEVER

Antibiotic, Miscellaneous

Antibiotic, Quinolone

Antibiotic, Tetracycline Derivative

SHIGELLA

Antibiotic, Cephalosporin (Third Generation)

Antibiotic, Penicillin

Antibiotic, Quinolone

Antibiotic, Sulfonamide Derivative

SPOROTRICHOSIS

Antifungal Agent, Systemic

STAPHYLOCOCCAL INFECTION

Antibiotic, Macrolide

STAPHYLOCOCCUS AUREUS (METHICILLIN RESISTANT)

Antibiotic, Aminoglycoside

Antibiotic, Miscellaneous

Antibiotic, Sulfonamide Derivative

STAPHYLOCOCCUS AUREUS (METHICILLIN SENSITIVE)

Antibiotic, Aminoglycoside

Antibiotic, Anaerobic

Antibiotic, Carbacephem

Antibiotic, Cephalosporin (First Generation)

Antibiotic, Cephalosporin (Second Generation)

INDICATION/THERAPEUTIC CATEGORY INDEX

STRABISMUS

Ophthalmic Agent, Miotic

Ophthalmic Agent, Toxin

STREPTOCOCCUS (AEROBIC)

Antibiotic, Carbacephem

Antibiotic, Cephalosporin (First Generation)

Antibiotic, Cephalosporin (Second Generation)

Antibiotic, Macrolide

Corticosteroid, Topical (Medium/High Potency)

TINEA (CRURIS)

Antifungal Agent, Systemic

Antifungal Agent, Topical

Corticosteroid, Topical (Medium/High Potency)

TINEA (PEDIS)

Antifungal Agent, Systemic

Antifungal Agent, Topical

Antipyretic

Corticosteroid, Systemic

VASOACTIVE INTESTINAL PEPTIDE-SECRETING TUMOR (VIP)

Antisecretory Agent

VENTRICULAR CONTRACTIONS, PREMATURE

Antiarrhythmic Agent, Class Ia

Antiarrhythmic Agent, Class Ib

Antiarrhythmic Agent, Class Ic

Antiarrhythmic Agent, Class II

VERTIGO

Antiemetic

INDICATION/THERAPEUTIC CATEGORY INDEX

WHOOPING COUGH

Antibiotic, Macrolide
E.E.S.® Oral 175
E-Mycin® Oral 175
Eryc® Oral 175
EryPed® Oral 175
Ery-Tab® Oral 175
Erythrocin® Oral 175
erythromycin 175
Ilosone® Oral 175
PCE® Oral 175
Wyamycin® S Oral 175

Antibiotic, Sulfonamide Derivative
Bactrim™ 118
Bactrim™ DS 118
Cotrim® 118
Cotrim® DS 118
co-trimoxazole 118
Septra® 118
Septra® DS 118
Sulfamethoprim® 118
Sulfatrim® 118
Sulfatrim® DS 118
Uroplus® DS 118
Uroplus® SS 118

Immune Globulin
Hypertussis® 367
pertussis immune globulin, human
.... 367

Toxoid
Acel-Immune® 154
diphtheria and tetanus toxoids
and pertussis vaccine,
adsorbed 153
diphtheria, tetanus toxoids, and
acellular pertussis vaccine
.... 154
diphtheria, tetanus toxoids, and
whole-cell pertussis vaccine
and hemophilus b
conjugate vaccine 154
Tetramune® 154
Tri-Immunol® 153
Tripedia® 154

WILMS' TUMOR

Antineoplastic Agent, Antibiotic
Adriamycin PFS™ 161
Adriamycin RDF™ 161
Cosmegen® 125
dactinomycin 125
doxorubicin hydrochloride 161
Rubex® 161

Antineoplastic Agent, Miotic Inhibitor
Oncovin® Injection 496
Vincasar® PFS Injection 496
vincristine sulfate 496

WILSON'S DISEASE

Antidote, Copper Toxicity
Cuprimine® 359
Depen® 359
penicillamine 359

Syprine® 477
trientine hydrochloride 477

Chelating Agent, Oral
Syprine® 477
trientine hydrochloride 477

XANTHOMONAS MALTAPHILIA

Antibiotic, Penicillin
piperacillin sodium and
tazobactam sodium 379
ticarcillin and clavulanate
potassium 467
Timentin® 467
Zosyn™ 379

Antibiotic, Quinolone
ciprofloxacin hydrochloride 102
Cipro™ Injection 102
Cipro™ Oral 102
Floxin® Injection 343
Floxin® Oral 343
lomefloxacin hydrochloride 277
Maxaquin® Oral 277
ofloxacin 343

Antibiotic, Sulfonamide Derivative
Bactrim™ 118
Bactrim™ DS 118
Cotrim® 118
Cotrim® DS 118
co-trimoxazole 118
Septra® 118
Septra® DS 118
Sulfamethoprim® 118
Sulfatrim® 118
Sulfatrim® DS 118
Uroplus® DS 118
Uroplus® SS 118

XEROPHTHALMIA

Ophthalmic Agent, Miscellaneous
artificial tears 33
Isopto® Plain [OTC] 33
Isopto® Tears [OTC] 33
Tearisol® [OTC] 33

YAWS

Antibiotic, Miscellaneous
chloramphenicol 88
Chloromycetin® 88

Antibiotic, Penicillin
Bicillin® L-A Injection 360
penicillin g benzathine 360
Permapen® Injection 360

Antibiotic, Tetracycline Derivative
Achromycin® V Oral 458
Ala-Tet® Oral 458
Nor-tet® Oral 458
Panmycin® Oral 458
Robitet® Oral 458
Sumycin® Oral 458
Teline® Oral 458
Tetracap® Oral 458
tetracycline 458
Tetralan® Oral 458
Tetram® Oral 458

737